THIRD CANADIAN EDITION

FIT&WELL

CORE CONCEPTS AND LABS IN PHYSICAL FITNESS AND WELLNESS

Thomas D. Fahey
California State University, Chico

Paul M. Insel
Stanford University

Walton T. Roth
Stanford University

Ilsa Wong
University of Lethbridge

McGraw-Hill Ryerson
Connect. Learn. Succeed.

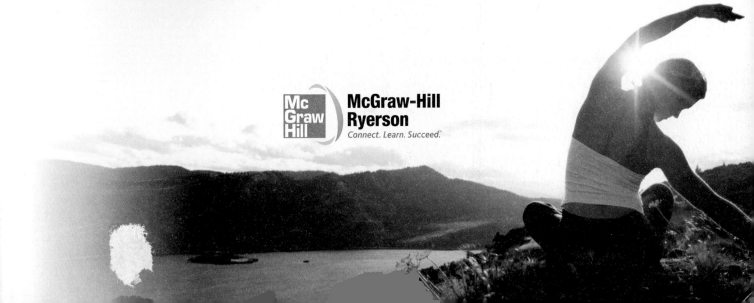

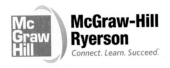
Fit & Well: Core Concepts and Labs in Physical Fitness and Wellness
Third Canadian Edition

1 2 3 4 5 6 7 8 9 10 DOW 1 9 8 7 6 5 4 3 2

ISBN: 0-07-105205-4
ISBN-13: 978-0-07-105205-4

Statistics Canada information is used with the permission of Statistics Canada. Users are forbidden to copy the data and redisseminate them, in an original or modified form, for commercial purposes, without permission from Statistics Canada. Information on the availability of the wide range of data from Statistics Canada can be obtained from Statistics Canada's Regional Offices, its World Wide Web site at www.statcan.gc.ca, and its toll-free access number 1-800-263-1136.

The Internet addresses listed in the text were accurate at the time of publication. The inclusion of a Web site does not indicate an endorsement by the authors or McGraw-Hill Ryerson, nor does McGraw-Hill Ryerson guarantee the accuracy of information presented at these sites.

Printed and bound in the United States.

Care has been taken to trace ownership of copyright material contained in this text; however, the publisher will welcome any information that enables them to rectify any reference or credit for subsequent editions.

Editorial Director: Rhondda McNabb
Publisher: Leanna MacLean
Marketing Manager: Stacey Metz
Developmental Editor: Daphne Scriabin
Senior Editorial Associate: Stephanie Giles
Supervising Editor: Graeme Powell
Copy Editor: Erin Moore
Permissions Editors: Elizabeth Kelly and Alison Derry
Production Coordinator: Sheryl MacAdam
Cover and Interior Design: Valid Design & Layout/Dave Murphy
Page Layout: Laserwords Private Limited
Printer: R. R. Donnelley/Willard (U.S.)

Library and Archives Canada Cataloguing in Publication

Fit & well: core concepts and labs in physical fitness and wellness/Thomas D. Fahey . . . [et al.].—3rd Canadian ed.

Includes bibliographical references and index.
ISBN 978-0-07-105205-4

1. Physical fitness—Textbooks. 2. Health—Textbooks.
I. Fahey, Thomas D. (Thomas Davin), 1947- II. Title: Fit and well.

GV481.F26 2013   613.7'043   C2012-904948-4

BRIEF CONTENTS

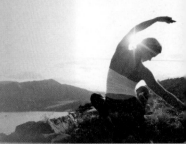

CONTENTS

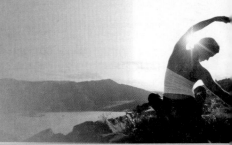

PREFACE

For today's fitness-conscious university/college student, the third Canadian edition of *Fit & Well* combines the best of two worlds. In the area of physical fitness, *Fit & Well* offers expert knowledge based on the latest findings in exercise physiology and sports medicine, along with tools for self-assessment and guidelines for becoming fit. In the area of wellness, it offers accurate, current information on today's most important health-related topics and issues, again with self-tests and guidelines for achieving wellness. The text provides comprehensive advice on wellness-related behaviour and practising a healthier way of life, as well as thorough coverage of health-related fitness and nutrition. *Fit & Well* provides the reader with comprehensive advice on making informed choices about food and promotes behavioural change throughout the text. Making informed choices is the *Fit & Well* difference.

CONTENT AND ORGANIZATION OF THE THIRD CANADIAN EDITION

In the third Canadian edition of *Fit & Well*, the organization of the text follows the format of fitness and wellness courses. Instructors do not have to jump around in the text to meet the needs of their course. Chapter 1 provides an introduction to fitness and wellness and explains the principles of behaviour change. Chapters 2–6 and 9 focus on the various areas of fitness. Chapter 2 provides an overview, discussing the components of fitness, the principles of physical training, and the factors involved in designing a well-rounded, personalized exercise program. Chapter 3 provides basic information on how the cardiorespiratory system functions, how the body produces energy for exercise, and how individuals can create successful cardiorespiratory fitness programs. Additional information has been added to Chapter 3 on the benefits of cardiorespiratory endurance exercise for children and adolescents. Chapters 4, 5, and 6 look at

muscular strength and endurance, flexibility and low-back health, and body composition. Sections include core strength training and the physiology of stretching, with added information on training with and without equipment. Chapters 7 and 8 investigate nutrition and weight management and their impact on the physical dimension of wellness. This edition includes information on alternate diets such as First Nations, Metis, and Inuit and the Vegetarian Food Guide Pyramid. Chapter 9 "puts it all together," describing the nature of a complete program that develops all the components of fitness. This chapter also includes complete sample exercise programs.

Chapter 10 is a key area of wellness promotion and lifestyle management that can have a profound effect on your participation in sport and physical activity: stress management. In this chapter, there is an additional **Take Charge** box on the topic of sleep. Chapters 11 and 12 focus on two of the most important reasons for making lifestyle changes: cardiovascular disease and cancer. Students learn the basic mechanisms of these diseases, how they are related to lifestyle, and what individuals can do to prevent them. Finally, Chapter 13 looks at four additional wellness topics: interpersonal relationships, aging, the health care system, and environmental health.

There are some significant changes to this third edition. A new **Career Options** box provides university/college students with a broad spectrum of careers related to a variety of topic areas in the book. In addition, chapters now include **Fitness Tips, Wellness Tips,** and **Personal Challenge** boxes that engage students in the topics in greater depth.

The third Canadian edition of *Fit & Well* has been completely revised to include updated Canadian examples, references, data, statistics, and bibliographical information. Coverage of the latest version of Canada's Food Guide has been included, along with Canada's Physical Activity Guide, physical fitness testing, and Canadian programs such as the Canadian Association for Health, Physical Education, Recreation and Dance (CAHPERD).

CHAPTER-BY-CHAPTER CHANGES

Chapter 1, Introduction to Wellness, Fitness, and Lifestyle Management

- The book's key message—that students need to take responsibility for their own fitness and wellness—has been given a new emphasis throughout this chapter, in strong but subtle terms. The **In Focus** feature ("Financial Wellness") complements the discussion of the six widely recognized dimensions of wellness and focuses on the importance of mastering basic personal financial skills. The feature has been expanded since the last edition, and includes especially relevant information for students on the dangers of becoming dependent on credit cards.
- The discussions of the National Wellness Goals have been refined to focus on the newest round of objectives and the latest statistics on Canadians' progress toward meeting those goals.
- All of the chapter's considerable statistical material has been updated to reflect the latest information on morbidity, mortality, and measures of quality of life.

Chapter 2, Basic Principles of Physical Fitness

- Includes the most recent statistics available from Statistics Canada and the Physical Activity Monitors on the physical activity and exercise habits of Canadians.
- The **Evidence for Exercise** feature ("Is Exercise Good for Your Brain?") has been revised to make it more relevant to students.
- The discussion of exercise recommendations has been refined to show how the Canadian Physical Activity Guidelines are in line with recommendations from other agencies.
- Significant new points have been added on the health benefits of weight training, weight training safety, and the effects of weight training on the body's metabolism.

Chapter 3, Cardiorespiratory Endurance

- All statistics have been updated to reflect the latest data from authoritative sources.
- New information has been added about the health benefits of combining strength training with aerobic conditioning.
- The chapter presents a wide variety of activities that benefit one's cardiorespiratory health, and challenges students to pick the activity that would best fit with their daily routine.

Chapter 4, Muscular Strength and Endurance

- The chapter presents several basic strength and endurance exercises that students can easily use to assess their fitness level, and challenges them to pick one exercise and set goals for improvement.
- Enumerates more ways than ever to develop muscular strength and endurance without going to the gym.
- Introduces weight training videos and discusses their usefulness.
- Discusses the specific benefits of doing multiple sets of weight-training exercises.

Chapter 5, Flexibility and Low-Back Health

- Reflects the latest recommendations for the minimum and maximum amounts of time to hold a stretch.
- Includes new statistics on the prevalence of osteoporosis and low bone mass.
- Presents a set of basic exercises one can do at home to strengthen the lower back and prevent or alleviate back pain.

Chapter 6, Body Composition

- Makes further distinctions between overweight and obesity.
- Includes newly updated statistics from Statistics Canada on the prevalence of overweight and obesity in Canada.

- Includes new information that expands the definition of metabolic syndrome.
- Explains the potential link between obesity and infertility.
- Provides new statistics on the prevalence of all types of diabetes, including prevalence among specific ethnic groups.
- Challenges students to record their weight every day, especially if they are trying to lose weight.

Chapter 7, Nutrition
- The overview of nutrients has been expanded and several key terms have been added.
- The entire chapter has been updated, where applicable, to discuss the Food and Nutrition Board, and Health Canada's Guidelines for Canadians.
- The discussion of sodium intake has been updated to reflect Health Canada's latest recommendation that most Canadians—not just those with risk factors for heart disease—reduce their sodium intake to 1500 mg per day.
- The discussion of Canada's Food Guide has been complemented by the addition of the First Nations, Metis, and Inuit Food Guide, and the Vegetarian Food Guide Pyramid.
- The discussion of dietary supplements has been expanded to help students understand when supplements may be necessary and when they can be most effective.

Chapter 8, Weight Management
- Reiterates the latest statistics on overweight and obesity in Canada, and discusses the health implications of overweightness and obesity.
- Challenges students to examine their own weight, think of reasons they may have gained weight, and list ways they can begin reducing their weight right away.
- Provides new data about the effects of exercise on metabolic rate and resting calorie consumption among university/college-age men.
- Explains how very simple, small steps—such as cutting back on soda—can have a direct impact on weight loss.
- Discusses high-tech weight management tools and how students can incorporate them into a weight loss program.

- Introduces new data on the impact of psychosocial factors on weight loss among university/college students.

Chapter 9, Putting Together a Complete Fitness Program
- Introduces research indicating that runners may benefit from including stretches in their pre-workout warm-up, contrary to other research indicating stretching should be done after working out.
- Provides new sources and updated data on the benefits and drawbacks of incorporating a stability ball into one's training program.
- Promotes the use of resistance bands as an easy way to incorporate weight training into a total workout program.
- Introduces a variety of motivational programs for use with smart phones, which can help beginning exercisers stick with a program.
- Provides updated research into the benefits and drawbacks of drinking bottled water, and the product's effects on the environment.

Chapter 10, Stress
- The definition of stress has been clarified and simplified.
- The chapter more clearly defines and differentiates the concepts of acute stress and chronic stress.
- New art illustrates the mechanics of sleep apnea.
- Explains the effects of chronic stress on the body's aging process.
- Expands the discussion of stress's effect on the body's immune system.
- Explores the way our personal and intimate relations with others can be a significant source of stress in our lives.

Chapter 11, Cardiovascular Health
- All statistics have been updated to reflect the latest data from authoritative sources, including the Heart and Stroke Foundation Statistics, 2011.
- Introduces easy-to-use and inexpensive digital blood pressure monitors and heart rate monitors that anyone can use at home.
- Provides warnings about the negative effects of weight training on blood pressure.
- Expanded discussions of heart disease risk factors such as C-reactive protein.

FOR FURTHER EXPLORATION

Organizations, Hotlines, and Websites

The Internet addresses (also called uniform resource locators, or URLs) listed here were accurate at the time of publication.

FOR FURTHER EXPLORATION

For Further Exploration sections offer suggestions for student resources that can be found online to build fitness and wellness. These sections also list recommended books, newsletters, organizations, hotlines, and websites.

HANDS-ON LABORATORY ACTIVITIES

To help students apply the principles of fitness and wellness to their own lives, *Fit & Well* includes **laboratory activities** for classroom use. These hands-on activities

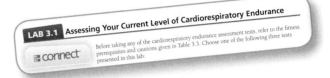

give students the opportunity to assess their current level of fitness and wellness, to create plans for changing their lifestyle to reach wellness, and to monitor their progress. They can assess their daily physical activity, for example, or their level of cardiorespiratory endurance; they can design a program to improve muscular strength or meet weight-loss goals; and they can explore their risk of developing cardiovascular disease or cancer. Many labs end with a section labelled "Using Your Results," which guides students in evaluating their scores, setting goals for change, and moving forward. Labs are found at the end of each chapter and are also available in an interactive format online.

Exercise photos demonstrate exactly how to perform exercises correctly.

QUICK-REFERENCE APPENDICES

Included at the end of the book are three appendices containing vital information in an easy-to-use format.

Appendix A, **Nutritional Content of Common Foods,** allows students to assess their daily diet in terms of 11 nutrient categories, including protein, fat, saturated fat, fibre, cholesterol, and sodium.

Appendix B, **Nutritional Content of Popular Items from Fast-Food Restaurants,** provides links to the websites of fast-food restaurants and their nutritional information guides.

Appendix C, **Monitoring Your Progress,** is a log that enables students to record and summarize the results of

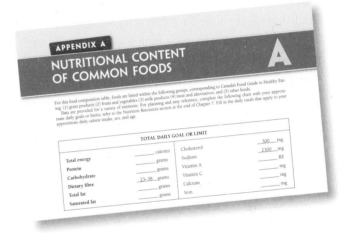

the assessment tests they complete as part of the laboratory activities. With space for preprogram and postprogram assessment results, the log provides an easy way to track the progress of a behaviour change program.

A bonus appendix, **Injury Prevention and Personal Safety,** is available online. This appendix is a reference guide to preventing common injuries, whether at home, at work, at play, or on the road. It also provides information on giving emergency care when someone else's life is in danger.

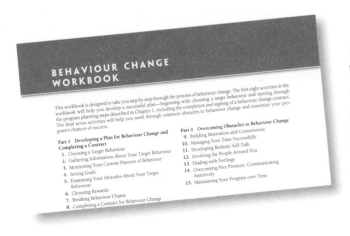

BUILT-IN BEHAVIOUR CHANGE WORKBOOK

The **built-in Behaviour Change Workbook** contains 15 separate activities that complement the lifestyle management model presented in Chapter 1. The workbook guides students in developing a successful program by walking them through each of the steps of behaviour change—from choosing a target behaviour to completing and signing a contract. It also includes activities to help students overcome common obstacles to behaviour change.

TEACHING AND LEARNING TOOLS

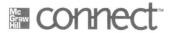

McGraw-Hill Connect™ is a web-based assignment and assessment platform that gives students the means to better connect with their coursework, with their instructors, and with the important concepts that they will need to know for success now and in the future.

With Connect, instructors can deliver assignments, quizzes, and tests online. Instructors can edit existing questions and author entirely new problems. They can track individual student performance—by question, by assignment, or in relation to the class overall—with detailed grade reports. They can integrate grade reports easily with Learning Management Systems (LMS) such as WebCT and Blackboard.

By choosing Connect, instructors are providing their students with a powerful tool for improving academic performance and truly mastering course material. Connect allows students to practise important skills at their own pace and on their own schedule. Importantly, students' assessment results and instructors' feedback are all saved online—so students can continually review their progress and plot their course to success.

Connect also provides 24/7 online access to an eBook—an online edition of the text—to aid students in successfully completing their work, wherever and whenever they choose.

KEY FEATURES

Simple Assignment Management

With Connect, creating assignments is easier than ever, so you can spend more time teaching and less time managing.

- Create and deliver assignments easily with new banks of homework questions and test bank material to assign online.

- Streamline lesson planning, student progress reporting, and assignment grading to make classroom management more efficient than ever.
- Go paperless with the eBook and online submission and grading of student assignments.

Smart Grading

When it comes to studying, time is precious. Connect helps students learn more efficiently by providing feedback and practice material when they need it, where they need it.

- Automatically score assignments, giving students immediate feedback on their work and side-by-side comparisons with correct answers.
- Access and review each response, and manually change grades or leave comments for students to review.
- Reinforce classroom concepts with practice tests and instant quizzes.

Instructor Library

The Connect Instructor Library is your course creation hub. It provides all the critical resources you'll need to build your course, just how you want to teach it.

- Assign eBook readings and draw from a rich collection of textbook-specific assignments
- Access instructor resources, including ready-made PowerPoint® presentations and media to use in your lectures.
- View assignments and resources created for past sections.
- Post your own resources for students to use.

eBook

Connect reinvents the textbook learning experience for the modern student. Every Connect subject area is seamlessly integrated with Connect eBooks, which are designed to keep students focused on the concepts key to their success.

- Provide students with a Connect eBook, allowing for anytime, anywhere access to the textbook.
- Merge media, animation, and assessments with the text's narrative to engage students and improve learning and retention.
- Pinpoint and connect key concepts in a snap using the powerful eBook search engine.
- Manage notes, highlights, and bookmarks in one place for simple, comprehensive review.

LearnSmart™

No two students are alike. McGraw-Hill LearnSmart™ is an intelligent learning system that uses a series of adaptive questions to pinpoint each student's knowledge gaps. LearnSmart then provides an optimal learning path for each student, so that they spend less time in areas they already know and more time in areas they don't. The result is LearnSmart's adaptive learning path helps students retain more knowledge, learn faster, and study more efficiently.

INSTRUCTOR RESOURCES

- *Instructor's Manual.* The Instructor's Manual contains learning objectives, key terms and definitions, a lecture outline, a list of resources, notes on the lab activities, Internet activities, Internet resources, and recommendations for in-class activities, discussion questions, or assignments.
- *Test Bank in Rich Text Format.* The Test Bank features multiple-choice, true/false, and essay questions. Each question is accompanied by an answer and a page reference in the text.
- *Computerized Test Bank.* This flexible and easy-to use electronic testing program allows instructors

to create tests from book-specific items. It accommodates a wide range of question types, and instructors may add their own questions. Multiple versions of the test can be created and printed.

- *Microsoft PowerPoint Slides.* These presentations offer high quality visuals to bring key concepts to life.

NUTRITIONCALC PLUS CANADIAN™

NutritionCalc Plus Canadian is a dietary analysis program with an easy-to-use interface that allows users to track their nutrient and food group intakes, energy expenditures, and weight control goals. It generates a variety of personalized reports and graphs for analysis, which can be emailed or downloaded into Excel or Word. The Canadian Edition of NutritionCalc Plus is populated with Canadian food choices and Canadian recommended activity levels and daily intakes for essential nutrients, vitamins, and minerals, and uses metric measurements. The Canadian Nutrient File includes ethnic foods, supplements, fast foods, and convenience foods, and users can add their own foods or recipes to the food list. NutritionCalc Plus is available online at **nutritioncalc.ca**.

SUPERIOR LEARNING SOLUTIONS AND SUPPORT

The McGraw-Hill Ryerson team is ready to help you assess and integrate any of our products, technology, and services into your course for optimal teaching and learning performance. Whether it's helping your students improve their grades, or putting your entire course online, the McGraw-Hill Ryerson team is here to help you do it. Contact your *iLearning Sales Specialist* today to learn how to maximize all of McGraw-Hill Ryerson's resources!

For more information on the latest technology and Learning Solutions offered by McGraw-Hill Ryerson and its partners, please visit us online: **www.mcgrawhill.ca/he/solutions**.

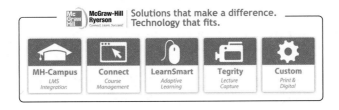

ACKNOWLEDGMENTS

Extensive feedback from numerous reviews and the valuable suggestions provided through that process helped to develop this Third Canadian Edition. Thank you to the following colleagues for their invaluable advice:

Bart Arnold, *University of Saskatchewan*

Tony Bauer, *Lakehead University*

Larry Cook, *Loyalist College*

Jarold Cosby, *Brock University*

Martin Dubuc, *Laurentian University*

Graham Fletcher, *University Fraser Valley*

Martin Gallo, *University of British Columbia*

Alain Gauthier, *Laurentian University*

Fred Gutoski, *University of Winnipeg*

Lauren Jawno, *Centennial College*

Jennifer Kuk, *York University*

Richard Montreuil, *Dawson College*

Anna Morrison, *Sault College*

Julie Rissler, *Algonquin College*

Anna Schulha, *Red Deer College*

Kim Soroka, *Concordia University*

Anne Marie Sullivan, *Memorial University*

Laurel Waterman, *George Brown College*

Many thanks to the McGraw-Hill Ryerson team of Leanna MacLean, Publisher; Daphne Scriabin, Developmental Editor; Kara Stahl, Supervising Editor; Erin Moore, Copy Editor; and Stacey Metz, Marketing Manager, whose various roles have been instrumental in putting this edition into print.

Ilsa Wong
University of Lethbridge

CHAPTER 1

INTRODUCTION TO WELLNESS, FITNESS, AND LIFESTYLE MANAGEMENT

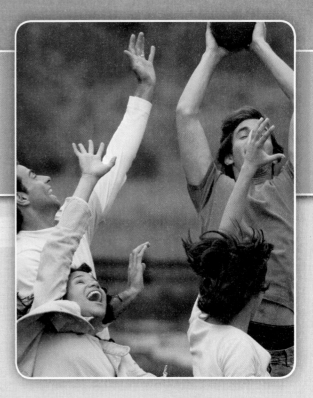

LEARNING OBJECTIVES

After reading this chapter, you should be able to

LO1 Describe the dimensions of wellness

LO2 Identify the major health problems in Canada today, and discuss their causes

LO3 Describe the behaviours that are part of a fit and well lifestyle

LO4 Explain the steps in creating a behaviour management plan to change a wellness-related behaviour

LO5 Discuss the available sources of wellness information and how to think critically about them

TEST YOUR KNOWLEDGE

1. **Which of the following lifestyle factors is the leading preventable cause of death for Canadians?**

    a. excess alcohol consumption
    b. cigarette smoking
    c. poor dietary habits
    d. lack of exercise

2. **More than two-thirds of all university/college students make which of the following positive lifestyle choices?**

    a. using safety belts
    b. not drinking and driving
    c. eating two or fewer high-fat foods per day
    d. not smoking cigarettes

3. **Which of the following health-related issues affects the greatest number of university/college students each year?**

    a. stress
    b. colds/flu/sore throat
    c. sleep problems
    d. concern for a friend or family member

ANSWERS

1. **B.** Smoking contributes to more than 37 000 deaths per year; poor diet and inactivity are responsible for about 21 000; and alcohol, about 6500.

2. **ALL FOUR.** However, the majority of students do not exercise regularly, do not wear bicycle helmets, and eat few fruits and vegetables. There are many areas in which college and university students can change their behaviour to improve their health.

3. **A.** About 27% of university/college students suffer so much stress that it affects their academic performance. High stress levels affect overall health and wellness, making it important to learn effective stress management techniques.

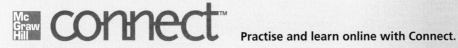

Practise and learn online with Connect.

A university/college student sets the following goals for herself:

- To join in new social circles and make new friends whenever possible
- To exercise every day
- To clean up trash and plant trees in blighted neighbourhoods in her community

These goals may differ, but they have one thing in common. Each contributes, in its own way, to this student's health and well-being. Not satisfied merely to be free of illness, she wants more. She has decided to live actively and fully—not just to be healthy but to pursue a state of overall wellness.

1.1 WELLNESS: THE NEW HEALTH GOAL

It is generally thought that the word **health** refers to the overall condition of a person's body or mind and as the World Health Organization defines is "A state of complete physical, mental and social well-being, and not merely the absence of disease." **Wellness** is a relatively new concept that expands our idea of health. Beyond the simple presence or absence of disease, wellness refers to optimal health and vitality—to living life to its fullest. Although we use the words *health* and *wellness* interchangeably, there are two important differences between them:

- Health—or some aspects of it—can be determined or influenced by factors beyond your control, such as your genes, age, and family history. For example, consider a man with a strong family history of prostate cancer. These factors place this man at a higher-than-average risk for developing prostate cancer himself.
- Wellness is largely determined by the decisions you make about how you live. That same man can reduce his risk of cancer by eating sensibly, exercising, and having regular screening tests. Even if he develops the disease, he may still rise above its effects to live a rich, meaningful life. This means choosing not only to care for himself physically but to maintain a positive outlook, keep up his relationships with others, challenge himself intellectually, and nurture other aspects of his life.

Enhanced wellness, therefore, involves making conscious decisions to control **risk factors** that contribute to disease or injury. Age and family history are risk factors you cannot control. Behaviours such as smoking, exercising, and eating a healthy diet are well within your control.

The overall goals of this text are to help you understand each of the areas of your life that you can control and make decisions that will enable you to reduce those risks.

LO1 The Dimensions of Wellness

Experts have defined six dimensions of wellness:

- Physical
- Emotional
- Intellectual
- Interpersonal
- Spiritual
- Environmental

Each dimension of wellness affects the others. Further, the process of achieving wellness is constant and dynamic (Figure 1.1), involving change and growth. Ignoring any dimension of wellness can have harmful effects on your life. The following sections briefly introduce the dimensions of wellness. Table 1.1 lists some of the specific qualities and behaviours associated with each dimension. Lab 1.1 will help you learn what wellness means to you and where you fall on the wellness continuum.

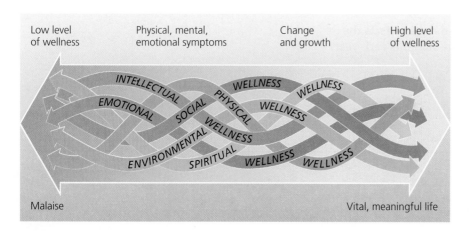

FIGURE 1.1 The wellness continuum.   The concept of wellness includes vitality in six interrelated dimensions, all of which contribute to overall wellness.

TABLE 1.1 Examples of Qualities and Behaviours Associated with the Dimensions of Wellness

Physical	Emotional	Intellectual
• Eating well	• Optimism	• Openness to new ideas
• Exercising	• Trust	• Capacity to question
• Avoiding harmful habits	• Self-esteem	• Ability to think critically
• Practising safer sex	• Self-acceptance	• Motivation to master new skills
• Recognizing symptoms of disease	• Self-confidence	• Sense of humour
• Getting regular checkups	• Ability to understand and accept one's feelings	• Creativity
• Avoiding injuries	• Ability to share feelings with others	• Curiosity
• Being active		• Lifelong learning
Interpersonal	**Spiritual**	**Environmental**
• Communication skills	• Capacity for love	• Having abundant, clean natural resources
• Capacity for intimacy	• Compassion	• Maintaining sustainable development
• Ability to establish and maintain satisfying relationships	• Forgiveness	• Recycling whenever possible
• Ability to cultivate support system of friends and family	• Altruism	• Reducing pollution and waste
	• Joy	
	• Fulfillment	
	• Caring for others	
	• Sense of meaning and purpose	
	• Sense of belonging to something greater than oneself	

PHYSICAL WELLNESS   Your physical wellness includes not just your body's overall condition and the absence of disease but your fitness level and your ability to care for yourself. The higher your fitness level (which is discussed throughout this book), the higher your level of physical wellness will be. Similarly, as you develop the ability to take care of your own physical needs, you ensure a greater level of physical wellness. To achieve optimum physical wellness, you need to make choices that will help you avoid illnesses and injuries. The decisions you make now, and the habits you develop over your lifetime, will largely determine the length and quality of your life.

EMOTIONAL WELLNESS   Your emotional wellness reflects your ability to understand and deal with your feelings. Emotional wellness involves attending to your own thoughts and feelings, monitoring your reactions, and identifying obstacles to emotional stability. Achieving this type of wellness means finding solutions to emotional problems, with professional help if necessary.

INTELLECTUAL WELLNESS   Those who enjoy intellectual (or mental) wellness constantly challenge their minds. An active mind is essential to wellness because it detects problems, finds solutions, and directs behaviour. People who enjoy intellectual wellness never stop learning; they continue trying to learn new things throughout their lifetime. They seek out and relish new experiences and challenges.

INTERPERSONAL WELLNESS   Your interpersonal (or social) wellness is defined by your ability to develop and maintain satisfying and supportive relationships. Such relationships are essential to physical and emotional health. Social wellness requires participating in and contributing to your community, country, and world.

SPIRITUAL WELLNESS   To enjoy spiritual health is to possess a set of guiding beliefs, principles, or values that give meaning and purpose to your life, especially during difficult times. The spiritually well person focuses on the positive aspects of life and finds spirituality to be an antidote for negative feelings such as cynicism, anger, and pessimism. Organized religions help many people develop spiritual health. Religion, however, is not the only source or form of spiritual wellness. Many people find meaning and purpose in their lives on their own—through nature, art, meditation, political action, or good works—or with their loved ones.

ENVIRONMENTAL WELLNESS Your environmental wellness is defined by the livability of your surroundings. Personal health depends on the health of the planet—from the safety of the food supply to the degree of violence in society. Your physical environment either supports your wellness or diminishes it. To improve your environmental wellness, you can learn about and protect yourself against hazards in your surroundings and work to make your world a cleaner and safer place.

OTHER ASPECTS OF WELLNESS Many experts consider occupational wellness and financial wellness to be additional important dimensions of wellness. *Occupational wellness* refers to the level of happiness and fulfillment you gain through your work. Although high salaries and prestigious titles are nice, they alone generally do not bring about occupational wellness. An occupationally well person truly likes his or her work, feels a connection with others in the workplace, and has opportunities to learn and be challenged. Other aspects of occupational wellness include enjoyable work, job satisfaction, and recognition from managers and colleagues. An ideal job draws on your interests and passions, as well as your vocational or professional skills, and allows you to feel that you are contributing to society in your everyday work.

To achieve occupational wellness, set career goals that reflect your personal values. For example, a career in sales might be a good choice for someone who values financial security, whereas a career in teaching or nursing might be a good choice for someone who values service to others.

Financial wellness refers to your ability to live within your means and manage your money in a way that gives you peace of mind. It includes balancing your income and expenditures, staying out of debt, saving for the future, and understanding your emotions about money. For more on this topic, see the box "Financial Wellness."

LO2 New Opportunities, New Responsibilities

Wellness is a relatively recent concept. A century ago, people considered themselves lucky just to survive to adulthood. A child born in 1900, for example, could expect to live only about 57 years. Many people died as a result of common **infectious diseases** (pneumonia, tuberculosis, diarrhea) and poor environmental conditions (unrefrigerated food, poor sanitation, air and water pollution). However, since 1900, the average life expectancy has gradually increased, thanks largely to the development of vaccines and antibiotics to prevent and fight infectious diseases and to public health campaigns to improve environmental conditions.

But a different set of diseases has emerged as our major health threat, and heart disease, cancer, and stroke are three of the leading causes of death for North Americans today (Table 1.2). Treating these and other **chronic diseases** is enormously expensive and extremely difficult.

The good news is that people do have some control over whether they develop chronic diseases. People make choices every day that either increase or decrease their risks for such diseases. These lifestyle choices include behaviours such as exercise, diet, smoking, and alcohol use. As Figure 1.2 shows, lifestyle factors contribute to our risk of chronic disease, and people can make good choices in an effort to profoundly influence and reduce their own health risks. Wellness cannot be prescribed; physicians and other health care professionals can provide information, advice, and encouragement—but the rest is up to each of us.

VITAL STATISTICS

TABLE 1.2 Leading Causes of Death in Canada

Rank	Cause of Death	Number of Deaths
1	Malignant neoplasms (cancers)	70 588
2	Diseases of heart (heart disease)	50 722
3	Cerebrovascular diseases (stroke)	13 870
4	Chronic lower respiratory diseases	10 923
5	Accidents (unintentional injuries)	10 234
6	Diabetes mellitus (diabetes)	7 521
7	Alzheimer's disease	6 573
8	Influenze and pneumonia	5 386
9	Nephritis, nephrotic syndrome, and nephrosis (kidney disease)	3 846
10	Intentional self-harm (suicide)	3 705

SOURCE: Adapted from Statistics Canada, Health Statistics Division, Leading Causes of Death, by sex, 2008 (Table 102-0561). Reproduced and distributed on an "as is" basis with the permission of Statistics Canada.

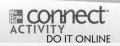

Financial Wellness

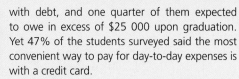

With the news full of stories of home mortgage rates, credit card debt, and personal bankruptcies, it has become painfully clear that many Canadians do not know how to manage their finances. Are such stressful experiences inevitable in today's world? Not at all. You can avoid them—and gain financial peace of mind—by developing the skills that contribute to financial wellness.

What exactly is financial wellness? Basically, it means having a healthy relationship with money. It involves such skills as knowing how to manage your money, using self-discipline to live within your means, using credit cards wisely, staying out of debt, meeting your financial obligations, and having a long-range financial plan. It also includes managing your emotional relationship with money and being in charge of your financial decisions. If you haven't developed these skills yet, now is the time to start.

Learn to Budget

Although the word *budget* may conjure up thoughts of deprivation, a budget is really just a way of tracking where your money goes and making sure you're spending it on the things that are most important to you. Basic budgeting worksheets are available online, but you can also just use a notebook with lined paper. On one page, list your monthly income by source (for example, job, stipend, parental aid), and on another, list your expenditures. If you're not sure where you spend your money, track your expenditures for a few weeks or a month. Then organize them into categories, such as housing (rent, utilities), food (groceries, eating out), transportation (car, insurance, parking, public transportation), entertainment (movies, music, cable TV, parties), services (cellphone, Internet service provider), personal care (haircuts, cosmetics), clothes, books and school supplies, health care, credit card and loan payments, and miscellaneous. These are suggestions; use categories that reflect the way you actually spend your money. Knowing where your money goes is the first step in gaining control of it.

Now total your income and expenditures. Are you taking in more than you spend, or are you spending more than you're taking in? Are you spending your money where you want to spend it, or are you surprised by your spending patterns? Use what you find out to set guidelines and goals for yourself. If your expenditures exceed your income, identify ways to make some cuts. If morning lattes are adding up, consider making coffee at home. If you have both a cellphone and a land line, consider whether you can give one up. If you're spending money on movies and restaurants, consider less expensive options like having a game night with friends or organizing a potluck.

Be realistic about what you can cut, but also realize that you may have to adjust your mind-set about what you can afford. Once you have a balance between income and expenses, don't stop there. Try to have a little left over each month for an emergency fund or savings. You may be surprised by how much peace of mind you can gain by living within your means!

Be Wary of Credit Cards

One recent financial study found that 58% of Canada's postsecondary students aged 18 to 24 are worried about money. Sixty-four percent of the students surveyed expect to graduate

with debt, and one quarter of them expected to owe in excess of $25 000 upon graduation. Yet 47% of the students surveyed said the most convenient way to pay for day-to-day expenses is with a credit card.

The best way to avoid credit card debt is to have just one card, to use it only when necessary, and to pay off the entire balance every month. Make sure you understand terms like *APR* (annual percentage rate—the interest you're charged on your balance), *credit limit* (the maximum amount you can borrow at any one time), *minimum monthly payment* (the smallest payment your creditor will accept each month), *grace period* (the number of days you have to pay your bill before interest, late fees, or other penalties are charged), and *over-the-limit* and *late fees* (the amount you'll be charged if your payment is late or you go over your credit limit). Banks make most of their money from fees. Read the fine print!

To see what you really do or don't know about credit cards, take the credit card quiz at www.fcac-acfc.gc.ca/eng/resources/toolCalculator/CreditCard/quiz/CreditCardQuiz-eng.asp?sn=0.

Get Out of Debt

If you do have credit card debt, stop using your cards and start paying them off. If you can't pay the whole balance, at least try to pay more than the minimum payment each month. Most people are surprised by how long it will take to pay off a loan by making only the minimum payments. For example, to pay off a credit card balance of $2000 at 10% interest with monthly payments of $20 would take 203 months—17 years. To see for yourself, check out an online credit card calculator like www.fcac-acfc.gc.ca/iTools-iOutils/CreditCardCalculator-eng.aspx (credit card payment calculator tool). By carrying a balance and incurring finance charges, you are also paying back much more than your initial loan—money you could be putting to other uses.

Some experts recommend choosing one card—the one with the largest balance or the highest interest—and paying off as much as you can every month. Others recommend paying off one or two cards with smaller balances to give yourself a sense of accomplishment and motivation to continue. Whatever your choice, if you have credit card debt, make it a priority to pay it off as soon as you can.

Become Financially Literate

Although modern life requires financial literacy—which includes everything from basics like balancing a chequebook to more sophisticated endeavours like developing a long-term financial plan—most Canadians have not received any kind of education in financial skills. The consensus is that developing lifelong financial skills should begin in early adulthood, during the university/college years, if not earlier.

If you want to improve your financial literacy, a good way to start is to take a course in personal finance or financial management skills. There are also many magazines that focus on money management, and of course a wealth of information can be found online. Make it a priority to achieve financial wellness, and start now. Money may not buy you love, but having control over your money can buy you a lot of peace of mind.

SOURCES: Federal Deposit Insurance Corporation. 2010. *Money Smart: A Financial Education Program* (http://www.fdic.gov/consumers/consumer/moneysmart/young.html; retrieved June 23, 2011); Plymouth State University. 2011. *Student Monetary Awareness and Responsibility Today!* (http://www.plymouth.edu/finaid/smart; retrieved June 23, 2011); U.S. Financial Literacy and Education Commission. 2010. *Do You Want to Learn How to Save, Manage, and Invest Your Money Better?* (http://www.mymoney.gov; retrieved June 23, 2011).

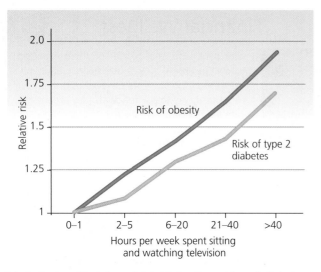

(a) **Sedentary lifestyle and risk of obesity and type 2 diabetes**

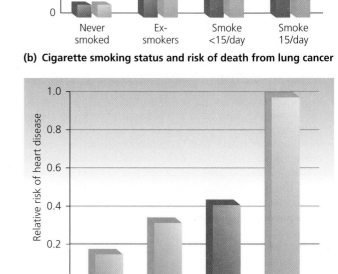

(b) **Cigarette smoking status and risk of death from lung cancer**

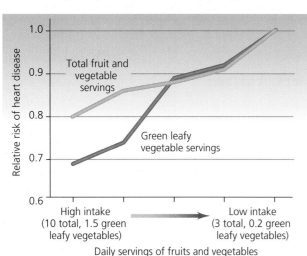

(c) **Fruit and vegetable intake and risk of heart disease**

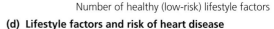

(d) **Lifestyle factors and risk of heart disease**

FIGURE 1.2 Lifestyle and risk of chronic disease. The research results shown above are just a few recent findings linking lifestyle behaviours to rates of disease and death. They indicate that (a) people who spend more time watching television are more likely to be obese and to develop type 2 diabetes; (b) people who smoke are much more likely to die of lung cancer than people who have never smoked or who have quit; (c) people who consume diets rich in fruits and vegetables, particularly green leafy vegetables, reduce their risk of heart disease; and (d) people who engage in a combination of healthy lifestyle behaviours have an 82% lower risk of heart disease than those who do not engage in such behaviours. The five lifestyle factors examined in this study were the participation in regular physical activity, the avoidance of smoking, and the maintenance of a healthy diet, body weight, and level of alcohol consumption.

SOURCES: Based on (a) Hu, F. B., et al. 2003. Television watching and other sedentary behaviours in relation to risk of obesity and type 2 diabetes mellitus in women. *Journal of the American Medical Association* 289(14): 1785–1791. (b) Prescott, E., et al. 1998. Mortality in women and men in relation to smoking. *International Epidemiological Association* 27: 27–32. (c) Joshipura, K. J., et al. 2001. The effect of fruit and vegetable intake on risk for coronary heart disease. *Annals of Internal Medicine* 134: 1106–1114. (d) Stampfer, M. J., et al. 2000. Primary prevention of coronary heart disease in women through diet and lifestyle. *New England Journal of Medicine* 343(1): 16–22.

This chapter provides an overview of a lifestyle that contributes to wellness and describes a method that can help you make lasting changes in your life to promote good health. The chapters that follow provide more detailed information about physical activity, healthy eating habits, and other components of a wellness lifestyle. The book as a whole is designed to be used to help you take charge of your behaviour and improve the quality of your life—to become fit and well.

National Wellness Goals

You may think of health and wellness as personal concerns, goals that you strive for on your own for your own benefit. But the Canadian government also has a vital interest in the health of all Canadians. A healthy population is the nation's greatest resource, the source of its vigour and wealth. Poor health, in contrast, drains the nation's resources and raises national health care costs. In fact, Canada's health care spending was estimated to be $191 billion in 2010, with

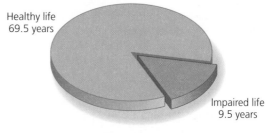
projections to rise in future years.[1] As the embodiment of our society's values, the federal government also has a humane interest in people's health. See Figure 1.3.

The Canadian government first began to recognize the importance of health promotion with the 1986 Ottawa Charter for Health Promotion. The Charter not only identified resources and strategies for health promotion, but ultimately lead to a challenge of "health for all" by the year 2000. This challenge was based upon the Framework for Health Promotion that enabled many of the provinces (particularly those in Western Canada) to create community-based health promotion projects or centres.

Of additional impact has been the Action Statement for Health Promotion (1996) that refocused attention onto the need for Canadians to value health. The Statement recognized the many dimensions of wellness and their overall impact on health; in addition, seven specific strategies for development were outlined:

1. Health promotion addresses health issues in context. It recognizes that many individual, social, and environmental factors interact to influence health. It searches for ways to explain how these factors interact in order to plan and act for the greatest health gain.

2. Health promotion supports a holistic approach that recognizes and includes the physical, mental, social, ecological, cultural, and spiritual aspects of health.

3. Health promotion requires a long-term perspective. It takes time to create awareness and build understanding of health determinants. This is true for organizations as well as for individuals.

4. Health promotion supports a balance between centralized and decentralized decision-making on policies that affect people where we live, work, and play.

5. Health promotion is multisectoral. While program initiatives often originate in the health sector, little can be done to change unhealthy living conditions and improve lifestyles without the support of other people, organizations, and policy sectors.

6. Health promotion draws on knowledge from a variety of sources. It depends on formal knowledge from the social, economic, political, medical, and environmental sciences. It also depends on the experiential knowledge of people.

7. Health promotion emphasizes public accountability. Those providing health promotion activities need to be accountable and to be able to expect the same commitment from other individuals and organizations.

More recently, the Canadian government identified goals and objectives in an effort to increase physical activity levels by 10% in the year 2010.[2]

Monitoring of these government initiatives is handled through the Physical Activity Benchmarks and Monitors which are produced by the Canadian Fitness and Lifestyle Research Institute (www.cflri.ca). The CFLRI 2008 Physical Activity Monitors suggest that all regions of Canada, with the exception of the North, are within reach of the goal of a 10% increase in physical activity levels. In fact, the Monitors suggest that Manitoba is only 1% from its target.

In an effort to carry out these strategies and achieve their goals for 2010, the Canadian government (Public Health Agency of Canada) in conjunction with the Canadian Society for Exercise Physiology (CSEP) has created Canada's Physical Activity Guide to Healthy Active Living (2002). These tools identify expectations for levels of physical activity that put Canadians of all ages (there are

Healthy life
69.5 years

Impaired life
9.5 years

Life expectancy
79.3 years

VITAL STATISTICS

FIGURE 1.3 Quantity of life versus quality of life. Years of healthy life as a proportion of life expectancy in the Canadian population.

SOURCE: Statistics Canada, 2008.

guides specific to children, youth, and older adults) on a path to wellness. Some provinces have begun to use these and other tools in the development of curriculum directed at increasing healthy lifestyle habits in students at the high school level and beyond.

LO3 Behaviours That Contribute to Wellness

A lifestyle based on good choices and healthy behaviours maximizes the quality of life. It helps people avoid disease, remain strong and fit, and maintain their physical and mental health as long as they live. The most important behaviours and habits are introduced briefly here and described in detail in later chapters.

BE PHYSICALLY ACTIVE The human body is designed to work best when it is active. It readily adapts to nearly any level of activity and exertion; in fact, **physical fitness** is defined as a set of physical attributes that allows the body to respond or adapt to the demands and stress of physical effort. The more we ask of our bodies, the stronger and more fit they become. When our bodies are not kept active, however, they deteriorate. Bones lose their density, joints stiffen, muscles become weak, and cellular energy systems begin to degenerate. To be truly well, human beings must be active. Unfortunately, a **sedentary** lifestyle is common among Canadians today; with close to 69% of Canadians' waking hours spent in sedentary pursuits.[3] Today, options for physical activity are vast and range from the traditional sports and physical activities (e.g., walking, jogging), to increased activity through video games (e.g., Nintendo Wii) and movement activities (e.g., yoga).

The benefits of physical activity are both physical and mental, immediate and long-term (Figure 1.4). In the short term, being physically fit makes it easier to do everyday tasks, such as lifting; it provides reserve strength for emergencies; and it helps people look and feel good. In the long term, being physically fit confers protection against chronic diseases and lowers the risk of dying prematurely (see the box "Does Being Physically Active Make a Difference in How Long You Live?"). Physically active people are less likely to develop or die from heart disease, respiratory disease, high blood pressure, cancer, osteoporosis, and type 2 diabetes (the most common form of diabetes).[4] As they get older, they may be able to avoid weight gain, muscle and bone loss, fatigue, and other problems associated with aging.

CHOOSE A HEALTHY DIET In addition to being sedentary, many Canadians have a diet that is too high in calories, unhealthy fats, and added sugars, and too low in fibre, complex carbohydrates, fruits, and vegetables. Like physical inactivity, this diet is linked to a number of chronic diseases. A healthy diet promotes wellness in both the short and long term. It provides necessary nutrients and sufficient energy without also providing too much of the dietary substances linked to diseases. See Chapter 7 for more detailed discussion of North American diets.

MAINTAIN A HEALTHY BODY WEIGHT Overweight and obesity are strongly associated with a number of disabling and potentially fatal conditions and diseases, including heart disease, cancer, and type 2 diabetes. Recent data show that in a 15-year span (1985–2000) there was a 72% increase in the number of Canadians who died as a result of obesity.[5] By comparison, similar statistics show a larger estimated increase (115%) in American death rates over an approximately 25-year (1980–2004) span.[6] Healthy body weight is an important part of wellness—but short-term dieting is not part of a fit and well lifestyle. Maintaining a healthy body weight requires a lifelong commitment to regular exercise, a healthy diet, and effective stress management.

MANAGE STRESS EFFECTIVELY Many people cope with stress by eating, drinking, or smoking too much. Others don't deal with it at all. In the short term, inappropriate stress management can lead to fatigue, sleep disturbances, and other unpleasant symptoms. Over longer periods of time, poor management of stress can lead to less efficient functioning of the immune system and increased susceptibility to disease. Learning to incorporate effective stress management techniques into daily life is an important part of a fit and well lifestyle. See Chapter 10 for a greater understanding of stress, how it affects us, and mechanisms to reduce the effects of stress.

AVOID TOBACCO AND DRUG USE AND LIMIT ALCOHOL CONSUMPTION Tobacco use is a risk factor for many of the leading causes of death among Canadians. It is estimated to kill over 37 000 Canadians[7] (444 000 Americans[8]) each year, more than any other behavioural or environmental factor. A hundred years ago,

- Increased endurance, strength, and flexibility
- Healthier muscles, bones, and joints
- Increased energy (calorie) expenditure
- Improved body composition
- More energy
- Improved ability to cope with stress
- Improved mood, higher self-esteem, and a greater sense of well-being
- Improved ability to fall asleep and sleep well

- Reduced risk of dying prematurely from all causes
- Reduced risk of developing and/or dying from heart disease, diabetes, high blood pressure, and colon cancer
- Reduced risk of becoming obese
- Reduced anxiety, tension, and depression
- Reduced risk of falls and fractures
- Reduced spending for health care

FIGURE 1.4 Benefits of regular physical activity.

How much of your leisure time do you spend doing nothing? It's easy to figure out: Just keep a simple log (like the one shown here) for a full week. Log the number of minutes of free time you have each day, and list your activities during those times. For our purposes, "free time" means exactly that; it doesn't include time you spend studying.

Day 1: _____
(minutes)

_____
(activities)

Day 2: _____
(minutes)

_____
(activities)

Day 3: _____
(minutes)

_____
(activities)

Day 4: _____
(minutes)

_____
(activities)

Day 5: _____
(minutes)

_____
(activities)

Day 6: _____
(minutes)

_____
(activities)

Day 7: _____
(minutes)

_____
(activities)

Based on this information, do you spend less than 30 minutes of your daily free time engaged in some type of physical activity? If so, look at your log and consider switching some of your current leisure-time activities for moderate-intensity exercise (like a brisk walk or a short bike ride).

Remember: you don't need to exercise for 30 minutes at a time to get the benefits of daily activity. You can break your exercise routine into three 10-minute chunks to make exercise fit your schedule and still enjoy all the health benefits of daily activity.

before cigarette smoking was widespread, lung cancer was considered a rare disease. Today, with over 20% of the Canadian population smoking,[9] lung cancer is the most common cause of cancer death among both men and women and one of the leading causes of death overall.

Certain forms of alcohol consumption can be linked to a shortened lifespan and even death. In 2002, approximately 4300 Canadians lost their lives to alcohol-related diseases and/or accidents.[10] Alcohol or drug intoxication is an especially notable factor in the death and disability of young people, particularly through **unintentional injuries** (such as drownings and car crashes caused by drunken driving) and violence.

PROTECT YOURSELF FROM DISEASE AND INJURY
The most effective way of dealing with disease and injury is to prevent them. Many of the lifestyle strategies discussed here help protect you against chronic illnesses. In addition, you can take specific steps to avoid infectious diseases, particularly those that are sexually transmitted.

THE ROLE OF OTHER FACTORS IN WELLNESS Heredity, the environment, and adequate health care are other important influences on health. These factors can interact in ways that raise or lower the quality of a person's life and the risk of developing particular diseases. For example, a sedentary lifestyle combined with a genetic predisposition for diabetes can greatly increase a person's risk for developing the disease. If this person also lacks adequate health care, he or she is much more likely to suffer dangerous complications from diabetes.

But in many cases, behaviour can tip the balance toward health even if heredity or environment is a negative factor. Breast cancer, for example, can run in families, but it is also associated with overweight and a sedentary lifestyle. A woman with a family history of breast cancer is less likely to die from the disease if she controls her weight, exercises, performs regular breast self-exams, and consults with her physician about mammograms. Lab 1.2 will help you evaluate your behaviours as they relate to wellness.

TERMS

physical fitness   A set of physical attributes that allows the body to respond or adapt to the demands and stress of physical effort.

sedentary   Physically inactive; literally, "sitting."

unintentional injury   An injury that occurs without harm being intended.

Does Being Physically Active Make a Difference in How Long You Live?

THE EVIDENCE FOR EXERCISE

Most of us know that being physically active makes us feel better and look better, but how do we know that physical activity and exercise are good for our health? To answer this question, the U.S. Department of Health and Human Services charged a committee with the task of reviewing the scientific literature to discover whether there is sufficient evidence to support physical activity recommendations to the public. The committee's report, the *Physical Activity Guidelines Advisory Committee Report, 2008*, summarizes the scientific evidence for the health benefits of habitual physical activity and the risks of sedentary behaviour. The report provides the rationale for government physical activity guidelines.

The first question the committee addressed was whether being physically active would help people live longer. The committee investigated the link between physical activity and all-cause mortality—deaths from all causes—by looking at 73 studies dating from 1995 to 2008. The subjects of the studies were both men and women, from all age groups (16 to 65+), and from different racial and ethnic groups. The review included studies conducted in countries in North America, Europe, the Middle East, Asia, and Australia. Follow-up time (the time from the study to the examination of mortality data) ranged from 10 months to 28 years, with a median time of 11.7 years. (The only exception to this was a Finnish study of former Olympic athletes, in which follow-up time was 71 years!)

The data from these studies strongly support an *inverse relation* between physical activity and all-cause mortality—that is, physically active individuals were less likely to die during the follow-up period. The review found that active people have about a 30% lower risk of dying compared with inactive people. These inverse associations were found not just for healthy adults but also for older adults (age 65 and older) for people with coronary artery disease and diabetes, for people with impaired mobility, and for people who were overweight or obese. Poor fitness and low physical activity levels were found to be better predictors of premature death than smoking, diabetes, or obesity. The committee found that about 150 minutes (2 to 2.5 hours) of physical activity per week is sufficient to decrease all-cause mortality (see Chapter 2 for more details). It appears that it is the overall volume of energy expended, regardless of what kinds of activities produce the energy expenditure, that makes a difference in risk of premature death.

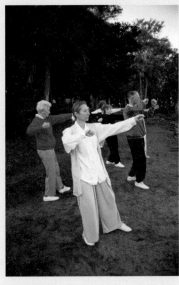

The committee also looked at whether there is a *dose-response* relation between physical activity and all-cause mortality—that is, whether more activity results in a greater reduction in death rates. Again, the studies showed an inverse relation between these two variables. This means not only that more activity above and beyond 150 minutes per week produces greater benefits but also that, for inactive people, benefits are seen at levels below 150 minutes per week. In fact, any increase in physical activity resulted in reduced risk of death. The committee refers to this as the "some is good; more is better" message. A target of 150 minutes per week is recommended, but any level of activity below the target is encouraged for inactive individuals.

Looking more closely at this relationship, the committee found that the greatest risk reduction is seen at the lower end of the physical activity spectrum (30 to 90 minutes per week). In fact, sedentary people who become more active have the greatest potential for improving health and reducing the risk of premature death. Additional risk reduction occurs as physical activity increases, but at a slower rate. For example, individuals who engaged in physical activity 90 minutes per week had a 20% reduction in mortality risk compared with inactive people, and individuals who were active 150 minutes per week, as noted earlier, had a 30% reduction in risk. But to achieve a 40% reduction in mortality, individuals had to be physically active 420 minutes per week (7 hours).

The message from the research is clear: It doesn't matter what activity you choose or even how much time you can devote to it per week as long as you get moving! The life you save will be your own!

SOURCE: Physical Activity Guidelines Advisory Committee. 2008. *Physical Activity Guidelines Advisory Committee Report, 2008*. Washington, D.C.: U.S. Department of Health and Human Services.

1.2 REACHING WELLNESS THROUGH LIFESTYLE MANAGEMENT

As you consider this description of behaviours that contribute to wellness—being physically active, choosing a healthy diet, and so on—you may be doing a mental comparison with your own behaviours. If you are like most young adults, you probably have some healthy habits and some habits that place your health at risk. For example, you may be physically active and have a healthy diet but indulge in binge drinking on weekends. You may be careful to wear your seat belt in your car but smoke cigarettes or use chewing tobacco. Moving in the direction of wellness means cultivating healthy behaviours and working to overcome unhealthy ones. This approach to lifestyle management is sometimes called **behaviour change.**

As you may already know from experience, changing an unhealthy habit can be harder than it looks. When you embark on a behaviour change plan, it may seem like too much work at first. But as you make progress, you will gain confidence in your ability to take charge of your life. You will also experience the benefits of wellness—more energy, greater vitality, deeper feelings of appreciation and curiosity, and a higher quality of life.

The rest of this chapter outlines a general process for changing unhealthy behaviours that is backed by research and that has worked for many people. You will also find many specific strategies and tips for change. For additional support, work through the activities in the Behaviour Change Workbook at the end of the text.

Use the information in this chapter along with Chapters 2–6 to put together a program that suits your goals for lifestyle development. Chapter 9 assists you in 'putting it all together'!

Getting Serious About Your Health

Before you can start changing a wellness-related behaviour, you have to know that the behaviour is problematic and that you *can* change it. To make good decisions, you need information about relevant topics and issues, including what resources are available to help you change.

EXAMINE YOUR CURRENT HEALTH HABITS Have you considered how your current lifestyle is affecting your health today and how it will affect your health in the future? Do you know which of your current habits enhance your health and which detract from it? Begin your journey toward wellness with self-assessment: Think about your own behaviour, complete the self-assessment in Lab 1.2, and talk with friends and family members about what they've noticed about your lifestyle and your health.

CHOOSE A TARGET BEHAVIOUR Changing any behaviour can be demanding. This is why it's a good idea to start small, by choosing one behaviour you want to change—called a **target behaviour**—and working on it until you succeed. Your chances of success will be greater if your first goal is simple, such as resisting the urge to snack between classes. As you change one behaviour, make your next goal a little more significant, and build on your success.

LEARN ABOUT YOUR TARGET BEHAVIOUR Once you've chosen a target behaviour, you need to know its risks and benefits for you—both now and in the future. Ask these questions:

- How is your target behaviour affecting your level of wellness today?
- What diseases or conditions does this behaviour place you at risk for?
- What effect would changing your behaviour have on your health?

As a starting point, use material from this text and from the resources listed in the For Further Exploration section at the end of each chapter; refer to the box "Evaluating Sources of Health Information" for additional guidelines.

FIND HELP Have you identified a particularly challenging target behaviour or mood, something like alcohol addiction, binge eating, or depression, that interferes with your ability to function or places you at a serious health risk? Help may be needed to change behaviours or conditions that may be too deeply rooted or too serious for self-management. Don't be discouraged by the seriousness or extent of the problem; many resources are available to help you solve it. On campus, the student health centre or campus counselling centre can provide assistance. To locate community resources, consult the yellow pages, your physician, or the Internet.

LO4 Building Motivation to Change

Knowledge is necessary for behaviour change, but it isn't usually enough to make people act. Millions of people have sedentary lifestyles, for example, even though they know it's bad for their health. This is particularly true of young adults, who may not be motivated to change because they feel well despite engaging in unhealthy behaviours (see the box "Wellness Matters for University/College Students"). To succeed at behaviour change, you need strong motivation.

EXAMINE THE PROS AND CONS OF CHANGE Health behaviours have short-term and long-term benefits and costs. Consider the benefits and costs of an inactive lifestyle:

- Short-term, such a lifestyle allows you more time to watch TV and hang out with friends, but it leaves you less physically fit and less able to participate in recreational activities.
- Long-term, it increases the risk of heart disease, cancer, stroke, and premature death.

WELLNESS TIP

If you're overweight, losing as little as 5 pounds can significantly reduce your risk of developing diabetes. To learn more, visit the Canadian Diabetes Association's website at www.diabetes.ca/.

behaviour change   A lifestyle management process that involves cultivating healthy behaviours and working to overcome unhealthy ones.

target behaviour   An isolated behaviour selected as the object of a behaviour change program.

TERMS

CRITICAL CONSUMER

General Strategies

A key first step in sharpening your critical thinking skills is to look carefully at your sources of wellness information. Critical thinking involves knowing where and how to find relevant information, how to separate fact from opinion, how to recognize faulty reasoning, how to evaluate information, and how to assess the credibility of sources.

- *Go to the original source.* Media reports often simplify the results of medical research. Find out for yourself what a study really reported, and determine whether it was based on good science. (You'll find additional strategies for evaluating research studies in Chapter 11.)

- *Watch for misleading language.* Reports that feature "breakthroughs" or "dramatic proof" are probably hype. Some studies will find that a behaviour "contributes to" or is "associated with" an outcome; this does not imply a proven cause-and-effect relationship.

- *Distinguish between research reports and public health advice.* If a study finds a link between a particular vitamin and cancer, that should not necessarily lead you to change your behaviour. But if Health Canada or the Canadian Cancer Society advises you to eat less fat or quit smoking, you can assume that many studies point in this direction and that this is advice you should follow.

- *Remember that anecdotes are not facts.* Just because your cousin Bertha lost 10 pounds on Dr. Amazing's new protein diet doesn't mean it's a safe, effective way for you to lose weight. Before you make a big change in your lifestyle, verify the information with your physician or other reliable sources.

- *Be skeptical and use your common sense.* If a report seems too good to be true, it probably is.

- *Make choices that are right for you.* Your roommate swears by swimming; you prefer aerobics. Friends and family members can be a great source of ideas and inspiration, but each of us needs to find a wellness lifestyle that works for us.

Internet Resources

Evaluating health information from online sources poses special challenges; when reviewing a health-related website, ask the following questions:

- *What is the source of the information? Who is the author or sponsor of the Webpage?*

- *How often is the site updated?*

- *What is the purpose of the page? Does the site promote particular products or procedures? Are there obvious reasons for bias?*

- *What do other sources say about a topic?*

- *Does the site conform to any set of guidelines or criteria for quality and accuracy?*

To successfully change your behaviour, you must believe that the benefits of change outweigh the costs.

Carefully examine the pros and cons of continuing your current behaviour and of changing to a healthier one. Focus on the effects that are most meaningful to you, including those that are tied to your personal identity and values. For example, if you see yourself as an active person who is a good role model for others, then adopting behaviours such as engaging in regular physical activity and getting adequate sleep will support your personal identity. If you value independence and control over your life, then quitting smoking would be consistent with your values and goals. To complete your analysis, ask friends and family members about the effects of your behaviour on them. For example, a younger sister may tell you that your smoking habit influenced her decision to take up smoking.

The short-term benefits of behaviour change can be an important motivating force. Although some people are motivated by long-term goals, such as avoiding a disease that may hit them in 30 years, most are more likely to be moved to action by shorter-term, more personal goals. Feeling better, doing better in school, improving at a sport, reducing stress, and increasing self-esteem are common short-term benefits of health behaviour change. Many wellness behaviours are associated with immediate improvements in quality of life. For example, surveys have found that nonsmokers feel healthy and full of energy more days each month than do smokers, and they report fewer days of sadness and troubled sleep; the same is true when physically active people are compared with sedentary people. Over time, these types of differences add up to a substantially greater quality of life for people who engage in healthy behaviours.

BOOST SELF-EFFICACY   When you start thinking about changing a health behaviour, a big factor in your eventual success is whether you have confidence in yourself and in your ability to change. **Self-efficacy** refers to your belief in your ability to successfully take action and perform a specific task. Strategies for boosting self-efficacy include developing an internal locus of control, using visualization and self-talk, and obtaining encouragement from supportive people.

FITNESS TIP

Visualization is such a powerful technique that Olympic athletes learn how to harness it for peak performance. It works for average people, too. Set a small fitness goal, then imagine yourself doing it—as clearly and as often as you can. Visualization can help you believe in yourself, and belief can be a step toward success!

Wellness Matters for University/College Students

If you are like most university/college students, you probably feel pretty good about your health right now. Most university/college students are in their late teens or early twenties, lead active lives, have plenty of friends, and look forward to a future filled with opportunity. With all these things going for you, why shouldn't you feel good?

A Closer Look

Although most university/college-age people look healthy, appearances can be deceiving. Each year, thousands of students lose productive academic time to physical and emotional health problems—some of which can continue to plague them for life.

The following table shows the top 10 health issues affecting students' academic performance, according to the 2008 National College Health Assessment II.

HEALTH ISSUE	STUDENTS AFFECTED (%)
Stress	27.2
Sleep difficulties	19.3
Anxiety	18.2
Cold/flu/sore throat	15.4
Work	13.1
Concern for a troubled friend or family member	11.3
Depression	11.2
Internet use/computer games	10.8
Relationship difficulties	10.7
Extracurricular activities	10.3

Each of these issues is related to one or more of the six dimensions of wellness, and most can be influenced by choices students make daily. Although some troubles—such as the death of a friend—cannot be controlled, other physical and emotional concerns can be minimized by choosing healthy behaviours. For example, there are many ways to manage stress, the top health issue affecting students. By reducing unhealthy choices (such as using alcohol to relax) and by increasing healthy choices (such as using time management techniques), even busy students can reduce the impact of stress on their life.

The survey also estimated that, based on students' reporting of their height and weight, more than 31% of university/college students are either overweight or obese. Although heredity plays a role in determining one's weight, lifestyle is also a factor in weight and weight management. In many studies over the past few decades, a large percentage of students have reported behaviours such as these:

- Overeating
- Snacking on junk food
- Frequently eating high-fat foods
- Using alcohol and binge drinking

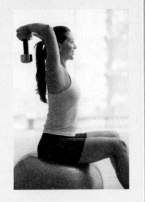

Clearly, eating behaviours are often a matter of choice. Although students may not see (or feel) the effects of their dietary habits today, the long-term health risks are significant. Overweight and obese persons run a higher-than-normal risk of developing diabetes, heart disease, and cancer later in life. We now know with certainty that improving one's eating habits, even a little, can lead to weight loss and improved overall health.

Other Choices, Other Problems

Students commonly make other unhealthy choices. Here are some examples from the 2004 Canadian Campus Survey:

- Nearly 62% of students spent money on at least one gambling activity since the school year began.
- About 32% of students had engaged in hazardous or harmful drinking patterns in the past year.
- Almost 17% of students had used cannabis at least once during the past month.

What choices do you make in these situations? Remember: It's never too late to change. The sooner you trade an unhealthy behaviour for a healthy one, the longer you'll be around to enjoy the benefits.

The Transition to University/College

Embarking on a new academic path can often mean moving far away from home, family, and friends and starting anew. A new environment, new academic expectations, and many more responsibilities for first-year students often means new challenges. Keup and Stolzenberg's (2004) Your First College Year survey reported that one third of the student sample reported feeling "frequently overwhelmed by all they had to do" during their transition to university/college. In addition, more than one third felt "frequently" or "occasionally" lonely or homesick and worried about meeting new people.

It has recently been suggested that one way to ease the challenges of the transition to university/college is to focus some of your wellness energies on your intrapersonal skills, interpersonal skills, adaptability, stress management skills, and general mood. Enhancing these emotional and social skills have been shown to positively alter academic success and academic retention (Parker & Duffy, 2005). Look for specialized programs run by your university/college student groups or counselling centres.

SOURCES: Adlaf, E.M., Demers, A., Gliksman, L. (Eds.). 2005. *Canadian Campus Survey 2004.* Centre for Addiction and Mental Health, Toronto, ON: CAMH; American College Health Association. 2009. *American College Health Association—National College Health Assessment II: Reference Group Data Report Fall 2008.* Baltimore, Md.: American College Health Association; and Parker, J.D.A., & Duffy, J.M. (2005, January 12). *Making a Successful Transition During the First Year of College: Does Emotional Intelligence Matter?* Retrieved October 20, 2011, from University of South Carolina: http://www.sc.edu/fye/resources/assessment/newessay/author/parkerduffy.html.

Locus of Control Who do you believe is controlling your life? Is it your parents, friends, or school? Is it "fate"? Or is it you? **Locus of control** refers to the figurative "place" a person designates as the source of responsibility for the events in his or her life. People who believe they are in control of their own lives are said to have an internal locus of control. Those who believe that factors beyond their control—heredity, friends and family, the environment, fate, luck, or other outside forces—are more important in determining the events of their lives are said to have an external locus of control.

For lifestyle management, an internal locus of control is an advantage because it reinforces motivation and commitment. An external locus of control can sabotage efforts to change behaviour. For example, if you believe you are destined to die of breast cancer because your mother died from the disease, you may view monthly breast self-exams and regular checkups as a waste of time. In contrast, if you believe you can take action to reduce your hereditary risk of breast cancer, you will be motivated to follow guidelines for early detection of the disease.

If you find yourself attributing too much influence to outside forces, gather more information about your wellness-related behaviours. List all the ways that making lifestyle changes will improve your health. If you believe you'll succeed, and if you recognize and accept that you are in charge of your life, you're on your way to wellness.

Visualization and Self-Talk One of the best ways to boost your confidence and self-efficacy is to visualize yourself successfully engaging in a new, healthier behaviour. Imagine yourself going for a regular after-dinner walk or choosing healthier snacks. Also visualize yourself enjoying all the short-term and long-term benefits that your lifestyle change will bring. Create a new self-image: What will you and your life be like when you become a regular exerciser or a healthy eater?

You can also use **self-talk,** the internal dialogue you carry on with yourself, to increase your confidence in your ability to change. Counter any self-defeating patterns of thought with more positive or realistic thoughts: "I am a strong, capable person, and I can maintain my commitment to change." Refer to Chapter 10 for more on self-talk.

Role Models and Other Supportive Individuals Social support can make a big difference in your level

of motivation and your chances of success. Perhaps you know people who have reached the goal you are striving for; they could be role models or mentors for you, providing information and support for your efforts. Gain strength from their experiences, and tell yourself, "If they can do it, so can I." In addition, find a buddy who wants to make the same changes you do and who can take an active role in your behaviour change program. For example, an exercise buddy can provide companionship and encouragement for times when you might be tempted to skip your workout.

IDENTIFY AND OVERCOME BARRIERS TO CHANGE Don't let past failures at behaviour change discourage you; they can be a great source of information you can use to boost your chances of future success. Make a list of the problems and challenges you faced in your previous behaviour change attempts; to this, add the short-term costs of behaviour change that you identified in your analysis of the pros and cons of change. Once you've listed these key barriers to change, develop a practical plan for overcoming each one. For example, if you always smoke when you're with certain friends, decide in advance how you will turn down the next cigarette you are offered.

Enhancing Your Readiness to Change

The transtheoretical, or "stages of change," model has been shown to be an effective approach to lifestyle self-management. According to this model, you move through distinct stages as you work to change your target behaviour. It is important to determine what stage you are in now so that you can choose appropriate strategies for progressing through the cycle of change. This approach can help you enhance your readiness and intention to change. Read the following sections to determine what stage you are in for your target behaviour. For ideas on changing stages, see the box "Tips for Moving Forward in the Cycle of Behaviour Change."

PRECONTEMPLATION People at this stage do not think they have a problem and do not intend to change their behaviour. They may be unaware of the risks associated with their behaviour or may deny them. They may have tried unsuccessfully to change in the past and may now feel demoralized and think the situation is hopeless. They may also blame other people or external factors for their problems. People in the precontemplation stage believe that there are more reasons or more important reasons not to change than there are reasons to change.

CONTEMPLATION People at this stage know they have a problem and intend to take action within 6 months. They acknowledge the benefits that behaviour change will have for them but are also very aware of the costs of changing—to be successful, people must believe that the benefits of change outweigh the costs. People in the contemplation stage wonder about possible courses of action but don't know how to proceed. There may also be specific barriers to change that appear too difficult to overcome.

PREPARATION People at this stage plan to take action within a month or may already have begun to make small changes in their behaviour. They may be engaging in their new, healthier behaviour, but not yet regularly or consistently. They may have created a plan for change but may be worried about failing.

ACTION During the action stage, people outwardly modify their behaviour and their environment. The action stage usually requires the greatest commitment of time and energy, and people in this stage are at risk for reverting to old, unhealthy patterns of behaviour.

MAINTENANCE People at this stage have maintained their new, healthier lifestyle for at least 6 months. Lapses may have occurred, but people in maintenance have been successful in quickly reestablishing the desired behaviour. The maintenance stage can last for months or years.

TERMINATION For some behaviours, a person may reach the sixth and final stage of termination. People at this stage have exited the cycle of change and are no longer tempted to lapse back into their old behaviour. They have a new self-image and total self-efficacy with regard to their target behaviour.

Dealing with Relapse

People seldom progress through the stages of change in a straightforward, linear way; rather, they tend to move to a certain stage and then slip back to a previous stage before resuming their forward progress. Research suggests that most people make several attempts before they successfully change a behaviour; four out of five people experience some degree of backsliding. For this reason, the stages of change are best conceptualized as a spiral, in which people cycle back through previous stages but are further along in the process each time they renew their commitment (Figure 1.5).

If you experience a lapse—a single slip—or a relapse—a return to old habits—don't give up. Relapse can be demoralizing, but it is not the same as failure; failure means stopping before you reach your goal and never changing your target behaviour. During the early stages of the change process, it's a good idea to plan for relapse so you can avoid guilt and self-blame and get back on track quickly. Follow these steps:

1. *Forgive yourself.* A single setback isn't the end of the world, but abandoning your efforts to change could have negative effects on your life.

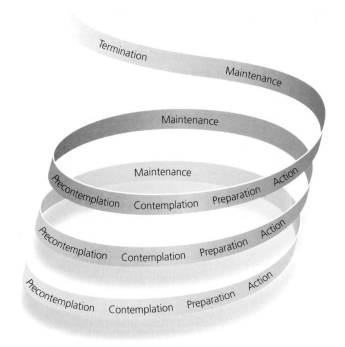

FIGURE 1.5 **The stages of change: A spiral model.**

SOURCE: Adapted from Prochaska, J. O., C. C. Diclemente, and J. C. Norcross. 1992. In search of how people change. *American Psychologist* 47(9): 1102–1114. Copyright © 1992 by the American Psychological Association. Reprinted by permission.

2. *Give yourself credit for the progress you have already made.* You can use that success as motivation to continue.

3. *Move on.* You can learn from a relapse and use that knowledge to deal with potential setbacks in the future.

If relapses keep occurring or if you can't seem to control them, you may need to return to a previous stage of the behaviour change process. If this is necessary, reevaluate your goals and your strategy. A different or less stressful approach may help you avoid setbacks when you try again.

Developing Skills for Change: Creating a Personalized Plan

Once you are committed to making a change, it's time to put together a plan of action. Your key to success is a well-thought-out plan that sets goals, anticipates problems, and includes rewards.

1. MONITOR YOUR BEHAVIOUR AND GATHER DATA Keep a record of your target behaviour and the circumstances surrounding it. Record this information for at least a week or two. Keep your notes in a health journal or notebook or on your computer (see the sample journal entries in Figure 1.6). Record each occurrence of your behaviour, noting the following:

- What the activity was
- When and where it happened
- What you were doing
- How you felt at that time

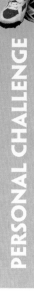

Picking Target Behaviours

When starting out on any behaviour change plan, the hardest part can be deciding what behaviour you want to change. But it doesn't have to be hard; as mentioned in the chapter, you'll probably have the greatest success if you start small. Use the following list to identify five health-related behaviours that you would like to change. List them in order, starting with the behaviour you think would be easiest to change and ending with the most difficult.

1. _____

2. _____

3. _____

4. _____

5. _____

The real challenge of this activity is thinking. Examine your lifestyle thoroughly, and consider the things you do (or don't do) every day that may be having a negative effect on your health or wellness. Don't worry if it takes some time to come up with a list, and don't be surprised if you shuffle the items around a few times. The goal is to come up with a list that is doable and realistic for you.

If your goal is to start an exercise program, track your activities to determine how to make time for workouts. A blank log is provided in Activity 3 in the Behaviour Change Workbook at the end of this text.

2. ANALYZE THE DATA AND IDENTIFY PATTERNS
After you have collected data on the behaviour, analyze the data to identify patterns. When are you most likely to overeat? What events trigger your appetite? Perhaps you are especially hungry at midmorning or when you put off eating dinner until 9 o'clock at night. Perhaps you overindulge in food and drink when you go to a particular restaurant or when you're with certain friends. Note

the connections between your feelings and such external cues as time of day, location, situation, and the actions of others around you.

3. BE "SMART" ABOUT SETTING GOALS
If your goals are too challenging, you will have trouble making steady progress and will be more likely to give up altogether. If, for example, you are in poor physical condition, it will not make sense to set a goal of being ready to run a marathon within 2 months. If you set goals you can live with, it will be easier to stick with your behaviour change plan and be successful.

Date	November 5				Day	M	TU	W	TH	F	SA	SU			

Time of day	M/S	Food eaten	Cals.	H	Where did you eat?	What else were you doing?	How did someone else influence you?	What made you want to eat what you did?	Emotions and feelings?	Thoughts and concerns?
7:30	M	1 C Corn Flakes cereal 1/2 C skim milk coffee, black 1 C orange juice	110 40 — 120	3	home	reading newspaper	alone	I always eat cereal in the morning	a little keyed up & worried	thinking about quiz in class today
10:30	S	1 apple	90	1	hall outside classroom	studying	alone	felt tired & wanted to wake up	tired	worried about next class
12:30	M	1 C chili 1 roll 1 pat butter 1 orange 2 oatmeal cookies 1 pop	290 120 35 60 120 150	2	campus food court	talking	eating w/ friends; we decided to eat at the food court	wanted to be part of group	excited and happy	interested in hearing everyone's plans for the weekend

M/S = Meal or snack   H = Hunger rating (0–3)

FIGURE 1.6 Sample health journal entries.

Precontemplation

- **Raise your awareness.** Research your target behaviour and its effects.

- **Be self-aware.** Look at the mechanisms you use to resist change, such as denial or rationalization. Find ways to counteract these mechanisms.

- **Seek social support.** Friends and family members can help you identify target behaviours and understand their impact on the people around you.

- **Identify helpful resources.** These might include exercise classes or stress-management workshops offered by your school.

Contemplation

- **Keep a journal.** A record of your target behaviour and the circumstances that elicit the behaviour can help you plan a change program.

- **Do a cost–benefit analysis.** Identify the costs and benefits (both current and future) of maintaining your behaviour and of changing it. Costs can be monetary, social, emotional, and so on.

- **Identify barriers to change.** Knowing these obstacles can help you overcome them.

- **Engage your emotions.** Watch movies or read books about people with your target behaviour. Imagine what your life will be like if you don't change.

- **Create a new self-image.** Imagine what you'll be like after changing your target behaviour. Try to think of yourself in new terms right now.

- **Think before you act.** Learn why you engage in the target behaviour. Determine what "sets you off," and train yourself not to act reflexively.

Preparation

- **Create a plan.** Include a start date, goals, rewards, and specific steps you will take to change your behaviour.

- **Make change a priority.** Create and sign a contract with yourself.

- **Practise visualization and self-talk.** These techniques can help prepare you mentally for challenging situations.

- **Take short steps.** Successfully practising your new behaviour for a short time—even a single day—can boost your confidence and motivation.

Action

- **Monitor your progress.** Keep up with your journal entries.

- **Change your environment.** Make changes that will discourage the target behaviour—for example, getting rid of snack foods or not stocking the refrigerator with beer.

- **Find alternatives to your target behaviour.** Make a list of things you can do to replace the behaviour.

- **Reward yourself.** Rewards should be identified in your change plan. Give yourself lots of praise, and focus on your success.

- **Involve your friends.** Tell them you want to change, and ask for their help.

- **Don't get discouraged.** Real change is difficult.

Maintenance

- **Keep going.** Continue using the positive strategies that worked in earlier stages.

- **Be prepared for lapses.** Don't let slip-ups set you back.

- **Be a role model.** Once you have successfully changed your behaviour, you may be able to help someone else do the same thing.

Experts suggest that your goals meet the "SMART" criteria; that is, your behaviour change goals should be:

- *Specific:* Avoid vague goals like "eat more fruits and vegetables." Instead, state your objectives in specific terms, such as "eat 2 cups of fruit and 3 cups of vegetables every day."

- *Measurable.* Recognize that your progress will be easier to track if your goals are quantifiable, so give your goal a number. You might measure your goal in terms of time (such as "walk briskly for 20 minutes a day"), distance ("run 3 km, 3 days per week"), or some other amount ("drink 8 glasses of water every day").

- *Attainable.* Set goals that are within your physical limits. For example, if you are a poor swimmer, it might not be possible for you to meet a short-term fitness goal by swimming laps. Walking or biking might be better options.

- *Realistic.* Manage your expectations when you set goals. For example, it may not be possible for a long-time smoker to quit cold turkey. A more realistic approach might be to use nicotine-replacement patches or gum for several weeks while getting help from a support group.

- *Time frame–specific.* Give yourself a reasonable amount of time to reach your goal, state the time frame in your behaviour change plan, and set your agenda to meet the goal within the time frame.

Using these criteria, a sedentary person who wanted to improve his health and build fitness might set a goal of being able to run 5 km in 30 minutes, to be achieved within a time frame of 6 months. To work toward that goal, he might set a number of smaller, intermediate goals that are easier to achieve. For example, his list of goals might look like this:

Week	Frequency (days/week)	Activity	Duration (minutes)
1	3	Walk < 1.6 km	10–15
2	3	Walk 1.6 km	15–20
3	4	Walk 1.6–3 km	20–25
4	4	Walk 3–5 km	25–30
5–7	3–4	Walk/run 1.6 km	15–20
. . .			
21–24	4–5	Run 3–5 km	25–30

Of course, it may not be possible to meet these goals, but you never know until you try. As you work toward meeting your long-term goal, you may find it necessary to adjust your short-term goals. For example, you may find that you can start running sooner than you thought, or you may be able to run farther than you originally estimated. In such cases, it may be reasonable to make your goals more challenging. Otherwise, you may want to make them easier in order to stay motivated.

For some goals and situations, it may make more sense to focus on something other than your outcome goal. If you are in an early stage of change, for example, your goal may be to learn more about the risks associated with your target behaviour or to complete a cost-benefit analysis. If your goal involves a long-term lifestyle change, such as reaching a healthy weight, it is better to focus on developing healthy habits than to target a specific weight loss. Your goal in this case might be exercising for 30 minutes every day, reducing portion sizes, or eliminating late-night snacks.

4. DEVISE A PLAN OF ACTION   Develop a strategy that will support your efforts to change. Your plan of action should include the following steps:

Get What You Need   Identify campus and community resources that can help you. For example, you can join a community walking club or sign up for a smoking cessation program. You may also need to buy some new running shoes or nicotine replacement patches. Get the items you need right away; waiting can delay your progress.

Modify Your Environment   If there are cues in your environment that trigger your target behaviour, try to control them. For example, if you normally have alcohol at home, getting rid of it can help prevent you from indulging. If you usually study with a group of friends in an environment that allows smoking, try moving to a nonsmoking area. If you always buy a snack at a certain vending machine, change your route to avoid it.

Control Related Habits   You may have habits that contribute to your target behaviour; modifying these

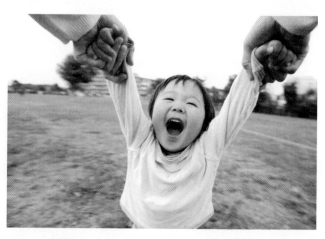

Your environment contains powerful cues for both positive and negative lifestyle choices. Identifying and using the healthier options available to you throughout the day is a key part of a successful behaviour change program.

habits can help change the behaviour. For example, if you usually plop down on the sofa while watching TV, try putting an exercise bike in front of the set so you can burn calories while watching your favourite programs.

Reward Yourself   Giving yourself instant, real rewards for good behaviour will reinforce your efforts. Plan your rewards; decide in advance what each one will be and how you will earn it. Tie rewards to achieving specific goals or subgoals. For example, you might treat yourself to a movie after a week of avoiding snacks. Make a list of items or events to use as rewards; they should be special to you and preferably unrelated to food or alcohol.

Involve the People Around You   Tell family and friends about your plan and ask them to help. To help them respond appropriately to your needs, create a specific list of dos and don'ts. For example, ask them to support you when you set aside time to exercise or avoid second helpings at dinner.

Plan for Challenges   Think about situations and people that might derail your program, and develop ways to cope with them. For example, if you think it will be hard to stick to your usual exercise program during exams, schedule short bouts of physical activity (such as a brisk walk) as stress-reducing study breaks.

5. MAKE A PERSONAL CONTRACT   A serious personal contract—one that commits you to your word—can result in a higher chance of follow-through than a casual, off-hand promise. Your contract can help prevent procrastination by specifying the important dates and can also serve as a reminder of your personal commitment to change.

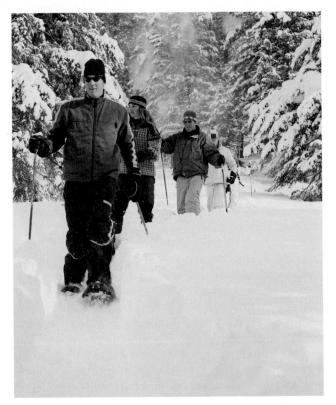

A convenient setting and a friendly companion help make exercise a satisfying and pleasurable experience. Choosing the right activity and doing it the right way are important elements in a successful behaviour change program.

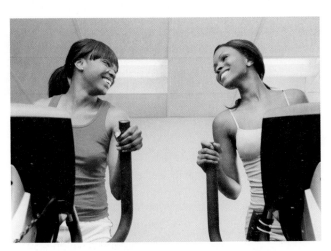

Help from a committed friend can ensure the success of any behaviour change program, whether you want to eat better, lose weight, stop smoking, or exercise more.

Your contract should include a statement of your goal and your commitment to reaching it. The contract should also include details, such as the following:

- The date you will start
- The steps you will take to measure your progress
- The strategies you plan to use to promote change
- The date you expect to reach your final goal

Have someone— preferably someone who will be actively helping you with your program—sign your contract as a witness.

Figure 1.7 shows a sample behaviour change contract for someone who is committing to eating more fruit every day. A blank contract is included as Activity 8 in the Behaviour Change Workbook.

Putting Your Plan into Action

The starting date has arrived, and you are ready to put your plan into action. This stage requires commitment, the resolve to stick with the plan no matter what temptations you encounter. Remember all the reasons you have to make the change—and remember that *you* are the boss. Use all your strategies to make your plan work. Make sure your environment is change-friendly, and obtain as much support and encouragement from others as possible. Keep track of your progress in your health journal, and give yourself regular rewards. And don't forget to give yourself a pat on the back—congratulate yourself, notice how much better you look or feel, and feel good about how far you've come and how you've gained control of your behaviour.

Staying With It

As you continue with your program, don't be surprised when you run up against obstacles; they're inevitable. In fact, it's a good idea to expect problems and give yourself

---

Behaviour Change Contract

1. I, _____, agree to increase my consumption of fruit from   1 cup per week to 2 cups per day.

2. I will begin on ____10/5____ and plan to reach my goal of __2 cups__ of fruit per day   by __12/7__

3. To reach my final goal, I have devised the following schedule of mini-goals. For each step in my program, I will give myself the reward listed.

   I will begin to have ½ cup   10/5   see movie
   of fruit with breakfast
   I will begin to have ½ cup   10/26   new cd
   of fruit with lunch
   I will begin to substitute fruit   11/16   concert
   juice for soda 1 time per day

   My overall reward for reaching my goal will be _trip to beach_

4. I have gathered and analyzed data on my target behaviour and have identified the following strategies for changing my behaviour: _Keep the fridge stocked with easy-to-carry fruit. Pack fruit in my backpack every day. Buy lunch at place that serves fruit._

5. I will use the following tools to monitor my progress toward my final goal: Chart on fridge door
   Health journal

   I sign this contract as an indication of my personal commitment to reach my goal: ____Tammy Lau____ ____9/28____

   I have recruited a helper who will witness my contract and also increase his consumption of fruit; eat lunch with me twice a week.
   ____Eric March____ ____9/28____

FIGURE 1.7 A sample behaviour change contract.

time to step back, see how you're doing, and make some changes before going on. If your program is grinding to a halt, identify what is blocking your progress. It may come from one of the sources described in the following sections.

SOCIAL INFLUENCES   Take a hard look at the reactions of the people you're counting on, and see if they're really supporting you. If they come up short, connect and network with others who will be more supportive.

A related trap is trying to get your friends or family members to change *their* behaviours. The decision to make a major behaviour change is something people come to only after intensive self-examination. You may be able to influence someone by tactfully providing facts or support, but that's all. Focus on yourself. If you succeed, you may become a role model for others.

LEVELS OF MOTIVATION AND COMMITMENT   You won't make real progress until an inner drive leads you to the stage of change at which you are ready to make a personal commitment to the goal. If commitment is your problem, you may need to wait until the behaviour you're dealing with makes your life more unhappy or unhealthy; then your desire to change it will be stronger. Or you may find that changing your goal will inspire you to keep going. For more ideas, refer to Activity 9 in the Behaviour Change Workbook at the end of the text.

CHOICE OF TECHNIQUES AND LEVEL OF EFFORT   If your plan is not working as well as you thought it would, make changes where you're having the most trouble. If you've lagged on your running schedule, for example, maybe it's because you don't like running. An aerobics class might suit you better. There are many ways to move toward your goal. Or you may not be trying hard enough. You do have to push toward your goal. If it were easy, you wouldn't need to have a plan.

STRESS BARRIER   If you've hit a wall in your program, look at the sources of stress in your life. If the stress is temporary, such as catching a cold or having a term paper due, you may want to wait until it passes before strengthening your efforts. If the stress is ongoing, find healthy ways to manage it (see Chapter 10 for ideas like taking a half-hour walk after lunch or beginning a yoga class). You may even want to make stress management your highest priority for behaviour change.

PROCRASTINATING, RATIONALIZING, AND BLAMING
Be alert to games you might be playing with yourself, so you can stop them. Such games include the following:

- *Procrastinating*. If you tell yourself, "It's Friday already; I might as well wait until Monday to start," you're procrastinating. Break your plan into smaller steps that you can accomplish one day at a time.
- *Rationalizing*. If you tell yourself, "I wanted to go swimming today but wouldn't have had time to wash my hair afterward," you're making excuses.

- *Blaming*. If you tell yourself, "I couldn't exercise because Dave was hogging the elliptical trainer," you're blaming others for your own failure to follow through. Blaming is a way of taking your focus off the real problem and denying responsibility for your own actions.

BE FIT AND WELL FOR LIFE   Your first attempts at making behaviour changes may never go beyond the contemplation or preparation stage. But as you experience some success, you'll start to have more positive feelings about yourself. You may discover new physical activities and sports you enjoy and you may encounter new situations and meet new people. Perhaps you'll surprise yourself by accomplishing things you didn't think were possible— breaking a longstanding nicotine habit, competing in a race, climbing a mountain, developing a leaner body. Most of all, you'll discover the feeling of empowerment that comes from taking charge of your health. Being healthy takes extra effort, but the paybacks in energy and vitality are priceless.

Once you've started, don't stop. Assume that health improvement is forever. Take on the easier problems first, and then use what you learn to tackle more difficult problems later. When you feel challenged, remind yourself that you are creating a lifestyle that minimizes your health risks and maximizes your enjoyment of life. You *can* take charge of your health in a dramatic and meaningful way. *Fit and Well* will show you how.

TIPS FOR TODAY AND THE FUTURE

You are in charge of your health! Many of the decisions you make every day have an impact on the quality of your life, both now and in the future.

RIGHT NOW YOU CAN

- Go for a 15-minute walk.
- Have a piece of fruit for a snack.
- Call a friend and arrange for a time to catch up with each other.
- Start thinking about whether you have a health behaviour you'd like to change. If you do, consider the elements of a behaviour change strategy. For example,
  - Begin a mental list of the pros and cons of the behaviour.
  - Create a format for a log to monitor your target behaviour.
  - Talk to someone who can support you in your attempts to make a behaviour change.

IN THE FUTURE YOU CAN

- Stay current on health- and wellness-related news and issues.
- Participate in health awareness and promotion campaigns in your community—for example, support smoking restrictions in local venues.
- Be a role model for someone else who is working on a health behaviour you have successfully changed.

- Wellness is the ability to live life fully, with vitality and meaning. Wellness is dynamic and multidimensional; it incorporates physical, emotional, intellectual, spiritual, interpersonal and social, and environmental dimensions.

- People today have greater control over and greater responsibility for their health than ever before.

- Behaviours that promote wellness include being physically active; choosing a healthy diet; maintaining a healthy body weight; managing stress effectively; avoiding use of tobacco and limiting alcohol use; and protecting oneself from disease and injury.

- Although heredity, environment, and health care all play roles in wellness and disease, behaviour can mitigate their effects.

- To make lifestyle changes, you need information about yourself, your health habits, and resources available to help you change.

- You can increase your motivation for behaviour change by examining the benefits and costs of change, boosting self-efficacy, and identifying and overcoming key barriers to change.

- The stages of change model describes six stages that people may move through as they try to change their behaviour: precontemplation, contemplation, preparation, action, maintenance, and termination.

- A specific plan for change can be developed by (1) collecting data on your behaviour and recording it in a journal; (2) analyzing the recorded data; (3) setting specific goals; (4) devising strategies for obtaining information, modifying the environment, rewarding yourself, involving others, and planning ahead; and (5) making a personal contract.

- To start and maintain a behaviour change program you need commitment, a well-developed and manageable plan, social support, and strong stress management techniques. It is also important to monitor the progress of your program, revising it as necessary.

Organizations, Hotlines, and Websites

The Internet addresses (also called uniform resource locators, or URLs) listed here were accurate at the time of publication.

Centers for Disease Control and Prevention. Through phone, fax, and the Internet, the CDC provides a wide variety of health information.
   800-311-3435; 888-CDC-FAXX (CDC Fax)
   http://www.cdc.gov

Canadian Institute for Health Information:
   http://www.cihi.ca

The Canadian Women's Health Network:
   http://www.cwhn.ca

Coalition for Active Living in Canada:
   http://www.activeliving.ca

Many other government websites provide access to health-related materials:

Health Canada:
   http://www.hc-sc.gc.ca

Healthy Living Unit–Public Health Agency of Canada:
   http://www.phac-aspc.gc.ca/pau-uap/fitness/

Physical Activity Guides:
   http://www.phac-aspc.gc.ca/pau-uap/paguide/

Women's Health Matters:
   http://www.womenshealthmatters.ca

Go Ask Alice. Sponsored by the Columbia University Health Service, this site provides answers to student questions about stress, sexuality, fitness, and many other wellness topics.
   http://www.goaskalice.columbia.edu

National Health Information Centre (NHIC). Puts consumers in touch with the organizations that are best able to provide answers to health-related questions.
   800-336-4797
   http://www.health.gov/nhic

Student Counseling Virtual Pamphlet Collection. Provides links to more than 400 pamphlets produced by different student counselling centres; topics include relationships, family issues, substance abuse, anger management, and study skills.
   http://counseling.uchicago.edu/vpc

World Health Organization (WHO). Provides information about WHO activities and about many health topics and issues affecting people around the world.
   http://www.who.int

The following are just a few of the many sites that provide consumer-oriented information on a variety of health issues:
   Family Doctor.Org: http://www.familydoctor.org
   InteliHealth: http://www.intelihealth.com
   Mayo Clinic: http://www.mayoclinic.com
   WebMD: http://webmd.com
   CNN Health: http://www.cnn.com/health
   MedlinePlus News: http://www.nlm.nih.gov/medlineplus/newsbydate.html
   Yahoo Health News: http://news.yahoo.com/health

Newsletters

Center for Science in the Public Interest Nutrition Action Health Letter (http://www.cspinet.org/nah/index.htm)

Consumer Reports on Health (800-274-7596; http://www .consumerreports.org/oh/index.htm)

Harvard Health Letter (877-649-9457; http://www.health.harvard .edu)

Harvard Men's Health Watch (877-649-9457)

Harvard Women's Health Watch (877-649-9457)

Mayo Clinic Housecall (http://www.mayoclinic.com/health/house call/HouseCall)

Tufts University Health & Nutrition Newsletter (http://www .tuftshealthletter.com)

University of California at Berkeley Wellness Letter (800-829-9170; http://www.wellnessletter.com)

Name _____   Section _____   Date _____

LAB 1.1 Your Wellness Profile

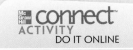

Consider how your lifestyle, attitudes, and characteristics relate to each of the six dimensions of wellness. Fill in your strengths for each dimension (examples of strengths are listed with each dimension). Once you've completed your lists, choose what you believe are your five most important strengths and circle them.

Physical wellness: To maintain overall physical health and engage in appropriate physical activity (e.g., stamina, strength, flexibility, healthy body composition).

_____

_____

_____

Intellectual wellness: To pursue and retain knowledge, think critically about issues, make sound decisions, identify problems, and find solutions (e.g., common sense, creativity, curiosity).

_____

_____

_____

Spiritual wellness: To develop a set of beliefs, principles, or values that give meaning or purpose to one's life; to develop faith in something beyond oneself (e.g., religious faith, service to others).

_____

_____

_____

Emotional wellness: To have a positive self-concept, deal constructively with your feelings, and develop positive qualities (e.g., optimism, trust, self-confidence, determination).

_____

_____

_____

Interpersonal/social wellness: To develop and maintain meaningful relationships with a network of friends and family members, and to contribute to your community (e.g., friendly, good-natured, compassionate, supportive, good listener).

_____

_____

_____

Environmental wellness: To protect yourself from environmental hazards and to minimize the negative impact of your behaviour on the environment (e.g., carpooling, recycling).

_____

_____

_____

Next, think about where you fall on the wellness continuum for each of the dimensions of wellness. Indicate your placement for each—physical, emotional, intellectual, spiritual, interpersonal/social, and environmental—by placing Xs on the continuum below.

| Low level of wellness | Physical, psychological, emotional symptoms | Change and growth | High level of wellness |

Based on both your current lifestyle and your goals for the future, what do you think your placement on the wellness continuum will be in 10 years? What new health behaviours would you have to adopt to achieve your goals? Which of your current behaviours would you need to change to maintain or improve your level of wellness in the future?

Does the description of wellness given in this chapter encompass everything you believe is part of wellness for you? Write your own definition of wellness, and include any additional dimensions that are important to you. Then rate your level of wellness based on your own definition.

Using Your Results

How did you score? Are you satisfied with your current level of wellness—overall and in each dimension? In which dimension(s) would you most like to increase your level of wellness?

What should you do next? As you consider possible target behaviours for a behaviour change program, choose things that will maintain or increase your level of wellness in one of the dimensions you listed as an area of concern. Remember to consider health behaviours such as smoking or eating a high-fat diet that may threaten your level of wellness in the future. Below, list several possible target behaviours and the wellness dimensions that they influence.

For additional guidance in choosing a target behaviour, complete the lifestyle self-assessment in Lab 1.2.

Name _____ Section _____ Date _____

LAB 1.2 Lifestyle Evaluation

connect ACTIVITY DO IT ONLINE

How does your current lifestyle compare with the lifestyle recommended for wellness? For each question, choose the answer that best describes your behaviour; then add up your score for each section.

	Almost Always	Sometimes	Never
Exercise/Fitness			
1. I engage in moderate exercise, such as brisk walking or swimming, for 20–60 minutes, three to five times a week.	4	1	0
2. I do exercises to develop muscular strength and endurance at least twice a week.	2	1	0
3. I spend some of my leisure time participating in individual, family, or team activities, such as gardening, bowling, or softball.	2	1	0
4. I maintain a healthy body weight, avoiding overweight and underweight.	2	1	0

Exercise/Fitness Score: _____

Nutrition			
1. I eat a variety of foods each day, including 5 or more servings of fruits and/or vegetables.	3	1	0
2. I limit the amount of total fat and saturated and trans fat in my diet.	3	1	0
3. I avoid skipping meals.	2	1	0
4. I limit the amount of salt and sugar I eat.	2	1	0

Nutrition Score: _____

Tobacco Use

If you never use tobacco, enter a score of 10 for this section and go to the next section.

	Almost Always	Sometimes	Never
1. I avoid using tobacco.	2	1	0
2. I smoke only a pipe or cigars, *or* I use smokeless tobacco.	2	1	0

Tobacco Use Score: _____

Alcohol and Drugs			
1. I avoid alcohol, or I drink no more than 1 (women) or 2 (men) drinks a day.	4	1	0
2. I avoid using alcohol or other drugs as a way of handling stressful situations or the problems in my life.	2	1	0
3. I am careful not to drink alcohol when taking medications (such as cold or allergy medications) or when pregnant.	2	1	0
4. I read and follow the label directions when using prescribed and over-the-counter drugs.	2	1	0

Alcohol and Drugs Score: _____

Emotional Health			
1. I enjoy being a student, and I have a job or do other work that I enjoy.	2	1	0
2. I find it easy to relax and express my feelings freely.	2	1	0
3. I manage stress well.	2	1	0
4. I have close friends, relatives, or others whom I can talk to about personal matters and call on for help when needed.	2	1	0
5. I participate in group activities (such as community or spiritual organizations) or hobbies that I enjoy.	2	1	0

Emotional Health Score: _____

	Almost Always	Sometimes	Never

Safety

1. I wear a seat belt while riding in a car. 2 1 0

2. I avoid driving while under the influence of alcohol or other drugs. 2 1 0

3. I obey traffic rules and the speed limit when driving. 2 1 0

4. I read and follow instructions on the labels of potentially harmful products or substances, such as household cleaners, poisons, and electrical appliances. 2 1 0

5. I avoid smoking in bed. 2 1 0

Safety Score: _____

Disease Prevention

1. I know the warning signs of cancer, heart attack, and stroke. 2 1 0

2. I avoid overexposure to the sun and use sunscreen. 2 1 0

3. I get recommended medical screening tests (such as blood pressure and cholesterol checks and Pap tests), immunizations, and booster shots. 2 1 0

4. I practise monthly skin and breast/testicle self-exams. 2 1 0

5. I am not sexually active or I have sex with only one mutually faithful, uninfected partner or I always engage in "safer sex" (using condoms). 2 1 0

2 1 0

Disease Prevention Score: _____

Scores of 9 and 10 Excellent! Your answers show that you are aware of the importance of this area to your health. More important, you are putting your knowledge to work for you by practising good health habits. As long as you continue to do so, this area should not pose a serious health risk.

Scores of 6 to 8 Your health practices in this area are good, but there is room for improvement.

Scores of 3 to 5 Your health risks are showing.

Scores of 0 to 2 You may be taking serious and unnecessary risks with your health.

Using Your Results

How did you score? In which areas did you score the lowest? Are you satisfied with your scores in each area? In which areas would you most like to improve your scores?

What should you do next? To improve your scores, look closely at any item to which you answered "sometimes" or "never." Identify and list at least three possible targets for a health behaviour change program. (If you are aware of other risky health behaviours you currently engage in, but which were not covered by this assessment, you may include those in your list.) For each item on your list, identify your current "stage of change" and one strategy you could adopt to move forward. Possible strategies might be obtaining information about the behaviour, completing an analysis of the pros and cons of change, or beginning a written record or your target behaviour.

Behaviour	**Stage**	**Strategy**
1. _____	_____	_____
2. _____	_____	_____
3. _____	_____	_____

SOURCE: Adapted from *Healthstyle: A Self-Test,* developed by the U.S. Public Health Service. The behaviours covered in this test are recommended for most North Americans, but some may not apply to people with certain chronic diseases or disabilities or to pregnant women, who may require special advice from their physician.

CHAPTER 2

BASIC PRINCIPLES OF PHYSICAL FITNESS

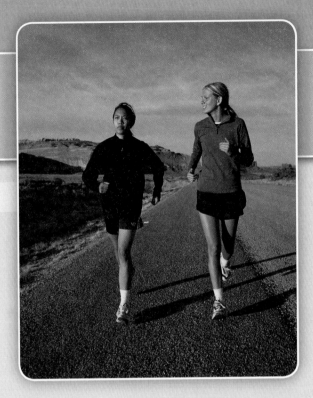

LEARNING OBJECTIVES

After reading this chapter, you should be able to

LO1 Describe how much exercise is recommended for developing health and fitness

LO2 Identify the components of physical fitness and the way each component affects wellness

LO3 Explain the goal of physical training and the basic principles of training

LO4 Describe the principles involved in designing a well-rounded exercise program

LO5 Discuss the steps that can be taken to make an exercise program safe, effective, and successful

TEST YOUR KNOWLEDGE

1. **To improve your health, you must do high-intensity exercise.**

   True or false?

2. **Which of the following activities uses about 150 calories?**

   a. washing a car for 45–60 minutes
   b. shooting a basketball for 30 minutes
   c. jumping rope for 15 minutes

3. **Regular exercise can make a person smarter.**

   True or false?

ANSWERS

1. **FALSE.** Even moderate physical activity—walking the dog, taking the stairs, or doing yard work—has significant health benefits.

2. **ALL THREE.** The more intense an activity is, the more calories it burns in a given amount of time. This is one reason that people who exercise vigorously can get the same benefits in less time than people who exercise at a moderate intensity.

3. **TRUE.** Regular exercise (even moderate-intensity exercise) benefits the human brain and nervous system in a variety of ways. For example, exercise improves cognitive function—that is, the brain's ability to learn, remember, think, and reason.

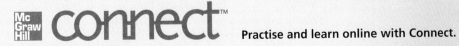

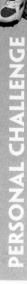

To Work Out. . . Or Not to Work Out?

What reasons do you have for not exercising—or not exercising more? Forget about superficial excuses such as "I couldn't run today because a SpongeBob marathon was on." Focus on *real* reasons that consistently interfere with your ability to be physically active. List the top three reasons, in order of significance:

Reason #1: _____

Reason #2: _____

Reason #3: _____

Now, focus on a real solution to each of the three problems. What can you do to prevent these issues from interfering with your ability to exercise in the future? Don't worry about one-time solutions; think about real, permanent solutions that will make these reasons for not exercising go away. List the solutions in the same order as the reasons you listed above:

Solution #1: _____

Solution #2: _____

Solution #3: _____

Think of this as more than just a list. Think of it as a commitment to resolve issues that keep you from meeting your fitness goals. That's the challenging part: Apply your solutions and stay active!

Any list of the benefits of physical activity is impressive. Although people vary greatly in physical fitness and performance ability, the benefits of regular physical activity are available to everyone.

This chapter provides an overview of physical fitness. It explains how lifestyle physical activity and more formal exercise programs contribute to wellness. It describes the components of fitness, the basic principles of physical training, and the essential elements of a well-rounded exercise program. Chapters 3–6 provide an in-depth look at each of the elements of a fitness program; Chapter 9 will help you put all these elements together into a complete, personalized program.

2.1 PHYSICAL ACTIVITY AND EXERCISE FOR HEALTH AND FITNESS

Despite the fact that two-thirds of Canadians strongly agree that leading a healthy lifestyle can lead to long-term health benefits, levels of physical inactivity in Canada are still too high. According to Statistics Canada's Health Reports (2009), only 52.5% of Canadian adults are moderately active during their leisure time.

The 2008 Physical Activity Monitors[1] (sponsored by the Canadian Fitness and Lifestyle Research Institute) report that factors such as gender, age, and income level may impact our level of physical activity.

- Women of all age groups are less likely to be physically active than men and the older women become, the wider the gap between the genders.
- Those with higher incomes are more likely to be at least moderately active than those with lower incomes.

Possible barriers to increased activity include lack of time and resources, social and environmental influences, and—most important—lack of motivation and commitment (see Lab 2.2 for more on barriers). Some people also fear injury. Although physical activity carries some risks, the risks of inactivity are far greater. Increased physical activity may be the single most important lifestyle behaviour change for promoting health and well-being.

Physical Activity on a Continuum

Physical activity is a movement carried out by the skeletal muscles and requiring energy. Different types of physical activity can vary by ease of intensity. Standing up or walking down a hallway require little energy or effort. More intense, sustained activities such as cycling 10 kilometres or running in a race require considerably more.

Exercise refers to a planned, structured, repetitive movement intended specifically to improve or maintain physical fitness. As discussed in Chapter 1, physical fitness is a set of physical attributes that allows the body to respond or adapt to the demands and stress of physical effort—to perform moderate-to-vigorous levels of physical activity without becoming overly tired. Levels of fitness depend on such physiological factors as the heart's ability to pump blood and the energy-generating capacity of the cells. These factors depend on genetics—a person's inborn potential for physical fitness—and behaviour—getting enough physical activity to stress the body and cause long-term physiological changes.

physical activity Body movement carried out by the skeletal muscles that requires energy.

exercise Planned, structured, repetitive movement intended to improve or maintain physical fitness.

Is Exercise Good for Your Brain?

We have long known that exercise is good for the muscles, bones, and heart. But what about the brain? Can exercise improve your brain's health and function? Can it ward off dementia? Can exercise even make you smarter? A growing body of research indicates that the answer to all these questions may be yes.

Some scientists, in fact, are now calling exercise the new "brain food." A variety of studies—including large-scale studies funded by the U.S. National Institute on Aging—show that even moderate physical activity can improve brain health and function and may delay the decline in cognitive function that occurs for many people as they age. Recent evidence shows that regular physical activity has the following positive effects on the human brain:

- Exercise improves cognitive function—that is, the brain's ability to learn, remember, think, and reason.

- Exercise can be used to overcome the negative effects of a poor diet (for example, a diet high in saturated fats) on brain health.

- Exercise promotes the creation of new nerve cells (neurons) in the brain and throughout the nervous system. By promoting this process (called *neurogenesis*), exercise provides some protection against injury and degenerative conditions that can destroy neurons.

- Exercise enhances the entire nervous system's plasticity—that is, its ability to change and adapt. In the brain, spinal cord, and nerves, this can mean developing new or different pathways for transmitting sensory information or motor commands.

- Exercise appears to have a protective effect on the brain as people age, helping to delay or even prevent the onset of neurodegenerative disorders such as Alzheimer's disease.

Although most people consider brain health to be a concern for the elderly, it is vital to wellness throughout life. For this reason, many studies on exercise and brain health include children as well as older adults. Targeted research has also focused on the impact of exercise on people with disorders such as cerebral palsy, multiple sclerosis, and developmental disabilities. Generally speaking, these studies all reach a similar conclusion: Exercise enhances brain health, at least to some degree, in people of all ages and a wide range of health statuses.

Along with the brain's physical health, exercise has a positive effect on mental health. The 2008 *Physical Activity*

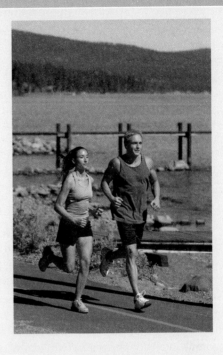

Guidelines Advisory Committee Report cited numerous studies on the relationship between physical activity and mental health (see Chapter 10 for more on this relationship). The overall message was that exercise—even modest activity such as taking a daily walk—can help combat a variety of mental health disorders.

It's hard to understate the impact of physical and mental disorders related to brain health. According to the Alzheimer's Society, half a million Canadians currently suffer from Alzheimer's disease and the number is increasing at a rate of one person every five minutes. People with depression, anxiety, or other mental disorders are more likely to suffer from chronic physical conditions. Taken together, these and other brain-related disorders cost untold millions of dollars in health care costs and lost productivity, as well as thousands of years of productive lifetime lost.

So, for the sake of your brain—as well as your muscles, bones, and heart—start creating your exercise program soon. You'll be healthier, and you may even feel a little smarter.

SOURCES: Garber, C. E., et al. 2011. Quantity and quality of exercise for developing and maintaining cardiorespiratory, musculoskeletal, and neuromotor fitness in apparently healthy adults: guidance for prescribing exercise. *Medicine and Science in Sports and Exercise* 43(7): 1334–1359; Physical Activity Guidelines Advisory Committee. 2008. *Physical Activity Guidelines Advisory Committee Report, 2008.* Washington, D.C.: U.S. Department of Health and Human Services; Stranahan, A. M., and M. P. Mattson. 2011. Bidirectional metabolic regulation of neurocognitive function. *Neurobiology of Learning and Memory* January (epub); Ploughman, M. 2008. Exercise is brain food: The effects of physical activity on cognitive function. *Developmental Neurorehabilitation* 11(3): 236–240; van Praag, H. 2009. Exercise and the brain: Something to chew on. *Trends in Neurosciences* 32(5): 283–290.

Physical activity is essential to health and confers wide-ranging health benefits, but exercise is necessary to significantly improve physical fitness. This important distinction between physical activity, which improves health and wellness, and exercise, which improves fitness, is a key concept in understanding the guidelines discussed in this section.

LIFESTYLE PHYSICAL ACTIVITY FOR HEALTH PROMOTION The Public Health Agency of Canada recently approved a review of physical activity guidelines for Canadians. This review was undertaken by the Canadian Society for Exercise Physiology (CSEP) and concluded that optimal health benefits were within reach for Canadians if

Classifying Activity Levels

Assessing your physical activity level is easier if you know how to classify different kinds of activities. Fitness experts categorize activities into the following three levels:

- *Light activity* includes the routine tasks associated with typical day-to-day life, such as vacuuming, walking slowly, shopping, or stretching. You probably perform dozens of light activities every day without even thinking about it. You can gain significant health benefits by turning light activities into moderate activities—by walking briskly instead of slowly, for example.

- *Moderate activity* causes your breathing and heart rate to accelerate but still allows for comfortable conversation, such as walking at 4–6 km per hour. It is sometimes described as activity that can be performed comfortably for about 45 minutes. Examples of moderate physical activity include brisk walking, social dancing, and cycling moderately on level terrain.

- *Vigorous activity* elevates your heart and breathing rates considerably and has other physical effects that improve your fitness level. Examples include jogging, hiking uphill, swimming laps, and playing most competitive sports.

---

they achieved minimum standards for physical activity. The Canadian Physical Activity Guidelines suggest that each age demographic should attain the following levels of physical activity:

- Children aged 5–11 years and youth aged 12–17 should accumulate at least 60 minutes of moderate-to-vigorous intensity physical activity daily.

- Adults aged 18 and older should accumulate at least 150 minutes of moderate-to-vigorous intensity aerobic physical activity per week, in bouts of 10 minutes or more.

In addition to guidelines for the amount of physical activity that Canadians should be achieving, CSEP also recommended that each group participate in muscle and bone strengthening activities. The guidelines can be downloaded for free at www.csep.ca/english/view .asp?x=804.

In the lifestyle approach to physical activity, people can choose activities that they find enjoyable and that fit into their daily routine; everyday tasks at school, work, and home can be structured to contribute to the daily activity total. The daily total of lifestyle activity can be accumulated in multiple short bouts—for example, two 10-minute bicycle rides to and from class and a brisk 15-minute walk to the post office. Figure 2.1 provides

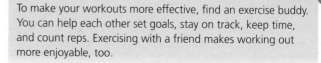

FITNESS TIP

To make your workouts more effective, find an exercise buddy. You can help each other set goals, stay on track, keep time, and count reps. Exercising with a friend makes working out more enjoyable, too.

more examples of activities that Canadians can perform in achieving acceptable levels of physical activity. See also "Classifying Activity Levels" above.

By increasing lifestyle physical activity, people can expect to significantly improve their health and well-being. If all the Canadians who are now completely sedentary were to adopt a more active lifestyle, there would be enormous benefit to the public's health and to individual well-being.

LO1 How Much Physical Activity Is Enough?

Some experts feel that people get most of the health benefits of an exercise program simply by becoming more active over the course of the day; the amount of activity needed depends on an individual's health status and

Very light effort	Light effort	Moderate effort	Vigorous effort	Maximum effort
	60 Minutes	30–60 Minutes	20–30 Minutes	
• Strolling • Dusting	• Light walking • Easy gardening • Stretching	• Brisk walking • Biking • Raking leaves • Swimming • Dancing • Water aerobics	• Aerobics • Jogging • Hockey • Basketball • Fast swimming • Fast dancing	• Sprinting • Racing
	Range Needed to Stay Healthy			

FIGURE 2.1 Activities to increase Canadians' physical activity.

SOURCE: Based on the ParticipAction Get Moving Program http://www.participaction.com/ get-moving/easy-ways-to-start-2/.

goals. Other experts feel that the activity goal set by the lifestyle approach is too low; they argue that people should exercise long enough and intensely enough to improve their body's capacity for exercise—that is, to improve physical fitness. There is probably truth in both of these positions.

Regular physical activity, regardless of the intensity, makes you healthier and can help protect you from many chronic diseases. Although you get many of the health benefits of exercise simply by being more active, you obtain even more benefits when you are physically fit. In addition to long-term health benefits, fitness also significantly contributes to quality of life. Fitness can give you freedom to move your body the way you want. Fit people have more energy and better body control. They can enjoy a more active lifestyle than their more sedentary counterparts. Even if you don't like sports, you need physical energy and stamina in your daily life and for many nonsport leisure activities—visiting museums, playing with children, gardening, and so on.

Where does this leave you? Most experts agree that some physical activity is better than none, but that more—as long as it does not result in injury—is probably better than some. To set a personal goal for physical activity and exercise, consider your current activity level, your health status, and your goals. At the very least, strive to become more active and get 30 minutes of moderate-intensity activity at least 5 days per week.. Choose to be active whenever you can. If weight management is a concern for you, begin by achieving the goal of 30 minutes of activity per day and then look to raise your activity level further, to 45–60 minutes per day or more. For even better health and well-being, participate in a structured exercise program that develops physical fitness. Any increase in physical activity will contribute to your health and well-being, now and in the future.

LO2 2.2 HEALTH-RELATED COMPONENTS OF PHYSICAL FITNESS

Some components of fitness are related to specific activities, and others relate to general health. **Health-related fitness** includes the following components:

- Cardiorespiratory endurance
- Muscular strength
- Muscular endurance
- Flexibility
- Body composition

Health-related fitness contributes to your capacity to enjoy life, helps your body withstand physical and psychological challenges, and protects you from chronic disease.

Cardiorespiratory Endurance

Cardiorespiratory endurance is the ability to perform prolonged, large-muscle, dynamic exercise at moderate-to-high levels of intensity. It depends on such factors as the ability of the lungs to deliver oxygen from the environment to the bloodstream, the capacity of the heart to pump blood, the ability of the nervous system and blood vessels to regulate blood flow, and the capability of the body's chemical systems to use oxygen and process fuels for exercise.

When levels of cardiorespiratory fitness are low, the heart has to work very hard during normal daily activities and may not be able to work hard enough to sustain high-intensity physical activity in an emergency. As cardiorespiratory fitness improves, related physical functions also improve. For example:

- The heart pumps more blood per heartbeat.
- Resting heart rate slows.
- Blood volume increases.
- Blood supply to tissues improves.
- The body can cool itself better.
- Resting blood pressure decreases.

A healthy heart can better withstand the strains of everyday life, the stress of occasional emergencies, and the wear and tear of time.

Endurance training also improves the functioning of the chemical systems, particularly in the muscles and liver, thereby enhancing the body's ability to use energy supplied by food and to do more exercise with less effort from the oxygen transport system.

health-related fitness Physical capacities that contribute to health: cardiorespiratory endurance, muscular strength, muscular endurance, flexibility, and body composition.

cardiorespiratory endurance The ability of the body to perform prolonged, large-muscle, dynamic exercise at moderate to high levels of intensity.

TERMS

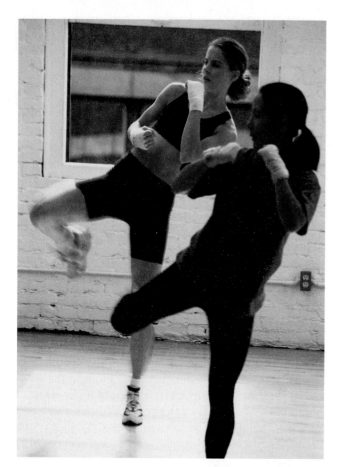

Cardiorespiratory endurance is a key component of health-related fitness. These participants in a kickboxing class are conditioning their hearts and lungs as well as gaining many other health benefits.

Cardiorespiratory endurance is a central component of health-related fitness because the functioning of the heart and lungs is so essential to overall good health. A person can't live very long or very well without a healthy heart. Poor cardiorespiratory fitness is linked with heart disease, type 2 diabetes, colon cancer, stroke, depression, and anxiety. A moderate level of cardiorespiratory fitness can even help compensate for certain health risks, including excess body fat: People who are lean but who have low cardiorespiratory fitness have been found to have higher death rates than people with higher levels of body fat who are otherwise fit.[2]

You can develop cardiorespiratory endurance through activities that involve continuous, rhythmic movements of large-muscle groups, such as the legs. Such activities include walking, jogging, cycling, and aerobic dancing.

muscular strength The amount of force a muscle can produce with a single maximum effort.

metabolism The sum of all the vital processes by which food energy and nutrients are made available to and used by the body.

muscular endurance The ability of a muscle to remain contracted or to contract repeatedly for a long period of time.

flexibility The ability to move joints through their full range of motion.

Muscular Strength

Muscular strength is the amount of force a muscle can produce with a single maximum effort. It depends on such factors as the size of muscle cells and the ability of nerves to activate muscle cells. Strong muscles are important for the smooth and easy performance of everyday activities, such as climbing stairs, as well as for emergency situations. They help keep the skeleton in proper alignment, preventing back and leg pain and providing the support necessary for good posture. Muscular strength has obvious importance in recreational activities. Strong people can hit a tennis ball harder, kick a soccer ball farther, and ride a bicycle uphill more easily.

Muscle tissue is an important element of overall body composition. Greater muscle mass means a higher rate of **metabolism** and faster energy use. Training to build muscular strength can also help people manage stress and boost their self-confidence.

Maintaining strength and muscle mass is vital for healthy aging. Older people tend to experience a decrease in both number and size of muscle cells; a condition called *sarcopenia*. Many of the remaining muscle cells become slower, and some become nonfunctional because they lose their attachment to the nervous system. Strength training (also known as *resistance training* or *weight training*) helps maintain muscle mass and function and possibly helps decrease the risk of osteoporosis (bone loss) in older people, which greatly enhances their quality of life and prevents life-threatening injuries.

Muscular Endurance

Muscular endurance is the ability to resist fatigue and sustain a given level of muscle tension—that is, to hold a muscle contraction for a long period of time or to contract a muscle over and over again. It depends on such factors as the size of muscle cells, the ability of muscles to store fuel, and the blood supply to muscles.

Muscular endurance is important for good posture and for injury prevention. For example, if abdominal and back muscles can't hold the spine correctly, the chances of low-back pain and back injury are increased. Good muscular endurance in the trunk muscles is more important than muscular strength for preventing back pain. Muscular endurance helps people cope with daily physical demands and enhances performance in sports and work.

Flexibility

Flexibility is the ability to move the joints through their full range of motion. It depends on joint structure, the length and elasticity of connective tissue, and nervous system activity. Flexible, pain-free joints are important for good health and well-being. Inactivity causes the joints to become stiffer with age. Stiffness, in turn, often causes older people to assume unnatural body postures that can

TERMS

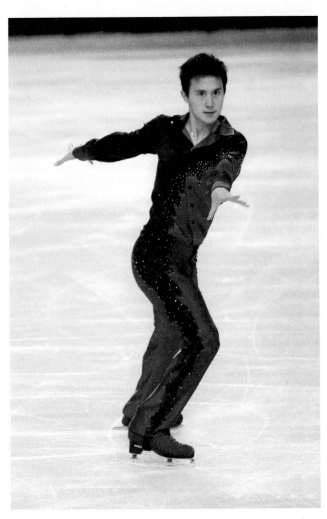

Elite athletes like Patrick Chan demonstrate sport-specific skills such as speed, power, agility, coordination, and reaction time.

stress joints and muscles. Stretching exercises can help ensure a healthy range of motion for all major joints.

Body Composition

Body composition refers to the proportion of fat and **fat-free mass** (muscle, bone, and water) in the body. Healthy body composition involves a high proportion of fat-free mass and an acceptably low level of body fat, adjusted for age and gender. A person with excessive body fat—especially fat in the abdomen—is more likely to experience a variety of health problems, including heart disease, insulin resistance, high blood pressure, stroke, joint problems, type 2 diabetes, gallbladder disease, blood vessel inflammation, some types of cancer, and back pain.

The best way to lose fat is through a lifestyle that includes a sensible diet and exercise. The best way to add muscle mass is through resistance training. Large changes in body composition aren't necessary to improve health; even a small increase in physical activity and a small decrease in body fat can lead to substantial health improvements.

Skill-Related Components of Fitness

In addition to the five health-related components of physical fitness, the ability to perform a particular sport or activity may depend on **skill-related fitness** components such as the following:

- *Speed:* The ability to perform a movement in a short period of time.
- *Power:* The ability to exert force rapidly, based on a combination of strength and speed.
- *Agility:* The ability to change the position of the body quickly and accurately.
- *Balance:* The ability to maintain equilibrium while moving or while stationary.
- *Coordination:* The ability to perform motor tasks accurately and smoothly using body movements and the senses.
- *Reaction time:* The ability to respond or react quickly to a stimulus.

Skill-related fitness tends to be sport-specific and is best developed through practice. For example, the speed, coordination, and agility needed to play basketball can be developed by playing basketball. Some fitness experts contend that some sports don't contribute to all the health-related components of physical fitness. However, engaging in sports is fun and can help you build fitness and contribute to other areas of wellness.

LO3   2.3 PRINCIPLES OF PHYSICAL TRAINING: ADAPTATION TO STRESS

The human body is very adaptable. The greater the demands made on it, the more it adjusts to meet those demands. Over time, immediate, short-term adjustments

body composition   The proportion of fat and fat-free mass (muscle, bone, and water) in the body.

fat-free mass   The nonfat component of the human body, consisting of skeletal muscle, bone, and water.

skill-related fitness   Physical capacities that contribute to performance in a sport or an activity: speed, power, agility, balance, coordination, and reaction time.

TERMS

DIMENSIONS OF DIVERSITY

Physical fitness and athletic achievement are not limited to the able-bodied. People with disabilities can also attain high levels of fitness and performance, as shown by the elite athletes who compete in the Paralympics. The premier event for athletes with disabilities, the Paralympics are held in the same year and city as the Olympics. The performance of these skilled athletes makes it clear that people with disabilities can be active, healthy, and extraordinarily fit; just like able-bodied athletes, athletes with disabilities strive for excellence and can serve as role models.

Currently, some 4.4 million Canadians are estimated to have chronic, significant disabilities.[3] Some disabilities are the result of injury, such as spinal cord injuries sustained in car crashes. Other disabilities result from illness, such as the blindness that sometimes occurs as a complication of diabetes or the joint stiffness that accompanies arthritis. And some disabilities are present at birth, as in the case of congenital limb deformities or cerebral palsy.

Exercise and physical activity are as important for people with disabilities as for able-bodied individuals—if not more important. Being active helps prevent secondary conditions that may result from prolonged inactivity, such as circulatory or muscular problems. It provides an emotional boost that helps support a positive attitude as well as opportunities to make new

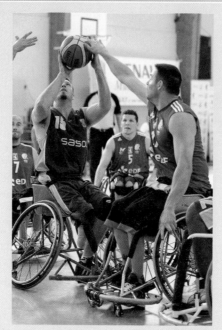

friends, increase self-confidence, and gain a sense of accomplishment. Canadians with a disability are less likely to be physically active than other Canadians.

People with disabilities don't have to be elite athletes to participate in sports and lead an active life. Some health clubs and fitness centres offer activities and events geared for people of all ages and types of disabilities. They may have modified aerobics classes, special weight training machines, classes involving mild exercise in warm water, and other activities adapted for people with disabilities. Popular sports and recreational activities include adapted horseback riding, golf, swimming, and skiing. Competitive sports are also available—for example, there are wheelchair versions of billiards, tennis, hockey, and basketball, as well as sports for people with hearing, visual, or mental impairments. For those who prefer to get their exercise at home, special videos are available geared to individuals who use wheelchairs or who have arthritis, hearing impairments, or many other disabilities.

If you have a disability and want to be more active, check with your physician about what's appropriate for you. Call your local community centre, YMCA/YWCA, independent living centre, or fitness centre to locate potential facilities; look for a facility with experienced personnel and appropriate adaptive equipment. For specialized videos, check with hospitals and health associations that are geared to specific disabilities, such as the Arthritis Society.

SOURCES: Fahey, Insel, and Walton (2013). *Fit & Well: Core Concepts and Labs in Physical Fitness and Wellness.* New York: McGraw-Hill, p. 38; and Active Living Alliance for Canadians with a Disability (http://www.ala.ca).

---

translate into long-term changes and improvements. When breathing and heart rate increase during exercise, for example, the heart gradually develops the ability to pump more blood with each beat. Then, during exercise, it doesn't have to beat as fast to meet the cells' demands for oxygen. The goal of **physical training** is to produce these long-term changes and improvements in the body's functioning. Although people differ in the maximum levels of physical fitness and performance they can achieve through training, the wellness benefits of exercise are available to everyone (see the box "Fitness and Disability").

Particular types and amounts of exercise are most effective in developing the various components of fitness.

TERMS

physical training The performance of different types of activities that cause the body to adapt and improve its level of fitness.

specificity The training principle that the body adapts to the particular type and amount of stress placed on it.

To put together an effective exercise program, you should first understand the basic principles of physical training, including the following:

- Specificity
- Progressive overload
- Reversibility
- Individual differences

All of these rest on the larger principle of adaptation.

Specificity—Adapting to Type of Training

To develop a particular fitness component, exercises must be performed that are specifically designed for that component. This is the principle of **specificity.** Weight training, for example, develops muscular strength but is less effective for developing cardiorespiratory endurance or flexibility. Specificity also applies to the skill-related fitness components—to improve at tennis, you must practise tennis—and to the different parts of the body—to develop stronger arms, you must exercise your arms. A well-rounded exercise program includes exercises geared to each component of fitness, to different parts of the body, and to specific activities or sports.

Progressive Overload—Adapting to Amount of Training and the FITT Principle

The body adapts to the demands of exercise by improving its functioning. When the amount of exercise (also called *overload* or *stress*) is increased progressively, fitness continues to improve. This is the principle of **progressive overload.**

The amount of overload is very important. Too little exercise will have no effect on fitness (although it may improve health); too much may cause injury and problems with the body's immune system and hormone levels. The point at which exercise becomes excessive is highly individual; it occurs at a much higher level in an Olympic athlete than in a sedentary person. For every type of exercise, there is a training threshold at which fitness benefits begin to occur, a zone within which maximum fitness benefits occur, and an upper limit of safe training.

The amount of exercise needed depends on the individual's current level of fitness, the person's genetically determined capacity to adapt to training, his or her fitness goals, and the component being developed. A novice, for example, might experience fitness benefits from jogging a kilometre in 6 minutes, but this level of exercise would cause no physical adaptations in a trained distance runner. Beginners should start at the lower end of the fitness benefit zone; fitter individuals will make more rapid gains by exercising at the higher end of the fitness benefit zone. Progression is critical because fitness increases only if the volume and intensity of workouts increase. Exercising at the same intensity every training session will maintain fitness but will not increase it, because the training stress is below the threshold required to produce adaptation.

The amount of overload needed to maintain or improve a particular level of fitness for a particular fitness component is determined through four dimensions, represented by the acronym FITT:

- *F*requency—how often
- *I*ntensity—how hard
- *T*ime—how long (duration)
- *T*ype—mode of activity

Some experts use the acronym FITTE, where the *E* stands for enjoyment—a key component of a successful, long-term fitness program. Chapters 3, 4, and 5 show you how to apply the FITT principle to exercise programs for cardiorespiratory endurance, muscular strength and endurance, and flexibility, respectively.

FREQUENCY Developing fitness requires regular exercise. Optimum exercise frequency, expressed in number

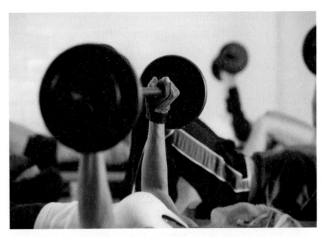

Progressive overload is important because fitness increases only when the volume and intensity of exercise increases. The body adapts to overload by becoming more fit.

of days per week, varies with the component being developed and the individual's fitness goals. For most people, a frequency of 3–5 days per week for cardiorespiratory endurance exercise and for resistance and flexibility training should be the goal of a general fitness program.

An important consideration in determining appropriate exercise frequency is recovery time, which is also highly individual and depends on factors such as training experience, age, and intensity of training. For example, 24 hours of rest between highly intensive workouts that involve heavy weights or track sprints is not enough recovery time for safe and effective training. Intense workouts need to be spaced out during the week to allow sufficient recovery time. On the other hand, you can exercise every day if your program consists of moderate-intensity walking or cycling. Learn to "listen to your body" to obtain a sufficient amount of rest between workouts. Chapters 3–5 provide more detailed information about training techniques and recovery periods for workouts focused on different fitness components.

INTENSITY Fitness benefits occur when a person exercises harder than his or her normal level of activity. The appropriate exercise intensity varies with each fitness component. To develop cardiorespiratory endurance, for example, a person must raise his or her heart rate above normal. To develop muscular strength, you must lift a heavier weight than normal; to develop flexibility, a person must stretch muscles beyond their normal length.

TIME (DURATION) Fitness benefits occur when you exercise for an extended period of time.

> **progressive overload** The training principle that placing increasing amounts of stress on the body causes adaptations that improve fitness.

- For cardiorespiratory endurance exercise, 30–60 minutes is recommended. Exercise can take place in a single session or in several sessions of 10 or more minutes. The greater the intensity of exercise, the less time needed to obtain fitness benefits.
- For high-intensity exercise, such as running, for example, 30–40 minutes is appropriate.
- For more moderate-intensity exercise, such as walking, 45–60 minutes may be needed. High-intensity exercise poses a greater risk of injury than lower-intensity exercise, so if you are a nonathletic adult, it's probably best to emphasize lower-to-moderate-intensity activity of longer duration.

To build muscular strength, muscular endurance, and flexibility, similar amounts of time are advisable, but these exercises are more commonly organized in terms of a specific number of repetitions of particular exercises. For resistance training, for example, a recommended program includes one or more sets of 8–12 repetitions of 8–10 different exercises that work the major muscle groups.

TYPE (MODE OF ACTIVITY)   The type of exercise in which you should engage varies with each fitness component and with your personal fitness goals. To develop cardiorespiratory endurance, you need to engage in continuous activities involving large-muscle groups—walking, jogging, cycling, or swimming, for example. Resistive exercises develop muscular strength and endurance, while stretching exercises build flexibility. The frequency, intensity, and time of the exercise will be different for each type of activity. See the section "Guidelines for Training" later in the chapter for more on choosing appropriate activities for your fitness program.

Reversibility—Adapting to a Reduction in Training

Fitness is a reversible adaptation. The body adjusts to lower levels of physical activity the same way it adjusts to higher levels. This is the principle of **reversibility.** When a person stops exercising, some fitness improvements are lost in as little as 2 weeks' time.[4] However, not all fitness levels reverse at the same rate. Strength fitness is very resilient, so a person can maintain strength fitness by doing resistive exercise as infrequently as once a week. On the other hand, cardiovascular and cellular fitness reverse themselves more quickly—sometimes within just a few days or weeks. Thus, if a training schedule must be curtailed temporarily, fitness improvements are best maintained by keeping the intensity of your workouts constant and while reducing their frequency or duration.

TERMS

reversibility   The training principle that fitness improvements are lost when demands on the body are lowered.

Individual Differences—Limits on Adaptability

Anyone watching the Olympics, can see that, from a physical standpoint, we are not all created equal. There are large individual differences in our ability to improve fitness, achieve a desirable body composition, and learn and perform sports skills. Some people are able to run longer distances, or lift more weight, or kick a soccer ball more skillfully than others will ever be able to, no matter how much they train. There are limits on the adaptability—the potential for improvement—of any human body. The body's ability to transport and use oxygen, for example, can be improved by only about 5–25% through endurance training.[5] An endurance athlete must therefore inherit a large metabolic capacity in order to reach competitive performance levels. In the past few years, scientists have identified specific genes that influence body fat, strength, and endurance.

However, physical training improves fitness regardless of heredity. For the average person, the body's adaptability is enough to achieve reasonable fitness goals.

LO4   2.4 DESIGNING YOUR OWN EXERCISE PROGRAM

Physical training works best when you have a plan. A plan helps you make gradual but steady progress toward your goals. Once you've determined that exercise is safe for you, planning for physical fitness consists of assessing how fit you are now, determining where you want to be, and choosing the right activities to help you get there.

Getting Medical Clearance

People of any age who are not at high risk for serious health problems can safely exercise at a moderate intensity (60% or less of maximum heart rate) without a prior medical evaluation (see Chapter 3 for a discussion of maximum heart rate). Likewise, if you are male and under 40 or female and under 50 and in good health, exercise is probably safe for you. If you do not fit into these age groups or have health problems—especially high blood pressure, heart disease, muscle or joint problems, or obesity—see your physician before starting a vigorous exercise program. The Canadian Society for Exercise

Heart disease and diabetes aren't the only reasons to get a doctor's approval before starting an exercise program. If you are severely overweight, have a family history of some chronic disease, or have just never exercised before, it could be advisable to talk to your doctor before becoming physically active.

Think about your current health status and your family history. If you think of any issues that might interfere with being physically active—or that might make exercise dangerous for you—list them below:

_____

_____

_____

_____

_____

If you write down anything, even *one* thing, make an appointment to see your doctor as soon as possible. Ask your doctor for an overall health evaluation, review your family history, and make sure the doctor knows you want to start being physically active on a regular basis. Then address the specific issues you listed above.

If your physician offers any specific advice, follow it. But if you can be physically active, even with some restrictions, make a commitment and get started on your exercise plan. And see your doctor regularly to make sure physical activity is working for you.

Physiology has developed the Physical Activity Readiness Questionnaire (PAR-Q) to help evaluate exercise safety; it is included in Lab 2.1. Completing it should alert you to any potential problems you may have. If a physician isn't sure whether exercise is safe for you, she or he may recommend an **exercise stress test** or a **graded exercise test (GXT)** to see whether you show symptoms of heart disease during exercise. For most people, however, it's far safer to exercise than to remain sedentary. For more information, see the box "Exercise and Cardiac Risk."

Assessing Yourself

The first step in creating a successful fitness program is to assess your current level of physical activity and fitness for each of the five health-related fitness components. The results of the assessment tests will help you set specific fitness goals and plan your fitness program. Lab 2.3 gives you the opportunity to assess your current overall level of activity and determine if it is appropriate. Assessment tests in Chapters 3–6 will help you evaluate your cardiorespiratory endurance, muscular strength, muscular endurance, flexibility, and body composition.

Before you begin assessing your level of physical activity and fitness, it is important to ensure that you are healthy enough to begin testing. Some may need to receive medical clearance before beginning.

Setting Goals

The ultimate general goal of every health-related fitness program is the same—wellness that lasts a lifetime. Whatever your specific goals, they must be important enough to you to keep you motivated. Most sports psychologists believe that setting and achieving goals is the most effective way to stay motivated about exercise (refer to Chapter 1 for more on goal setting, as well as the

Common Questions Answered at the end of this chapter). After you complete the assessment tests in Chapters 3–6, you will be able to set goals directly related to each fitness component, such as working toward a 5-km jog or doing 20 push-ups. First, though, think carefully about your overall goals, and be clear about why you are starting a program.

Choosing Activities for a Balanced Program

An ideal fitness program combines a physically active lifestyle with a systematic exercise program to develop and maintain physical fitness. This basis for a program is detailed in Canada's Physical Activity Guidelines for Canadians (see the guidelines for adults in Figure 2.2). Full details for all age groups can be found on the Public Health Agency website (www.phac-aspc.gc.ca/hp-ps/hl-mvs/pa-ap/03paap-eng.php). If you are currently sedentary, your goal is to focus on activities that will gradually increase the amount of moderate-intensity physical activity in your daily life. Appropriate activities include brisk walking, climbing stairs, yard work, and washing your car. You don't have to exercise vigorously, but you should experience a moderate increase in your heart and breathing rates. As described earlier, your activity time can be broken up into small blocks over the course of a day.

exercise stress test   A test usually administered on a treadmill or cycle ergometer that involves analysis of the changes in electrical activity in the heart from an electrocardiogram (EKG or ECG) taken during exercise. Used to determine if any heart disease is present and to assess current fitness level.

graded exercise test (GXT)   An exercise test that starts at an easy intensity and progresses to maximum capacity.

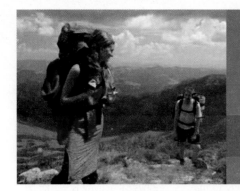

Tips to Get Active

> Physical Activity Tips for Adults (18-64 years)

Physical activity plays an important role in your health, well-being and quality of life. Improve your health by being active as part of a healthy lifestyle.

1 Be active at least **2.5 hours a week** to achieve health benefits.

2 Focus on **moderate to vigorous aerobic activity** throughout each week, broken into sessions of 10 minutes or more.

3 Get stronger by adding activities **that target your muscles and bones** at least two days per week.

Tips to help you get active

- ☑ **Choose a variety of physical activities you enjoy.** Try different activities until you find the ones that feel right for you.
- ☑ **Get into a routine** — go to the pool, hit the gym, join a spin class or set a regular run and do some planned exercise. Make it social by getting someone to join you.

- ☑ **Limit the time you spend watching TV** or sitting in front of a computer during leisure time.
- ☑ **Move yourself** — use active transportation to get places. Whenever you can, walk, bike, or run instead of taking the car.

- ☑ **Spread your sessions of moderate to vigorous aerobic activity throughout the week.** Do at least 10 minutes of physical activity at a time.
- ☑ **Join a team** — take part in sports and recreation activities in groups. You'll make new friends and get active at the same time.

FIGURE 2.2 Canada's physical activity guidelines. These physical activity guidelines show the components of a balanced fitness program, and emphasizes the importance of daily moderate-intensity physical activity.

SOURCE: Canadian Physical Activity Guidelines. Tips to Get Active: Physical Activity Tips for Adults (18-64 years). Canadian Society for Exercise Physiology/Public Health Agency of Canada, 2011. Reproduced with permission from the Minister of Health, 2012.

These guidelines have proven to be universal and are included in CSEP's Canadian Physical Activity, Fitness, and Lifestyle Approach (CPAFLA) protocols for Canadians to follow (Table 2.1). A balanced program includes activities to develop all the health-related components of fitness:

- *Cardiorespiratory endurance* is developed by continuous rhythmic movements of large-muscle groups in activities such as walking, jogging, cycling, swimming, and aerobic dance and other forms of group exercise. Choose activities that you enjoy and that are convenient. Other popular choices are inline skating, dancing, and backpacking.

Start-and-stop activities such as tennis, racquetball, and soccer can also develop endurance if your skill level is sufficient to enable periods of continuous play. Training for cardiorespiratory endurance is discussed in Chapter 3.

- *Muscular strength and endurance* can be developed through resistance training—training with weights or performing calisthenic exercises such as push-ups and curl-ups. Training for muscular strength and endurance is discussed in Chapter 4.
- *Flexibility* is developed by stretching the major muscle groups, regularly and with proper technique. Flexibility is discussed in Chapter 5.

Canadian Physical Activity, Fitness, and Lifestyle Approach (CPAFLA)

The CPAFLA is a health-related fitness assessment protocol created by the Canadian Society for Exercise Physiologists (CSEP) that is administered on over a million Canadians every year. The protocol uses a unique approach in examining three key elements of our lives. These elements are our Healthy Physical Activity, our Healthy Lifestyle (with a *Health/Fitness Counsellor*), and our Health-Related Fitness (with a *Fitness Appraiser*).

There are many levels of assessment and counselling to choose from as the CPAFLA is a client-centred approach. For example, you could complete a full appraisal, a partial appraisal, or seek advice only. The focus of the CPAFLA is on health enhancement and creating a guideline for a physical activity/exercise program. In addition, active living and lifestyle habits that relate to overall health status are examined, and in many cases an individualized exercise program can be prescribed (with a *Personal Trainer*).

Many of the physical assessments in this text are adapted from the CPAFLA protocols and when considering your initial assessment results, you may want to consider a full appraisal (or even a partial appraisal) from a CSEP-certified professional. At the very least, a visit with a CSEP-certified personal trainer may aid you in developing a program that is right for you.

Qualifications

A CSEP-certified health/fitness professional (i.e., a CSEP Certified Personal Trainer® or CSEP Certified Exercise Physiologist®) is all three: Health/Fitness Counsellor, Fitness Appraiser, and a Personal Trainer. They are the only fitness professionals in Canada that have acquired their skills, knowledge/abilities, and training through some formal academic training, i.e., university/college coursework. The CSEP has further qualified their professional status by having candidates complete a vigorous examination process in the subject matter. To contact a CSEP professional (CSEP-CPT or CSEP-CEP) in your area, search the CSEP Online Member Directory (www.csep.ca/english/view.asp?x=887), or contact one of their provincial/regional offices.

SOURCE: Canadian Society for Exercise Physiologists http://www.csep.ca/english/view.asp?x=585.

TABLE 2.1 Exercise Recommendations for Fitness Development in Healthy Adults

Exercise to Develop and Maintain Cardiorespiratory Endurance and Body Composition

Frequency of training	4–7 days per week.
Intensity of training	55/65–90% of maximum heart rate or 40/50–85% of maximum oxygen uptake reserve.* For average individuals, intensities of 70–85% of maximum heart rate are appropriate. For unfit individuals, the lower intensity values (55–64% of maximum heart rate and 40–49% of maximum oxygen uptake reserve) are most applicable.
Time (duration) of training	30–60 total minutes of continuous, or intermittent (in sessions lasting 10 or more minutes) aerobic activity. Duration is dependent on the intensity of activity; thus, lower-intensity activity should be conducted over a longer period of time (40 minutes or more). Lower-to-moderate-intensity activity of longer duration is recommended for the nonathletic adult.
Type (mode) of activity	Any activity that uses large-muscle groups, can be maintained continuously, and is rhythmic and aerobic in nature, for example, walking-hiking, running-jogging, cycling-bicycling, cross-country skiing, aerobic dance and other forms of group exercise, rope skipping, rowing, stair climbing, swimming, skating, and endurance game activities.

Exercise to Develop and Maintain Muscular Strength and Endurance, Flexibility, and Body Composition

Resistance training	One set of 8–10 exercises that condition the major muscle groups should be performed 2–4 days per week. Most people should complete 8–12 repetitions of each exercise; for older and more frail people (approximately 50–60 years of age and above), 10–15 repetitions with a lighter weight may be more appropriate. Multiple-set regimens will provide greater benefits if time allows.
Flexibility training	Stretches for the major muscle groups should be performed 4–7 days per week; at least 4 repetitions held for 10–30 seconds should be completed.

*Instructions for calculating target heart rate intensity for cardiorespiratory endurance exercise are presented in Chapter 3.

SOURCE: Adapted from Pollock, M., G. Gaesser, and J. Butcher, et al., ACSM Position Stand: The recommended quantity and quality of exercise for developing and maintaining cardiorespiratory and muscular fitness, and flexibility in healthy adults. Position paper. *Medicine and Science in Sports and Exercise* 30(6): 975–991.

• *Healthy body composition* can be developed through a sensible diet and a program of regular exercise. Cardiorespiratory endurance exercise is best for reducing body fat; resistance training builds muscle mass, which, to a small extent, helps increase metabolism. Body composition is discussed in Chapter 6 and weight management in Chapter 8.

There are as many different fitness programs as there are individuals. The key for each of us is to find an adequate or more-than-adequate fitness program that fits into our busy daily routine. Chapter 9 contains guidelines to help you choose activities and put together a complete exercise program that suits your goals and preferences. (Refer to Figure 2.3 for a summary of the health and fitness benefits of different levels of physical activity.)

Although sedentary activities are often unavoidable—attending class, studying, working in an office, and so on—many people choose inactivity over activity during their leisure time. Change sedentary patterns by becoming more active whenever you can. Move more and sit less.

CAREER OPTIONS FOR . . .

Principles of Physical Training

FITNESS AND WELLNESS: personal fitness consultant, strength and conditioning specialist, health club director.

RECREATION: sport and fitness program coordinator, community sports administrator, special event coordinator.

REHABILITATION: athletic injury trainer, kinesiologist, special population adaptive specialist.

SOURCE: Physical and Health Education Canada (http://www.phecanada.ca).

	Lifestyle physical activity	Moderate exercise program	Vigorous exercise program
Description	Moderate physical activity (150 minutes per week; muscle-strengthening exercises 2 or more days per week)	Cardiorespiratory endurance exercise (20–60 minutes, 3–5 days per week); strength training (2–3 nonconsecutive days per week); and stretching exercises (2 or more days per week)	Cardiorespiratory endurance exercise (20–60 minutes, 3–5 days per week); interval training; strength training (3–4 nonconsecutive days per week); and stretching exercises (5–7 days per week)
Sample activities or program	• Walking to and from work, 15 minutes each way • Cycling to and from class, 10 minutes each way • Doing yard work for 30 minutes • Dancing (fast) for 30 minutes • Playing basketball for 20 minutes • Muscle exercises such as push-ups, squats, or back exercises	• Jogging for 30 minutes, 3 days per week • Weight training, 1 set of 8 exercises, 2 days per week • Stretching exercises, 3 days per week	• Running for 45 minutes, 3 days per week • Intervals, running 400 m at high effort, 4 sets, 2 days per week • Weight training, 3 sets of 10 exercises, 3 days per week • Stretching exercises, 6 days per week
Health and fitness benefits	Better blood cholesterol levels, reduced body fat, better control of blood pressure, improved metabolic health, and enhanced glucose metabolism; improved quality of life; reduced risk of some chronic diseases Greater amounts of activity can help prevent weight gain and promote weight loss	All the benefits of lifestyle physical activity, plus improved physical fitness (increased cardiorespiratory endurance, muscular strength and endurance, and flexibility) and even greater improvements in health and quality of life and reductions in chronic disease risk	All the benefits of lifestyle physical activity and a moderate exercise program, with greater increases in fitness and somewhat greater reductions in chronic disease risk Participating in a vigorous exercise program may increase risk of injury and overtraining

FIGURE 2.3 Health and fitness benefits of different amounts of physical activity and exercise.

Exercise and Cardiac Risk

Participating in exercise and sports is usually a wonderful experience that improves wellness in both the short and long term. In rare instances, however, vigorous exertion is associated with sudden death. It may seem difficult to understand that although regular exercise protects people from heart disease, it also increases the risk of sudden death.

Congenital heart defects (heart abnormalities present at birth) are the most common cause of exercise-related sudden death in people under 35. In nearly all other cases, coronary artery disease is responsible. In this condition, fat and other substances build up in the arteries that supply blood to the heart. Death can result if an artery becomes blocked or if the heart's rhythm and pumping action are disrupted. Exercise, particularly intense exercise, may trigger a heart attack in someone with underlying heart disease.

A study of jogging deaths in Rhode Island found that there was one death per 396 000 hours of jogging, or about one death per 7620 joggers per year—an extremely low risk for each individual jogger. Another study of men involved in a variety of physical activities found one death per 1.51 million hours of exercise. This 12-year study of more than 21 000 men found that those who didn't exercise vigorously were 74 times more likely to die suddenly from cardiac arrest during or shortly after exercise. It is also important

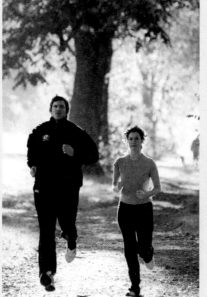

to note that people are much safer exercising than engaging in many other common activities, including driving a car.

Although quite small, the risk does exist and may lead some people to wonder why exercise is considered such an important part of a wellness lifestyle. Exercise causes many positive changes in the body—in healthy people as well as those with heart disease— that more than make up for the slightly increased short-term risk of sudden death. Training slows or reverses the fatty buildup in arteries and helps protect people from deadly heart rhythm abnormalities. People who exercise regularly have an overall risk of sudden death only about two-thirds that of nonexercisers. Active people who stop exercising can expect their heart attack risk to increase by 300%.

Obviously, someone with underlying coronary artery disease is at greater risk than someone who is free from the condition. However, many cases of heart disease go undiagnosed. The riskiest scenario may involve the middle-aged or older individual who suddenly begins participating in a vigorous sport or activity after being sedentary for a long time. This finding provides strong evidence for the recommendation that people increase their level of physical activity gradually and engage in regular, rather than sporadic, activity.

SOURCES: Fahey, T. D., and G. D. Swanson. 2008. A model for defining the optimal amount of exercise contributing to health and avoiding sudden cardiac death. *Medicina Sportiva* 12(4): 124–128; Albert, C. M., et al. 2000. Trigger of sudden death from cardiac causes by vigorous exertion. *New England Journal of Medicine* 343(19): 1355–1361.

LO5   Guidelines for Training

The following guidelines will make your exercise program more effective and successful.

TRAIN THE WAY YOU WANT YOUR BODY TO CHANGE
Stress your body such that it adapts in the desired direction. To have a more muscular build, lift weights. To be more flexible, do stretching exercises. To improve performance in a particular sport, practise that sport or the movements used in it.

TRAIN REGULARLY   Consistency is the key to improving fitness. Fitness improvements are lost if too much time is allowed to pass between exercise sessions.

START SLOWLY AND GET IN SHAPE GRADUALLY   As Figure 2.4 shows, an exercise program can be divided into three phases:

- *Beginning phase.* The body adjusts to the new type and level of activity.

- *Making progress phase.* Fitness increases.
- *Maintenance phase.* The targeted level of fitness is sustained over the long term.

When beginning a program, start slowly to give your body time to adapt to the stress of exercise. Choose activities carefully according to your fitness status. If you have been sedentary or are overweight, try an activity such as walking or swimming that won't jar the body or strain the joints.

WELLNESS TIP

Moderation is important, especially if you're just starting to get physically active. Work at a pace that's comfortable and enjoyable, with a goal of making gradual improvements. This will help you get into the habit of being active, and will help you avoid burnout.

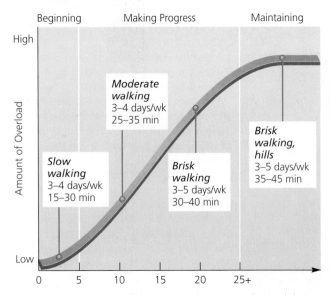

Beginning   Making Progress   Maintaining

High

Moderate walking
3–4 days/wk
25–35 min

Slow walking
3–4 days/wk
15–30 min

Brisk walking, hills
3–5 days/wk
35–45 min

Brisk walking
3–5 days/wk
30–40 min

Amount of Overload

Low

0   5   10   15   20   25+

Time Since Beginning an Exercise Program (in Weeks)

FIGURE 2.4 Progression of an exercise program. This figure shows how the amount of overload is increased gradually over time in a sample walking program. Regardless of the activity chosen, it is important that an exercise program begin slowly and progress gradually. Once you achieve the desired level of fitness, you can maintain it by exercising 3–5 days a week.

SOURCE: Progression data from American College of Sports Medicine. 2009. *ACSM's Guidelines for Exercise Testing and Prescription,* 8th ed. Philadelphia: Lippincott Williams and Wilkins.

As you progress, increase duration and frequency before increasing intensity. If you train too much or too intensely, you are more likely to suffer injuries or become **overtrained,** a condition characterized by lack of energy, aching muscles and joints, and decreased physical performance. Injuries and overtraining slow down an exercise program and impede motivation. The goal is not to get in shape as quickly as possible but to gradually become and remain physically fit.

WARM UP BEFORE EXERCISE Warming up can decrease your chances of injury by helping your body gradually progress from rest to activity. A good warm-up can increase muscle temperature, reduce joint stiffness, bathe the joint surfaces in lubricating fluid, and increase blood flow to the muscles, including the heart. Some studies suggest that warming up may also enhance muscle metabolism and mentally prepare you for a workout.

A warm-up should include low-intensity, whole-body movements similar to those used in the activity that will follow. For example, runners may walk and jog slowly

TERMS

overtraining A condition caused by training too much or too intensely, characterized by lack of energy, decreased physical performance, fatigue, depression, aching muscles and joints, and susceptibility to injury.

prior to running at full-speed. A tennis player might hit forehands and backhands at a low intensity before playing a vigorous set of tennis. It is important to note that a warm-up is not the same thing as a stretching workout. For safety and effectiveness, it is best to stretch *after* an endurance or strength-training workout, when muscles are warm—and not as part of a warm-up. Appropriate and effective warm-ups are discussed in greater detail in Chapters 3–5.

COOL DOWN AFTER EXERCISE During exercise, as much as 90% of circulating blood is directed to the muscles and skin, up from as little as 20% during rest. If you suddenly stop moving after exercise, the amount of blood returning to your heart and brain may be insufficient, and you may experience dizziness, a drop in blood pressure, or other problems. Cooling down at the end of a workout helps safely restore circulation to its normal resting condition. So, don't sit or lie down or jump into the shower after exercise without cooling down first. Cool down by continuing to move at a slow pace—walking, for example—for 5–10 minutes, as your heart and breathing rate slowly return to normal. At the end of the cool-down period, do stretching exercises while your muscles are still warm. Cool down longer after intense exercise sessions. Chapters 3–5 provide you with more information about the cool down.

EXERCISE SAFELY Physical activity can cause injury or even death if you don't consider safety. For example, you should always:

- Wear a helmet when biking, skiing, or rock climbing.
- Wear eye protection when playing racquetball or squash.
- Wear bright clothing when exercising on a public street.
- Walk or run with a partner in a park or on a deserted track.
- Give vehicles plenty of leeway, even when you have the right of way.

Overloading your muscles and joints can lead to serious injury, so train within your capacity. Use high-quality equipment and keep it in good repair. Report broken gym equipment to the health club manager.

LISTEN TO YOUR BODY AND GET ADEQUATE REST Rest can be as important as exercise for improving fitness. Fitness reflects an adaptation to the stress of exercise. Building fitness involves a series of exercise stresses, recuperation, and adaptation leading to improved fitness, followed by further stresses. Build rest into your training program, and don't exercise if it doesn't feel right. Sometimes you need a few days of rest to recover enough to train with the intensity required for improving fitness. Getting enough sleep is an important part of the recovery

Vary Your Activities

Do you have a hard time thinking of new activities to try? Check the boxes next to the activities listed here that interest you. Then look for resources and facilities on your campus or in your community.

Outdoor Exercises

- ☐ Walking
- ☐ Inline skating
- ☐ Hiking
- ☐ Running

- ☐ Swimming
- ☐ Horseback riding
- ☐ Fly fishing
- ☐ Skateboarding

- ☐ Cycling
- ☐ Rowing
- ☐ Ice skating
- ☐ Backpacking

Exercises You Can Do at Home and Work

- ☐ Desk exercises
- ☐ Yard work
- ☐ Painting the walls
- ☐ Calisthenics

- ☐ Sweeping the walkway
- ☐ Walking the dog
- ☐ Gardening
- ☐ Exploring on foot

- ☐ Shopping
- ☐ Housework
- ☐ Entering a walk-a-thon
- ☐ Shovelling snow

Sports and Games

- ☐ Basketball
- ☐ Softball
- ☐ Bowling
- ☐ Golf
- ☐ Soccer

- ☐ Tennis
- ☐ Hockey
- ☐ Surfing
- ☐ Badminton
- ☐ Ultimate Frisbee

- ☐ Volleyball
- ☐ Windsurfing
- ☐ Dancing
- ☐ Snow skiing
- ☐ Gymnastics

Health Club Exercises

- ☐ Weight training
- ☐ Ski machine
- ☐ Elliptical trainer
- ☐ Treadmill
- ☐ Stationary bike

- ☐ Circuit training
- ☐ Supine bike
- ☐ Medicine ball
- ☐ Plyometrics
- ☐ Water aerobics

- ☐ Group exercise
- ☐ Rowing machine
- ☐ Rope skipping
- ☐ Punching bag
- ☐ Racquetball

process. On the other hand, you can't train sporadically, either. If you listen to your body and it always tells you to rest, you won't make any progress.

CYCLE THE VOLUME AND INTENSITY OF YOUR WORKOUTS To add enjoyment and variety to your program, and to further improve fitness, don't train at the same intensity during every workout. Train intensely on some days and train lightly on others. Proper management of the level of workout intensity is a key to improved physical fitness. Use cycle training, also known as *periodization,* to provide enough recovery for intense training; By training lightly one workout, you can train harder the next. However, take care to increase the volume and intensity of your program gradually—never more than 10% per week.

VARY YOUR ACTIVITIES Change your exercise program from time to time to keep things fresh and help develop a higher degree of fitness. The body adapts quickly to an exercise stress, such as walking, cycling, or swimming. Gains in fitness in a particular activity become more difficult with time. Varying the kinds of exercises in your program allows you to adapt to many types of exercise and develops fitness in a variety of activities (see the box "Vary Your Activities"). Changing activities may also help reduce your risk of injury.

TRAIN WITH A PARTNER Training partners can motivate and encourage each other through rough spots and help each other develop proper exercise techniques. Training with a partner can make exercising seem easier

Digital Workout Aids

When you're just starting to get physically active, you can wind up with a lot of questions. How many kilometres did I walk? How many sit-ups did I do? How many minutes did I run? When your mind is completely focused on just *doing* an activity, it's easy to lose count of time, distance, and reps. But it's important to keep track of these things: Move too little and you won't see any progress; move too much and you run the risk of injury or burnout. Either outcome is bad news for your exercise program.

Luckily, we live in a digital age, and the fitness industry is providing an ever-growing array of tools that can track your progress for you. If you like to walk or run, digital pedometers can track your distance and the number of steps you take. Advanced trackers can even record any hills you encounter during your workout. If calisthenics are your choice, there are gaming systems and smartphone apps that work for specific exercises to count reps, assess your form, and challenge you to push yourself harder.

You can track more than just your exercise habits with digital assistance. Electronic devices and smart programs are available to help with many aspects of wellness, including the following:

- Dietary habits
- Calories consumed and burned
- Stress management
- Meditation and spirituality
- Heart rate and respiration
- Menstrual cycles
- Family medical history
- Journalling

And that's just to name a few. We'll introduce a variety of these digital devices and apps in later chapters, in the new "Wellness in the Digital Age" feature box like this one. You may find one or more digital apps (many of which are free) that appeal to you and can help you make progress toward your own fitness and wellness goals.

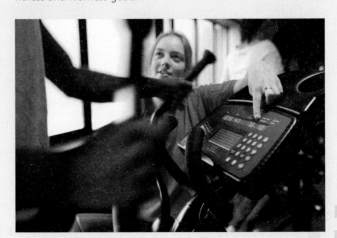

and more fun. It can also help you keep motivated and on track. A commitment to a friend is a powerful motivator.

TRAIN YOUR MIND Becoming fit requires commitment, discipline, and patience. These qualities come from understanding the importance of exercise and having clear and reachable goals. Use the lifestyle management techniques discussed in Chapter 1 to keep your program on track. Believe in yourself and your potential—and you *will* achieve your goals!

FUEL YOUR ACTIVITY APPROPRIATELY Good nutrition, including rehydration and resynthesis of liver and muscle carbohydrate stores, is part of optimal recuperation from exercise. Consume enough calories to support your exercise program without gaining body fat. Many studies show that consuming carbohydrates and protein before or after exercise promotes restoration of stored fuels and helps heal injured tissues so that you can exercise intensely again shortly. Nutrition for exercise is discussed in greater detail in Chapters 3 and 7.

HAVE FUN You are more likely to stick with an exercise program if it's fun. Choose a variety of activities that you enjoy. Some people like to play competitive sports, such as tennis, golf, or volleyball. Competition can boost motivation, but remember: Sports are competitive, whereas training for fitness is not. Other people like more solitary activities, such as jogging, walking, or swimming. Still others like high-skill individual sports, such as skiing, surfing, or skateboarding. Many activities can help you get fit, so choose the ones you enjoy. You can also boost your enjoyment and build your social support network by exercising with friends and family.

TRACK YOUR PROGRESS Monitoring the progress of your program can help keep you motivated and on track. Depending on the activities you've included in your program, you may track different measures of your program—minutes of jogging, kilometres of cycling, laps of swimming, number of push-ups, amount of weight lifted, and so on. If your program is focused on increasing daily physical activity, consider using an inexpensive pedometer to monitor the number of steps you take each day (see Lab 2.3 for more information on setting goals and monitoring activity with a pedometer). Specific examples of program monitoring can be found in the labs for Chapters 3–5.

Fitness centres can provide you with many benefits—motivation and companionship are among the most important. A fitness centre may also offer expert instruction and supervision as well as access to better equipment than you could afford on your own. If you're thinking of joining a fitness centre, here are some guidelines to help you choose a club that's right for you.

Trained Personnel

- Determine if the personal trainers and fitness instructors are certified by a recognized professional association such as the Canadian Society for Exercise Physiology (CSEP). All personal trainers are not equal—many organizations certify trainers and few of these require much formal training. Trainers with degrees in exercise physiology or physical education are usually the most knowledgeable.

- Find out if the club has a trained exercise physiologist on staff, someone with a degree in exercise physiology, kinesiology, or exercise science. If the facility offers nutritional counselling, it should employ someone who is a registered dietitian (R.D.) or who has other formal training.

- Ask how much experience the instructors have. Clubs may employ people because they were good athletes or look fit; by themselves, these are not good reasons to hire someone. Ideally, trainers should have both academic preparation and practical experience.

Convenience

- Look for an established facility that's within 10–15 minutes of your home or work. If it's farther away, your chances of sticking to an exercise regimen start to diminish.

- Check out the facility's hours, then visit it at the time you would normally exercise. Will you have easy access to the equipment and exercise classes you want at that time?

Atmosphere

- Look around to see if there are other members who are your age and at about your fitness level. (If everyone seems close in age or fitness level, then the club may cater to a certain age group or lifestyle—for example, hard-core bodybuilders.)

- If you like to exercise to music, make sure you like the music played there, both its type and volume.

- Observe how the members dress. Will you fit in, or will you be uncomfortable?

- Check to see that the facility is clean, including showers and lockers. Make sure the facility is climate controlled and well ventilated.

- For some, accessibility may be an important criteria for selection. Be sure to check all areas of the club to ensure that your needs will be met.

Safety

- Find out if the facility offers basic fitness testing that includes cardiovascular screening.

- Determine if there is emergency equipment on the premises and if personnel are trained in CPR.

- Ask if at least one staff member on each shift is trained in first aid.

- Find out if the club has an Emergency Action Plan in the event that a member has a heart attack or serious injury (many clubs do not).

Cost

- Pay for only what you need and can afford. If you want to use only workout equipment, you may not need a club that has racquetball courts and saunas.

- Check the contract. Choose the one that covers the shortest period of time possible, especially if it's your first fitness club experience.

- Make sure the contract permits you to extend your membership if you have a prolonged illness or go on vacation.

- Try out the club. Ask for a free trial workout, or a 1-day pass, or an inexpensive 1- or 2-week trial membership.

- Find out whether there is an extra charge for the particular services you want.

Effectiveness

- Tour the facility. Does it offer what the brochure says it does?

- Check the equipment. A good club will have treadmills, bikes, stair-climbers, resistance machines, and weights.

- Make sure these machines are up-to-date and well maintained. Make sure the facility is certified. Look for the displayed names Fitness Industry Council of Canada (FIC), American College of Sports Medicine (ACSM), or American Council on Exercise (ACE).

- Don't get cheated. Check with your Better Business Bureau or Consumer Affairs office to see if others have complained.

KEEP YOUR EXERCISE PROGRAM IN PERSPECTIVE As important as physical fitness is, it is only part of a well-rounded life. You have to have time for work and school, family and friends, relaxation and hobbies. Some people become overinvolved in exercise and neglect other parts of their lives. They think of themselves as runners, dancers, swimmers, or triathletes rather than as people who participate in those activities. Balance and moderation are the key ingredients of a fit and well life.

I have asthma. Is it OK for me to start an exercise program?

Probably, but you should see your doctor before you start exercising, especially if you have been sedentary up to this point. Your personal physician can advise you on the type of exercise program that is best for you, given the severity of your condition, and how to avoid suffering exercise-related asthma attacks.

What should my fitness goals be?

Begin by thinking about your general overall goals—the benefits you want to obtain by increasing your activity level and/or beginning a formal exercise program. Examples of long-term goals include reducing your risk of chronic diseases, increasing your energy level, and maintaining a healthy body weight.

To help shape your fitness program, you need to also set specific, short-term goals based on measurable factors. These specific goals should be an extension of your overall goals—the specific changes to your current activity and exercise habits needed to achieve your general goals. In setting short-term goals, be sure to use the SMART criteria described in Chapter 1. As noted there, your goals should be Specific, Measurable, Attainable, Realistic, and Time frame–specific (SMART).

You need information about your current levels of physical activity and physical fitness in order to set appropriate goals. The labs in this chapter will help you determine your physical activity level—for example, how many minutes per day you engage in moderate or vigorous activity or how many daily steps you take. Using this information, you can set goals for lifestyle physical activity to help you meet your overall goals. For example, if your general long-term goals are to reduce the risk of chronic disease and prevent weight gain, the Dietary Guidelines recommend 60 minutes of moderate physical activity daily. If you currently engage in 30 minutes of moderate activity daily, then your behaviour change goal would be to add 30 additional minutes of daily physical activity (or an equivalent number of additional daily steps—about 3500–4000); your time frame for the change might be 8–12 weeks.

Labs in Chapters 3–6 provide opportunities to specifically assess your fitness status for all the health-related components of fitness. The results of these assessments can guide you in setting specific fitness goals. For instance, if the labs in Chapter 4 indicate that you have good muscular strength and endurance in your lower body but poor strength and endurance in your upper body, then setting a specific goal for improving upper-body muscle fitness would be an appropriate goal—increasing the number of push-ups you can do from 22 to 30, for example. Chapters 3–6 include additional advice for setting appropriate goals.

Once you start your behaviour change program, you may discover that your goals aren't quite appropriate—perhaps you were overly optimistic, or maybe you set the bar too low. There are limits to the amount of fitness you can achieve, but within the limits of your genes and health status, you can make significant improvements in fitness. Adjust your goals as needed.

How can I fit my exercise program into my day?

Good time management is an important skill in creating and maintaining an exercise program. Choose a regular time to exercise, preferably the same time every day. Don't tell yourself you'll exercise "sometime during the day" when you have free time—that free time may never come. Schedule your workout, and make it a priority. Include alternative plans in your program to account for circumstances like bad weather or vacations.

Where can I get help and advice about exercise?

One of the best places to get help is an exercise class. If you join a health club or fitness centre, follow the guidelines in the box "Choosing a Fitness Centre." There, expert instructors can help you learn the basics of training and answer your questions. Make sure the instructor is certified by a recognized professional organization and/or has formal training in exercise physiology. Read articles by credible experts in fitness magazines. Many of these magazines include articles by leading experts in exercise science written at a layperson's level.

A qualified personal trainer can also help you get started in an exercise program or a new form of training. Make sure this person has proper qualifications, such as certification by CSEP, National Strength and Conditioning Association (NSCA), or American Council on Exercise (ACE). Don't seek out a person for advice simply because he or she looks fit. UCLA researchers found that 60% of the personal trainers in their study couldn't pass a basic exam on training methods, exercise physiology, or biomechanics. Trainers who performed best had university/college degrees in exercise physiology, physical education, or physical therapy. So choose your trainer carefully and don't get caught up with fads or appearances.

Should I follow my exercise program if I'm sick?

If you have a mild head cold or feel one coming on, it is probably OK to exercise moderately. Just begin slowly and see how you feel. However, if you have symptoms of a more serious illness—fever, swollen glands, nausea, extreme tiredness, muscle aches—wait until you have fully recovered before resuming your exercise program. Continuing to exercise while suffering from an illness more serious than a cold can compromise your recovery and may even be dangerous.

Where Do You Go from Here?

Now that you have an awareness of the basics behind lifestyle change, take some time to learn about the physical changes that can happen when you engage in a fitness training program. Chapters 3–5 will guide you through the development of specific programs for the cardiovascular, muscle, and flexibility systems while Chapter 6 helps you to understand the overall effect that these systems can have on our body composition. Use Chapters 1 and 2 to then help create an overall general fitness training program in Chapter 9.

SUMMARY

- Moderate daily exercise contributes substantially to good health. Even without a formal, vigorous exercise program, you can get many of the same health benefits by becoming more physically active.
- If you are already active, you benefit even more by increasing the intensity or duration of your activity.
- The five components of physical fitness most important for health are cardiorespiratory endurance, muscular strength, muscular endurance, flexibility, and body composition.
- Physical training is the process of producing long-term improvements in the body's functioning through exercise. All training is based on the fact that the body adapts to physical stress.
- According to the principle of *specificity,* bodies change specifically in response to the type of training received.
- Bodies also adapt to *progressive overload.* Therefore, when we progressively increase the frequency,

intensity, and time (duration) of the right type of exercise, we become increasingly fit.
- Bodies adjust to lower levels of activity by losing fitness, a principle known as *reversibility.* To counter the effects of reversibility we should keep training at the same intensity, even if we reduce the number or length of sessions.
- According to the principle of *individual differences,* people vary in the maximum level of fitness they can achieve.
- When designing an exercise program, determine if medical clearance is needed, assess your current level of fitness, set realistic goals, and choose activities that develop all components of fitness.
- Train regularly, get in shape gradually, warm up and cool down, maintain a structured but flexible program, exercise safely, consider training with a partner, train your mind, have fun, and keep exercise in perspective.

FOR FURTHER EXPLORATION

Journals

ACSM Health and Fitness Journal (401 West Michigan Street, Indianapolis, IN 46202; http://www.acsm-healthfitness.org)

Applied Physiology, Nutrition and Metabolism (http://www.nrcresearch press.com/loi/apnm)

Physician and Sportsmedicine (4530 W. 77th Street, Minneapolis, MN 55435; many of the articles are also available online at http://www.physsportsmed.com)

Organizations, Hotlines, and Websites

American College of Sports Medicine (ACSM). The principal professional organization for sports medicine and exercise science. Provides brochures, publications, and audio- and videotapes.
   317-637-9200
   http://www.acsm.org

American Council on Exercise (ACE). Promotes exercise and fitness; the website features fact sheets on many consumer topics, including choosing shoes, cross-training, and steroids.

800-825-3636

http://www.acefitness.org

Canada's Physical Activity Guide. Offers many suggestions for incorporating physical activity into everyday life; also includes the Physical Activity Readiness Questionnaire (PAR-Q).

http://www.phac-aspc.gc.ca/pau-uap/paguide/

Canadian Association for Health, Physical Education, Recreation, and Dance (CAHPERD). A professional organization dedicated to promoting quality health and physical education programs.

800-213-7193

http://www.cahperd.org

Canadian Kinesiology Alliance.

http://www.cka.ca

Canadian Society for Exercise Physiology. Promotes human performance through research related to exercise physiology.

http://www.csep.ca

Certified Personal Trainers Network.

http://www.cptn.com

CDC Physical Activity Information. Provides information on the benefits of physical activity and suggestions for incorporating moderate physical activity into daily life.

http://www.cdc.gov/nccdphp/dnpa/physical

Georgia State University: Exercise and Physical Fitness Page. Provides information about the benefits of exercise and how to get started on a fitness program.

http://www2.gsu.edu/~wwwfit/

MedlinePlus: Exercise and Physical Fitness. Provides links to news and reliable information about fitness and exercise from government agencies and professional associations.

http://www.nlm.nih.gov/medlineplus/exercisephysical
fitness.html

The following provide links to sites with information on a wide variety of activities and fitness issues; evaluate commercial sites carefully.

Fitness Partner Connection Jumpsite: http://primusweb.com/
fitnesspartner/

NetSweat: The Internet's Fitness Resource: http://www.netsweat
.com/

Yahoo!Fitness: dir.yahoo.com/Health/Fitness

LAB 2.1   Safety of Exercise Participation

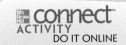

Physical Activity Readiness
Questionnaire - PAR-Q
(revised 2002)

PAR-Q & YOU

(A Questionnaire for People Aged 15 to 69)

Regular physical activity is fun and healthy, and increasingly more people are starting to become more active every day. Being more active is very safe for most people. However, some people should check with their doctor before they start becoming much more physically active.

If you are planning to become much more physically active than you are now, start by answering the seven questions in the box below. If you are between the ages of 15 and 69, the PAR-Q will tell you if you should check with your doctor before you start. If you are over 69 years of age, and you are not used to being very active, check with your doctor.

Common sense is your best guide when you answer these questions. Please read the questions carefully and answer each one honestly: check YES or NO.

YES	NO		
☐	☐	**1.**	**Has your doctor ever said that you have a heart condition <u>and</u> that you should only do physical activity recommended by a doctor?**
☐	☐	**2.**	**Do you feel pain in your chest when you do physical activity?**
☐	☐	**3.**	**In the past month, have you had chest pain when you were not doing physical activity?**
☐	☐	**4.**	**Do you lose your balance because of dizziness or do you ever lose consciousness?**
☐	☐	**5.**	**Do you have a bone or joint problem (for example, back, knee or hip) that could be made worse by a change in your physical activity?**
☐	☐	**6.**	**Is your doctor currently prescribing drugs (for example, water pills) for your blood pressure or heart condition?**
☐	☐	**7.**	**Do you know of <u>any other reason</u> why you should not do physical activity?**

If

you

answered

YES to one or more questions

Talk with your doctor by phone or in person BEFORE you start becoming much more physically active or BEFORE you have a fitness appraisal. Tell your doctor about the PAR-Q and which questions you answered YES.

- You may be able to do any activity you want — as long as you start slowly and build up gradually. Or, you may need to restrict your activities to those which are safe for you. Talk with your doctor about the kinds of activities you wish to participate in and follow his/her advice.
- Find out which community programs are safe and helpful for you.

NO to all questions

If you answered NO honestly to <u>all</u> PAR-Q questions, you can be reasonably sure that you can:
- start becoming much more physically active — begin slowly and build up gradually. This is the safest and easiest way to go.
- take part in a fitness appraisal — this is an excellent way to determine your basic fitness so that you can plan the best way for you to live actively. It is also highly recommended that you have your blood pressure evaluated. If your reading is over 144/94, talk with your doctor before you start becoming much more physically active.

DELAY BECOMING MUCH MORE ACTIVE:
- if you are not feeling well because of a temporary illness such as a cold or a fever — wait until you feel better; or
- if you are or may be pregnant — talk to your doctor before you start becoming more active.

PLEASE NOTE: If your health changes so that you then answer YES to any of the above questions, tell your fitness or health professional. Ask whether you should change your physical activity plan.

<u>Informed Use of the PAR-Q</u>: The Canadian Society for Exercise Physiology, Health Canada, and their agents assume no liability for persons who undertake physical activity, and if in doubt after completing this questionnaire, consult your doctor prior to physical activity.

No changes permitted. You are encouraged to photocopy the PAR-Q but only if you use the entire form.

NOTE: If the PAR-Q is being given to a person before he or she participates in a physical activity program or a fitness appraisal, this section may be used for legal or administrative purposes.

"I have read, understood and completed this questionnaire. Any questions I had were answered to my full satisfaction."

NAME _____

SIGNATURE _____   DATE _____

SIGNATURE OF PARENT _____   WITNESS _____
or GUARDIAN (for participants under the age of majority)

Note: This physical activity clearance is valid for a maximum of 12 months from the date it is completed and becomes invalid if your condition changes so that you would answer YES to any of the seven questions.

   © Canadian Society for Exercise Physiology   Supported by: 🍁 Health Santé
Canada Canada   continued on other side...

Part II General Health Profile

To help further assess the safety of exercise for you, complete as much of this health profile as possible.

General Information

Age: _____ Total cholesterol: _____ Blood pressure: _____ / _____

Height: _____ HDL: _____ Triglycerides: _____

Weight: _____ LDL: _____ Blood glucose level: _____

Are you currently trying to _____ gain or _____ lose weight? (check one if appropriate)

Medical Conditions/Treatments

Check any of the following that apply to you and add any other conditions that might affect your ability to exercise safely.

_____ heart disease _____ depression, anxiety, or another psychological disorder _____ other injury or joint problem: _____

_____ lung disease _____ substance abuse problem

_____ diabetes _____ eating disorder _____ other: _____

_____ allergies _____ back pain _____ other: _____

_____ asthma _____ arthritis _____ other: _____

_____ Do you have a family history of cardiovascular disease (CVD) (a parent, sibling, or child who had a heart attack or stroke before age 55 for men or 65 for women)?

List any medications or supplements you are taking or any medical treatments you are undergoing. Include the name of the substance or treatment and its purpose. Include both prescription and over-the-counter drugs and supplements.

Lifestyle Information

Check any of the following that is true for you, and fill in the requested information.

_____ I usually eat high-fat foods (fatty meats, cheese, fried foods, butter, full-fat dairy products) every day.

_____ I consume fewer than 5 servings of fruits and vegetables on most days.

_____ I smoke cigarettes or use other tobacco products. If true, describe your use of tobacco (type and frequency): _____

_____ I regularly drink alcohol. If true, describe your typical weekly consumption pattern: _____

_____ I often feel as if I need more sleep. (I need about hours _____ per day; I get about _____ hours per day.)

_____ I feel as though stress has reduced my level of wellness during the past year.

Describe your current activity pattern. What types of moderate physical activity do you engage in on a daily basis? Are you involved in a formal exercise program or do you regularly participate in sports or recreational activities?

Using Your Results

How did you score? Did the PAR-Q indicate that exercise is likely to be safe for you? Is there anything in your health profile that you think may affect your ability to exercise safely? Have you had any problems with exercise in the past?

What should you do next? If the assessments in this lab indicate that you should see your physician before beginning an exercise program, or if you have any questions about the safety of exercise for you, make an appointment to talk with your health care provider to address your concerns.

LAB 2.2 Overcoming Barriers to Being Active

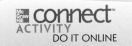

Barriers to Being Active Quiz

Directions: Listed below are reasons that people give to describe why they do not get as much physical activity as they think they should. Please read each statement and indicate how likely you are to say each of the following statements:

How likely are you to say this?	Very likely	Somewhat likely	Somewhat unlikely	Very unlikely
1. My day is so busy now, I just don't think I can make the time to include physical activity in my regular schedule.	3	2	1	0
2. None of my family members or friends like to do anything active, so I don't have a chance to exercise.	3	2	1	0
3. I'm just too tired after work to get any exercise.	3	2	1	0
4. I've been thinking about getting more exercise, but I just can't seem to get started.	3	2	1	0
5. I'm getting older so exercise can be risky.	3	2	1	0
6. I don't get enough exercise because I have never learned the skills for any sport.	3	2	1	0
7. I don't have access to jogging trails, swimming pools, bike paths, etc.	3	2	1	0
8. Physical activity takes too much time away from other commitments—like work, family, etc.	3	2	1	0
9. I'm embarrassed about how I will look when I exercise with others.	3	2	1	0
10. I don't get enough sleep as it is. I just couldn't get up early or stay up late to get some exercise.	3	2	1	0
11. It's easier for me to find excuses not to exercise than to go out and do something.	3	2	1	0
12. I know of too many people who have hurt themselves by overdoing it with exercise.	3	2	1	0
13. I really can't see learning a new sport at my age.	3	2	1	0
14. It's just too expensive. You have to take a class or join a club or buy the right equipment.	3	2	1	0
15. My free times during the day are too short to include exercise.	3	2	1	0
16. My usual social activities with family or friends do not include physical activity.	3	2	1	0
17. I'm too tired during the week and I need the weekend to catch up on my rest.	3	2	1	0
18. I want to get more exercise, but I just can't seem to make myself stick to anything.	3	2	1	0

How likely are you to say this?	Very likely	Somewhat likely	Somewhat unlikely	Very unlikely
19. I'm afraid I might injure myself or have a heart attack.	3	2	1	0
20. I'm not good enough at any physical activity to make it fun.	3	2	1	0
21. If we had exercise facilities and showers at work, then I would be more likely to exercise.	3	2	1	0

Scoring

- Enter the circled number in the spaces provided, putting the number for statement 1 on line 1, statement 2 on line 2, and so on.

- Add the three scores on each line. Your barriers to physical activity fall into one or more of seven categories: lack of time, social influence, lack of energy, lack of willpower, fear of injury, lack of skill, and lack of resources. A score of 5 or above in any category shows that this is an important barrier for you to overcome.

$$\underline{\quad}_{1} + \underline{\quad}_{8} + \underline{\quad}_{15} = \underline{\qquad}_{\text{Lack of time}}$$

$$\underline{\quad}_{2} + \underline{\quad}_{9} + \underline{\quad}_{16} = \underline{\qquad}_{\text{Social influences}}$$

$$\underline{\quad}_{3} + \underline{\quad}_{10} + \underline{\quad}_{17} = \underline{\qquad}_{\text{Lack of energy}}$$

$$\underline{\quad}_{4} + \underline{\quad}_{11} + \underline{\quad}_{18} = \underline{\qquad}_{\text{Lack of willpower}}$$

$$\underline{\quad}_{5} + \underline{\quad}_{12} + \underline{\quad}_{19} = \underline{\qquad}_{\text{Fear of injury}}$$

$$\underline{\quad}_{6} + \underline{\quad}_{13} + \underline{\quad}_{20} = \underline{\qquad}_{\text{Lack of skill}}$$

$$\underline{\quad}_{7} + \underline{\quad}_{14} + \underline{\quad}_{21} = \underline{\qquad}_{\text{Lack of resources}}$$

Using Your Results

How did you score? How many key barriers did you identify? Are they what you expected?

What should you do next? For your key barriers, try the strategies listed on the following pages and/or develop additional strategies that work for you. Check off any strategy that you try.

Suggestions for Overcoming Physical Activity Barriers

Lack of Time

_____ Identify available time slots. Monitor your daily activities for 1 week. Identify at least three 30-minute time slots you could use for physical activity.

_____ Add physical activity to your daily routine. For example, walk or ride your bike to work or shopping, organize social activities around physical activity, walk the dog, exercise while you watch TV, park farther from your destination, etc.

_____ Make time for physical activity. For example, walk, jog, or swim during your lunch hour, or take fitness breaks instead of coffee breaks.

_____ Other: _____

Social Influence

_____ Explain your interest in physical activity to friends and family. Ask them to support your efforts.

_____ Invite friends and family members to exercise with you. Plan social activities involving exercise.

_____ Develop new friendships with physically active people. Join a group, such as the YMCA or a hiking club.

_____ Other: _____

Lack of Energy

_____ Schedule physical activity for times in the day or week when you feel energetic.

_____ Convince yourself that if you give it a chance, exercise will increase your energy level; then, try it.

_____ Other: _____

Lack of Willpower

_____ Plan ahead. Make physical activity a regular part of your daily or weekly schedule and write it on your calendar.

_____ Invite a friend to exercise with you on a regular basis and write it on *both* your calendars.

_____ Join an exercise group or class.

_____ Other: _____

Fear of Injury

_____ Learn how to warm up and cool down to prevent injury.

_____ Learn how to exercise appropriately considering your age, fitness level, skill level, and health status.

_____ Choose activities involving minimal risk.

_____ Other: _____

Lack of Skill

_____ Select activities requiring no new skills, such as walking, climbing stairs, or jogging.

_____ Exercise with friends who are at the same skill level as you are.

_____ Find a friend who is willing to teach you some new skills.

_____ Take a class to develop new skills.

_____ Other: _____

Lack of Resources

_____ Select activities that require minimal facilities or equipment, such as walking, jogging, jumping rope, or calisthenics.

_____ Identify inexpensive, convenient resources available in your community (community education programs, park and recreation programs, worksite programs, etc.).

_____ Other: _____

Are any of the following additional barriers important for you? If so, try some of the strategies listed here or invent your own.

Weather Conditions

_____ Develop a set of regular activities that are always available regardless of weather (indoor cycling, aerobic dance, indoor swimming, calisthenics, stair climbing, rope skipping, mall walking, dancing, gymnasium games, etc.).

_____ Look on outdoor activities that depend on weather conditions (cross-country skiing, outdoor swimming, outdoor tennis, etc.) as "bonuses"—extra activities possible when weather and circumstances permit.

_____ Other: _____

Travel

_____ Put a jump rope in your suitcase and jump rope.

_____ Walk the halls and climb the stairs in hotels.

_____ Stay in places with swimming pools or exercise facilities.

_____ Join the YMCA or YWCA (ask about reciprocal membership agreement).

_____ Visit the local shopping mall and walk for half an hour or more.

_____ Bring a small tape recorder and your favourite aerobic exercise tape.

_____ Other: _____

Family Obligations

_____ Trade babysitting time with a friend, neighbour, or family member who also has small children.

_____ Exercise with the kids—go for a walk together, play tag or other running games, get an aerobic dance or exercise DVD for kids (there are several on the market) and exercise together. You can spend time together and still get your exercise.

_____ Hire a babysitter and look at the cost as a worthwhile investment in your physical and mental health.

_____ Jump rope, do calisthenics, ride a stationary bicycle, or use other home gymnasium equipment while the kids watch TV or when they are sleeping.

_____ Try to exercise when the kids are not around (e.g., during school hours or their nap time).

_____ Other: _____

Retirement Years

_____ Look on your retirement as an opportunity to become more active instead of less. Spend more time gardening, walking the dog, and playing with your grandchildren. Children with short legs and grandparents with slower gaits are often great walking partners.

_____ Learn a new skill you've always been interested in, such as ballroom dancing, square dancing, or swimming.

_____ Now that you have the time, make regular physical activity a part of every day. Go for a walk every morning or every evening before dinner. Treat yourself to an exercycle and ride every day during a favourite TV show.

_____ Other: _____

SOURCE: CDC Division of Nutrition and Physical Activity. 1999. *Promoting Physical Activity: A Guide for Community Action.* Champaign, Ill.: Human Kinetics.

LAB 2.3 Using a Pedometer to Track Physical Activity

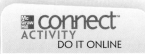

How physically active are you? Would you be more motivated to increase daily physical activity if you had an easy way to monitor your level of activity? If so, consider wearing a pedometer to track the number of steps you take each day—a rough but easily obtainable reflection of daily physical activity.

Determine Your Baseline

Wear the pedometer for a week to obtain a baseline average daily number of steps.

	M	Tu	W	Th	F	Sa	Su	Average
Steps								

Set Goals

Set an appropriate goal for increasing steps. The goal of 10 000 steps per day is widely recommended, but your personal goal should reflect your baseline level of steps. For example, if your current daily steps are far below 10 000, a goal of walking 2000 additional steps each day might be appropriate. If you are already close to 10 000 steps per day, choose a higher goal. Also consider the physical activity goals in the 2005 Dietary Guidelines:

- To reduce the risk of chronic disease, aim to accumulate at least 30 minutes of moderate physical activity per day.
- To help manage body weight and prevent gradual, unhealthy weight gain, engage in 60 minutes of moderate-to-vigorous-intensity activity on most days of the week.
- To sustain weight loss, engage daily in at least 60–90 minutes of moderate-intensity physical activity.

To help gauge how close you are to meeting these time-based physical activity goals, you might walk for 10–15 minutes while wearing your pedometer to determine how many steps correspond with the time-based goals from the Dietary Guidelines.

Once you have set your overall goal, break it down into several steps. For example, if your goal is to increase daily steps by 2000, set mini-goals of increasing daily steps by 500, allowing 2 weeks to reach each mini-goal. Smaller goals are easier to achieve and can help keep you motivated and on track. Having several interim goals also gives you the opportunity to reward yourself more frequently. Note your goals below:

Mini-goal 1: _____ Target date: _____ Reward: _____

Mini-goal 2: _____ Target date: _____ Reward: _____

Mini-goal 3: _____ Target date: _____ Reward: _____

Overall goal: _____ Target date: _____ Reward: _____

Develop Strategies for Increasing Steps

What can you do to become more active? Your text includes a variety of suggestions, including walking when you do errands, getting off one stop from your destination on public transportation, parking an extra block or two away from your destination, and doing at least one chore every day that requires physical activity. If weather or neighbourhood safety is an issue, look for alternative locations to walk. For example, find an indoor gym or shopping mall or even a long hallway. Check out locations that are near or on the way to your campus, workplace, or residence. If you think walking indoors will be dull, walk with friends or family members or wear headphones (if safe) and listen to music or audiobooks.

Are there any days of the week for which your baseline steps are particularly low and/or it will be especially difficult because of your schedule to increase your number of steps? Be sure to develop specific strategies for difficult situations.

Below, list at least five strategies for increasing daily steps:

_____

_____

_____

Track Your Progress

Based on the goals you set, fill in your goal portion of the progress chart with your target average daily steps for each week. Then wear your pedometer every day and note your total daily steps. Track your progress toward each mini-goal and your final goal. Every few weeks, stop and evaluate your progress. If needed, adjust your plan and develop additional strategies for increasing steps. In addition to the chart in this worksheet, you might also want to graph your daily steps to provide a visual reminder of how you are progressing toward your goals. Make as many copies of this chart as you need.

Week	Goal	M	Tu	W	Th	F	Sa	Su	Average
1									
2									
3									

Progress Checkup

How close are you to meeting your goal? How do you feel about your program and your progress?

If needed, describe changes to your plan and additional strategies for increasing steps:

Week	Goal	M	Tu	W	Th	F	Sa	Su	Average
4									
5									
6									

Progress Checkup

How close are you to meeting your goal? How do you feel about your program and your progress?

If needed, describe changes to your plan and additional strategies for increasing steps:

Week	Goal	M	Tu	W	Th	F	Sa	Su	Average
7									
8									
9									

Progress Checkup

How close are you to meeting your goal? How do you feel about your program and your progress?

If needed, describe changes to your plan and additional strategies for increasing steps:

CHAPTER 3

CARDIORESPIRATORY ENDURANCE

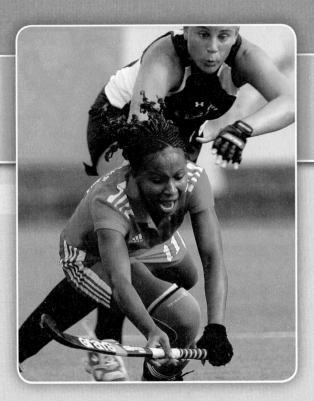

LEARNING OBJECTIVES

After reading this chapter, you should be able to

LO1 Describe how the body produces the energy it needs for exercise

LO2 List the major effects and benefits of cardiorespiratory endurance exercise

LO3 Explain how cardiorespiratory endurance is measured and assessed

LO4 Describe how frequency, intensity, time (duration), and type of exercise affect the development of cardiorespiratory endurance

LO5 Explain the best ways to prevent and treat common exercise injuries

TEST YOUR KNOWLEDGE

1. **Compared to sedentary people, those who engage in regular moderate endurance exercise are likely to**

   a. have fewer colds
   b. be less anxious and depressed
   c. fall asleep more quickly and sleep better
   d. be more alert and creative

2. **About how much blood does the heart pump during each minute of aerobic exercise?**

   a. 4–5 litres
   b. 8–10 litres
   c. 18–20 litres

3. **During an effective 30-minute cardiorespiratory endurance workout, you should lose 1–2 pounds.**

   True or false?

ANSWERS

1. **ALL FOUR.** Endurance exercise has many immediate benefits that affect all the dimensions of wellness and improve overall quality of life.

2. **C.** During exercise, cardiac output increases to 18–20 litres or more per minute, compared to 4–5 litres at rest.

3. **FALSE.** Any weight loss during an exercise session is due to fluid loss that needs to be replaced to prevent dehydration and enhance performance. It is best to drink enough during exercise to match fluid loss in sweat; weigh yourself before and after a workout to make sure that you are drinking enough.

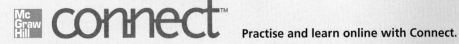

Practise and learn online with Connect.

Cardiorespiratory endurance—the ability of the body to perform prolonged, large-muscle, dynamic exercise at moderate-to-high levels of intensity—is a key health-related component of fitness. As explained in Chapter 2, a healthy cardiorespiratory system is essential to high levels of fitness and wellness.

This chapter reviews the short- and long-term effects and benefits of cardiorespiratory endurance exercise. It then describes several tests that are commonly used to assess cardiorespiratory fitness. Finally, it provides guidelines for creating your own cardiorespiratory endurance program, one that is geared to your current level of fitness and built around activities you enjoy.

3.1 BASIC PHYSIOLOGY OF CARDIORESPIRATORY ENDURANCE EXERCISE

A basic understanding of the body processes involved in cardiorespiratory endurance exercise can help you design a safe and effective fitness program.

The Cardiorespiratory System

The **cardiorespiratory system** consists of the heart, the blood vessels, and the respiratory system (air passages, trachea, bronchi, and lungs). The cardiorespiratory system circulates blood through the body, transporting oxygen, nutrients, and other key substances to the organs and tissues that need them. It also carries away waste products so they can be used or expelled.

THE HEART The heart is a four-chambered, fist-sized muscle located just beneath the ribs under the sternum (breastbone). Its role is to pump oxygen-poor blood to the lungs and oxygenated (oxygen-rich) blood to the rest of the body. Blood actually travels through two separate circulatory systems: The right side of the heart pumps blood to the lungs in what is called **pulmonary circulation,** and the left side pumps blood through the rest of the body in **systemic circulation.** A person weighing 70 kg has about 5 litres of blood, which are circulated through the cardiovascular system about once every minute.

The following steps describe the path blood follows as it travels through the heart and the cardiorespiratory system (Figure 3.1):

1. Waste-laden, oxygen-poor blood travels through large vessels, called **venae cavae,** into the heart's right upper chamber, or **atrium.**

2. After the right atrium fills, it contracts and pumps blood into the heart's right lower chamber, or **ventricle.**

3. When the right ventricle is full, it contracts and pumps blood through the pulmonary artery into the lungs.

4. In the lungs, blood picks up oxygen and discards carbon dioxide.

5. The cleaned, oxygenated blood flows from the lungs through the pulmonary veins into the heart's left atrium.

6. After the left atrium fills, it contracts and pumps blood into the left ventricle.

7. When the left ventricle is full, it pumps blood through the **aorta**—the body's largest artery—for distribution to the rest of the body's blood vessels.

The period of the heart's contraction is called **systole;** the period of relaxation is called **diastole.** During systole, the atria contract first, pumping blood into the ventricles. A fraction of a second later, the ventricles contract, pumping blood to the lungs and the body. During diastole, blood flows into the heart.

Blood pressure, the force exerted by blood on the walls of the blood vessels, is created by the pumping action of the heart. Blood pressure is greater during systole than during diastole. Normal blood pressure readings for a young, healthy male are approximately 120 mm Hg (systolic) and 80 mm Hg (diastolic). Women typically display blood pressure readings (both systolic and diastolic) that average 10 to 20 mm HG below that of men. These differences are likely related to height; blood pressure is higher in taller individuals and males are typically taller than females.[1] Regular monitoring is an important step in the process of managing and reducing the risk for cardiovascular disease (see Chapter 11).

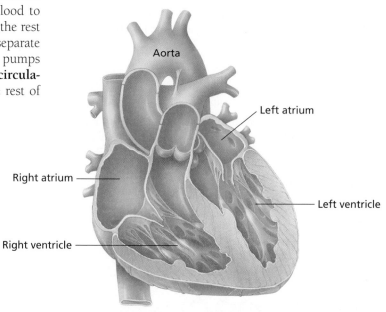

FIGURE 3.1 Chambers of the heart.

The heartbeat—the split-second sequence of contractions of the heart's four chambers—is controlled by nerve impulses. These signals originate in a bundle of specialized cells in the right atrium called the *pacemaker* or *sinoatrial (SA) node*. Unless it is speeded up or slowed down by the brain in response to such stimuli as danger or the tissues' need for more oxygen, the heart produces nerve impulses at a steady rate.

THE BLOOD VESSELS Blood vessels are classified by size and function. **Veins** carry blood to the heart. **Arteries** carry it away from the heart. Veins have thin walls, but arteries have thick elastic walls that enable them to expand and relax with the volume of blood being pumped through them.

After leaving the heart, the aorta branches into smaller and smaller vessels. The smallest arteries branch still further into **capillaries,** tiny vessels only one cell thick. The capillaries deliver oxygen and nutrient-rich blood to the tissues and pick up oxygen-poor, waste-laden blood. From the capillaries, this blood empties into small veins (*venules*) and then into larger veins that return it to the heart to repeat the cycle.

Blood pumped through the heart doesn't reach the cells of the heart, so the organ has its own network of arteries, veins, and capillaries. Two large vessels, the right and left coronary arteries, branch off the aorta and supply the heart muscle with oxygenated blood. Blockage of a coronary artery is a leading cause of heart attacks (see Chapter 11).

THE RESPIRATORY SYSTEM The **respiratory system** supplies oxygen to the body and carries off carbon dioxide—a waste product of body processes—and helps regulate acid produced during metabolism. Air passes in and out of the lungs as a result of pressure changes brought about by the contraction and relaxation of the diaphragm and rib muscles. As air is inhaled, it passes through the nasal passages, the throat, larynx, trachea (windpipe), and bronchi into the lungs. The lungs consist of many branching tubes that end in tiny, thin-walled air sacs called **alveoli.**

Carbon dioxide and oxygen are exchanged between alveoli and capillaries in the lungs. Carbon dioxide passes from blood cells into the alveoli, where it is carried up and out of the lungs (exhaled). Oxygen from inhaled air is passed from the alveoli into blood cells; these oxygen-rich blood cells then return to the heart and are pumped throughout the body. Oxygen is an important component of the body's energy-producing system, so the cardiorespiratory system's ability to pick up and deliver oxygen is critical for the functioning of the body.

THE CARDIORESPIRATORY SYSTEM AT REST AND DURING EXERCISE At rest and during light activity, the cardiorespiratory system functions at a fairly steady pace. Your heart beats at a rate of about 50–90 beats per minute, and you take about 12–20 breaths per minute.

During exercise, the demands on the cardiorespiratory system increase. Body cells, particularly working muscles, need to obtain more oxygen and fuel and to eliminate more waste products. To meet these demands, your body makes the following changes:

- Heart rate increases, up to 170–210 beats per minute during intense exercise.
- The heart's **stroke volume** increases, meaning that the heart pumps out more blood with each beat.
- The heart pumps and circulates more blood per minute as a result of the faster heart rate and greater stroke volume. During exercise, this **cardiac output** increases to 18–23 litres per minute, compared to about 4.5–6 litres per minute at rest.
- Blood flow changes, so as much as 85–90% of the blood may be delivered to working muscles. At rest, about 15–20% of blood is distributed to the skeletal muscles.
- Systolic blood pressure increases, while diastolic blood pressure holds steady or declines slightly. A typical exercise blood pressure might be 175/65.
- To oxygenate this increased blood flow, you take deeper breaths and breathe faster, up to 40–60 breaths per minute.

cardiorespiratory system The system that circulates blood through the body; consists of the heart, blood vessels, and respiratory system.

pulmonary circulation The part of the circulatory system that moves blood between the heart and the lungs; controlled by the right side of the heart.

systemic circulation The part of the circulatory system that moves blood between the heart and the rest of the body; controlled by the left side of the heart.

venae cavae The large veins through which blood is returned to the right atrium of the heart.

atrium One of the two upper chambers of the heart in which blood collects before passing to the ventricles (pl. atria).

ventricle One of the two lower chambers of the heart, from which blood flows through arteries to the lungs and other parts of the body.

aorta The body's large artery; receives blood from the left ventricle and distributes it to the body.

systole Contraction of the heart.

diastole Relaxation of the heart.

blood pressure The force exerted by the blood on the walls of the blood vessels; created by the pumping action of the heart.

veins Vessels that carry blood to the heart.

arteries Vessels that carry blood away from the heart.

capillaries Very small blood vessels that distribute blood to all parts of the body.

respiratory system The lungs, air passages, and breathing muscles; supplies oxygen to the body and removes carbon dioxide.

alveoli Tiny air sacs in the lungs that allow the exchange of oxygen and carbon dioxide between the lungs and blood.

stroke volume The amount of blood the heart pumps with each beat.

cardiac output The amount of blood pumped by the heart each minute; a function of heart rate and stroke volume.

All of these changes are controlled and coordinated by special centres in the brain, which use the nervous system and chemical messengers to control the process.

LO1 Energy Production

Metabolism is the sum of all the chemical processes necessary to maintain the body. Energy is required to fuel vital body functions—to build and break down tissue, contract muscles, conduct nerve impulses, regulate body temperature, and so on.

The rate at which your body uses energy—its **metabolic rate**—depends on your level of activity. At rest, you have a low metabolic rate; if you begin to walk, your metabolic rate increases. If you jog, your metabolic rate may increase more than 800% above its resting level. Olympic-calibre distance runners can increase their metabolic rate by 2000% or more.

ENERGY FROM FOOD The body converts chemical energy from food into substances that cells can use as fuel. These fuels can be used immediately or stored for later use. The body's ability to store fuel is critical, because if all the energy from food were released immediately, much of it would be wasted.

The three classes of energy-containing nutrients in food are carbohydrates, fats, and proteins. During digestion, most carbohydrates are broken down into the simple sugar **glucose**. Some glucose remains circulating in the blood ("blood sugar"), where it can be used as a quick source of fuel to produce energy. Glucose may also be converted to **glycogen** and stored in the liver, muscles, and kidneys. If glycogen stores are full and the body's immediate need for energy is met, the remaining glucose

is converted to fat and stored in the body's fatty tissues. Excess energy from dietary fat is also stored as body fat. Protein in the diet is used primarily to build new tissue, but it can be broken down for energy or incorporated into fat stores. Glucose, glycogen, and fat are important fuels for the production of energy in the cells; protein is a significant energy source only when other fuels are lacking. (See Chapter 7 for more on the other roles of carbohydrate, fat, and protein in the body.)

ATP: THE ENERGY "CURRENCY" OF CELLS The basic form of energy used by cells is **adenosine triphosphate, or ATP.** When a cell needs energy, it breaks down ATP, a process that releases energy in the only form the cell can use directly. Cells store a small amount of ATP; when they need more, they create it through chemical reactions that utilize the body's stored fuels—glucose, glycogen, and fat. When you exercise, your cells need to produce more energy. Consequently, your body mobilizes its stores of fuel to increase ATP production.

Exercise and the Three Energy Systems

The muscles in your body use three energy systems to create ATP and fuel cellular activity. These systems use different fuels and chemical processes and perform different, specific functions during exercise (Table 3.1).

THE IMMEDIATE ENERGY SYSTEM The **immediate ("explosive") energy system** provides energy rapidly but for only a short period of time. It is used to fuel activities that last for about 10 or fewer seconds—examples in sports include weight lifting and shot-putting; examples in daily life include rising from a chair or picking

---

TABLE 3.1 Characteristics of the Body's Energy Systems

	Anaerobic-Alactic (Immediate)	Energy System* Anaerobic-Lactic	Oxidative (Aerobic)
Duration of activity for which system predominates	0–10 seconds	10 seconds–2 minutes	>2 minutes
Intensity of activity for which system predominates	High	High	Low to moderately high
Rate of ATP production	Immediate, very rapid	Rapid	Slower, but prolonged
Fuel	Adenosine triphosphate (ATP), creatine phosphate (CP)	Muscle stores of glycogen and glucose	Body stores of glycogen, glucose, fat, and protein
Oxygen used?	No	No	Yes
Sample activities	Weight lifting, picking up a bag of groceries	400-metre run, running up several flights of stairs	1500-metre run, 30-minute walk, standing in line for a long time

*For most activities, all three systems contribute to energy production; the duration and intensity of the activity determine which system predominates.

SOURCE: Adapted from Brooks, G. A., et. al. 2005. *Exercise Physiology. Human Bioenergetics and its Applications,* 4th ed. New York: McGraw-Hill. Copyright © 2005 The McGraw-Hill Companies. Reproduced with permission of The McGraw-Hill Companies.

up a bag of groceries. The components of this energy system include existing cellular ATP stores and creatine phosphate (CP), a chemical that cells can use to make ATP. CP levels are depleted rapidly during exercise, so the maximum capacity of this energy system is reached within a few seconds. Cells must then switch to the other energy systems to restore levels of ATP and CP. (Without adequate ATP, muscles will stiffen and become unusable.)

THE NONOXIDATIVE ENERGY SYSTEM The **nonoxidative (anaerobic) energy system** is used at the start of an exercise session and for high-intensity activities lasting for about 10 seconds to 2 minutes, such as the 400-metre run. During daily activities, this system may be called on to help you run to catch a bus or dash up several flights of stairs. This nonoxidative energy system creates ATP by breaking down glucose and glycogen. This system doesn't require oxygen to produce energy, which is why it is referred to as the **anaerobic** system. This system's capacity to produce energy is limited, but it can generate a great deal of ATP in a short period of time. For this reason, it is the most important energy system for very intense exercise.

There are two key limiting factors for the anaerobic-lactic energy system. First, the body's supply of glucose and glycogen is limited. If these are depleted, a person may experience fatigue and dizziness, and judgment may be impaired. (The brain and nervous system rely on carbohydrates as fuel.) Second, increases in hydrogen and potassium ions (which are thought to interfere with metabolism and muscle contraction) cause fatigue. During heavy exercise, such as sprinting, large increases in hydrogen and potassium ions cause muscles to fatigue rapidly. The anaerobic energy system also creates metabolic acids. Fortunately, exercise training increases the body's ability to cope with metabolic acid. Improved fitness allows you to exercise at higher intensities before the abrupt build-up of metabolic acids—a point that scientists call the *lactate threshold*. One metabolic acid, called **lactic acid** (lactate), is often linked to fatigue during intense exercise. However, lactic acid is an important fuel at rest and during exercise.

THE OXIDATIVE ENERGY SYSTEM The **oxidative (aerobic) energy system** is used during any physical activity that lasts longer than about 2 minutes, such as distance running, swimming, hiking, or even standing in line. The oxidative system requires oxygen to generate ATP, which is why it is considered an **aerobic** system. The oxidative system cannot produce energy as quickly as the other two systems, but it can supply energy for much longer periods of time. It provides energy during most daily activities.

In the oxidative energy system, ATP production takes place in cellular structures called **mitochondria**. Because mitochondria can use carbohydrates (glucose and glycogen) or fats to produce ATP, the body's stores of fuel for this system are much greater than those for the other two energy systems. The actual fuel used depends on the intensity and duration of exercise and on the fitness status of the individual. Carbohydrates are favoured during more intense exercise (over 65% of maximum capacity); fats, for mild, low-intensity activities. During a prolonged exercise session, carbohydrates are the predominant fuel at the start of the workout, but fat utilization increases over time. Fit individuals use a greater proportion of fat as fuel because increased fitness allows people to do activities at lower intensities. This is an important adaptation because glycogen depletion is one of the limiting factors for the oxidative energy system. Thus, by being able to use more fat as fuel, a fit individual can exercise for a longer time before glycogen is depleted and muscles become fatigued.

Oxygen is another limiting factor. The oxygen requirement of this energy system is proportional to the intensity of exercise. As intensity increases, so does oxygen consumption. There is a limit to the body's ability to increase oxygen use; this limit is referred to as **maximal oxygen consumption,** or $\dot{V}O_{2max}$. $\dot{V}O_{2max}$ is influenced by genetics, fitness status (power-generating capacity and fatigue resistance), gender, and age. It depends on many factors, including the capacity of blood to carry oxygen, the rate at which oxygen is transported to the tissues, and the amount of oxygen that cells extract from the blood. $\dot{V}O_{2max}$ determines how intensely a person can perform endurance exercise and for how long, and it is considered the best overall measure of the capacity of the cardiorespiratory system. Table 3.2 shows the different levels of $\dot{V}O_{2max}$ that those who participate and excel in a variety of physical activities may display. (The assessment tests described later in the chapter are designed to help you predict your $\dot{V}O_{2max}$.)

THE ENERGY SYSTEMS IN COMBINATION Your body typically uses all three energy systems when you exercise. The intensity and duration of the activity determine which system predominates. For example, when you play tennis, you use the immediate energy system when hitting the ball, but you replenish cellular energy stores using the nonoxidative and oxidative systems. When cycling, the oxidative system predominates. However, if you must suddenly exercise intensely—ride up a steep hill, for example—the other systems become important because the oxidative system is unable to supply ATP fast enough to sustain high-intensity effort.

PHYSICAL FITNESS AND ENERGY PRODUCTION Physically fit people can increase their metabolic rate substantially, generating the energy needed for powerful or sustained exercise. People who are not fit cannot respond to exercise in the same way. Their bodies are less capable of delivering oxygen and fuel to exercising muscles; they can't burn as many calories during or after exercise, and they are also less able to cope with lactic acid and other substances produced during intense physical activity that contribute to fatigue. Because of this, they become fatigued more rapidly; their legs hurt and they breathe heavily walking up a flight of stairs, for example. Regular physical training can substantially improve the body's ability to produce energy and meet the challenges of increased physical activity.

In designing an exercise program, focus on the energy system most important to your goals. Because improving the functioning of the cardiorespiratory system is critical to overall wellness, endurance exercise that utilizes the oxidative energy system—activities performed at moderate to high intensities for a prolonged duration—is a key component of any health-related fitness program.

TABLE 3.2	Maximal Oxygen Uptake (mL/kg/min) in Various Population Groups		
Non Athletes	**Age**	**Males**	**Females**
	10–19	47–56	38–46
	20–29	43–52	33–42
	30–39	39–48	30–38
	40–49	36–44	26–35
	50–59	34–41	24–33
	60–69	31–38	22–30
	70–79	28–35	20–27
Athletes			
Baseball/softball	18–32	48–56	52–57
Basketball	18–30	40–60	43–60
Bicycling	18–26	62–74	47–57
Canoeing	22–28	55–67	48–52
Football	20–36	42–60	
Gymnastics	18–22	52–58	36–50
Ice Hockey	10–30	50–63	
Jockey	20–40	50–60	
Orienteering	20–60	47–53	46–60
Racquetball	20–35	55–62	50–60
Rowing	20–35	60–72	58–65
Skiing, alpine	18–30	57–68	50–55
Skiing, nordic	20–28	65–94	60–75
Ski jumping	18–24	58–63	
Soccer	22–28	54–64	50–60
Speed skating	18–24	56–73	44–55
Swimming	10–25	50–70	40–60
Track & Field, discus	22–30	42–55	
Track & Field, running	18–39	60–85	50–75
	40–75	40–60	35–60
Track & Field, shot put	22–30	40–46	
Volleyball	18–22		40–56
Weightlifting	20–30	38–52	
Wrestling	20–30	52–65	

SOURCE: Reprinted with permission from W. L. Kenney, J. H. Wilmore, and D. C. Costill, 2012. *Physiology of Sport and Exercise,* 5th edition. (Champaign, IL: Human Kinetics). p. 269.

LO2 3.2 BENEFITS OF CARDIORESPIRATORY ENDURANCE EXERCISE

Cardiorespiratory endurance exercise helps the body become more efficient and better able to cope with physical challenges. It also lowers risk for many chronic diseases.

Ask Yourself

QUESTIONS FOR CRITICAL THINKING AND REFLECTION

When you think about the types of physical activity you engage in during your typical day or week, which ones use the immediate energy system? The nonoxidative energy system? The oxidative energy system? How can you increase activities that use the oxidative energy system?

Improved Cardiorespiratory Functioning

Earlier in this chapter, we described some of the major changes that occur in the cardiorespiratory system when you exercise, such as increases in cardiac output and blood pressure, breathing rate, and blood flow to the skeletal muscles. In the short term, all these changes help the body respond to the challenge of exercise. When performed regularly, endurance exercise also leads to permanent adaptations in the cardiorespiratory system (Figure 3.2). These improvements reduce the effort required to do everyday tasks and make the body better able to respond to physical challenges. This, in a nutshell, is what it means to be physically fit.

Endurance exercise enhances the heart's health by:

- Maintaining or increasing the heart's own blood and oxygen supply.
- Increasing the heart muscle's function, so it pumps more blood per beat. This improved function keeps the heart rate lower both at rest and during exercise.

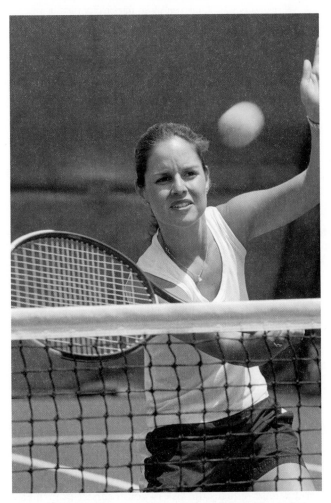

Exercise offers both long-term health benefits and immediate pleasures. Many popular sports and activities develop cardiorespiratory endurance.

The resting heart rate of a fit person is often 10–20 beats per minute lower than that of an unfit person. This translates into as many as 10 million fewer beats in the course of a year.

- Strengthening the heart's contractions and thus participating in an increase in overall cardiac output.
- Increasing the heart's cavity size (in young adults).
- Increasing blood volume so the heart pushes more blood into the circulatory system during each contraction.
- Reducing blood pressure.

Improved Cellular Metabolism

Regular endurance exercise also improves the body's metabolism, down to the cellular level, enhancing your ability to produce and use energy efficiently. Cardiorespiratory training improves metabolism by doing the following:

- Increasing the number of capillaries in the muscles. Additional capillaries supply the muscles with more fuel and oxygen and more quickly eliminate waste products. Greater capillary density also helps heal injuries and reduce muscle aches.
- Training muscles to make the most of oxygen and fuel so they work more efficiently.
- Increasing the size of and number of mitochondria in muscle cells, increasing cells' energy capacity.
- Preventing glycogen depletion and increasing the muscles' ability to use lactic acid and fat as fuels.

Regular exercise may also help protect your cells from chemical damage caused by agents called *free radicals*. (See Chapter 7 for more on free radicals and special enzymes the body uses to fight them.)

Fitness programs that best develop metabolic efficiency include both long-duration, moderately intense endurance exercise and brief periods of more intense effort. For example, climbing a small hill while jogging or cycling introduces the kind of intense exercise that leads to more efficient use of lactic acid and fats.

Reduced Risk of Chronic Disease

Regular endurance exercise lowers your risk of many chronic, disabling diseases. It can also help people with those diseases improve their health (see the box "Benefits of Exercise for Older Adults"). The most significant health benefits occur when someone who is sedentary becomes moderately active.

CARDIOVASCULAR DISEASE Sedentary living is a key contributor to cardiovascular disease (CVD). CVD is a general category that encompasses several diseases of the heart and blood vessels, including coronary heart disease (which can cause heart attacks), stroke, and high blood pressure. Sedentary people are significantly more likely to die of CVD than are fit individuals.

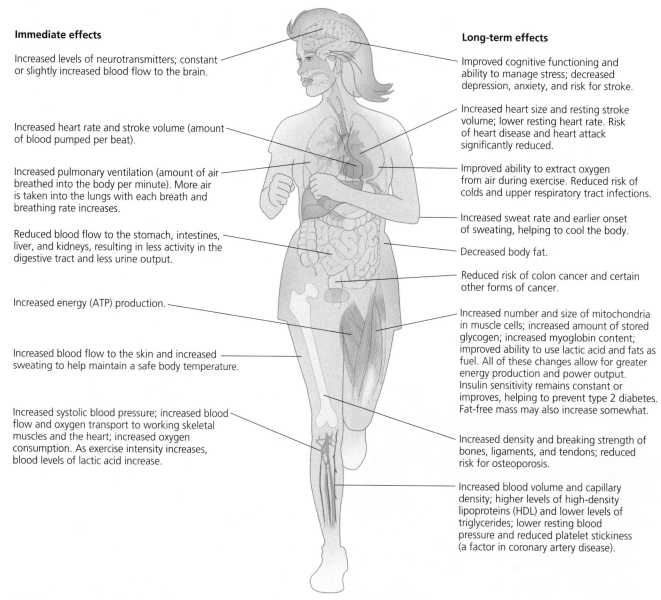

Immediate effects

Increased levels of neurotransmitters; constant or slightly increased blood flow to the brain.

Increased heart rate and stroke volume (amount of blood pumped per beat).

Increased pulmonary ventilation (amount of air breathed into the body per minute). More air is taken into the lungs with each breath and breathing rate increases.

Reduced blood flow to the stomach, intestines, liver, and kidneys, resulting in less activity in the digestive tract and less urine output.

Increased energy (ATP) production.

Increased blood flow to the skin and increased sweating to help maintain a safe body temperature.

Increased systolic blood pressure; increased blood flow and oxygen transport to working skeletal muscles and the heart; increased oxygen consumption. As exercise intensity increases, blood levels of lactic acid increase.

Long-term effects

Improved cognitive functioning and ability to manage stress; decreased depression, anxiety, and risk for stroke.

Increased heart size and resting stroke volume; lower resting heart rate. Risk of heart disease and heart attack significantly reduced.

Improved ability to extract oxygen from air during exercise. Reduced risk of colds and upper respiratory tract infections.

Increased sweat rate and earlier onset of sweating, helping to cool the body.

Decreased body fat.

Reduced risk of colon cancer and certain other forms of cancer.

Increased number and size of mitochondria in muscle cells; increased amount of stored glycogen; increased myoglobin content; improved ability to use lactic acid and fats as fuel. All of these changes allow for greater energy production and power output. Insulin sensitivity remains constant or improves, helping to prevent type 2 diabetes. Fat-free mass may also increase somewhat.

Increased density and breaking strength of bones, ligaments, and tendons; reduced risk for osteoporosis.

Increased blood volume and capillary density; higher levels of high-density lipoproteins (HDL) and lower levels of triglycerides; lower resting blood pressure and reduced platelet stickiness (a factor in coronary artery disease).

FIGURE 3.2 Immediate and long-term effects of regular cardiorespiratory endurance exercise.   When endurance exercise is performed regularly, short-term changes in the body develop into more permanent adaptations; these include improved ability to exercise, reduced risk of many chronic diseases, and improved psychological and emotional well-being.

Cardiorespiratory endurance exercise lowers your risk of CVD by doing the following:

- Promoting a healthy balance of fats in the blood. High concentrations of blood fats such as cholesterol and triglycerides are linked to CVD. Exercise raises levels of "good cholesterol" (high-density *lipoproteins*, or HDL) and may lower levels of "bad cholesterol" (low-density lipoproteins, or LDL).
- Reducing high blood pressure, which is a contributing factor to several kinds of CVD.
- Enhancing the function of the cells that line the arteries (endothelial cells).
- Reducing inflammation.
- Preventing obesity and type 2 diabetes, both of which contribute to CVD.

Details on various types of CVD, their associated risk factors, and lifestyle factors that can reduce your risk for developing CVD are discussed in Chapter 11.

CANCER   Although the findings are not conclusive, some studies have shown a relationship between increased physical activity and a reduction in a person's risk of cancer. Exercise reduces the risk of colon cancer in men and women[2] and there is promising data that it reduces the

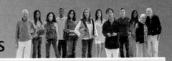

Benefits of Exercise for Older Adults

Research has shown that most aspects of physiological functioning peak when people are about 30 years old and then decline at a rate of about 0.5–1.0% a year. This decline in physical capacity is characterized by a decrease in maximal oxygen consumption, cardiac output, muscular strength, fat-free mass, joint mobility, and other factors. However, regular exercise can substantially alter the rate of decline in functional status, and it is associated with both longevity and improved quality of life.

Regular endurance exercise in older people can:

- Improve maximal oxygen consumption by up to 15–30%; the same degree of improvement seen in younger people. In fact, studies have shown that Masters athletes in their 70s have $\dot{V}O_{2max}$ values equivalent to those of sedentary 20-year-olds.

- Improve cardiorespiratory functioning, cellular metabolism, body composition, and psychological and emotional well-being.

- Improve balance, which can reduce the risk of injuries from falls.

- Reduce the risk of heart disease, cancer, diabetes, osteoporosis, and dementia.

Resistance training in older people can:

- Build strength and fat-free mass.

- Help to retain a level of independence.

- Boost spirits.

Flexibility training in older people can:

- Improve the range of motion in joints.

- Help to maintain functional independence.

Life expectancy in Canada has increased dramatically over the past century with Canadians enjoying an average of 69.5 healthy years. A lifetime of regular exercise is one of the best age-proofing strategies available; however, it's never too late to start. Even in people over 80, beginning an exercise program can improve physical functioning and quality of life. Most older adults are able to participate in a program that includes moderate walking and strengthening and stretching exercises, and modified programs can be created for people with chronic conditions and other special health concerns. The wellness benefits of exercise are available to people of all ages and levels of ability.

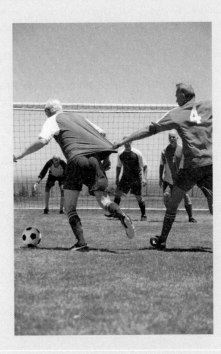

SOURCES: Brooks, G. A., et al. 2005. *Exercise Physiology: Human Bioenergetics and Its Applications,* 4th ed. New York: McGraw-Hill; and American College of Sports Medicine. 2001. *ACSM's Resource Manual for Guidelines for Exercise Testing and Prescription,* 4th ed. Philadelphia: Williams and Wilkins.

risk of cancer of the breast[3] and reproductive organs[4] in women. See Chapter 12 for more information on various types of cancer and the impact of exercise on our risk for suffering from cancer.

TYPE 2 DIABETES Regular exercise helps prevent the development of type 2 diabetes, the most common form of diabetes.[5] Exercise metabolizes (burns) excess sugar and makes cells more sensitive to the hormone insulin, which is involved in the regulation of blood sugar levels. Obesity is a key risk factor for diabetes, and exercise helps keep body fat at healthy levels. But even without fat loss, exercise improves control of blood sugar levels in many people with diabetes, and

physical activity is an important part of treatment. (See Chapter 6 for a more detailed discussion on diabetes and insulin resistance.)

OSTEOPOROSIS A special benefit of exercise, especially for women, is protection against osteoporosis, a disease that results in loss of bone density and poor bone strength. Weight-bearing exercise helps build bone during the teens and twenties. People with denser bones can better endure the bone loss that occurs with aging. With stronger bones and muscles and better balance, fit people are less likely to experience debilitating falls and bone fractures. (See Chapter 7 for more on osteoporosis.)

DIMENSIONS OF DIVERSITY

Why Is It Important to Combine Aerobic Exercise with Strength Training?

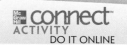

THE EVIDENCE FOR EXERCISE

For a variety of reasons, many people choose to focus on only one aspect of physical wellness or fitness. For example, many women concentrate on cardiorespiratory and flexibility exercises but ignore weight training for fear of developing bulky muscles. Many men, conversely, focus exclusively on resistance training in the hope of developing large, strong muscles. They often avoid cardio or flexibility workouts, fearing such exercises will result in loss of hard-earned muscle mass. While some exercise is better than none, it is best to include activities that develop all components of health-related fitness.

Emphasizing one aspect of fitness at the expense of others may be a special concern for weight trainers who don't do enough cardiorespiratory conditioning. Although exercise experts universally agree that resistance training is beneficial for a variety of reasons (as detailed in Chapter 4), it also has a downside.

A number of studies conducted around the world have tracked the impact of weight-training exercises on the cardiovascular system, to determine whether resistance training is helpful or harmful to the heart and blood vessels. These studies have shown that strength training poses short- and long-term risks to cardiovascular health and especially to arterial health. Aside from the risk of injury, lifting weights has been shown to have the following adverse effects on the cardiovascular system:

- Weight training promotes short-term stiffness of the blood vessels, which could promote hypertension (high blood pressure) over time and increase the load on the heart.

- Lifting weights (especially heavy weights) causes extreme short-term boosts in blood pressure; a Canadian study revealed that blood pressure can reach 480/350 mm Hg during heavy lifting. Over the long-term, sharp elevations in

blood pressure can damage arteries, even if each pressure increase lasts only a few seconds.

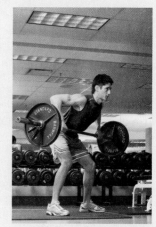

- Weight training places stress on the endothelial cells that line blood vessels. Because these cells secrete nitrous oxide (a chemical messenger involved in a variety of bodily functions), this stress can contribute to a wide range of negative effects, from erectile dysfunction to heart disease.

A variety of studies have shown that the best way to offset cardiovascular stress caused by strength training is to do cardiorespiratory endurance exercise (such as brisk walking or using an elliptical machine) immediately after a weight-training session. Ground-breaking Japanese research showed that following resistance training with aerobic exercise prevents the stiffening of blood vessels and its associated damage. In this 8-week study, participants did aerobics before lifting weights, after lifting weights, or not at all. The group that did aerobics after weight training saw the greatest positive impact on arterial health; participants who did aerobics before lifting weights did not see any improvement in the health of their blood vessels.

The bottom line of all this research? Resistance training and cardiorespiratory exercise are both good for you, if you do them in the right order. So, when you plan your workouts, be sure to do 15–60 minutes of aerobic exercise after each weight-training session.

SOURCES: Aagaard, P., and J. L. Andersen. 2010. Effects of strength training on endurance capacity in top-level endurance athletes. *Scandinavian Journal Medicine Science Sports.* 20(supplement 2): 39–47; Okamoto, T., M. Masuhara, and K. Ikuta. 2006. Effects of eccentric and concentric resistance training on arterial stiffness. *Journal of Human Hypertension* 20(5): 348–354; Okamoto, T., M. Masuhara, and K. Ikuta. 2007. Combined aerobic and resistance training and vascular function: Effect of aerobic exercise before and after resistance training. *Journal of Applied Physiology* 103(5): 1655–1661; and Physical Activity Guidelines Advisory Committee. 2008. *Physical Activity Guidelines Advisory Committee Report, 2008.* Washington, D.C.: U.S. Department of Health and Human Services.

DEATHS FROM ALL CAUSES   Physically fit people have a reduced risk of dying from all causes, with the greatest benefits found for people with the highest levels of fitness (see Figure 3.3 for the results of one recent study). Physical inactivity is a good predictor of premature death and is as important a risk factor as smoking, high blood pressure, obesity, and diabetes.

Better Control of Body Fat

Too much body fat is linked to a variety of health problems, including CVD, cancer, and type 2 diabetes. Healthy body composition can be difficult to achieve and maintain because a diet that contains all essential nutrients can be relatively high in calories, especially for someone who is sedentary. Excess calories are stored in the body as fat. Regular exercise increases daily calorie

expenditure so that a healthy diet is less likely to lead to weight gain. Endurance exercise burns calories directly and, if intense enough, continues to do so by raising resting metabolic rate for several hours following an exercise session. A higher metabolic rate means that it is easier for a person to maintain a healthy weight or to lose weight. Exercise alone cannot ensure a healthy body composition, however; as described in Chapters 6 through 8, you will lose more weight more rapidly and keep it off longer if you decrease your calorie intake as well as boost your calorie expenditure through exercise.

Improved Immune Function

Exercise can have either positive or negative effects on the immune system, the physiological processes that protect us from disease. Moderate endurance exercise boosts

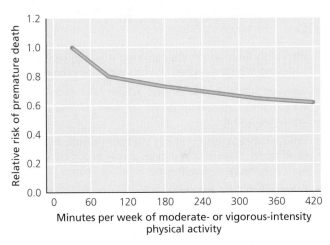

FIGURE 3.3 **Doing only 150 minutes of moderate-intensity physical activity per week provides significant health benefits.** As you exercise longer or more intensely, you reduce your risk of dying prematurely from a variety of causes.

SOURCE: Physical Activity Guidelines Advisory Committee. 2008. *Physical Activity Guidelines Advisory Committee Report, 2008.* Washington, D.C.: U. S. Department of Health and Human Services.

immune function, whereas excessive training (overtraining) depresses it. Physically fit people get fewer colds and upper respiratory tract infections than people who are not fit. Exercise affects immune function by influencing levels of specialized cells and chemicals involved in the immune response. In addition to regular moderate exercise, the immune system can be strengthened by eating a well-balanced diet, managing stress, and getting 7–8 hours of sleep every night.

Improved Psychological and Emotional Well-Being

Most people who participate in regular endurance exercise experience social, psychological, and emotional benefits. Performing physical activities provides proof of skill mastery and self-control, thus enhancing self-image. Recreational sports provide an opportunity to socialize, have fun, and strive to excel. Endurance exercise lessens anxiety, depression, stress, anger, and hostility, thereby improving mood and boosting cardiovascular health. Regular exercise also improves sleep. For more on the wellness benefits of regular endurance exercise, see the box "Exercise, Mood, and the Mind."

LO3 3.3 ASSESSING CARDIORESPIRATORY FITNESS

The body's ability to maintain a level of exertion (exercise) for an extended period of time is a direct reflection of cardiorespiratory fitness. It is determined by the body's ability to take up, distribute, and use oxygen during physical activity. As explained earlier, the best quantitative measure

of cardiorespiratory endurance is maximal oxygen consumption, expressed as $\dot{V}O_{2max}$ the amount of oxygen the body uses when a person reaches maximum ability to supply oxygen during exercise (measured in millilitres of oxygen used per minute for each kilogram of body weight). Maximal oxygen consumption can be measured precisely in an exercise physiology laboratory through analysis of the air a person inhales and exhales when exercising to a level of exhaustion (maximum intensity). This procedure can be expensive and time-consuming, making it impractical for the average person.

Choosing an Assessment Test

Fortunately, several simple assessment tests provide reasonably good estimates of maximal oxygen consumption (within ± 10–15% of the results of a laboratory test). Four commonly used assessments are the following:

- *The 1.6-km Walk Test.* The 1.6-km walk test estimates your level of cardiorespiratory fitness (maximal oxygen consumption) based on the amount of time it takes you to complete 1.6 kilometres of brisk walking and your exercise heart rate at the end of your walk. A fast time and a low heart rate indicate a high level of cardiorespiratory endurance.

- *The 3-minute Step Test.* The rate at which the pulse returns to normal after exercise is also a good measure of cardiorespiratory capacity; heart rate remains lower and recovers faster in people who are more physically fit. For the step test, you step continually at a steady rate and then monitor your heart rate during recovery.

- *The 2.4-km Run-Walk Test.* Oxygen consumption increases with speed in distance running, so a fast time on this test indicates high maximal oxygen consumption.

- *Leger's 20-metre Shuttle Run.* Capacity to efficiently use oxygen over time will be reflected in those who reach higher stages of this test. Those who reach higher stages are considered to be more physically fit individuals.

- *Enhanced creativity and intellectual functioning.* In studies of university and college students, physically active students score higher on tests of creativity than sedentary students. Exercise improves alertness and memory in the short term, and over time, exercise helps maintain reaction time, short-term memory, and nonverbal reasoning skills and enhances brain metabolism.

- *Improved work productivity.* Workers' quality of work, time-management abilities, and mental and interpersonal performance have been found to be better on days they exercise.

- *Increased opportunities for social interaction.* Exercise provides many opportunities for positive interaction with others.

Exercise, Mood, and the Mind

Although much of the discussion of the benefits of exercise focuses on improvements to physical wellness, many people discover that the best reason to become and stay active is the boost that regular exercise provides to the nonphysical dimensions of wellness. The following are just some of the effects of regular physical activity.

- *Reduced anxiety.* Exercise reduces symptoms of anxiety such as worry and self-doubt both in people who are anxious most of the time (trait anxiety) and in people who become anxious in response to a particular experience (state anxiety). Exercise is associated with a lower risk for panic attacks, generalized anxiety disorder, and social anxiety disorder.

- *Reduced depression and improved mood.* Exercise relieves feelings of sadness and hopelessness and can be as effective as psychotherapy in treating mild-to-moderate cases of depression. Exercise improves mood and increases feelings of well-being in both depressed and non-depressed people.

- *Improved sleep.* Regular physical activity helps people fall asleep more easily; it also improves the quality of sleep, making it more restful.

- *Reduced stress.* Exercise reduces the body's overall response to all forms of stressors and helps people deal more effectively with the stress they do experience (see Chapter 10).

- *Enhanced self-esteem, self-confidence, and self-efficacy.* Exercise can boost self-esteem and self-confidence by providing opportunities for people to succeed and excel; it also improves body image (see Chapters 6 and 8). Sticking with an exercise program increases people's belief in their ability to be active, thereby boosting self-efficacy.

How does exercise cause all these positive changes? A variety of mechanisms have been proposed. Physical activity stimulates the thought and emotion centres of the brain, producing improvements in mood and cognitive functioning. It increases alpha brain-wave activity, which is associated with a highly relaxed state. Exercise stimulates the release of chemicals such as endorphins, which may suppress fatigue, decrease pain, and produce euphoria; and phenylethylamine, which may boost energy, mood, and attention. Exercise decreases the secretion of hormones triggered by emotional stress and alters the levels of many other neurotransmitters, including serotonin, a brain chemical linked to mood.

Exercise also provides a distraction from stressful stimuli and an emotional outlet for feelings of stress, hostility, and aggression.

Lab 3.1 provides detailed instructions for each of these tests. An additional assessment, the 12-minute swim test, is also provided. To assess yourself, choose one among these methods based on your access to equipment, your current physical condition, and your own preference. Don't take any of these tests without checking with your physician if you are ill or have any of the risk factors for exercise discussed in Chapter 2 and Lab 2.1. Table 3.3 lists the fitness prerequisites and cautions recommended for each test.

Additional assessments for cardiorespiratory fitness include cycle ergometer and swimming tests and a distance test for people who use wheelchairs.

Monitoring Your Heart Rate

Each time your heart beats, it pumps blood into your arteries; this surge of blood causes a pulse that you can feel by holding your fingers against an artery. Counting your pulse to determine your exercise heart rate is a key part of most assessment tests for maximal oxygen consumption. Heart rate can also be used to monitor exercise

---

TABLE 3.3	Fitness Prerequisites and Cautions for the Cardiorespiratory Endurance Assessment Tests
Test	**Fitness Prerequisites/Cautions**
1.6-km walk test	Recommended for anyone who meets the criteria for safe exercise. Can be used by individuals who cannot perform other tests because of low fitness level or injury.
3-minute step test	If you suffer from joint problems in your ankles, knees, or hips or you are significantly overweight, check with your physician before taking this test. People with balance problems or for whom a fall would be particularly dangerous, including older adults and pregnant women, should use special caution or avoid this test.
2.4-km run-walk test	Recommended for people who are healthy and at least moderately active. If you have been sedentary, you should participate in a 4- to 8-week walk-run program before taking the test. Don't take this test in extremely hot or cold weather if you aren't used to exercising under those conditions.
Leger's 20-metre shuttle run	Recommended for people who are healthy and at least moderately active. If you have been sedentary or suffer from musculoskeletal problems, you should not take the test.

Note: The conditions for exercise safety given in Chapter 2 apply to all fitness assessment tests. If you answered yes to any question on the PAR-Q in Lab 2.1, see your physician before taking any assessment test. If you experience any unusual symptoms while taking a test, stop exercising and discuss your condition with your instructor.

intensity during a workout. (Intensity is described in more detail in the next section.)

The two most common sites for monitoring heart rate are the carotid artery in the neck and the radial artery in the wrist (See Figure 3.4). To take your pulse, press your index and middle fingers gently on the correct site. You may have to shift position several times to find the best place to feel your pulse. Do not use your thumb to check your pulse; it has a pulse of its own that can confuse your count. Be careful not to push too hard, particularly when taking your pulse in the carotid artery (strong pressure on this artery may cause a reflex that slows the heart rate).

Heart rates are usually assessed in beats per minute (bpm). But counting your pulse for an entire minute isn't practical when you're exercising. And because heart rate slows rapidly when you stop exercising, it can give inaccurate results. It's best to do a shorter count—10 seconds—and then multiply the result by 6 to get your heart rate in beats per minute. (You can also use a heart rate monitor to check your pulse. See the box "Heart Rate Monitors and GPS Devices" for more information.)

Interpreting Your Score

Once you've completed one or more of the assessment tests, use the table under "Rating Your Cardiovascular Fitness" at the end of Lab 3.1 to determine your current level of cardiorespiratory fitness. As you interpret your score, remember that field tests of cardiorespiratory fitness are not precise scientific measurements and do have a 10–15% margin of error.

You can use the assessment tests to monitor the progress of your fitness program by retesting yourself from time to time. Always compare scores for the *same* test: Your scores on different tests may vary considerably because of differences in skill and motivation and weaknesses in the tests themselves.

3.4 DEVELOPING A CARDIORESPIRATORY ENDURANCE PROGRAM

Cardiorespiratory endurance exercises are best for developing the type of fitness associated with good health, so they should serve as the focus of your exercise program. To create a successful endurance exercise program, follow these guidelines:

- Set realistic goals.
- Set your starting frequency, intensity, and duration of exercise at appropriate levels.
- Choose suitable activities.
- Warm up and cool down.
- Adjust your program as your fitness improves.

Setting Goals

You can use the results of cardiorespiratory fitness assessment tests to set a specific oxygen consumption goal for your cardiorespiratory endurance program. Your goal should be high enough to ensure a healthy cardiorespiratory system, but not so high that it will be impossible to achieve. Scores in the fair and good ranges for maximal

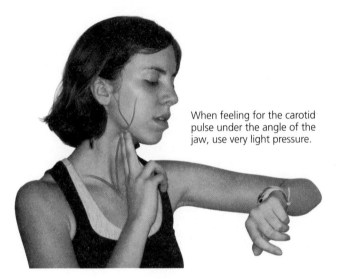

When feeling for the carotid pulse under the angle of the jaw, use very light pressure.

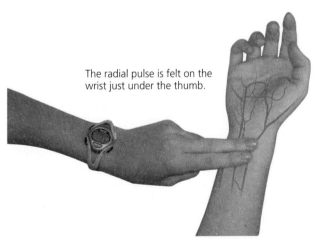

The radial pulse is felt on the wrist just under the thumb.

FIGURE 3.4 Checking your pulse. A pulse count can be used to determine exercise heart rate. The pulse can be taken at the carotid artery in the neck (top) or at the radial artery in the wrist (bottom).

Heart Rate Monitors and GPS Devices

A heart rate monitor is an electronic device that checks the user's pulse, either continuously or on demand. These devices make it easy to monitor your heart rate before, during, and after exercise. Some include global positioning system (GPS) receivers that help you track the distance you walk, run, or bike.

Wearable Monitors

Most consumer-grade monitors have two pieces—a strap that wraps around the user's chest and a wrist strap. The chest strap contains one or more small electrodes, which detect changes in the heart's electrical voltage. A transmitter in the chest strap sends this data to a receiver in the wrist strap. A small computer in the wrist strap calculates the wearer's heart rate and displays it on a small screen.

In a few low-cost monitors, the chest and wrist straps are connected together by a wire, but the most popular monitors use wireless technology to transmit data between the straps. In advanced wireless monitors, data is encoded so it cannot be read by any other monitors that may be nearby, as is often the case in a crowded gym. A one-piece (or "strapless") heart rate monitor does not include a chest strap; the wrist-worn device contains sensors that detect a pulse in the wearer's hand.

Monitors in Gym Equipment

Many pieces of workout equipment—including newer-model treadmills, stationary bikes, and elliptical trainers—feature built-in heart rate monitors. The monitor is usually mounted into the device's handles. To check your heart rate at any time while working out, simply grip the handles in the appropriate place; within a few seconds, your current heart rate will appear on the device's console.

Other Features

Heart rate monitors can do more than just check your pulse. For example, most monitors can tell you the following kinds of information:

- Highest and lowest heart rate during a session
- Average heart rate

- Target heart range, based on your age, weight, and other factors
- Time spent within the target range
- Number of calories burned during a session

Some monitors can upload their data to a computer, so information can be stored and analyzed. The analytical software can help you track your progress over a period of time or a number of workouts. Monitors with GPS option can record the distance you have travelled during a workout or over an entire day.

Advantages

Heart rate monitors are useful if very close tracking of heart rate is important in your program. They offer several advantages:

- They are accurate, and they reduce the risk of mistakes when checking your own pulse. (Note, however, that chest-strap monitors are considered more accurate than strapless models. If you use a monitor built into gym equipment, its accuracy will depend on how well the device is maintained.)
- They are easy to use, although a sophisticated, multifunction monitor may take some time to master.
- They do the monitoring for you, so you don't have to worry about checking your own pulse.

When shopping for a heart rate or exercise GPS monitor, do your homework. Quality, reliability, and warranties vary. Ask personal trainers in your area for their recommendations, and look for product reviews in consumer magazines or online.

---

oxygen consumption suggest good fitness; scores in the excellent and superior ranges indicate a high standard of physical performance.

Through endurance training, an individual may be able to improve maximal oxygen consumption $\dot{V}O_{2max}$ by about 10–30%. The amount of improvement possible depends on age, health status, and initial fitness level; people who start at a very low fitness level can improve by a greater percentage than elite athletes because the latter are already at a much higher fitness level, a level that may approach their genetic physical limits. If you are tracking $\dot{V}O_{2max}$ using the field tests described in this chapter, you may be able to increase your score by more than 30% due to improvements in other physical factors,

such as muscle power, which can affect your performance on the tests.

Another physical factor you can track to monitor progress is resting heart rate—your heart rate at complete rest, measured in the morning before you get out of bed and move around. Resting heart rate may decrease by as much as 10–15 beats per minute in response to endurance training. Changes in resting heart rate may be noticeable after only about 4–6 weeks of training.

You may want to set other types of goals for your fitness program. For example, if you walk, jog, or cycle as part of your fitness program, you may want to set a time or distance goal—working up to walking up to 10 km in one session, completing a 5 km run in 28 minutes, or cycling a total of 50 km per week. A more modest goal might be to achieve Health Canada's minimum activity level of doing at least 150 minutes of moderate to vigorous activity per week. Although it's best to base your program on "SMART" goals, you may also want to set some more qualitative goals, such as becoming more energetic, sleeping better, and improving the fit of your clothes.

LO4 Applying the FITT Equation

As described in Chapter 2, you can use the acronym FITT to remember key parameters of your fitness program: Frequency, Intensity, Time (duration), and Type of activity.

FREQUENCY OF TRAINING Accumulating at least 150 minutes per week of moderate to vigorous physical activity is enough to promote health. Most experts recommend that people exercise 3 to 5 days per week to build cardiorespiratory endurance. Training more than 5 days per week can lead to injury and isn't necessary for the typical person on an exercise program designed to promote wellness. It is safe to do moderate-intensity activity such as walking and gardening every day. Training fewer than 3 days per week makes it difficult to improve your fitness (unless exercise intensity is very high) or to use exercise to lose weight. Remember, however, that some exercise is better than none.

INTENSITY OF TRAINING Intensity is the most important factor for increasing aerobic fitness. You must exercise intensely enough to stress your body so that fitness improves. Three methods of monitoring exercise intensity are described below; choose the method that works best for you. Be sure to make adjustments in your intensity levels for environmental or individual factors. For example, on a hot and humid day or on your first day back to your program after an illness, you should decrease your intensity level.

Target Heart Rate Zone One of the best ways to monitor the intensity of cardiorespiratory endurance exercise is to measure your heart rate. It isn't necessary to exercise at your maximum heart rate to improve maximal oxygen consumption. Fitness adaptations occur at lower heart rates with a much lower risk of injury.

According to the American College of Sports Medicine, your **target heart rate zone**—rates at which you should exercise to experience cardiorespiratory benefits—is between 65% and 90% of your maximum heart rate. To calculate your target heart rate zone, follow these steps:

1. Estimate your maximum heart rate (MHR) by subtracting your age from 220, or have it measured precisely by undergoing an exercise stress test in a doctor's office, hospital, or sports medicine lab. (Note: Using the formula to estimate maximum heart rate can be very inaccurate for some people such as

those on certain medications; but particularly older adults and young children. If your exercise heart rate seems inaccurate—that is, exercise within your target zone seems either too easy or too difficult—then use the perceived exertion method described in the next section or have your maximum heart rate measured precisely.)

2. Multiply your MHR by 65% and 90% to calculate your target heart rate zone. (Note: Very unfit people should use 55% of MHR for their training threshold.)

For example, a 19-year-old would calculate her target heart rate zone as follows:

MHR = 220 − 19 = 201
65% training intensity = 0.65 × 201 = 131 bpm
90% training intensity = 0.90 × 201 = 181 bpm

To gain fitness benefits, the young woman in our example would have to exercise at an intensity that raises her heart rate to between 131 and 181 bpm.

An alternative method for calculating target heart rate uses **heart rate reserve,** the difference between maximum heart rate and resting heart rate. Using this method, target heart rate is equal to resting heart rate plus between 50% (40% for very unfit people) and 85% of heart rate reserve. Although some people will obtain more accurate results using this more complex method, both methods provide reasonable estimates of an appropriate target heart rate zone. Formulas for both methods of calculating target heart rate are given in Lab 3.2.

If you have been sedentary, start by exercising at the lower end of your target heart rate range (65% of maximum heart rate or 50% of heart rate reserve) for at least 4–6 weeks. Fast and significant gains in maximal oxygen consumption can be made by exercising closer to the top of the range, but you may increase your risk of injury and overtraining. You *can* achieve significant health benefits by exercising at the bottom of your target range, so don't feel pressured into exercising at an unnecessarily intense level. If you exercise at a lower intensity, you can increase the duration or frequency of training to obtain as much benefit to your health, as long as you are above the 65% training threshold. For people with a very low initial level of fitness, a lower training intensity, 55–64% of maximum heart rate or 40–49% of heart rate reserve, may be sufficient to achieve improvements in maximal oxygen consumption, especially at the start of an exercise program. Intensities of 70–85% of maximum heart rate are appropriate for average individuals.

target heart rate zone   The range of heart rates that should be reached and maintained during cardiorespiratory endurance exercise to obtain training effects.

heart rate reserve   The difference between maximum heart rate and resting heart rate; used in one method for calculating target heart rate range.

TABLE 3.4 Target Heart Rate Range and 10-Second Counts

Age (years)	Target Heart Rate Range (bpm)*	10-Second Count (beats)*
20–24	127–180	21–30
25–29	124–176	20–29
30–34	121–171	20–28
35–39	118–167	19–27
40–44	114–162	19–27
45–49	111–158	18–26
50–54	108–153	18–25
55–59	105–149	17–24
60–64	101–144	16–24
65+	97–140	16–23

*Target heart rates lower than those shown here are appropriate for individuals with a very low initial level of fitness. Ranges are based on the following formula: Target heart rate = 0.65 to 0.90 of maximum heart rate, assuming maximum heart rate = 220 – age. The heart rate range values shown here correspond to RPE values of about 12–18.

By monitoring your heart rate, you will always know if you are working hard enough to improve, not hard enough, or too hard. To monitor your heart rate during exercise, count your pulse while you're still moving or immediately after you stop exercising. Count beats for 10 seconds, and then multiply that number by 6 to see if your heart rate is in your target zone. If the young woman in our example were aiming for 144 bpm, she would want a 10-second count of 24 beats. Another way to monitor your heart rate is to either wear a monitor on your body or use the heart rate monitors that are sometimes found on aerobic equipment. Table 3.4 above shows target heart rate ranges and 10-second counts based on the maximum heart rate formula.

Ratings of Perceived Exertion Another way to monitor intensity is to monitor your perceived level of exertion. Repeated pulse counting during exercise can become a nuisance if it interferes with the activity. As your exercise program progresses, you will probably become familiar with the amount of exertion required to raise your heart rate to target levels. In other words, you will know how you feel when you have exercised intensely enough. If this is the case, you can use the

scale of **ratings of perceived exertion (RPE)** shown in Figure 3.5 to monitor the intensity of your exercise session without checking your pulse.

To use the RPE scale, select a rating that corresponds to your subjective perception of how hard you are exercising when you are training in your target heart rate zone. If your target zone is about 135–155 bpm, exercise intensely enough to raise your heart rate to that level, and then associate a rating—for example, "somewhat hard" or "hard" (14 or 15)—with how hard you feel you are working. To reach and maintain intensity in future workouts, exercise hard enough to reach what you feel is the same level of exertion. You should periodically check your RPE against your target heart rate zone to make sure it's correct. A simple way to check is to add a '0' to your RPE and the resulting number should fall in your target heart rate zone. Research has shown RPE to be an accurate means of monitoring exercise intensity, and you may find it easier and more convenient than pulse counting.

Talk Test Another easy method of monitoring exercise exertion—in particular, to prevent overly intense exercise—is the talk test. Although your breathing rate will increase during cardiorespiratory endurance exercise, you should not work out so intensely that you cannot

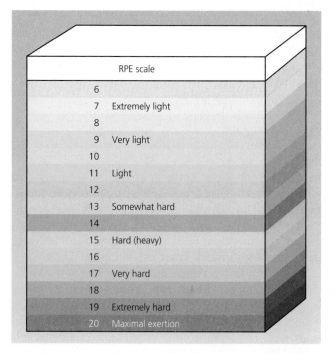

FIGURE 3.5 Ratings of perceived exertion (RPE). Experienced exercisers may use this subjective scale to estimate how near they are to their target heart rate zone. The scale was developed in the 1950s by Swedish exercise physiologist Gunnar Borg and is also known as the Borg scale.

SOURCE: *Psychology from Research to Practice* (1978), ed. H. L. Pick. Kluwer Academic/Plenum Publishing Corporation. Reprinted with permission of Springer Science and Business Media and the author.

speak comfortably. The talk test is an effective gauge of intensity for many types of activities.[6]

Table 3.5 provides a quick reference to each of the three methods of estimating exercise intensity discussed here.

TIME (DURATION) OF TRAINING A total duration of 30–60 minutes is recommended; exercise can take place in a single session or in multiple sessions lasting 10 or more minutes. The total duration of exercise depends on its intensity. To improve cardiorespiratory endurance during a low-to-moderate-intensity activity such as walking or slow swimming, you should exercise for 45–60 minutes. For high-intensity exercise performed at the top of your target heart rate zone, a duration of 20 minutes is sufficient.

Some studies have shown that 5–10 minutes of extremely intense exercise (greater than 90% of maximal oxygen consumption) improves cardiorespiratory endurance. However, training at this intensity, particularly during high-impact activities, increases the risk of injury, especially if no warm-up (or an inadequate warm-up) is performed. Also, because of the discomfort of high-intensity exercise, you are more likely to discontinue your exercise program. Longer-duration, low-to-moderate-intensity activities generally result in more gradual gains in maximal oxygen consumption. In planning your program, start with less vigorous activities and gradually increase intensity.

TYPE OF ACTIVITY Cardiorespiratory endurance exercises include activities that involve the rhythmic use of large muscle groups for an extended period of time, such as jogging, walking, cycling, aerobic dancing and other forms of group exercise, cross-country skiing, and swimming. Start-and-stop sports, such as tennis and racquetball, also qualify if you have enough skill to play continuously and intensely enough to raise your heart rate to target levels. Other important considerations are access to facilities, expense, equipment, and the time required to achieve an adequate skill level and workout.

TABLE 3.5 Estimating Exercise Intensity

Method	Moderate Intensity	Vigorous Intensity
Percent of maximum heart rate	55–69%	70–90%
Heart rate reserve	40–59%	60–85%
Rating of perceived exertion	12–13 (somewhat hard)	14–16 (hard)
Talk test	Speech with some difficulty	Speech limited to short phrases

Warming Up and Cooling Down

It's important to warm up before every session of cardiorespiratory endurance exercise and to cool down afterward. Because the body's muscles work better when their temperature is slightly above resting level, warming up enhances performance and decreases the chance of injury. It gives the body time to redirect blood to active muscles and the heart time to adapt to increased demands. Warming up also helps spread protective fluid throughout the joints, preventing injury to their surfaces.

A warm-up session should include low-intensity, whole-body movements similar to those in the activity that will follow, such as walking slowly before beginning a brisk walk, hitting forehands and backhands before a tennis match, and running a 6-minute kilometre before progressing to a 4-minute one. An active warm-up of 5–10 minutes is adequate for most types of exercise. However, warm-up time will depend on your level of fitness, experience, and individual preferences.

Do not use stretching as part of your preexercise warm-up. Warm-up stretches do not prevent injury and have little or no effect on postexercise muscle soreness. Stretching before exercise can increase the energy cost of your workout and adversely affect strength, power, balance, reaction time, and movement time. Stretching interferes with muscle and joint receptors that are vital to performance of sport and movement skills. For these reasons, it is best to stretch at the end of your workout, while your muscles are still warm and your joints are lubricated. (See Chapter 5 for a detailed discussion of stretching and flexibility exercises.)

Cooling down after exercise is important for returning the body to a non-exercising state. A cool down helps maintain blood flow to the heart and brain and redirects blood from working muscles to other areas of the body; it helps prevent a large drop in blood pressure, dizziness, and other potential cardiovascular complications. A cool-down, consisting of 5–10 minutes of reduced activity, should follow every workout to allow heart rate, breathing, and circulation to return to normal. Decrease the intensity of exercise gradually during your cool-down. For example, following a running workout, begin your cool-down by jogging at half speed for 30 seconds to a minute; then do several minutes of walking, reducing your speed slowly. A good rule of thumb is to cool down at least until your heart rate drops below 100 beats per minute.

The general pattern of a safe and successful workout for cardiorespiratory fitness is illustrated in Figure 3.6.

Building Cardiorespiratory Fitness

Building fitness is as much an art as a science. Your fitness improves when you overload your body. However, you must increase the intensity, frequency, and duration of exercise carefully to avoid injury and overtraining.

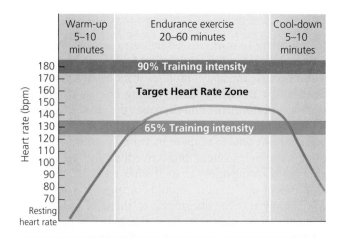

Warm-up 5–10 minutes | Endurance exercise 20–60 minutes | Cool-down 5–10 minutes

90% Training intensity

Target Heart Rate Zone

65% Training intensity

Frequency: 3–5 days per week

Intensity: 55/65–90% of maximum heart rate, 40/50–85% of heart rate reserve plus resting heart rate, or an RPE rating of about 12–18 (lower intensities—55–64% of maximum heart rate and 40–49% of heart rate reserve—are applicable to people who are quite unfit; for average individuals, intensities of 70–85% of maximum heart rate are appropriate)

Time (duration): 20–60 minutes (one session or multiple sessions lasting 10 or more minutes)

Type of activity: Cardiorespiratory endurance exercises, such as walking, jogging, biking, swimming, cross-country skiing, and rope skipping

FIGURE 3.6 The FITT principle for a cardiorespiratory endurance workout. Longer-duration exercise at lower intensities can often be as beneficial for promoting health as shorter-duration, high-intensity exercise.

TABLE 3.6 Sample Progression for an Endurance Program

Stage/Week	Frequency (days/week)	Intensity* (beats/minute)	Time (duration in minutes)
Initial stage			
1	3	120–135	20
2	3	120–135	25
3	4	135–150	25
4	4	135–150	30
Improvement stage			
5–7	3–4	150–160	25–30
8–10	3–4	150–160	30–35
11–13	3–4	155–170	30–35
14–16	4–5	155–170	30–35
17–20	4–5	155–170	35–40
21–24	4–5	160–180	35–40
Maintenance stage			
25+	3–5	160–180	30–45

*The target heart rates shown here are based on calculations for a healthy 20-year-old; the program progresses from an initial target heart rate of 50% to a maintenance range of 70–85% of maximum heart rate.

SOURCE: Adapted from American College of Sports Medicine. 2009. *ACSM's Guidelines for Exercise Testing and Prescription,* 8th ed. Philadelphia: Lippincott Williams and Wilkins. Reprinted with permission from the publisher.

For the initial phase of your program, which may last anywhere from 3 to 6 weeks, exercise at the low end of your target heart rate zone. Begin with a frequency of 3–4 days per week, and choose a duration appropriate for your fitness level: 12–15 minutes if you are very unfit, 20 minutes if you are sedentary but otherwise healthy, and 30–40 minutes if you are an experienced exerciser. Use this phase of your program to allow both your body and your schedule to adjust to your new exercise routine. Once you can exercise at the upper levels of frequency (4–5 days per week) and duration (30–40 minutes) without excessive fatigue or muscle soreness, you are ready to progress.

The next phase of your program is the improvement phase, lasting from 4 to 6 months. During this phase, slowly and gradually increase the amount of overload until you reach your target level of fitness (see the sample training progression in Table 3.6). Take care not to increase overload too quickly. It is usually best to avoid increasing intensity and duration during the same session or all three training variables in one week. Increasing duration in increments of 5–10 minutes every 2–3 weeks is usually appropriate. Signs of a too rapid progression in overload include muscles aches and pains, lack of usual interest in exercise, extreme fatigue, and inability to complete a workout. Keep an exercise log or training diary to help monitor your workouts and progress.

Maintaining Cardiorespiratory Fitness

You will not improve your fitness indefinitely. The more fit you become, the harder you have to work to improve (see the box "Interval Training: Pros and Cons"). There are limits to the level of fitness you can achieve, and if you increase intensity and duration indefinitely, you are likely to become injured or overtrained. After a progression phase of 4–6 months, you may reach your goal of an acceptable level of fitness. You can then maintain fitness by continuing to exercise at the same intensity at least 3 nonconsecutive days every week. If you stop exercising, you lose your gains in fitness fairly rapidly. If you take time off for any reason, start your program again at a lower level and rebuild your fitness in a slow and systematic way.

When you reach the maintenance phase, you may want to set new goals for your program and make some adjustments to maintain your motivation. Adding variety to your program can be a helpful strategy. Engaging in multiple types of endurance activities, an approach

Many people who practise formal exercise programs do less activity during the rest of the day, which partially defeats the purpose of the exercise program. Below are some ideas for becoming more active during the day. Check which one you can work into your lifestyle:

1. **Exercise before dinner:** Pre-meal exercise decreases appetite and promotes a feeling of fullness.

2. **Enter a charity walk-a-thon:** Many charities make money by getting people to sign up as sponsors in walk-a-thons and fun runs. These events help charities and make you look better in a bikini.

3. **Do errands by bike or on foot:** You are not chained to your car. Buy a grocery cart and walk to the store. Carts are small, so you won't buy as much food and will increase fitness at the same time.

4. **Take the dog for a walk:** Do your dog and yourself a favour and go for a walk together.

5. **Hit softballs or baseballs at the batting cage:** Hitting balls is a great way to get ready for springtime softball games and is a terrific total body exercise.

6. **Hit a bucket of balls at the golf course:** Many people think golf is a less-active sport. Hit a couple of hundred balls at the driving range and see how you feel the next day. This is a great way to burn calories and improve your game.

7. **Do aerobics 30 to 90 minutes a day:** People who walk only 30 minutes, 5 times per week will lose an average of 5 pounds in 6 to 12 months—without dieting, watching what they eat, or exercising intensely.

8. **Do calisthenics first thing in the morning:** Calisthenics are resistive exercises that use body weight as resistance. These are excellent for a person who wants to develop muscle strength but is unwilling to join a health club or devote too much time to the activity. Examples include push-ups, squats, curl-ups, chair dips, crunches, and jumping jacks.

9. **Exercise in the housework gym:** A vacuum cleaner is actually a lunge machine. Use a little creativity and you can turn simple household chores into a weight and aerobics workout. Try wearing a weighted vest while you sweep or mop the floor. Don't walk up the stairs— run. Jog in place as you wash the dishes. Stretch while putting away the dishes.

10. **Active shopping:** Go on a window-shopping hike. Walk through the mall and check out every single shop. If you live in a small town, check out each store twice. If you live near the West Edmonton Mall, cover the stores in four days.

11. **Trim the hedge:** Go to the hardware store and purchase hand hedge trimmers. This garden chore burns calories and builds chest, shoulder, leg, and core muscles.

12. **Sweep the walkway:** Try interval sweeping: Pick a 10-m strip of cement and sweep as fast and as hard as you can. Also, try lunge sweeping: Do a lunge every time you sweep the broom—first your left leg, then your right.

By themselves, few of these methods will make you physically fit. But combining two or three of these techniques gives you powerful tools that will help you build fitness and keep the fat off.

---

known as **cross-training**, can help boost enjoyment and prevent some types of injuries. For example, someone who has been jogging 5 days a week may change her program so that she jogs 3 days a week, plays tennis 1 day a week, and goes for a bike ride 1 day a week.

LO5 3.5 EXERCISE SAFETY AND INJURY PREVENTION

Exercising safely and preventing injuries are two important challenges for people who engage in cardiorespiratory endurance exercise. This section provides basic safety guidelines that can be applied to a variety of fitness activities. Chapters 4 and 5 include additional advice specific to strength training and flexibility training.

Hot Weather and Heat Stress

Human beings require a relatively constant body temperature to survive. A change of just a few degrees in body temperature can quickly lead to distress and even death.

If you lose too much water or if your body temperature gets too high, you may suffer from heat stress. Problems associated with heat stress include dehydration, heat cramps, heat exhaustion, and heatstroke.

In a high-temperature environment, exercise safety depends on the body's ability to dissipate heat and maintain blood flow to active muscles. The body releases heat from exercise through the evaporation of sweat. This process cools the skin and the blood circulating near the body's surface. Sweating is an efficient process as long as the air is relatively dry. As humidity increases, however, the sweating mechanism becomes less efficient because extra moisture in the air inhibits the evaporation of sweat from the skin. This is why it takes longer to cool down in humid weather than in dry weather.

cross-training   Alternating two or more activities to improve a single component of fitness.

TERMS

Interval Training: Pros and Cons

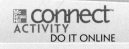
Few exercise techniques are more effective at improving fitness rapidly than *high-intensity interval training (HIT)*—a series of very brief, high-intensity exercise sessions interspersed with short rest periods. The four components of interval training are distance, repetition, intensity, and rest, defined as follows:

- *Distance* refers to either the distance or the time of the exercise interval.

- *Repetition* is the number of times the exercise is repeated.

- *Intensity* is the speed at which the exercise is performed.

- *Rest* is the time spent recovering between exercises.

Canadian researchers found that 6 sessions of high-intensity interval training on a stationary bike increased muscle oxidative capacity by almost 50%, muscle glycogen by 20%, and cycle endurance capacity by 100%. The subjects made these amazing improvements by exercising only 15 minutes in 2 weeks. Each workout consisted of 4 to 7 repetitions of high-intensity exercise (each repetition consisted of 30 seconds at near maximum effort) on a stationary bike. A follow-up study in moderately active women using the same training method showed that interval training increased the entire body's capacity for burning fat during exercise. These studies (and more than 20 others) showed the value of high-intensity training for building aerobic capacity and endurance.

You can use interval training in your favourite aerobic exercises, including ground or treadmill running, stair climbing, elliptical training, swimming, or cycling. In fact, the type of exercise you select is not important as long as you exercise at a high intensity. HIT training can even be used to help develop sports skills. For example, a runner might do 4 to 8 repetitions of 200-metre sprints at near-maximum effort. A tennis player might practise volleys against a wall as fast as possible for 4 to 8 repetitions lasting 30 seconds each. A swimmer might

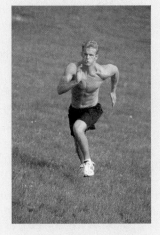

swim 4 to 8 repetitions of 50 metres at 100% effort. It is important to rest from 3 to 5 minutes between repetitions, regardless of the type of exercise being performed.

If you add HIT to your exercise program, do not practise interval training more than 3 days per week. Intervals are exhausting and easily lead to injury. Let your body tell you how many days you can tolerate. If you become overly tired after doing interval training 3 days per week, cut back to 2 days. If you feel good, try increasing the intensity or volume of intervals (but not the number of days per week) and see what happens. As with any kind of exercise program, begin HIT training slowly and progress conservatively. Although the Canadian studies showed that HIT training produced substantial fitness improvements by themselves, it is best to integrate HIT into your total exercise program. You should not be so tired from doing intervals that you cannot function during the rest of the day or perform other parts of your regular exercise program.

One additional form of training that will aid in improving cardiorespiratory fitness once you have developed a strong base is **Fartlek training.** This method introduces periods of more intense training, e.g., sprint training or hills, into your cardiorespiratory routine. It may be incorporated into a longer, less intense cardiorespiratory workout by simply using environmental conditions such as hills or stairs. In addition to accelerating your cardiorespiratory fitness level, this method also works to add variety to your training routine.

You can avoid significant heat stress by staying fit, avoiding overly intense or prolonged exercise for which you are not prepared, drinking adequate fluids before and during exercise, and wearing clothes that allow heat to dissipate.

DEHYDRATION Your body needs water to carry out many chemical reactions and to regulate body temperature. Sweating during exercise depletes your body's water supply and can lead to **dehydration** if fluids aren't replaced. Although dehydration is most common in hot weather, it can occur even in comfortable temperatures if fluid intake is insufficient.

TERMS

Fartlek training   Incorporating relatively more intense training into a less intense training session. Use existing environmental conditions, i.e., hills and stairs, and plan the training session to include them on the running/ jogging route.

dehydration   Excessive loss of body fluid.

Dehydration increases body temperature and decreases sweat rate, plasma volume, cardiac output, maximal oxygen consumption, exercise capacity, muscular strength, and stores of liver glycogen. You may begin to feel thirsty when you have a fluid deficit of about 1% of total body weight.

Drinking fluids before and during exercise is important to prevent dehydration and enhance performance. Thirst receptors in the brain make you want to drink fluids, but during heavy or prolonged exercise or exercise in hot weather, thirst alone isn't a good indication of how much you need to drink. As a rule of thumb, drink at least 2 cups (475 ml) of fluid 2 hours before exercise, and then drink enough during exercise to match fluid loss in sweat. Drink at least 1 cup of fluid every 20–30 minutes during exercise, more in hot weather or if you sweat heavily. To determine if you're drinking enough fluid, weigh yourself before and after an exercise session—any weight loss is due to fluid loss that needs to be replaced.

Very rarely, athletes consume too much water and develop *hyponatremia,* a condition characterized by lung congestion, muscle weakness, and nervous system problems. Following the guidelines presented here can help prevent this condition.

Bring a water bottle when you exercise so you can replace your fluids when they're being depleted. For exercise sessions lasting less than 60–90 minutes, cool water is an excellent fluid replacement. For longer workouts, choose a sports drink that contains water and small amounts of electrolytes (sodium, potassium, and magnesium) and simple carbohydrates ("sugar," usually in the form of sucrose, glucose, lactate, or glucose polymers). Electrolytes, which are lost from the body in sweat, are important because they help regulate the balance of fluids in body cells and the bloodstream. The carbohydrates in typical sports drinks are rapidly digestible and can thus help maintain blood glucose levels. Choose a beverage with no more than 8 grams of simple carbohydrate per 100 millilitres. See Chapter 7 for more on diet and fluid recommendations for active people.

HEAT CRAMPS Involuntary cramping and spasms in the muscle groups used during exercise are sometimes called **heat cramps.** While depletion of sodium and potassium from the muscles is involved with the problem, the primary cause of cramps is muscle fatigue. Children are particularly susceptible to heat cramps, but the condition can also occur in adults, even those who are fit. The best treatment for heat cramps is a combination of gentle stretching, replacement of fluid and electrolytes, and rest.

HEAT EXHAUSTION Symptoms of **heat exhaustion** include the following:

- A rapid, weak pulse
- Low blood pressure
- Headache
- Faintness, weakness, dizziness
- Profuse sweating
- Pale face
- Psychological disorientation (in some cases)
- Normal or slightly elevated core body temperature

Heat exhaustion occurs when an insufficient amount of blood returns to the heart because so much of the body's blood volume is being directed to working muscles (for exercise) and to the skin (for cooling). Treatment for heat exhaustion includes resting in a cool area, removing excess clothing, applying cool or damp towels to the body, and drinking fluids. An affected individual should rest for the remainder of the day and drink plenty of fluids for the next 24 hours.

HEATSTROKE **Heatstroke** is a major medical emergency involving the failure of the brain's temperature regulatory centre. The body does not sweat enough, and body temperature rises dramatically to extremely dangerous levels. In addition to high body temperature, symptoms can include the following:

- Hot, flushed skin (dry or sweaty), red face
- Chills, shivering
- Very high or very low blood pressure
- Confusion, erratic behaviour
- Convulsions, loss of consciousness

A heatstroke victim should be cooled as rapidly as possible and immediately transported to a hospital. To lower body temperature, get out of the heat, remove excess clothing, drink cold fluids, and apply cool or damp towels to the body or immerse the body in cold water.

Cold Weather

In extremely cold conditions, problems can occur if a person's body temperature drops or if particular parts of the body are exposed. If the body's ability to warm itself through shivering or exercise can't keep pace with heat loss, the core body temperature begins to drop. This condition, known as **hypothermia**, depresses the central nervous system, resulting in sleepiness and a lower metabolic rate. As metabolic rate drops, body temperature declines even further, and coma and death can result.

Frostbite—the freezing of body tissues—is another potential danger of exercise in extremely cold conditions. Frostbite most commonly occurs in exposed body parts like earlobes, fingers, and the nose, and it can cause permanent circulatory damage. Hypothermia and frostbite both require immediate medical treatment.

To exercise safely in cold conditions, don't stay out in very cold temperatures for too long. Take both the temperature and the wind into account when planning your exercise session. Frostbite is possible within 30 minutes in calm conditions when the temperature is colder than −20°C or in windy conditions (50 km/h) if the temperature is below −12°C. **Wind chill** values that reflect both the temperature and the wind speed are available as part of a local weather forecast and from Environment Canada (http://www.weatheroffice.gc.ca/canada_e.html).

> **heat cramps**   Sudden muscle spasms and pain associated with intense exercise in hot weather.
>
> **heat exhaustion**   Heat illness resulting from exertion in hot weather.
>
> **heatstroke**   A severe and often fatal heat illness characterized by significantly elevated core body temperature.
>
> **hypothermia**   Low body temperature due to exposure to cold conditions.
>
> **frostbite**   Freezing of body tissues characterized by pallor, numbness, and a loss of cold sensation.
>
> **wind chill**   A measure of how cold it feels based on the rate of heat loss from exposed skin caused by cold and wind; the temperature that would have the same cooling effect on a person as a given combination of temperature and wind speed.

TERMS

Appropriate clothing provides insulation and helps trap warm air next to the skin. Dress in layers so you can remove them as you warm up and can put them back on if you get cold. A substantial amount of heat loss comes from the head and neck, so keep these areas covered. In subfreezing temperatures, protect the areas of your body most susceptible to frostbite—fingers, toes, ears, nose, and cheeks—with warm socks, mittens or gloves, and a cap, hood, or ski mask. Wear clothing that breathes and will wick moisture away from your skin to avoid being cooled or overheated by trapped perspiration. Many types of comfortable, lightweight clothing that provide good insulation are available. It's also important to warm up thoroughly and to drink plenty of fluids.

Poor Air Quality

Air pollution can decrease exercise performance and negatively affect health, particularly if you smoke or have respiratory problems such as asthma, bronchitis, or emphysema. The effects of smog are worse during exercise than at rest because air enters the lungs faster. Polluted air may also contain carbon monoxide, which displaces oxygen in the blood and reduces the amount of oxygen available to working muscles. In a 2007 study, the ACSM found that exercise in polluted air could decrease lung function to the same extent as heavy smoking. Symptoms of poor air quality include eye and throat irritations, difficulty breathing, and possibly headache and malaise.

Do not exercise outdoors during a smog alert or if air quality is very poor. If you have any type of cardiorespiratory difficulty, you should also avoid exertion outdoors when air quality is poor. You can avoid some smog and air pollution by exercising in indoor facilities, in parks, near water (riverbanks, lakeshores, and ocean beaches), or in residential areas with less traffic (areas with stop-and-go traffic will have lower air quality than areas where traffic moves quickly). Air quality is also usually better in the early morning and late evening, before and after the commute hours.

Exercise Injuries

Most injuries are annoying rather than serious or permanent. However, an injury that isn't cared for properly can escalate into a chronic problem, sometimes serious enough to permanently curtail the activity. It's important to learn how to deal with injuries so they don't derail your fitness program. Strategies for the care of common exercise injuries and discomforts appear in Table 3.7; some general guidelines are given below.

TABLE 3.7 Care of Common Exercise Injuries and Discomforts

Injury	Symptoms	Treatment
Blister	Accumulation of fluid in one spot under the skin	Don't pop or drain it unless it interferes too much with your daily activities. If it does pop, clean the area with antiseptic and cover with a bandage. Do not remove the skin covering the blister.
Bruise (contusion)	Pain, swelling, and discoloration	R-I-C-E: rest, ice, compression, elevation.
Fracture and/or dislocation	Pain, swelling, tenderness, loss of function, and deformity	Seek medical attention, immobilize the affected area, and apply cold.
Joint sprain	Pain, tenderness, swelling, discoloration, and loss of function	R-I-C-E; apply heat when swelling has disappeared. Stretch and strengthen affected area.
Muscle cramp	Painful, spasmodic muscle contractions	Gently stretch for 15–30 seconds at a time and/or massage the cramped area. Drink fluids and increase dietary salt intake if exercising in hot weather.
Muscle soreness or stiffness	Pain and tenderness in the affected muscle	Stretch the affected muscle gently; exercise at a low intensity; apply heat. Nonsteroidal anti-inflammatory drugs, such as ibuprofen, help some people.
Muscle strain	Pain, tenderness, swelling, and loss of strength in the affected muscle	R-I-C-E; apply heat when swelling has disappeared. Stretch and strengthen the affected area.
Plantar fasciitis	Pain and tenderness in the connective tissue on the bottom of your feet	Apply ice, take nonsteroidal anti-inflammatory drugs, and stretch. Wear night splints when sleeping.
Shin splint	Pain and tenderness on the front of the lower leg; sometimes also pain in the calf muscle	Rest; apply ice to the affected area several times a day and before exercise; wrap with tape for support. Stretch and strengthen muscles in the lower legs. Purchase good-quality footwear and run on soft surfaces.
Side stitch	Pain on the side of the abdomen	Stretch the arm on the affected side as high as possible; if that doesn't help, try bending forward while tightening the abdominal muscles.
Tendinitis	Pain, swelling, and tenderness of the affected area	R-I-C-E; apply heat when swelling has disappeared. Stretch and strengthen the affected area.

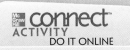
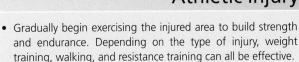

- Reduce the initial inflammation using the R-I-C-E principle (see text).

- After 36–48 hours, apply heat *if the swelling has disappeared completely*. Immerse the affected area in warm water or apply warm compresses, a hot water bottle, or a heating pad. As soon as it's comfortable, begin moving the affected joints slowly. If you feel pain, or if the injured area begins to swell again, reduce the amount of movement. Continue gently stretching and moving the affected area until you have regained normal range of motion.

- Gradually begin exercising the injured area to build strength and endurance. Depending on the type of injury, weight training, walking, and resistance training can all be effective.

- Gradually reintroduce the stress of an activity until you can return to full intensity. Don't progress too rapidly or you'll reinjure yourself. Before returning to full exercise participation, you should have a full range of motion in your joints, normal strength and balance among your muscles, normal coordinated patterns of movement (with no injury compensation movements, such as limping), and little or no pain.

TAKE CHARGE

WHEN TO CALL A PHYSICIAN   Some injuries require medical attention. Consult a physician for the following:

- Head and eye injuries
- Possible ligament injuries
- Broken bones
- Internal disorders: chest pain, fainting, elevated body temperature, intolerance to hot weather

Also seek medical attention for ostensibly minor injuries that do not get better within a reasonable amount of time. You may need to modify your exercise program for a few weeks to allow an injury to heal.

MANAGING MINOR EXERCISE INJURIES   For minor cuts and scrapes, stop the bleeding and clean the wound. Treat injuries to soft tissue (muscles and joints) with the R-I-C-E principle: Rest, Ice, Compression, and Elevation.

- *Rest:* Stop using the injured area as soon as you experience pain. Avoid any activity that causes pain.
- *Ice:* Apply ice to the injured area to reduce swelling and alleviate pain. Apply ice immediately for 10–20 minutes, and repeat every few hours until the swelling disappears. Let the injured part return to normal temperature between icings, and do not apply ice to one area for more than 20 minutes. An easy method for applying ice is to freeze water in a paper cup, peel some of the paper away, and rub the exposed ice on the injured area. If the injured area is large, you can surround it with several bags of crushed ice or ice cubes, or bags of frozen vegetables. Place a thin towel between the bag and your skin. If you use a cold gel pack, limit application time to 10 minutes. Apply ice regularly for 36–48 hours or until the swelling is gone; it may be necessary to apply ice for a week or more if swelling persists.
- *Compression:* Wrap the injured area firmly with an elastic or compression bandage between icings. If the area starts throbbing or begins to change colour, the bandage may be wrapped too tightly. Do not sleep with the wrap on.

- *Elevation:* Raise the injured area above heart level to decrease the blood supply and reduce swelling. Use pillows, books, or a low chair or stool to raise the injured area.

The day after the injury, some experts recommend also taking an over-the-counter medication such as aspirin, ibuprofen, or naproxen to decrease inflammation. To rehabilitate your body, follow the steps listed in the box "Rehabilitation Following a Minor Athletic Injury."

PREVENTING INJURIES   The best method for dealing with exercise injuries is to prevent them. If you choose activities for your program carefully and follow the training guidelines described here and in Chapter 2, you should be able to avoid most types of injuries. Important guidelines for preventing athletic injuries include the following:

- Train regularly and stay in condition.
- Gradually increase the intensity, duration, or frequency of your workouts.
- Avoid or minimize high-impact activities; alternate them with low-impact activities.
- Get proper rest between exercise sessions.
- Drink plenty of fluids.
- Warm up thoroughly before you exercise and cool down afterward.
- Achieve and maintain a normal range of motion in your joints.
- Use proper body mechanics when lifting objects or executing sports skills.
- Don't exercise when you are ill or overtrained.
- Use proper equipment, particularly shoes, and choose an appropriate exercise surface. If you exercise on a grass field, soft track, or wooden floor, you are less likely to be injured than on concrete or a hard track. (For information on athletic shoes, see the box "Choosing Exercise Footwear.")
- Don't return to your normal exercise program until any athletic injuries have healed. Restart your program at a lower intensity and gradually increase the amount of overload.

Choosing Exercise Footwear

Footwear is perhaps the most important item of equipment for almost any activity. Shoes protect and support your feet and improve your traction. When you jump or run, you place as much as six times more force on your feet than when you stand still. Shoes can help cushion against the stress that this additional force places on your lower legs, thereby preventing injuries. Some athletic shoes are also designed to help prevent ankle rollover, another common source of injury.

General Guidelines

When choosing athletic shoes, first consider the activity you've chosen for your exercise program. Shoes appropriate for different activities have very different characteristics.

Foot type is another important consideration. If your feet tend to roll inward excessively, you may need shoes with additional stability features on the inner side of the shoe to counteract this movement. If your feet tend to roll outward excessively, you may need highly flexible and cushioned shoes that promote foot motion. Most women will get a better fit if they choose shoes that are specifically designed for women's feet rather than downsized versions of men's shoes.

Successful Shopping

For successful shoe shopping, keep the following strategies in mind:

- Shop late in the day or, ideally, following a workout. Your foot size increases over the course of the day and after exercise.
- Wear socks like those you plan to wear during exercise.
- Try on both shoes and wear them around for 10 or more minutes. Try walking on a noncarpeted surface. Approximate the movements of your activity: walk, jog, run, jump, and so on.

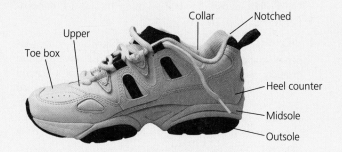

Toe box · Upper · Collar · Notched · Heel counter · Midsole · Outsole

- Check the fit and style carefully:
  - Is the toe box roomy enough? Your toes will spread out when your foot hits the ground or you push off. There should be at least one thumb's width of space from the longest toe to the end of the toe box.
  - Do the shoes have enough cushioning? Do your feet feel supported when you bounce up and down? Try bouncing on your toes and on your heels.
  - Do your heels fit snugly into the shoe? Do they stay put when you walk, or do they slide up?
  - Are the arches of your feet right on top of the shoes' arch supports?
  - Do the shoes feel stable when you twist and turn on the balls of your feet? Try twisting from side to side while standing on one foot.
  - Do you feel any pressure points?
  - If you exercise at dawn or dusk, choose shoes with reflective sections for added visibility and safety.
- Replace athletic shoes about every 3 months or 500–800 km of jogging or walking.

TIPS FOR TODAY AND THE FUTURE

Regular, moderate exercise, even in short bouts spread through the day, can build and maintain cardiorespiratory fitness.

RIGHT NOW YOU CAN

- Assess your cardiorespiratory fitness by using one of the methods discussed in this chapter and in Lab 3.1.
- Do a short bout of endurance exercise: 10–15 minutes of walking, jogging, cycling, or another endurance activity.
- If you have physical activity planned for later in the day, drink some fluids now to make sure you are fully hydrated for your workout.

- Consider the exercise equipment, including shoes, you currently have on hand. If you need new equipment, start gathering the information you'll need to get the best equipment you can afford.

IN THE FUTURE YOU CAN

- Graduate to a different, more challenging fitness assessment as your cardiorespiratory fitness improves.
- Incorporate different types of exercises into your cardiorespiratory endurance training to keep yourself challenged and motivated.

Do I need a special diet for my endurance exercise program?

No. For most people, a nutritionally balanced diet contains all the energy and nutrients needed to sustain an exercise program. Don't waste your money on unnecessary vitamins, minerals, and protein supplements. (Chapter 7 has information about putting together a healthy diet.)

How can I measure how far I walk or run?

The simplest and cheapest way to measure distance is with a pedometer, which counts your steps. A pedometer's accuracy depends on how precisely you measure your stride length; follow the instructions that come with your pedometer to set this measure. Although stride length varies among individuals, 2000 steps typically equals about 1.6 km, and 10 000 steps equals about 8 km. To track your distance and your progress using a pedometer, follow the guidelines in Lab 2.3. For advice on purchasing a pedometer that meets your needs, check consumer and fitness magazines and websites (http://www.webwalking.com).

Will interval training develop cardiorespiratory endurance (CRE)?

Interval training refers to short bouts of high intensity exercise alternated with short periods of rest or light activity.

An example of a workout based on interval training is a 400-metre run followed by a 200-metre walk, with the cycle repeated 2 to 10 times. You will develop CRE more quickly doing interval training. However, intervals are also more uncomfortable and increase your risk of injury and overtraining. Don't perform interval training more than 2–3 days per week.

How can I safely increase exercise intensity to build fitness?

For both athletes and nonathletes, it is extremely important to increase intensity very gradually and to rest between exercise sessions. If you train too hard and/or don't rest enough, you are more likely to be injured—and be discouraged from continuing with your fitness program. For endurance training, overload techniques such as interval training and wind sprints can help you build fitness quickly but also pose a greater risk of injury or overtraining. Start off with a few high intensity bouts of exercise and build up gradually. Don't practise interval training or wind sprints more than 2–3 days per week unless you have a high fitness level.

Increase intensity or duration by about 1–3% in a single workout; rest the following day and then do your typical workout. Repeat the more difficult workout after another day of rest. Adjust your progress according to how you feel. You can't increase fitness in a few days. Be patient—with gradual increases in intensity and plenty of rest

between workouts, you will be able to move to a higher level of fitness without injury.

If I plan to include both cardiorespiratory endurance training and strength training in a single workout, which should I do first?

It depends on your goals. If the primary goal of your fitness program is conditioning your cardiorespiratory system, then do your endurance workout first. If your fitness program is focused on large gains in strength and you plan to lift relatively heavy weights, then do your strength training workout first. You are likely to make the most rapid gains in fitness in whichever activity you engage in first, when you are fresh.

Is it all right to participate in cardiorespiratory endurance exercise while menstruating?

Yes. There is no evidence that exercise during menstruation is unhealthy or that it has negative effects on performance. If you have headaches, backaches, and abdominal pain during menstruation, you may not feel like exercising; for some women, exercise helps relieve these symptoms. Listen to your body, and exercise at whatever intensity is comfortable for you.

SUMMARY

- The cardiorespiratory system consists of the heart, blood vessels, and respiratory system; it picks up and transports oxygen, nutrients, and waste products.
- The body takes chemical energy from food and uses it to produce ATP and fuel cellular activities. ATP is stored in the body's cells as the basic form of energy.
- During exercise, the body supplies ATP and fuels cellular activities by combining three energy

systems: immediate, for short periods of energy; non-oxidative (anaerobic), for intense activity; and oxidative (aerobic), for prolonged activity. Which energy system predominates depends on the duration and intensity of the activity.

- Cardiorespiratory endurance exercise improves cardiorespiratory functioning and cellular metabolism; it reduces the risk of chronic disease such as heart disease, cancer, type 2 diabetes, obesity, and osteoporosis; and it improves immune function and psychological and emotional well-being.

- Cardiorespiratory fitness is measured by seeing how well the cardiorespiratory system transports and uses oxygen. The upper limit of this measure is called maximal oxygen consumption, or $\dot{V}O_{2max}$.

- $\dot{V}O_{2max}$ can be measured precisely in a laboratory, or it can be estimated reasonably well through less expensive assessment tests.

- To have a successful exercise program, set realistic goals; choose suitable activities; begin slowly; always warm up and cool down; and as fitness improves, exercise more often, longer, and/or harder.

- Intensity of training can be measured through target heart rate zone and ratings of perceived exertion.

FOR FURTHER EXPLORATION

Books

American College of Sports Medicine. 2003. *ACSM Fitness Book.* 3d ed. Champaign, Ill.: Human Kinetics. *Includes fitness assessment tests and advice on creating a complete fitness program.*

Barough, N. 2004. *Walking for Fitness.* New York: DK. *Provides advice on putting together a walking program that matches your fitness goals.*

Coffman, S. 2007. *Successful Programs for Fitness and Health Clubs.* Champaign, Ill.: Human Kinetics. *Presents more than 100 ready-to-use programs for use in fitness centers, group exercise studios, pools, gyms, and classrooms.*

Fenton, M. 2008. *The Complete Guide to Walking, New and Revised: For Health, Weight Loss, and Fitness.* Guilford, Conn.: Lyons Press. *Discusses walking as a fitness method and a way to avoid diseases such as diabetes.*

Heyward, V. 2002. *Advanced Fitness Assessment and Exercise Prescription.* 4th ed. Champaign, Ill.: Human Kinetics. *Provides information and ratings for a large number of fitness tests as well as guidelines for putting together a successful program.*

Marcus, B. H., and L. A. Forsyth. 2009. *Motivating People to be Physically Active,* 2nd ed. Champaign, Ill.: Human Kinetics. *Describes methods for helping people increase their level of physical activity.*

McArdle, W.D., Katch, F.L., & Katch, V.L. (2007). *Exercise Physiology: Energy, Nutrition, and Human Performance.* New York, NY: Lippincott Williams & Wilkins,. *Provides an extensive overview of the physiology involved in exercise.*

National Institute on Aging. 2003. *Fitness Over Fifty: An Exercise Guide from the National Institute on Aging.* Long Island City, N.Y.: Hatherleigh Press. *Includes information on a safe and effective fitness program.*

Nieman, D.C. 2007. *Exercise Testing and Prescription: A Health-Related Approach,* 6th ed. New York: McGraw-Hill. *A comprehensive discussion of the effect of exercise and exercise testing and prescription.*

Noakes, T. 2003. *Lore of Running.* 4th ed. Champaign, Ill.: Human Kinetics. *Provides detailed information on physiology, training, racing, and injury prevention.*

Organizations and Websites

Canadian Society for Exercise Physiology. Presents information on a variety of topics related to the study of exercise physiology, exercise biochemistry, fitness and health.
http://www.csep.ca

Cardiovascular Training Among Children. Online reference for devising a cardiovascular training program for children and adolescents.
http://www.nasmpro.com/nasmpro/library/showarticle.aspx?id=9514

Franklin Institute Science Museum/The Heart: An Online Exploration. An online museum exhibit with information on the structure and function of the heart, blood vessels, and respiratory system.
http://www.fi.edu/biosci/heart.html

Georgia State University: Exercise and Physical Fitness Page. Provides information about the benefits of exercise and how to get started on a fitness program.
http://www.gsu.edu/~ wwwfit

Health Canada. Look up the latest statistics on Canadian participation levels, information on risk factors and the cardiovascular system.
http://www.hc-sc.gc.ca/index-eng.php

Heart and Stroke Foundation of Canada. Provides information on the benefits of exercise for a healthy heart.
http://www.heartandstroke.ca

Industry Canada—Office of Consumer Affairs. Provides practical information for consumers interested in purchasing fitness equipment.
http://strategis.ic.gc.ca/

MedlinePlus: Exercise and Physical Fitness. Provides links to news and reliable information about fitness from government agencies and professional associations.
http://www.nlm.nih.gov/medlineplus/exercisephysicalfitness.html

Runner's World Online. Contains a wide variety of information about running, including tips for beginning runners, advice about training, and a shoe buyer's guide.
http://www.runnersworld.com

University of Florida: Keeping Fit. Provides useful information about fitness in a question-and-answer format; an extensive set of links is also provided.
http://www.hhp.ufl.edu/index.php

Women's Sports Foundation. Provides information and links about training and about many specific sports activities.
http://www.womenssportsfoundation.org/cgi-bin/iowa/

Yahoo/Recreation. Contains links to many sites with practical advice on many sports and activities.
http://dir.yahoo.com/recreation/sports

See also the listings in Chapters 2 and 11.

LAB 3.1 Assessing Your Current Level of Cardiorespiratory Endurance

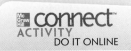

Before taking any of the cardiorespiratory endurance assessment tests, refer to the fitness prerequisites and cautions given in Table 3.3. Choose one of the following three tests presented in this lab:

- 1.6-km walk test
- 3-minute step test
- 2.4-km run-walk test
- Leger's 20-metre shuttle run

For best results, don't exercise strenuously or consume caffeine the day of the test, and don't smoke or eat a heavy meal within about 3 hours of the test.

The 1.6-km Walk Test

Equipment

1. A track or course that provides a measurement of 1.6 kilometres
2. A stopwatch, clock, or watch with a second hand
3. A weight scale

Preparation

Measure your body weight (in kilograms) before taking the test.

Body weight: _____ lbs

Instructions

1. Warm up before taking the test. Do some walking, easy jogging, or calisthenics and some stretching exercises.
2. Cover the 1.6-km course as quickly as possible. Walk at a pace that is brisk but comfortable. You must raise your heart rate above 120 beats per minute (bpm).
3. As soon as you complete the distance, note your time and take your pulse for 10 seconds.

    Walking time: _____ min _____ sec

    10-second pulse count: _____ beats
4. Cool down after the test by walking slowly for several minutes.

Determining Maximal Oxygen Consumption

1. Convert your 10-second pulse count into a value for exercise heart rate by multiplying it by 6.

    Exercise heart rate: _____ × 6 = _____ bpm
                    10-sec pulse count
2. Convert your walking time from minutes and seconds to a decimal figure. For example, a time of 14 minutes and 45 seconds would be 14 + (45/60), or 14.75 minutes.

    Walking time: _____ min + (_____ sec ÷ 60 sec/min) = _____ min
3. Insert values for your age, gender, weight, walking time, and exercise heart rate in the following equation, where

    W = your weight (in pounds)

    A = your age (in years)

    G = your gender (male = 1; female = 0)

    T = your time to complete the 1.6-km course (in minutes)

    H = your exercise heart rate (in beats per minute)

    $$\dot{V}O_{2max} = 132.853 - (0.0769 \times W) - (0.3877 \times A) + (6.315 \times G) - (3.2649 \times T) - (0.1565H)$$

For example, a 20-year-old, 190-pound male with a time of 14.75 minutes and an exercise heart rate of 152 bpm would calculate maximal oxygen consumption as follows:

$$\dot{V}O_{2max} = 132.853 - (0.0769 \times 190) - (0.3877 \times 20) + (6.315 \times 1) - (3.2649 \times 14.75) - (0.1565 \times 152)$$
$$= 45 \ ml/kg/min$$

$$\dot{V}O_{2max} = 132.853 - (0.0769 \times \underline{\hspace{2cm}}) - (0.3877 \times \underline{\hspace{2cm}}) + (6.315 \times \underline{\hspace{2cm}})$$
$$\text{weight (lb)} \qquad \text{age (years)} \qquad \text{Gender}$$
$$- (3.2649 \times \underline{\hspace{2cm}}) - (0.1565 \times \underline{\hspace{2cm}}) = \underline{\hspace{2cm}} ml/kg/min$$
$$\text{walking time (min)} \qquad \text{exercise heart rate (bpm)}$$

4. Copy this value for $\dot{V}O_{2max}$ into the appropriate place in the chart on the final page of this lab.

The 3-Minute Step Test

Equipment

1. A step, bench, or bleacher step that is 16.25 inches from ground level
2. A stopwatch, clock, or watch with a second hand
3. A metronome

Preparation

Practise stepping up onto and down from the step before you begin the test. Each step has four beats: up-up-down-down. Males should perform the test with the metronome set for a rate of 96 beats per minute, or 24 steps per minute. Females should set the metronome at 88 beats per minute, or 22 steps per minute.

Instructions

1. Warm up before taking the test. Do some walking, easy jogging, and stretching exercises.
2. Set the metronome at the proper rate. Your instructor or a partner can call out starting and stopping times; otherwise, have a clock or watch within easy viewing during the test.
3. Begin the test and continue to step at the correct pace for 3 minutes.
4. Stop after 3 minutes. Remain standing and count your pulse for the 15-second period from 5 to 20 seconds into recovery. 15-second pulse count: _____ beats.
5. Cool down after the test by walking slowly for several minutes.

Determining Maximal Oxygen Consumption

1. Convert your 15-second pulse count to a value for recovery heart rate by multiplying by 4.

   Recovery heart rate: _____ × 4 = _____ bpm

   15-sec pulse count

2. Insert your recovery heart rate in the equation below, where

   H = recovery heart rate (in beats per minute)

   Males: $\dot{V}O_{2max} = 111.33 - (0.42 \times H)$

   Females: $\dot{V}O_{2max} = 65.81 - (0.1847 \times H)$

   For example, a man with a recovery heart rate of 162 bpm would calculate maximal oxygen consumption as follows:

   $$\dot{V}O_{2max} = 111.33 - (0.42 \times 162) = 43 \ ml/kg/min$$

   Males: $\dot{V}O_{2max} = 111.33 - (0.42 \times \underline{\hspace{2cm}}) = \underline{\hspace{2cm}} ml/kg/min$

   recovery heart rate (bpm)

   Females: $\dot{V}O_{2max} = 65.81 - (0.1847 \times \underline{\hspace{2cm}}) = \underline{\hspace{2cm}} ml/kg/min$

   recovery heart rate (bpm)

3. Copy this value for $\dot{V}O_{2max}$ into the appropriate place in the chart on the final page of this lab.

The 2.4-km Run-Walk Test

Equipment

1. A running track or course that is flat and provides exact measurements of up to 2.4 kilometres
2. A stopwatch, clock, or watch with a second hand

Preparation

You may want to practise pacing yourself prior to taking the test to avoid going too fast at the start and becoming prematurely fatigued. Allow yourself a day or two to recover from your practice run before taking the test.

Instructions

1. Warm up before taking the test. Do some walking, easy jogging, and stretching exercises.
2. Try to cover the distance as fast as possible without overexerting yourself. If possible, monitor your own time, or have someone call out your time at various intervals of the test to determine whether your pace is correct.
3. Record the amount of time, in minutes and seconds, it takes you to complete the 2.4-km distance. Running-walking time: _____ min _____ sec.
4. Cool down after the test by walking or jogging slowly for about 5 minutes.

Determining Maximal Oxygen Consumption

1. Convert your running time from minutes and seconds to a decimal figure. For example, a time of 14 minutes and 25 seconds would be 14 + (25/60), or 14.4 minutes.
   Running-walking time: _____ min + (_____ sec ÷ 60 sec/min) = _____ min
2. Insert your running time in the equation below, where

   T = running time (in minutes)

   $\dot{V}O_{2max} = (483 \div T) + 3.5$

   For example, a person who completes 2.4 kilometres in 14.4 minutes would calculate maximal oxygen consumption as follows:

   $\dot{V}O_{2max} = (483 \div 14.4) + 3.5 = 37\ ml/kg/min$

   $\dot{V}O_{2max} = (483 \div \underline{\hspace{3cm}}) + 3.5 = \underline{\hspace{3cm}}\ \textbf{ml/kg/min}$
   run-walk time (min)
3. Copy this value for $\dot{V}O_{2max}$ into the appropriate place in the chart on the final page of this lab.

Leger's 20-Metre Shuttle Run

Equipment

1. Marking cones
2. 20-metre measuring tape
3. Pre-recorded audio-tape, tape recorder, recording sheets

Preparation

The goal of this test is to complete the highest number of stages of the run as possible. Each stage is represented by a number of repetitions of the same speed. The tape provides you with a sample stage so that you can become familiar with the protocol.

Instructions

1. Warm up before taking the test. Do some walking, easy jogging, and stretching exercises.
2. In this test you will run back and forth between two lines spaced 20 metres apart, according to the taped cadence. In each instance you will touch the line at each end and wait for the next signal to begin running towards the other end.
3. The starting speed of the test is 8.5 km/h and increases 0.5 km/h each minute of the test. You will stop the test when you can no longer keep pace with the taped cadence.
4. Use the formula below to predict your $\dot{V}O_{2max}$ score using the speed of your last completed stage as your maximal aerobic velocity (MAV).

   $\dot{V}O_{2max}$ score $= -24.4 + (6.0 \times MAV)$

Once you have calculated your score, place your value in the table below and find your rating on the following chart. Place that rating in the table.

Rating Your Cardiovascular Fitness

Record your $\dot{V}O_{2max}$ score(s) and the corresponding fitness rating from the table below.

Women		Very Poor	Poor	Fair	Good	Excellent	Superior
Age:	18–29	Below 31.6	31.6–35.4	35.5–39.4	39.5–43.9	44.0–50.1	Above 50.1
	30–39	Below 29.9	29.9–33.7	33.8–36.7	36.8–40.9	41.0–46.8	Above 46.8
	40–49	Below 28.0	28.0–31.5	31.6–35.0	35.1–38.8	38.9–45.1	Above 45.1
	50–59	Below 25.5	25.5–28.6	28.7–31.3	31.4–35.1	35.2–39.8	Above 39.8
	60–69	Below 23.7	23.7–26.5	26.6–29.0	29.1–32.2	32.3–36.8	Above 36.8
Men							
Age:	18–29	Below 38.1	38.1–42.1	42.2–45.6	45.7–51.0	51.1–56.1	Above 56.1
	30–39	Below 36.7	36.7–40.9	41.0–44.3	44.4–48.8	48.9–54.2	Above 54.2
	40–49	Below 34.6	34.6–38.3	38.4–42.3	42.4–46.7	46.8–52.8	Above 52.8
	50–59	Below 31.1	31.1–35.1	35.2–38.2	38.3–43.2	43.3–49.6	Above 49.6
	60–69	Below 27.4	27.4–31.3	31.4–34.9	35.0–39.4	39.5–46.0	Above 46.0

SOURCE: Ratings based on norms from the Cooper Institute for Aerobics Research, Dallas, Texas, *The Physical Fitness Specialist Manual,* Revised 2002. Used with permission.

	$\dot{V}O_{2max}$	Cardiovascular Fitness Rating
1.6-km walk test		
3-minute step test		
2.4-km run-walk test		
Leger's 20-metre shuttle run		

Using Your Results

How did you score? Are you surprised by your rating for cardiovascular fitness? Are you satisfied with your current rating?

If you're not satisfied, set a realistic goal for improvement:

Are you satisfied with your current level of cardiovascular fitness as evidenced in your daily life—your ability to walk, run, bicycle, climb stairs, do yardwork, engage in recreational activities?

If you're not satisfied, set some realistic goals for improvement, such as completing a 5K run or 40K bike ride:

What should you do next? Enter the results of this lab in the Preprogram Assessment column in Appendix C. If you've set goals for improvement, begin planning your cardiorespiratory endurance exercise program by completing the plan in Lab 3.2. After several weeks of your program, complete this lab again, and enter the results in the Postprogram Assessment column of Appendix C. How do the results compare? (Remember, it's best to compare $\dot{V}O_{2max}$ scores for the same test.)

SOURCES: Kline, G. M., et al. 1987. Estimation of $\dot{V}O_{2max}$ from a one-mile track walk, gender, age, and body weight. *Medicine and Science in Sports and Exercise* 19(3): 253–259: McArdle, W. D., F. I. Katch, and V. L. Katch. 2007. *Exercise Physiology: Energy, Nutrition, and Human Performance.* Philadelphia: Lea and Febiger, pp. 225–226; Brooks, G. A., and T. D. Fahey. 1987. *Fundamentals of Human Performance.* New York: Macmillan; and Leger, L. and Gadoury, C, 1989. Validity of the 20m shuttle run test with 1 minute stages to predict $\dot{V}O_{2max}$ in adults. *Canadian Journal of Sport Science* (14)1: 21–26.

Name _____   Section _____   Date _____

LAB 3.2   Developing an Exercise Program for Cardiorespiratory Endurance

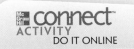

1. *Goals.* List the goals for your cardiorespiratory endurance exercise program. Your goals can be specific or general, short or long term. In the first section, include specific, measurable goals that you can use to track the progress of your fitness program. These goals might be things like raising your cardiorespiratory fitness rating from fair to good or swimming laps for 30 minutes without resting. In the second section, include long-term and more qualitative goals, such as improving self-confidence and reducing your risk for chronic disease.

Specific Goals: Current Status   Final Goal

_____   _____

_____   _____

_____   _____

Other goals: _____

_____

2. *Type of Activities.* Choose one or more endurance activities for your program. These can include any activity that uses large-muscle groups, can be maintained continuously, and is rhythmic and aerobic in nature. Examples include walking, jogging, cycling, group exercise such as aerobic dance, rowing, rope skipping, stair climbing, cross-country skiing, swimming, skating, and endurance game activities such as soccer and tennis. Choose activities that are both convenient and enjoyable. Fill in the activity names on the program plan.

3. *Frequency.* On the program plan, fill in how often you plan to participate in each activity; CSEP recommends participating in cardiorespiratory endurance exercise 3–5 days per week.

Program Plan									
Type of Activity	Frequency (check √)							*Intensity (bpm or RPE)*	*Time (min)*
	M	*Tu*	*W*	*Th*	*F*	*Sa*	*Su*		

4. *Intensity.* Determine your exercise intensity using one of the following methods, and enter it on the program plan. You should begin your program at a lower intensity and slowly increase intensity as your fitness improves, so select a range of intensities for your program.

  a. Target heart rate zone: Calculate target heart rate zone in beats per minute and then calculate the corresponding 10-second exercise count by dividing the total count by 6. For example, the 10-second exercise counts corresponding to a target heart rate zone of 122–180 bpm would be 20–30 beats.

  Maximum heart rate: $220 - \dfrac{}{\text{age (years)}} = \underline{\hspace{2cm}}$ bpm

  Maximum Heart Rate Method

  65% training intensity $= \dfrac{}{\text{maximum heart rate}}$ bpm $\times\ 0.65 = \underline{\hspace{2cm}}$ bpm

  90% training intensity $= \dfrac{}{\text{maximum heart rate}}$ bpm $\times\ 0.90 = \underline{\hspace{2cm}}$ bpm

  Target heart rate zone = _____ **to** _____ **bpm**   **10-second count =** _____ **to** _____

Heart Rate Reserve Method

Resting heart rate:_____ bpm (taken after 10 minutes of complete rest)

Heart rate reserve = $\underline{\hspace{2cm}}$ bpm − $\underline{\hspace{2cm}}$ bpm = _____ bpm
 maximum heart rate resting heart rate

50% training intensity = ($\underline{\hspace{2cm}}$ bpm × 0.50) + $\underline{\hspace{2cm}}$ bpm = _____ bpm
 heart rate reserve resting heart rate

85% training intensity = ($\underline{\hspace{2cm}}$ bpm × 0.85) + $\underline{\hspace{2cm}}$ bpm = _____ bpm
 heart rate reserve resting heart rate

Target heart rate zone = _____ to _____ bpm   **10-second count = _____ to _____**

    b. Ratings of perceived exertion (RPE): If you prefer, determine an RPE value that corresponds to your target heart rate range (see Table 3.4 and Figure 3.5).

5. *Time (Duration).* A total time of 30–60 minutes is recommended; your duration of exercise will vary with intensity. For developing cardiorespiratory endurance, higher-intensity activities can be performed for a shorter duration; lower intensities require a longer duration. Enter a duration (or a range of duration) on the program plan.

6. *Monitoring your program.* Complete a log like the one below to monitor your program and track your progress. Note the date on top, and fill in the intensity and time (duration) for each workout. If you prefer, you can also track other variables such as distance. For example, if your cardiorespiratory endurance program includes walking and swimming, you may want to track kilometres walked and metres swum in addition to the duration of each exercise session. For more extensive sets of logs, refer to the Daily Fitness and Nutrition Journal that accompanies your text.

Activity/Date													
1	Intensity												
	Time												
	Distance												
2	Intensity												
	Time												
	Distance												
3	Intensity												
	Time												
	Distance												
4	Intensity												
	Time												
	Distance												

7. *Making progress.* Follow the guidelines in the chapter and Table 3.5 to slowly increase the amount of overload in your program. Continue keeping a log, and periodically evaluate your progress.

Progress Check-Up: Week _____ of program

Goals: Original Status   *Current Status*

_____   _____

_____   _____

_____   _____

    List each activity in your program and describe how satisfied you are with the activity and with your overall progress. List any problems you've encountered or any unexpected costs or benefits of your fitness program so far.

CHAPTER 4

MUSCULAR STRENGTH AND ENDURANCE

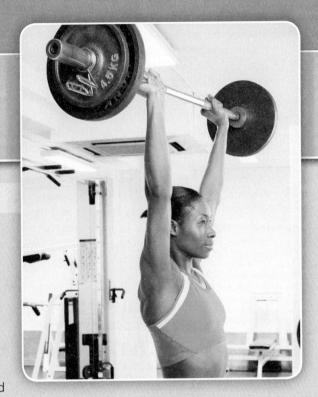

LEARNING OBJECTIVES

After reading this chapter, you should be able to

LO1 Describe the basic physiology of muscles and how strength training affects muscles

LO2 Identify the benefits of muscular strength and endurance and describe how they contribute to our wellness

LO3 Assess muscular strength and endurance

LO4 Apply the FITT principle to create a safe and successful strength training program

LO5 Describe the effects of supplements and drugs that are marketed to active people and athletes

LO6 Explain how to safely perform common strength training exercises using free weights and weight machines

TEST YOUR KNOWLEDGE

1. **For women, weight training typically results in which of the following?**

   a. bulky muscles
   b. significant increases in body weight
   c. improved body image

2. **To maximize strength gains, it is a good idea to hold your breath as you lift a weight.**

   True or false?

3. **Regular strength training is associated with which of the following benefits?**

   a. denser bones
   b. reduced risk of heart disease
   c. improved body composition
   d. fewer injuries
   e. improved metabolic health

ANSWERS

1. **C.** Because the vast majority of women have low levels of testosterone, they do not develop large muscles or gain significant amounts of weight in response to a moderate weight training program. Men have higher levels of testosterone, so they can build large muscles more easily.

2. **FALSE.** Holding one's breath while lifting weights, called the Valsalva manoeuvre, can significantly (and possibly dangerously) elevate blood pressure; it also reduces blood flow to the heart and may cause faintness. You should breathe smoothly and normally while weight training.

3. **All FIVE.** Regular strength training has many benefits for both men and women.

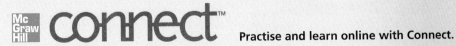

Practise and learn online with Connect.

Muscles make up more than 40% of your body mass. You depend on them for movement, and, because of their mass, they are the site of a large portion of the energy reactions (metabolism) that take place in your body. Strong, well-developed muscles help you perform daily activities with greater ease, protect you from injury, and enhance your well-being in other ways.

As described in Chapter 2, muscular strength is the ability to generate force during a maximal effort; muscular endurance is the ability to resist fatigue while holding or repeating a muscular contraction for a long time. This chapter explains the benefits of strength training (also called *resistance training* or *weight training*) and describes methods of assessing muscular strength and endurance. It then explains the basics of weight training and provides guidelines for setting up your own strength training program.

LO1 4.1 BASIC MUSCLE PHYSIOLOGY AND THE EFFECTS OF STRENGTH TRAINING

Muscles move the body and enable it to exert force because they move the skeleton. When a muscle contracts (shortens), it moves a bone by pulling on the tendon that attaches the muscle to the bone, as shown in Figure 4.1. When a muscle relaxes (lengthens), the tension placed on the tendon is released and the bone moves back to—or closer to—its starting position.

Muscle Fibres

Muscles consist of individual muscle cells, or **muscle fibres,** connected in bundles (Figure 4.1). A single muscle is made up of many bundles of muscle fibres and is covered by layers of connective tissue that hold the fibres together. Muscle fibres, in turn, are made up

of smaller units called **myofibrils.** Myofibrils are made up of a series of contractile units called *sarcomeres,* which are composed largely of actin and myosin molecules. Muscle cells contract when the myosin molecules glide across the actin molecules in a ratchetlike movement.

Strength training causes the size of individual muscle fibres to increase by increasing the number of myofibrils. Larger muscle fibres mean a larger and stronger muscle. The development of large muscle fibres is called **hypertrophy;** inactivity causes **atrophy,** the reversal of this process. In some species, muscles can increase in size through a separate process called **hyperplasia,** which involves an increase in the number of muscle fibres rather than the size of muscle fibres. In humans, hyperplasia is not thought to play a significant role in determining muscle size.

Muscle fibres are classified as slow-twitch, fast-twitch or intermediate fibres according to their strength, speed of contraction, and energy source.

- **Slow-twitch fibres (Type I fibres)** are relatively fatigue resistant, but they don't contract as rapidly or strongly as fast-twitch fibres. The principal energy system that fuels slow-twitch fibres is aerobic (oxidative) and given their resistance to fatigue, these fibres do not produce a great deal of force. Slow-twitch muscle fibres are typically reddish in colour.

- **Fast-twitch fibres (Type II fibres)** contract more rapidly and forcefully than slow-twitch fibres but fatigue more quickly. Although oxygen is important in the energy system that fuels fast-twitch fibres, they rely more on anaerobic (nonoxidative) metabolism than do slow-twitch fibres (see Chapter 3 for a discussion of energy systems). Fast-twitch muscle fibres are typically whitish in colour.

- **Intermediate fibres (Type IIb fibres)** contain a mixture of the qualities of both slow and fast-twitch fibres. These fibres are less quick to contract than fast-twitch but quicker than slow-twitch fibres. They also

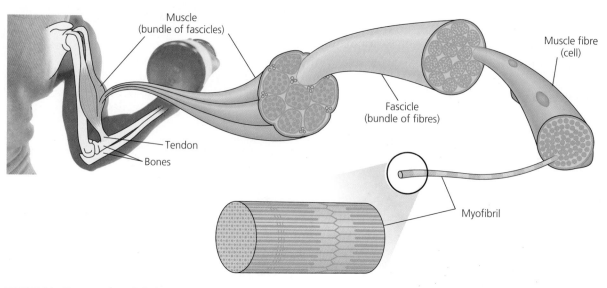

FIGURE 4.1 Components of skeletal muscle tissue.

TABLE 4.1 Physiological Changes and Benefits from Strength Training

Change	Benefits
Increased muscle mass* and strength	Increased muscular strength Improved body composition Higher rate of metabolism Toned, healthy-looking muscles Decreased risk of premature death Improved quality of life
Increased utilization of motor units during muscle contractions	Increased muscular strength and power
Improved coordination of motor units	Increased muscular strength and power
Increased strength of tendons, ligaments, and bones	Lower risk of injury to these tissues
Increased storage of fuel in muscles	Increased resistance to muscle fatigue
Increased size of fast-twitch muscle fibres (from a high-resistance program)	Increased muscular strength and power
Increased size of slow-twitch muscle fibres (from a high-repetition program)	Increased muscular endurance
Increased blood supply to muscles (from a high-repetition program) and improved blood vessel health	Increased delivery of oxygen and nutrients Increased elimination of wastes
Biochemical improvements (for example, increased sensitivity to insulin)	Enhanced metabolic health
Improved blood fat levels	Reduced risk of heart disease
Increased muscle endurance	Enhanced ability to exercise for long periods and maintain good body posture

*Due to genetic and hormonal differences, men will build more muscle mass than women, but both genders make about the same percent gains in strength through a good program.

endure longer than fast-twitch but not as long as slow-twitch fibres. Intermediate fibres rely on a combination of aneorobic and aerobic energy sources and produce less force than fast-twitch but more than slow-twitch.

Most muscle contains a mixture of the fibre types. The proportion of the types of fibres varies significantly among different muscles and different individuals, and that proportion is largely fixed at birth, although fibres can contract faster or slower following a period of training or a period of inactivity. The type of fibre that acts during a particular activity depends on the type of work required. Endurance activities like jogging tend to use slow-twitch fibres, whereas strength and **power** activities like sprinting use fast-twitch fibres. Strength training can increase the size and strength of both fast-twitch and slow-twitch fibres, although fast-twitch fibres are preferentially increased.

Motor Units

To exert force, the body recruits one or more motor units to contract. A **motor unit** is made up of a nerve connected to a number of muscle fibres. The number of muscle fibres in a motor unit varies from two to hundreds. When a motor nerve calls on its fibres to contract, all fibres contract to their full capacity. The number of motor units recruited depends on the amount of strength required: When a person picks up a small weight, he or she uses fewer motor units than when picking up a large weight.

Strength training improves the body's ability to recruit motor units—a phenomenon called **muscle learning**—which increases strength even before muscle size increases. The physiological changes and benefits that result from strength training are summarized in Table 4.1 above.

muscle fibre   A single muscle cell, usually classified according to strength, speed of contraction, and energy source.

myofibrils   Protein structures that make up muscle fibres.

hypertrophy   An increase in the size of a muscle fibre, usually stimulated by muscular overload.

atrophy   A decrease in the size of muscle cells.

hyperplasia   An increase in the number of muscle cells.

slow-twitch fibres   Red muscle fibres that are fatigue-resistant but have a slow contraction speed and a lower capacity for tension; usually recruited for endurance activities.

fast-twitch fibres   White muscle fibres that contract rapidly and forcefully but fatigue quickly; usually recruited for actions requiring strength and power.

intermediate fibres   A muscled fibre that responds somewhere in between the speed, endurance, and contractile force of slow- and fast-twitch fibres.

power   The ability to exert force rapidly.

motor unit   A motor nerve (one that initiates movement) connected to a number of muscle fibres.

muscle learning   The improvement in the body's ability to recruit motor units, brought about through strength training.

TERMS

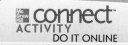
Does Muscular Strength Reduce the Risk of Premature Death?

Strength training can make you stronger, but can it also help you live longer? According to a growing body of evidence, the answer may be yes—especially for men.

A number of studies have associated greater muscular strength with lower rates of death from all causes, including cancer and cardiovascular disease. According to the results of a study released in 2008 (which followed nearly 9000 men over 18 years), the stronger a man is, the lower his risk of premature death from a variety of causes. This study gauged participants' strength through exercises such as bench and leg presses; other studies have measured strength using a handgrip test, with similar outcomes. The resulting data showed significant differences in death rates among the participants, with the strongest men having the lowest death rates. This effect was particularly important for older and overweight men.

When participants in the study died, researchers analyzed causes of death and correlated the numbers of dead and surviving participants with data about their muscular fitness, the amount of time they spent exercising, and other factors (such as metabolic data, cardiovascular health, smoking status, and age). The findings revealed that, compared to men with the greatest muscular strength, men with the lowest levels of muscular strength were

- 1.5 times more likely to die from all causes
- 1.6 times more likely to die from cardiovascular disease
- 1.25 times more likely to die from cancer

These correlations held across all age groups (ranging from age 20 to 82) and body mass indexes. They were particularly striking in older men (age 60 and older), who were more than four times more likely to die from cancer than similar-age men with greater muscular strength.

Similarly, a 2005 study of more than 3000 men demonstrated an inverse relationship between muscular strength and metabolic syndrome, a cluster of symptoms that includes high blood pressure, high blood glucose levels, high triglyceride levels, low HDL cholesterol levels, and abdominal obesity. Metabolic syndrome

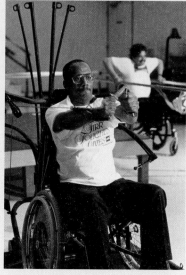

increases risk for diabetes, heart disease, and other illnesses. The results were true regardless of participants' age, weight, or waist circumference. The findings led researchers to suggest that weight training may be a valuable way for men to avoid metabolic syndrome. Protection against metabolic syndrome is also provided by cardiorespiratory fitness, according to a 2004 study of 8570 men, in which scientists measured each participant's level of muscular strength and cardiorespiratory fitness.

You don't have to be a power lifter or bodybuilder to enjoy the benefits of strength training. In the 2008 study, for example, participants were advised on basic fitness techniques and healthy lifestyle behaviours. Although participants were encouraged to incorporate weight training into their fitness routine, each man chose the type and amount of weight training he felt most comfortable doing. Many researchers believe that the basic minimum recommendation of doing weight training on 2 nonconsecutive days per week may be enough to lower the average male's risk of premature death, provided he is not obese and does not already have risk factors such as diabetes, hypertension, or preexisting cancer. At the same time, as noted in Chapter 3, strength training can have negative effects on the cardiovascular system in some men, at least temporarily, if not followed by aerobic exercise. To date, only small-scale studies have been performed on women, so more research is needed to see if the same conclusions apply to women.

SOURCES: Physical Activity Guidelines Advisory Committee. 2008. *Physical Activity Guidelines Advisory Committee Report, 2008.* Washington, D.C.: U.S. Department of Health and Human Services; Ruiz, J. R., et al. 2008. Association between muscular strength and mortality in men: Prospective cohort study. *BMJ* 337: a439; Ruiz, J. R., et al. 2009. Muscular strength and adiposity as predictors of adulthood cancer mortality in men. *Cancer Epidemiology, Biomarkers, and Prevention* 18: 1468; and Rantanen, T., et al. 2011. Midlife muscle strength and human longevity up to age 100 years: A 44-year prospective study among a decedent cohort. *Age* published online: DOI 10.1007/s11357-011-9256-y.

LO2 4.2 BENEFITS OF MUSCULAR STRENGTH AND ENDURANCE

Enhanced muscular strength and endurance can lead to improvements in the areas of performance, injury prevention, body composition, self-image, lifetime muscle and bone health, and chronic disease prevention. Most important, greater muscular strength and endurance reduce the risk of premature death. Stronger people have a lower death rate due to all causes, including cardiovascular disease and cancer (see the box "Does Muscular Strength Reduce the Risk of Premature Death?"). The link

between strength and death rate is independent of age, physical activity, smoking, alcohol intake, body composition, and family history of cardiovascular disease.

Improved Performance of Physical Activities

A person with a moderate-to-high level of muscular strength and endurance can perform everyday tasks—such as climbing stairs and carrying books or groceries—with ease. Increased strength can enhance your enjoyment of recreational sports by making it possible to achieve high levels of performance and to handle advanced techniques. Strength training also results in modest improvements in maximal oxygen consumption. People with poor muscle strength tire more easily and are less effective in both everyday and recreational activities.

Injury Prevention

Increased muscular strength and endurance help protect you from injury in two key ways:

- By enabling you to maintain good posture
- By encouraging proper body mechanics during everyday activities such as walking and lifting

Good muscle strength and, particularly, endurance in the abdomen, hips, lower back, and legs support the back in proper alignment and help prevent low-back pain, which two-thirds of Canadians report that they suffered in the last year alone.[1] (Prevention of low-back pain is discussed in Chapter 5.)

Training for muscular strength and endurance also makes the **tendons, ligaments,** and cartilage cells stronger and less susceptible to injury. Resistance exercise prevents injuries best when the strength training program is gradual and progressive and builds all the major muscle groups.

Improved Body Composition

As Chapter 2 explained, healthy body composition means that the body has a high proportion of fat-free mass (primarily composed of muscle) and a relatively small proportion of fat. Strength training improves body composition by increasing muscle mass, thereby tipping the body composition ratio toward fat-free mass and away from fat.

Building muscle mass through strength training also helps with losing fat because metabolic rate is related to muscle mass: The more muscle mass, the higher the metabolic rate. A high metabolic rate means that a nutritionally sound diet coupled with regular exercise will not lead to an increase in body fat. Strength training can boost resting metabolic rate by up to 15%,[2] depending on how hard you train. Resistance exercise also increases muscle temperature, which in turn slightly increases the rate at which you burn calories over the hours following a weight training session.

Enhanced Self-Image and Quality of Life

Strength training leads to an enhanced self-image in both men and women by providing stronger, firmer-looking muscles and a toned, healthy looking body. Men tend to build larger, stronger muscles. Women tend to lose inches, increase strength, and develop greater muscle definition. The larger muscles in men combine with high levels of the hormone **testosterone,** for a strong tissue-building effect; see the box "Gender Differences in Muscular Strength."

Because strength training involves measurable objectives (weight lifted, repetitions accomplished), a person can easily recognize improved performance, leading to

greater self-confidence and self-esteem. Strength training also improves quality of life by increasing energy, preventing injuries, and making daily activities easier and more enjoyable.

Improved Muscle and Bone Health with Aging

Research has shown that good muscle strength helps people live healthier lives. A lifelong program of regular strength training prevents muscle and nerve degeneration that can compromise the quality of life and increase the risk of hip fractures and other potentially life-threatening injuries.

In the general population people begin to lose muscle mass after age 30, a condition called *sarcopenia*. At first they may notice that they can't play sports as well as they could in high school. After more years of inactivity and strength loss, people may have trouble performing even the simple movements of daily life, such as walking up a flight of stairs, or doing yard work. By age 70 about 31% of older adults have difficulty lifting 10 pounds—about the weight of a bag of groceries.[3] Although aging contributes to decreased strength, inactivity causes most of the loss. Poor strength makes it much more likely that a person will be injured during everyday activities.

As a person ages, motor nerves can become disconnected from the portion of muscle they control. Aging and inactivity also cause muscles to become slower and therefore less able to perform quick, powerful movements. Strength training helps maintain motor nerve connections and the quickness of muscles.

Osteoporosis (bone loss) is common in people over age 50, with one in four postmenopausal women in Canada suffering from osteoporosis.[4] Osteoporosis leads to fractures that can be life-threatening. Hormonal changes from aging account for much of the bone loss that occurs, but lack of bone stress due to inactivity and a poor diet are contributing factors. Strength training can lessen bone loss even if it is taken up later in life, and if practised regularly, strength training can even build bone mass

tendon A tough band of fibrous tissue that connects a muscle to a bone or other body part and transmits the force exerted by the muscle.

ligament A tough band of tissue that connects the ends of bones to other bones or supports organs in place.

testosterone The principal male hormone, responsible for the development of secondary sex characteristics and important in increasing muscle size.

TERMS

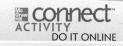

DIMENSIONS OF DIVERSITY

Gender Differences in Muscular Strength

Men are generally stronger than women because they typically have larger bodies overall and a larger proportion of their total body mass is made up of muscle. But when strength is expressed per unit of cross-sectional area of muscle tissue, men are only 1–2% stronger than women in the upper body and about equal to women in the lower body. (Men have a larger proportion of muscle tissue in the upper body, so it's easier for them to build upper-body strength than it is for women.) Individual muscle fibres are larger in men, but the metabolism of cells within those fibres is the same in both sexes.

Two factors that help explain these disparities between the sexes are testosterone levels and the speed of nervous control of muscle. Testosterone promotes the growth of muscle tissue in both males and females. Testosterone levels are about 6–10 times higher in men than in women, so men tend to have larger muscles. Also, because the male nervous system can activate muscles faster, men tend to have more power.

Women are often concerned that they will develop large muscles from strength training. Because of hormonal differences, most women do not develop big muscles unless they train intensely over many years or take anabolic steroids. Women do gain muscle and improve body composition through strength training, but they don't develop bulky muscles or gain significant

amounts of weight: A study of average women who weight trained 2–3 days per week for 8 weeks found that the women gained about 1.75 pounds of muscle and lost about 3.5 pounds of fat.

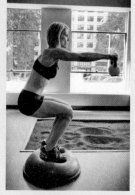

Losing muscle over time is a much greater health concern for women than small gains in muscle weight, especially because any gains in muscle weight are typically more than balanced with loss of fat weight. Both men and women lose muscle mass and power as they age, but because men start out with more muscle when they are young and don't lose power as quickly, older women tend to have greater impairment of muscle function than older men. This may partially account for the higher incidence of life-threatening falls in older women.

The bottom line is that both men and women can increase strength through strength training. Women may not be able to lift as much weight as men, but kilogram for kilogram of muscle, they have nearly the same capacity to gain strength as men.

in postmenopausal women and older men. Increased muscle strength can also help prevent falls, which are a major cause of injury in people with osteoporosis. (Additional strategies for preventing osteoporosis are described in Chapter 7.)

Metabolic and Heart Health

Strength training helps prevent and manage both cardiovascular disease (CVD) and diabetes by:

- Improving glucose metabolism.
- Increasing maximal oxygen consumption.
- Reducing blood pressure.
- Increasing HDL cholesterol and reducing LDL cholesterol (in some people).

Stronger muscles reduce the demand on the heart during ordinary daily activities such as lifting and carrying objects. The benefits of resistive exercise to the heart are so great that the Canadian Heart and Stroke Foundation recommends that healthy adults and many low-risk cardiac patients do strength training 2–4 days per week.[5] Resistance training may not be appropriate for people with some types of heart disease.

repetition maximum (RM) The maximum amount of resistance that can be moved a specified number of times; 1 RM is the maximum weight that can be lifted once. 5 RM is the maximum weight that can be lifted five times.

repetitions The number of times an exercise is performed continuously during one set.

LO3 4.3 ASSESSING MUSCULAR STRENGTH AND ENDURANCE

Muscular strength is usually assessed by measuring the maximum amount of weight a person can lift one time. This single maximal movement is referred to as a **repetition maximum (RM).** You can assess the strength of your major muscle groups by taking the one-repetition maximum (1 RM) tests for the bench press and by taking functional leg strength tests. You can measure 1 RM directly or estimate it by doing multiple repetitions with a submaximal (lighter) weight; this is referred to as an estimation of your 1 RM. CSEP has suggested an adapted protocol for estimating percentages of 1 RM based on the number of repetitions completed. See Lab 4.1 for the CSEP estimations.

It is best to train for at least several weeks before attempting a direct 1 RM test; once you have a baseline value, you can retest after 6–12 weeks to check your progress. Refer to Lab 4.1 for guidelines on taking these tests. Instructions for assessing grip strength using a dynamometer are also included in Lab 4.1. For more accurate results, avoid any strenuous weight training for 48 hours beforehand.

Muscular endurance is usually assessed by counting the maximum number of **repetitions** of a muscular contraction a person can do (such as in push-ups) or the maximum amount of time a person can hold a muscular contraction (such as in the flexed-arm hang). You can test

Tests of strength have challenged humans since the dawn of history. Strength is highly specific; one type of strength does not necessarily predict another. Strength tests help you determine your current fitness level and help you set achievable goals. You could test your capacity doing almost any exercise. Test your maximum performance on as many of the following tests as you can.

TEST	MAXIMUM REPETITIONS OR TIME	GOAL
Push-ups (Modified or regular)	_____	_____
Pull-ups or bent-arm bar hang	_____	_____
One-arm kettlebell snatches	_____	_____
Two-arm kettlebell swings	_____	_____
Bench press for reps (at a specific weight; e.g., 135 pounds, 225 pounds)	_____	_____

Write down your performance for each exercise in the second column of the list. (Note that you should wait at least a few minutes between tests.) If you aren't happy with the results, set a reasonable goal for each exercise in the third column. If you aren't sure what a reasonable goal would be, talk to your instructor or a certified personal trainer. Use these goals as a starting point for a broad-ranging strength training program.

the muscular endurance of major muscle groups in your body by taking the curl-up test, the push-up test, and the squat endurance test. See Lab 4.2 for complete instructions on taking these assessment tests.

4.4 CREATING A SUCCESSFUL STRENGTH TRAINING PROGRAM

When the muscles are stressed by a greater load than they are used to, they adapt and improve their function. The type of adaptation that occurs depends on the type of stress applied.

Static versus Dynamic Strength Training Exercises

Strength training exercises are generally classified as static or dynamic. Each involves a different way of using and strengthening muscles.

STATIC EXERCISE   Also called **isometric** exercise, **static exercise** involves a muscle contraction without a change in the length of the muscle or the angle in the joint on which the muscle acts. In isometrics, the muscle contracts, but there is no movement. To perform an isometric exercise, a person can use an immovable object like a wall to provide resistance, or just tighten a muscle while remaining still (for example, tightening the abdominal muscles while sitting at a desk). The spine extension and the side bridge are both isometric exercises.

Static exercises aren't as widely used as dynamic exercises because they don't develop strength throughout a joint's entire range of motion. During almost all movements, however, some muscles contract statically to support the skeleton so that other muscles can contract dynamically. For example, when you throw, hit a ball, or ski, the core muscles (in the abdomen and back) stabilize the spine. This stability allows more powerful contractions in the lower- and upper-body muscles. The core muscles contract statically during dynamic exercises, such as squats, lunges, and overhead presses.

Static exercises are useful in strengthening muscles after an injury or surgery, when movement of the affected joint could delay healing. Isometrics are also used to overcome weak points in an individual's range of motion. Statically strengthening a muscle at its weakest point will allow more weight to be lifted with that muscle during dynamic exercise. Certain types of calisthenics and Pilates exercises (described in more detail later in the chapter) also provide static contractions. For maximum strength gains, hold the isometric contraction maximally for 6 seconds; do 5–10 repetitions.

DYNAMIC EXERCISE   Also called **isotonic** exercise, **dynamic exercise** involves a muscle contraction with a change in the length of the muscle. Dynamic exercises are the most popular type of exercises for increasing muscle strength and seem to be most valuable for developing strength that can be transferred to other forms of physical activity. They can be performed with weight machines, free weights, or a person's own body weight (as in sit-ups or push-ups).

---

static (isometric) exercise   Exercise involving a muscle contraction without a change in the length of the muscle.

dynamic (isotonic) exercise   Exercise involving a muscle contraction with a change in the length of the muscle.

TERMS

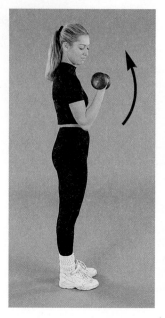
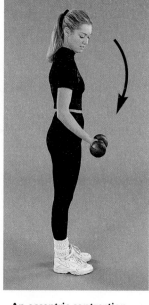

A concentric contraction   An eccentric contraction

There are two kinds of dynamic muscle contractions:

- A **concentric muscle contraction** occurs when the muscle applies enough force to overcome resistance and shortens as it contracts.
- An **eccentric muscle contraction** (also called a *plyometric contraction*) occurs when the resistance is greater than the force applied by the muscle and the muscle lengthens as it contracts.

For example, in an arm curl, the biceps muscle works concentrically as the weight is raised toward the shoulder and eccentrically as the weight is lowered.

Constant and Variable Resistance   Two of the most common dynamic exercise techniques are constant resistance exercise and variable resistance exercise.

- **Constant resistance exercise** uses a constant load (weight) throughout a joint's entire range of motion.

Training with free weights is a form of constant resistance exercise. A problem with this technique is that, because of differences in leverage, there are points in a joint's range of motion where the muscle controlling the movement is stronger and points where it is weaker. The amount of weight a person can lift is limited by the weakest point in the range.

- In **variable resistance exercise,** the load is changed to provide maximum load throughout the entire range of motion. This form of exercise uses machines that place more stress on muscles at the end of the range of motion, where a person has better leverage and is capable of exerting more force. The Nautilus pull-over machine is an example of a variable resistance exercise machine.

Constant and variable resistance exercises are both extremely effective for building strength and endurance.

Hydraulic strength training machines use air pressure for resistance and are popular in many gyms and health clubs. They build strength in beginners but are less effective for more advanced strength trainers. The machines provide resistance only during the concentric (muscle shortening) phase of the exercise and not during the eccentric (muscle lengthening) phase. Such machines do not preload the muscles with resistance; they provide resistance only after the movement has been started.

Other Dynamic Exercise Techniques

- **Eccentric (plyometric) loading** involves placing a load on a muscle as it lengthens. The muscle contracts eccentrically in order to control the weight. Eccentric loading is practised during most types of resistance training. For example, you are performing an eccentric movement as you lower the weight to your chest during a bench press in preparation for the active movement. You can also perform exercises designed specifically to overload muscle eccentrically, a technique called *negatives*.
- **Plyometrics** is the sudden eccentric loading and stretching of muscles followed by a forceful concentric contraction. An example would be the action of the lower-body muscles when jumping from a bench to the ground and then jumping back onto the bench. This type of exercise is used to develop explosive strength; it also helps build and maintain bone density.
- **Speed loading** involves moving a weight as rapidly as possible in an attempt to approach the speeds used in movements like throwing a softball or sprinting. In the bench press, for example, speed loading might involve doing 5 repetitions as fast as possible using a weight that is half the maximum load you can lift. You can gauge your progress by timing how fast you can perform the repetitions. Speed loading is not recommended for most people because of the risk of injury.

Training with **kettlebells** is a type of speed loading. Kettlebell training is highly ballistic, meaning that many exercises involve fast, pendulum-type motions, extreme decelerations, and high-speed eccentric muscle contractions. Kettlebell swings require dynamic concentric muscle contractions during the upward phase of the exercise followed by high-speed eccentric contractions to control the movement when returning to the starting position. Kettlebell training is very popular around the world, but more research is needed to better understand its effects on strength, power, and fitness.

- **Isokinetic** exercise involves exerting force at a constant speed against an equal force exerted by a special strength training machine. The isokinetic machine provides variable resistance at different points in the joint's range of motion, matching the effort applied by the individual, while keeping the speed of the movement constant. Isokinetic exercises are excellent for building strength and endurance.

COMPARE THE DIFFERENT TYPES OF EXERCISE Static exercises require no equipment, so they can be done virtually anywhere. They build strength rapidly and are useful for rehabilitating injured joints. On the other hand, they have to be performed at several different angles for each joint to improve strength throughout the joint's entire range of motion. Dynamic exercises can be performed without equipment (calisthenics) or with equipment (weight lifting). They are excellent for building strength and endurance, and they tend to build strength through a joint's full range of motion. Most people develop muscular strength and endurance using dynamic exercises. Ultimately, the type of exercise a person chooses depends on individual goals, preferences, and access to equipment.

Weight Machines versus Free Weights

Muscles get stronger if you make them work against a resistance. Resistance can be provided by free weights, your own body weight, or sophisticated exercise machines.

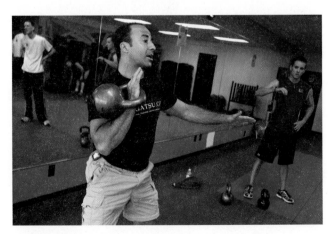

Kettlebells are growing in popularity. They provide a fast, effective workout when used properly.

Many people prefer weight machines because they are safe, convenient, and easy to use. You just set the resistance, sit down at the machine, and start working. Machines make it easy to isolate and work specific muscles. You don't need a **spotter**—someone who stands by to assist when free weights are used—and you don't have to worry about dropping a weight on yourself. Many machines provide support for the back.

Free weights require more care, balance, and coordination to use, but they strengthen your body in ways that are more adaptable to real life. They are also more popular with athletes for developing explosive strength for sports, especially sports that require a great deal of strength. Free weights are widely available, inexpensive, and convenient for home use.

Other Training Methods and Types of Equipment

You don't need a fitness centre or expensive equipment to strength train. If you prefer to train at home or like low-cost alternatives, consider the following options.

RESISTANCE BANDS Resistance or exercise bands are elastic strips or tubes of rubber material that are inexpensive, lightweight, and portable. They are available in a variety of styles and levels of resistance; some are sold with instructional guides or DVDs, and classes may be offered at fitness centres. Many free weight exercises can be adapted for resistance bands. For example, you can do biceps curls by standing on the centre of the band and holding one end of the band in each hand; resistance is provided when you stretch the band to perform the curl.

EXERCISE (STABILITY) BALLS The exercise or stability ball is an extra-large inflatable ball. It was originally developed for use in physical therapy but has become a popular piece of exercise equipment for use in the home or gym. It can be used to work the entire body, but it is particularly effective for working the core stabilizing muscles in the

kettlebell A large iron weight with a connected handle; used for ballistic weight training exercises such as swings and one-arm snatches.

isokinetic The application of force at a constant speed against an equal force.

spotter A person who assists with a weight training exercise done with free weights.

TERMS

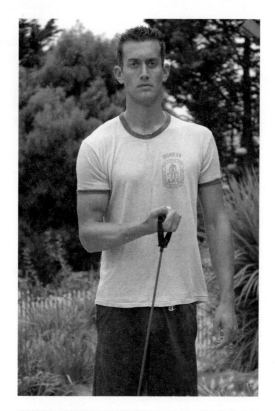

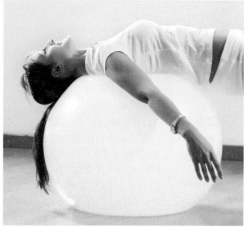

abdomen, chest, and back— muscles that are important for preventing back problems. The ball's instability forces the exerciser to use the stability muscles to balance the body, even when a person simply sits on the ball. Moves such as crunches have been found to be more effective when they are performed with an exercise ball.

When choosing a ball, make sure that your thighs are parallel to the ground when you sit on it; if you are a beginner or have back problems, choose a larger ball so that your thighs are at an angle, with hips higher than knees. Beginners should use caution until they feel comfortable with the movements and take care to avoid poor form due to fatigue. See Chapter 7 for more on incorporating stability balls into a fitness program.

PILATES   Pilates (*pil LAH teez*) was developed by German gymnast and boxer Joseph Pilates early in the twentieth century. It often involves the use of specially designed resistance training devices, although some classes feature just mat or floor work. Pilates focuses on strengthening and stretching the core muscles in the back, abdomen, and buttocks to create a solid base of support for whole-body movement; the emphasis is on concentration, control, movement flow, and breathing. Mat exercises can be done at home, but because there are hundreds of Pilates exercises, some of them strenuous, it is best to begin with some qualified instruction. The Pilates Association of Canada (http://www.pilatesassociationofcanada.ca) offers advice on finding a qualified teacher.

MEDICINE BALLS, SUSPENSION TRAINING, AND STONES
Almost anything that provides resistance to movement will develop strength. Rubber medicine balls weigh up

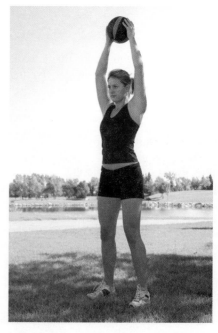

Medicine balls can be used in many ways to get an effective resistance workout.

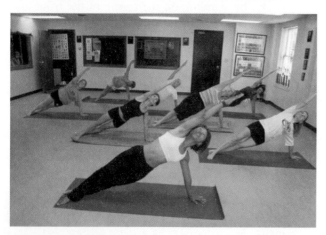

Resistance for strength training can be provided by many different techniques and types of equipment. Shown here are resistance bands (top), a stability ball (centre), and a Pilates mat exercise that uses body weight for resistance.

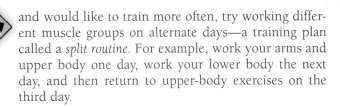

to 50 pounds and can be used for a variety of functional movements, such as squats and overhead throws. Suspension training uses body weight as the resistance and involves doing exercises with ropes or cords attached to a hook, bar, door jam, or sturdy tree branch. Stones can provide resistance to almost any movement, are free, and can be found in many shapes and sizes.

NO-EQUIPMENT CALISTHENICS   You can use your own body weight as resistance for strength training. Exercises such as curl-ups, push-ups, squats, step-ups, heel raises, chair dips, and lunges can be done anywhere.

LO4   Applying the FITT Principle: Selecting Exercises and Putting Together a Program

A complete weight training program works all the major muscle groups. It usually takes about 8–10 different exercises to get a complete workout. Use the FITT principle—frequency, intensity, time, and type—to set the parameters of your program.

FREQUENCY OF EXERCISE   For general fitness, Health Canada and the Canadian Society for Exercise Physiology (CSEP) recommend a frequency of 2–4 days per week for weight training. Allow your muscles at least 1 day of rest between workouts; if you train too often, your muscles won't be able to work at a high enough intensity to improve their fitness, and soreness and injury are more likely to result. If you enjoy weight training

and would like to train more often, try working different muscle groups on alternate days—a training plan called a *split routine*. For example, work your arms and upper body one day, work your lower body the next day, and then return to upper-body exercises on the third day.

INTENSITY OF EXERCISE: AMOUNT OF RESISTANCE
The amount of weight (resistance) you lift in weight training exercises is as important as intensity in cardio-respiratory endurance training (HR or RPE). It determines the way your body will adapt to weight training and how quickly these adaptations will occur. Choose weights based on your current level of muscular fitness and your fitness goals.

Choose a weight heavy enough to fatigue your muscles but light enough for you to complete the repetitions with good form. To build strength rapidly, you should lift weights as heavy as 80% of your maximum capacity (1 RM). If you're more interested in building endurance, choose a lighter weight (perhaps 40–60% of 1 RM) and do more repetitions.

For example, if your maximum capacity for the leg press is 100 kilograms, you might lift 80 kilograms to build strength and 50 kilograms to build endurance. For a general fitness program to develop both strength and endurance, choose a weight in the middle of this range, perhaps 70% of 1 RM. Or you can create a program that includes both higher-intensity exercise (80% of 1 RM for 8–10 repetitions) and lower-intensity exercise (60% of 1 RM for 15–20 repetitions); this routine will develop both fast-twitch and slow-twitch muscle fibres.

Because it can be tedious and time-consuming to continually reassess your maximum capacity for each exercise, you might find it easier to choose a weight based on the number of repetitions of an exercise you can perform with a given resistance.

TIME OF EXERCISE: REPETITIONS AND SETS   To improve fitness, you must do enough repetitions of each exercise to fatigue your muscles. The number of repetitions needed to cause fatigue depends on the amount of resistance: the heavier the weight, the fewer repetitions to reach fatigue. In general, a heavy weight and a low number of repetitions (5-6) build strength and overload primarily fast-twitch fibres, whereas a light weight and a high number of repetitions (15–20) build endurance and primarily overload slow-twitch fibres.

For a general fitness program to build both strength and endurance, try to do about 8–12 repetitions of each exercise; a few exercises, such as abdominal crunches and calf raises, may require more. Choose a weight heavy enough to fatigue your muscles but light enough for you to complete the repetitions with good form. To avoid risk of injury, older (approximately 50–60 years of age and above) and frailer people should perform more repetitions (10–15) using a lighter weight.

Improving Your Technique with Video

Want to get stronger? Then you need to focus on developing your skills at least as much as you focus on lifting more weight. Improving skill is the best way to increase strength during movements such as hitting a tennis ball or baseball, performing a bench press, driving a golf ball, skiing down a slope, or carrying a bag of groceries up a flight of stairs. In the world of weight training, skill means lifting weights with proper form; the better your form, the better your results.

The brain develops precise neural pathways as you learn a skill. As you improve, the pathways conduct nervous impulses faster and more precisely until the movement almost becomes reflexive. The best way to learn a skill is through focused practice that involves identifying mistakes, correcting them, and practising the refined movement many times. However, simply practising the skill is not enough if you want to improve and perform more powerful movements. You must perform the movements correctly instead of practising mistakes or poor form over and over again.

Here's where technology can help. Watch videos of people performing weight-training movements correctly. You may be able to borrow videos from your instructor, purchase low-cost training videos through magazines and sporting goods stores, or find them on the Internet. If you watch training videos online, however, make sure they were produced by an authoritative source on weight training. Otherwise, you may be learning someone else's mistakes.

Film your movements using a phone camera or inexpensive video camera. Compare your movements with those of a more skilled person performing them correctly. Make a note of poor movement patterns and try to change your technique to make it more mechanically correct. Share your videos with your instructor or a certified personal trainer, who can help you identify poor form and teach you ways to correct your form.

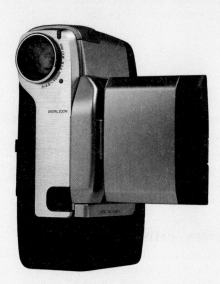

In weight training, a **set** refers to a group of repetitions of an exercise followed by a rest period. To develop strength and endurance for general fitness, you can make gains doing a single set of each exercise, provided you use enough resistance to fatigue your muscles. (You should just barely be able to complete the 8–12 repetitions—using good form—for each exercise.) Doing more than 1 set of each exercise will increase strength development, and most serious weight trainers do at least 3 sets of each exercise (see the section "More Advanced Strength Training Programs" for guidelines on more advanced programs).

If you perform more than 1 set of an exercise, you need to rest long enough between sets to allow your muscles to work at a high enough intensity to increase fitness. The length of the rest interval depends on the amount of resistance. In a program to develop a combination of strength and endurance for wellness, a rest period of 1–3 minutes between sets is appropriate; if you are lifting heavier loads to build maximum strength, rest 3–5 minutes between sets. You can save time in your workouts by alternating sets of different exercises. Each muscle group can rest between sets while you work on other muscles.

Training volume is one method of quantifying the total load lifted during weight training. Use this formula to calculate the training volume for a workout:

$$\text{repetitions} \times \text{weight} \times \text{sets}$$

For example, if you did 3 sets of 10 repetitions for biceps curls using 50 pounds, the training volume for the exercise would be 1500 pounds ($3 \times 10 \times 50 = 1500$). Do the same calculation for every exercise in your program and add the results together to determine the total training volume for the entire workout.

Overtraining—doing more exercise than your body can recover from—can occur in response to heavy resistance training. Possible signs of overtraining include lack of progress or decreased performance, chronic fatigue, decreased coordination, and chronic muscle soreness. The best remedy for overtraining is rest; add more days of recovery between workouts. With extra rest, chances are you'll be refreshed and ready to train again. Adding variety to your program, discussed later in the chapter, can also help with overtraining from resistance exercise.

TYPE OR MODE OF EXERCISE For overall fitness, you need to include exercises for your neck, upper back, shoulders, arms, chest, abdomen, lower back, thighs, buttocks, and calves—about 8–10 exercises in all. If you are also training for a particular sport, include exercises

TERMS

set A group of repetitions followed by a rest period.

to strengthen the muscles important for optimal performance *and* the muscles most likely to be injured. This chapter includes weight training programs for general fitness using both free weights and weight machines.

It is important to balance exercises between **agonist** and **antagonist** muscle groups When a muscle contracts, it is known as the agonist; the opposing muscle, which must relax and stretch to allow contraction by the agonist, is known as the antagonist. Whenever you do an exercise that moves a joint in one direction, also select an exercise that works the joint in the opposite direction. For example, if you do knee extensions to develop the muscles on the front of your thighs, also do leg curls to develop the antagonistic muscles on the back of your thighs.

The order of exercises can also be important. Do exercises for large-muscle groups or for more than one joint before you do exercises that use small-muscle groups or single joints. This allows for more effective overload of the larger, more powerful muscle groups. Small-muscle groups fatigue more easily than larger ones, and small-muscle fatigue limits your capacity to overload larger-muscle groups. For example, lateral raises, which work the shoulder muscles, should be performed after bench presses, which work the chest and arms in addition to the shoulders. If you fatigue your shoulder muscles by doing lateral raises first, you won't be able to lift as much weight and effectively fatigue all the key muscle groups used during the bench press.

Also, order exercises so that you work agonist and antagonist muscle groups in sequence, one after the other. For example, follow biceps curls, which work the biceps, with triceps extensions, which exercise the triceps—the antagonist muscle to the biceps.

The Warm-Up and Cool-Down

As with cardiorespiratory endurance exercise, you should warm up before every weight training session and cool down afterward (Figure 4.2). You should do both a general warm-up—several minutes of walking or easy jogging—and a warm-up for the weight training exercises you plan to perform. For example, if you plan to do 1 or more sets of 10 repetitions of bench presses with 125 pounds, you might do 1 set of 10 repetitions with 50 pounds as a warm-up. Do similar warm-up exercises for each exercise in your program.

To cool down after weight training, relax for 5–10 minutes after your workout. Although this is controversial, a few studies have suggested that including a period of postexercise stretching may help prevent muscle soreness; warmed-up muscles and joints make this a particularly good time to work on flexibility.

Getting Started and Making Progress

The first few sessions of weight training should be devoted to learning the movements and allowing your nervous system to practise communicating with your muscles so you

WELLNESS TIP

A standard push-up is equivalent to bench-pressing 60% of your body weight. A set of 12 push-ups is a quick, effective upper-body workout. No gym required!

Warm-up 5–10 minutes	Strength training exercises for major muscle groups (8–10 exercises)		Cool-down 5–10 minutes
	Sample program		
	Exercise	*Muscle group(s) developed*	
	Bench press	Chest, shoulders, triceps	
	Pull-ups	Lats, biceps	
	Shoulder press	Shoulders, trapezius, triceps	
	Upright rowing	Deltoids, trapezius	
	Biceps curls	Biceps	
	Lateral raises	Shoulders	
	Squats	Gluteals, quadriceps	
	Heel raises	Calves	
	Abdominal curls	Abdominals	
	Spine extensions	Low- and mid-back spine extensors	
Start	Side bridges	Obliques, quadratus lumborum	*Stop*

Frequency: 2–3 nonconsecutive days per week

Intensity/Resistance: Weights heavy enough to cause muscle fatigue when exercises are performed with good form for the selected number of repetitions

Time: Repetitions: 8–12 of each exercise (10–15 with a lower weight for people over age 50–60); **Sets:** 1 (doing more than 1 set per exercise may result in faster and greater strength gains); rest 1–2 minutes between exercises.

Type of activity: 8–10 strength training exercises that focus on major muscle groups

FIGURE 4.2   The FITT principle for a strength training workout.

can develop strength effectively. To start, choose a weight that you can move easily through 8–12 repetitions, and do only 1 set of each exercise and rest 1–2 minutes between exercises. Gradually add weight and (if you want) sets to your program over the first few weeks until you are doing 1–3 sets of 8–12 repetitions of each exercise.

As you progress, add weight according to the "two-for-two" rule: When you can perform 2 additional repetitions with a given weight on 2 consecutive training sessions, increase the load. For example, if your target is to perform

agonist   A muscle in a state of contraction, opposed by the action of another muscle, its *antagonist*.

antagonist   A muscle that opposes the action of another muscle, its *agonist*.

8–10 repetitions per exercise, and you performed 12 repetitions in your previous 2 workouts, it would be appropriate to increase your load. If adding weight means you can do only 7 or 8 repetitions, stay with that weight until you can again complete 12 repetitions per set. If you can do only 4–6 repetitions after adding weight, or if you can't maintain good form, you've added too much and should take some off.

You can add more resistance in large muscle exercises, such as squats and bench presses, than you can in smaller muscle exercises, such as curls. For example, when you can complete 12 repetitions of squats with good form, you may be able to add 10–20 pounds of additional resistance; for curls, on the other hand, you might add only 3–5 pounds. As a general guideline, try increases of approximately 5%, which is half a pound of additional weight for each 10 pounds you are currently lifting.

You can expect to improve rapidly during the first 6–10 weeks of training: a 10–30% increase in the amount of weight lifted. Gains will then come more slowly. Your rate of improvement will depend on how hard you work and how your body responds to resistance training. Factors such as age, motivation, and heredity will affect your progress.

After you have achieved the level of strength and muscularity that you want, you can maintain your gains by training 2–3 days per week. You can monitor the progress of your program by recording the amount of resistance and the number of repetitions and sets you perform on a workout card like the one shown in Figure 4.3.

More Advanced Strength Training Programs

The program just described is sufficient to develop and maintain muscular strength and endurance for general fitness. Performing more sets of a smaller number of repetitions with a heavier load will cause greater increases in strength. Such a program might include 3–5 sets of 4–6 repetitions each; the load used should be heavy enough to cause fatigue with the smaller number of repetitions. Rest long enough after a set (3–5 minutes) to allow your muscles to recover and to work intensely during the next set.

Experienced weight trainers often engage in some form of cycle training, also called *periodization,* in which the exercises, number of sets and repetitions, and intensity

WORKOUT CARD FOR ___Sara Lopez___

Exercise/Date		9/14	9/16	9/18	9/21	9/23	9/25	9/28	9/30	10/2	10/5	10/7	10/9	10/12	10/14	10/16										
Bench press	Wt.	45	45	45	50	50	50	60	60	60	65	65	65	70	70	70										
	Sets	1	1	1	1	1	1	1	1	1	1	1	1	1	1	1										
	Reps.	10	10	12	10	12	12	10	9	12	10	12	12	9	9	10										
Pull-ups (assisted)	Wt.	—	—	—	—	—	—	—	—	—	—	—	—	—	—	—										
	Sets	1	1	1	1	1	1	1	1	1	1	1	1	1	1	1										
	Reps.	5	5	5	6	6	6	7	7	7	8	8	8	9	9	10										
Shoulder press	Wt.	20	20	20	25	25	25	30	30	30	30	30	30	35	35	35										
	Sets	1	1	1	1	1	1	1	1	1	1	1	1	1	1	1										
	Reps.	10	10	12	10	12	12	8	10	9	10	12	12	10	10	10										
Upright rowing	Wt.	5	5	10	10	10	10	12	12	12	12	15	15	15	15	15										
	Sets	1	1	1	1	1	1	1	1	1	1	1	1	1	1	1										
	Reps.	12	12	8	10	11	12	9	10	10	12	8	8	8	9	10										
Biceps curls	Wt.	15	15	15	20	20	20	25	25	25	25	25	25	30	30	30										
	Sets	1	1	1	1	1	1	1	1	1	1	1	1	1	1	1										
	Reps.	10	10	10	10	12	12	8	10	10	10	12	12	9	10	12										
Lateral raise	Wt.	5	5	5	5	5	5	7.5	7.5	7.5	7.5	7.5	7.5	10	10	10										
	Sets	1	1	1	1	1	1	1	1	1	1	1	1	1	1	1										
	Reps.	8	8	10	10	12	12	8	10	10	10	12	12	8	8	9										
Squats	Wt.	—	—	—	45	45	45	55	55	55	65	65	65	75	75	75										
	Sets	1	1	1	1	1	1	1	1	1	1	1	1	1	1	1										
	Reps.	10	12	15	8	12	12	8	12	12	10	10	12	8	10	10										
Heel raises	Wt.	—	—	—	45	45	45	55	55	55	65	65	65	75	75	75										
	Sets	1	1	1	1	1	1	1	1	1	1	1	1	1	1	1										
	Reps.	15	15	15	8	12	12	10	12	12	10	12	12	10	12	12										
Abdominal curls	Wt.	—	—	—	—	—	—	—	—	—	—	—	—	—	—	—										
	Sets	1	1	1	1	1	1	1	1	1	1	1	1	1	1	1										
	Reps.	20	20	20	20	20	20	25	25	25	25	25	25	25	25	25										
Spine extensions	Wt.	—	—	—	—	—	—	—	—	—	—	—	—	—	—	—										
	Sets	1	1	1	1	1	1	1	1	1	1	1	1	1	1	1										
	Reps.	5	5	5	8	8	8	10	10	10	10	10	10	11	12	12										
Side bridge	Wt.	—	—	—	—	—	—	—	—	—	—	—	—	—	—	—										
	Sets	1	1	1	1	1	1	1	1	1	1	1	1	1	1	1										
	Seconds	60	60	60	65	65	70	70	70	70	76	75	80	80	80	80										

FIGURE 4.3 A sample workout card for a general fitness strength training program.

are varied within a workout and/or between workouts. For example, you might do a particular exercise more intensely during some sets or on some days than others; you might also vary the exercises you perform for particular muscle groups. For more detailed information on these more advanced training techniques, consult a strength coach certified by the National Strength and Conditioning Association or another reliable source. If you decide to adopt a more advanced training regimen, start off slowly to give your body a chance to adjust and to minimize the risk of injury.

CORE STRENGTH TRAINING   Most body movements involve several joints and many muscles, either as prime movers, assist muscles, stabilizers, or antagonists. The link and coordination among these movements is called the kinetic chain. The key to most linked movements is the *core,* also called the trunk or midsection, consisting of the abdominal muscles, deep lateral stabilizing muscles, and the spinal extensor muscles. The core is critical because it transmits forces between the lower and upper body and helps stabilize the spine. Building strength and endurance in these muscle groups is key to most sports movements, to many activities of daily living, and to a healthy lower back.

What exercises build core strength and endurance? You can build core strength by forcing the trunk muscles to stabilize the spine while standing, sitting, or lying down. Examples of simple, low-tech core strengthening exercises include sitting on an exercise ball and keeping from falling over and holding a push-up position on your forearms for 15 seconds. Whole body exercises are particularly effective; examples include curl-ups on an exercise ball, side bridges, spine extensions, squats, and standing bench presses on a crossover pulley. Pilates, a form of exercise discussed in this section, often focuses on the core muscles. For a complete program of core strengthening exercises, see the Mayo Clinic program at http://www.mayoclinic.com/health/core-strength/SM00047. In addition, the program of strength and stretching exercises for low-back health presented in Chapter 5 also features many exercises that help build core strength.

Weight Training Safety

Injuries happen in weight training. Maximum physical effort, elaborate machinery, rapid movements, and heavy weights can combine to make the weight room a dangerous place if proper precautions aren't taken. To help ensure that your workouts are safe and productive, follow the guidelines in the box "Safe Weight Training" and the following suggestions.

USE PROPER LIFTING TECHNIQUE   Every exercise has a proper technique that is important for obtaining maximum benefits and preventing injury. Your instructor or

---

FITNESS TIP

Doing three sets of resistance exercise is more anabolic than one set, meaning that doing multiple sets enhances muscle protein synthesis. If you're serious about strength training, do multiple sets of exercises to maximize muscle protein synthesis and muscle growth.

---

weight room attendant can help explain the specific techniques for different exercises and weight machines.

Perform exercises smoothly and with good form. The CSEP/ACSM suggests a moderate rate for each repetition—a 3-second concentric contraction and a 3-second eccentric contraction. Lift or push the weight forcefully during the active phase of the lift and then lower it slowly with control. Perform all lifts through the full range of motion.

USE SPOTTERS AND COLLARS WITH FREE WEIGHTS
Spotters are necessary when an exercise has potential for danger; a weight that is out of control or falls can cause a serious injury. A spotter can assist you if you cannot complete a lift or if the weight tilts. A spotter can also help you move a weight into position before a lift and provide help or additional resistance during a lift. Spotting requires practice and coordination between the lifter and the spotter(s).

Collars are devices that secure weights to a barbell or dumbbell. Although people lift weights without collars, doing so is dangerous. It is easy to lose your balance or to raise one side of the weight faster than the other. Without collars, the weights on one side of the bar will slip off and crash to the floor.

BE ALERT FOR INJURIES   Report any obvious muscle or joint injuries to your instructor or physician, and stop exercising the affected area. Training with an injured joint or muscle can lead to a more serious injury. Make sure you get the necessary first aid.

Consult a physician if you have any unusual symptoms during exercise or if you're uncertain whether weight training is a proper activity for you. Conditions such as heart disease and high blood pressure can be aggravated during weight training. Immediately report symptoms such as headaches; dizziness; laboured breathing; numbness; vision disturbances; and chest, neck, or arm pains.

LO5   A Caution About Natural Health Products and Drugs

Many active people use a wide variety of **natural health products (NHP)** and drugs in the quest for improved performance and appearance. Most of these substances

---

natural health products (NHP)   Any product set out by the Natural Health Products Regulations in the Food and Drug Act governed by Health Canada. These products are considered to be safe as over-the-counter products and do not require a prescription to be sold.

Safe Weight Training

General Guidelines

- When beginning a program or trying new exercises or equipment, ask an instructor for help doing exercises safely and with correct technique.

- Lift weights from a stabilized body position; keep weights as close to your body as possible.

- Protect your back by maintaining control of your spine and avoiding dangerous positions. Don't twist your body while lifting.

- Observe proper lifting techniques and good form at all times. Don't lift beyond the limits of your strength.

- Don't hold your breath while doing weight training exercises. Doing so causes a decrease in blood returning to the heart and can make you become dizzy and faint. It can also increase blood pressure to dangerous levels. Exhale when exerting the greatest force, and inhale when moving the weight into position for the active phase of the lift. Breathe smoothly and steadily.

- Don't use defective equipment. Be aware of broken collars or bolts, frayed cables, broken chains, or loose cushions.

- Don't exercise if you're ill, injured, or overtrained. Do not try to work through the pain.

Free Weights

- Make sure the bar is loaded evenly on both sides.

- When you pick a weight up from the ground, keep your back straight and your head level. Don't bend at the waist with straight legs.

- Lift weights smoothly; don't jerk them. Control the weight through the entire range of motion.

- Do most of your lifting with your legs. Keep your hips and buttocks tucked in. When doing standing lifts, maintain a good posture so that you protect your back. Bend at the hips, not with the spine. Feet should be shoulder-width

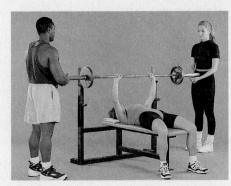

apart, heels and balls of the feet in contact with the floor, and knees slightly bent.

- Don't bounce weights against your body during an exercise.

Spotting

- Use spotters for free-weight exercises in which the bar crosses the face or head (e.g., the bench press), is placed on the back (e.g., squats), or is racked in front of the chest (e.g., overhead press from the rack).

- If one spotter is used, the spotter should stand behind the lifter; if two spotters are used, one spotter should stand at each end of the barbell.

- For squats with heavy resistance, use at least three spotters—one behind the lifter (hands near lifter's hips, waist, or torso) and one on each side of the bar.

- Spot dumbbell exercises at the forearms, as close to the weights as possible.

- For over-the-face and over-the-head lifts, the spotter should hold the bar with an alternate grip (one palm up and one palm down) inside the lifter's grip

- Ensure good communication between spotter and lifter by agreeing on verbal signals before the exercise.

---

are ineffective and expensive and many are dangerous. A balanced diet should be your primary nutritional strategy.

NATURAL HEALTH PRODUCT AND DRUG USE BY ACTIVE PEOPLE The variety and combinations of NHPs and drugs used by physically active people make it extremely difficult to determine the efficacy of these practices or to predict their side effects. Many medical studies describe catastrophic side effects from use of unsafe drugs and NHPs. Most NHPs simply don't work.

Keep in mind that no NHP or drug will change a weak, untrained person into a strong, fit person. Those changes require regular training that stresses the muscles, heart,

lungs, and metabolism and causes the body to adapt. They also require a healthy, balanced diet, as described in Chapter 7. The next section describes weight training exercises that can help you reach your goals.

Ask Yourself

QUESTIONS FOR CRITICAL THINKING AND REFLECTION

Do you think athletes should be allowed to use drugs and supplements to improve their sports performance? Would you be tempted to use a banned performance-enhancing drug if you thought you could get away with it? Why or why not?

Natural Health Products: A Consumer Dilemma

In January 2004, Canada's Department of Justice registered the Natural Health Products Regulations (NHPR) under its Food and Drugs Act. The NHPR are a regulatory framework from which consumers can gain a sense of confidence in the safety and quality of natural health products (NHP) sold in Canada. The NHPR include regulations stating that:

- To classify as an NHP, substances cannot be classified as Controlled Drugs and Substances by the Food and Drug Act. The Department of Justice provides a list of these drugs on its website at http://laws.justice.gc.ca/en/C-38.8/.

- All NHPs must be licensed by the Department of Justice before they can be sold in Canada. Licensure is by paper application and the NHP is not physically tested for its effects or potential benefits (whereas Controlled Drugs and Substances are physically tested).

- Manufacturers/distributors of licensed NHPs can make health claims about their products. The efficacy of these claims is the responsibility of the manufacturer/distributor.

Given that manufacturers/distributors of licensed NHPs can advertise their products by using health claims, it can be difficult to wade through the advertising hype when choosing an NHP. It's only human nature to want to feel, perform, and look as good as possible but there is no guarantee that advertising claims about NHPs are true.

When faced with the decision about which NHP might be helpful to you, consider the following questions:

- *Do you really need an NHP at all?* Nutritional authorities agree that most athletes and young adults can obtain all the necessary ingredients for health and top athletic performance by eating a well-balanced diet and training appropriately. There is no NHP that outperforms wholesome real food and a good training regimen. Remember, too, that athletic performance and appearance are not life and death issues. It's one thing to take a

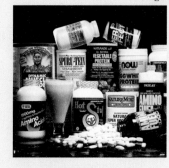

cancer chemotherapy drug with many known adverse effects if there is a reasonable chance that it will save your life. It's another to take a potentially dangerous dietary supplement that may not even work for you when your goal is to increase your sports performance.

- *Is the product safe and effective?* The fact that an NHP is available in your local store is no guarantee of safety. As described above, the Department of Justice doesn't regulate NHPs in the same way as drugs. The only way to determine if an NHP really works is to perform carefully controlled research on human subjects. Testimonials from individuals who claim to have benefited from the product don't count. Few NHPs have undergone careful human testing, so it is difficult to tell which of them may actually work. Reliable resources for information on NHPs include the FDA Center for Food Safety and Applied Nutrition (http://www.cfsan.fda.gov/~dms/supplmnt.html) and the Nutritional Supplements for Athletes website from Kansas State University (http://www.oznet.ksu.edu/nutrition/supplements.htm).

- *Can you be sure that the specific product is of high quality?* In 1999 the Government of Canada created the Natural Health Products Directorate (NHPD) whose "role is to ensure that Canadians have ready access to natural health products that are safe, effective and of high quality while respecting freedom of choice and philosophical and cultural diversity" (http://www.hc-sc.gc.ca/ahc-asc/branch-dirgen/hpfb-dgpsa/nhpd-dpsn/index_e.html).

LO6 4.5 WEIGHT TRAINING EXERCISES

A general book on fitness and wellness cannot include a detailed description of all weight training exercises. Here we present a basic program for developing muscle fitness using free weights and weight machines. Instructions for each exercise are accompanied by photographs and a listing of the muscles being trained. (Figure 4.4 is a diagram of the muscular system.) Table 4.2 lists alternative and additional exercises that can be performed on various machines or with free weights. If you are interested in learning how to do these exercises, ask your instructor, fitness consultant, or coach for assistance.

Labs 4.2 and 4.3 will help you assess your current level of muscular endurance and design your own weight training program. If you want to develop strength for a particular activity, your program should contain exercises for general fitness, exercises for the muscle groups most important for the activity, and exercises for muscle groups most often injured. Regardless of the goals of your program or the type of equipment you use, your program should be structured so that you obtain maximum results without risking injury.

WELLNESS TIP

Health Canada has issued several consumer warnings about dietary supplements—particularly the kinds that are marketed to people who want to build muscle and lose fat. A number of products have been pulled off store shelves after Health Canada found they were not safe. Talk to your doctor before considering any dietary supplement.

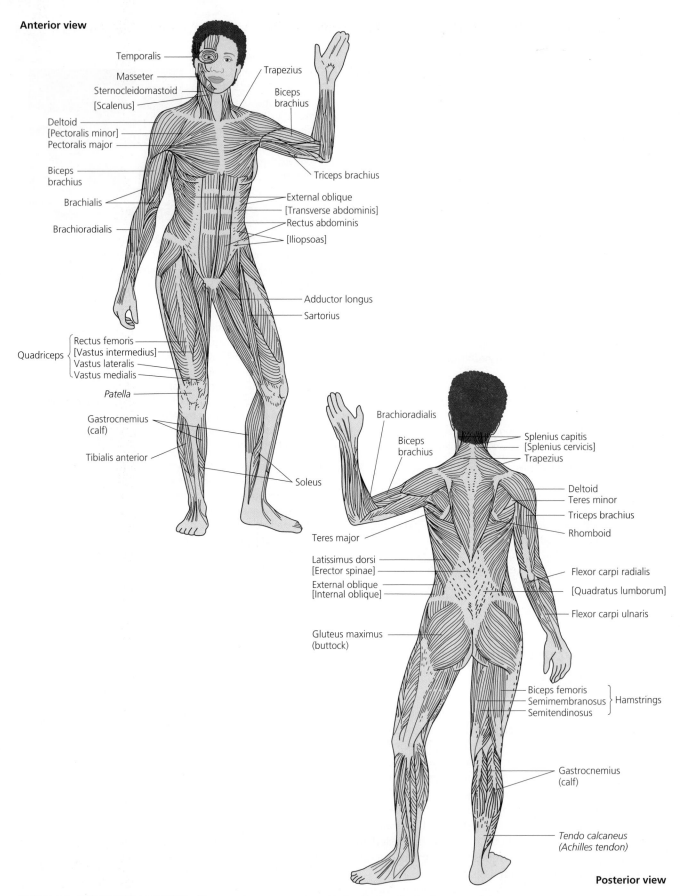

Anterior view

Temporalis

Masseter

Sternocleidomastoid

[Scalenus]

Deltoid

[Pectoralis minor]

Pectoralis major

Biceps brachius

Brachialis

Brachioradialis

Trapezius

Biceps brachius

Triceps brachius

External oblique

[Transverse abdominis]

Rectus abdominis

[Iliopsoas]

Adductor longus

Sartorius

Quadriceps
{
Rectus femoris
[Vastus intermedius]
Vastus lateralis
Vastus medialis
}

Patella

Gastrocnemius (calf)

Tibialis anterior

Soleus

Brachioradialis

Biceps brachius

Teres major

Latissimus dorsi

[Erector spinae]

External oblique

[Internal oblique]

Gluteus maximus (buttock)

Splenius capitis

[Splenius cervicis]

Trapezius

Deltoid

Teres minor

Triceps brachius

Rhomboid

Flexor carpi radialis

[Quadratus lumborum]

Flexor carpi ulnaris

Biceps femoris
Semimembranosus   } Hamstrings
Semitendinosus

Gastrocnemius (calf)

Tendo calcaneus (Achilles tendon)

Posterior view

FIGURE 4.4   THE MUSCULAR SYSTEM.   The muscle names enclosed in brackets refer to deep muscles.

TABLE 4.2 Weight Training Exercises for Machines, Free Weights, Exercise Bands, and No Equipment

Company	Legs	Arms	Shoulders and Chest	Torso
Cybex	Hip abduction Hip adduction Leg extension Leg press Leg curl Rotary calf	Arm curl Triceps extension	Chest press Incline press Overhead press	Ab crunch Pull-down Torso rotation
Hammer	Abductor Adductor Calf H squat Iso leg curl Iso leg extension Iso lateral leg press Leg curl Leg extension Leg press Seated calf raise	Behind-neck press Bench press Flat back chest Front military press Incline press Iso behind-neck press Iso incline press Iso wide chest Seated bicep Seated triceps	Bench press Flat back chest Iso wide chest Lateral raise Rear deltoid Rotator cuff Seated dip	Behind-neck pull-down Bilateral row Dead lift Front pull-down High row Iso pullover Low row Pullover Row Shrug
Nautilus	Calf raise Leg curl Leg extension Leg press	Biceps curl Preacher curl Triceps extension	10-degree chest 50-degree chest Bench press Incline press Lateral raise Military press Seated dip	Abdominal Compound row Hip and back Hip flexion Lat pull-down Pullover Rotary torso
Universal Gym	Abductor kick Adductor kick Calf raises (leg press) Knee extension Knee flexion Leg press	Biceps curl Dips Lat pull	Bench press Front raise Incline press Rip-up Shoulder press Upright row	Bent-over row Crunch Lat pull Pullover Pull-up Side bend
Free weights	Back squat Front squat Hack squat Leg curl Leg extension Leg press Lunges Seated calf Smith machine Step-ups	Barbell curl Dumbbell curl French curl Preacher curl	Bench press Decline press Dumbbell back raise Dumbbell flys Dumbbell front raise Dumbbell lateral raise Incline press Overhead press	Abdominal crunch Abdominal sit-ups Bent-over row Dead lift Incline lever row Lat pull-down Pullover Seated row Shrug Upright row
Exercise bands	Squats Lunges Hamstring curls Leg abduction Leg adduction Kick backs	Biceps curls Triceps extensions	Chest press Shoulder press Lateral raise Seated row	Trunk curl Reverse crunch Sit backs Back extensions Lat pull-down
Exercises without weights	Squats Overhead squats Lunges Side lunges Rear lunges Wall sits Step-ups	Isometric curls Isometric triceps extensions Chair dips 90° Bent-arm bar hang, supine grip	Push-ups Pull-ups Handstand press against wall	Curl-ups Bicycles Knee raises from bar Side bends Twists

SOURCE: Adapted from Fahey, T. D., 2007. *Basic Weight Training for Men and Women,* 6th ed. Copyright © 2007. The McGraw-Hill Companies, Inc. Reprinted with permission of The McGraw-Hill Companies, Inc.

WEIGHT TRAINING EXERCISES: Free Weights

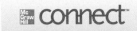

EXERCISE 1

Bench Press

Instructions:

(a) Lying on a bench on your back with your feet on the floor, grasp the bar with palms upward and hands shoulder-width apart. If the weight is on a rack, move the bar carefully from the supports to a point over the middle of your chest or slightly above it (at the lower part of the sternum).

(b) Lower the bar to your chest. Then press it in a straight line to the starting position. Don't arch your back or bounce the bar off your chest. You can also do this exercise with dumbbells.

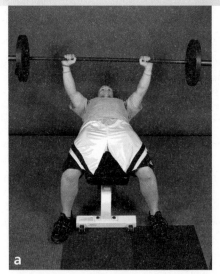

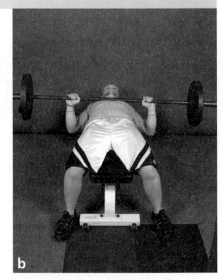

a b

Note: *To allow an optimal view of exercise technique, a spotter does not appear in these demonstration photographs; however, spotters should be used for most exercises with free weights.*

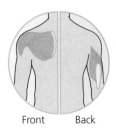

Front   Back

Muscles developed:

Pectoralis major, triceps, deltoids

EXERCISE 2   Pull-Up

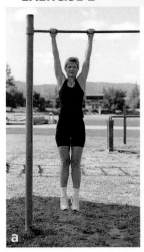

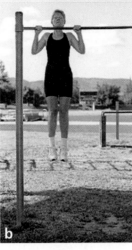

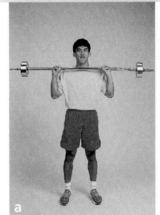

Assisted pull-up:

(c) This is done as described for a pull-up, except that a spotter assists the person by pushing upward at the waist, hips, or legs during the exercise.

Instructions:

(a) Begin by grasping the pull-up bar with both hands, palms facing forward and elbows extended fully.

(b) Pull yourself upward until your chin goes above the bar. Then return to the starting position.

Muscles developed:

Latissimus dorsi, biceps

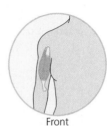

Front

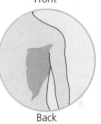

Back

EXERCISE 3   Shoulder Press (Overhead or Military Press)

Instructions: This exercise can be done standing or seated, with dumbbells or a barbell. The shoulder press begins with the weight at your chest, preferably on a rack.

(a) Grasp the weight with your palms facing away from you.

(b) Push the weight overhead until your arms are extended. Then return to the starting position (weight at chest). Be careful not to arch your back excessively.

If you are a more advanced weight trainer, you can "clean" the weight (lift it from the floor to your chest). The clean should be attempted only after instruction from a knowledgeable coach; otherwise, it can lead to injury.

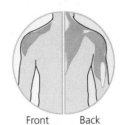

Front   Back

Muscles developed:

Deltoids, triceps, trapezius

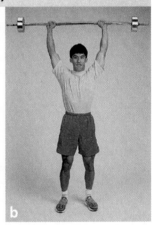

EXERCISE 4 — Upright Rowing

Instructions: From a standing position with arms extended fully, grasp a barbell with a close grip (hands about 6–12 inches apart) and palms toward the body. Raise the bar to about the level of your collarbone, keeping your elbows above bar level at all times. Return to the starting position.

This exercise can be done using dumbbells, a weighted bar (shown), or a barbell.

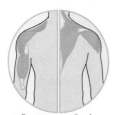

Front   Back

Muscles developed:
Trapezius, deltoids, biceps

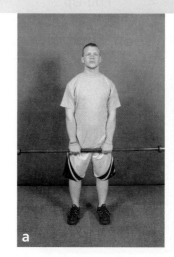
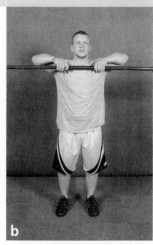

a   b

EXERCISE 5 — Biceps Curl

Instructions:

(a) From a standing position, grasp the bar with your palms upward and your hands shoulder-width apart.
(b) Keeping your upper body rigid, flex (bend) your elbows until the bar reaches a level slightly below the collarbone. Return the bar to the starting position.

This exercise can be done using dumbbells, a curl bar (shown), or a barbell; some people find that using a curl bar places less stress on the wrists.

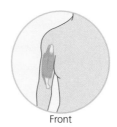

Front

Muscles developed:
Biceps, brachialis

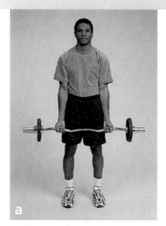
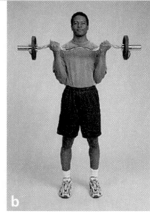

a   b

EXERCISE 6 — Lateral Raise

Instructions:

(a) Stand with feet shoulder-width apart and a dumbbell in each hand. Hold the dumbbells parallel to each other.
(b) With elbows slightly bent, slowly lift both weights until they reach shoulder level. Keep your wrists in a neutral position, in line with your forearms. Return to the starting position.

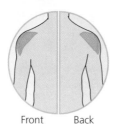

Front   Back

Muscles developed:
Deltoids

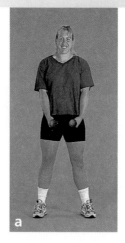
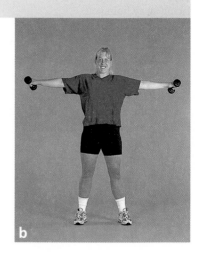

a   b

EXERCISE 7 — Squat

Instructions: If the bar is racked, place the bar on the fleshy part of your upper back and grasp the bar at shoulder width. Keeping your back neutral and head level, remove the bar from the rack and take a step back. Stand with feet slightly more than shoulder-width apart and toes pointed slightly outward.

(a) Rest the bar on the back of your shoulders, holding it there with hands facing forward.

(b) Keeping your head level and lower back straight and pelvis back, squat down until your thighs are below parallel with the floor. Let your thighs move laterally (outward) so that you "squat between your legs." This will help keep your back straight and keep your heels on the floor. Drive upward toward the starting position, hinging at the hips and keeping your back in a fixed position throughout the exercise.

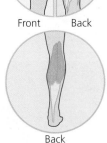
Front   Back

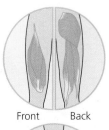
Back

Muscles developed:
Quadriceps, gluteus maximus, hamstrings, gastrocnemius

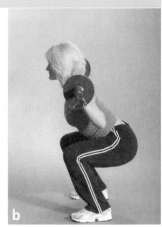
a   b

EXERCISE 8 — Heel Raise

Instructions: Stand with feet shoulder-width apart and toes pointed straight ahead.

(a) Rest the bar on the back of your shoulders, holding it there with hands facing forward.

(b) Press down with your toes while lifting your heels. Return to the starting position.

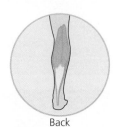
Back

Muscles developed:
Gastrocnemius, soleus

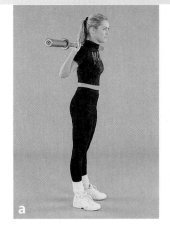
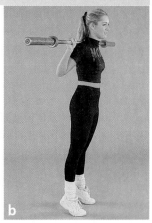
a   b

EXERCISE 9   Curl-Up or Crunch

Instructions:

(a) Lie on your back on the floor with your arms folded across your chest and your feet on the floor or on a bench.

(b) Curl your trunk up minimizing your head and shoulder movement. Lower to the starting position. Focus on using your abdominal muscles rather than the muscles in your shoulders, chest, and neck.

This exercise can also be done using an exercise ball.

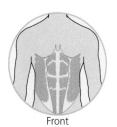

Front

Muscles developed:

Rectus abdominis, obliques

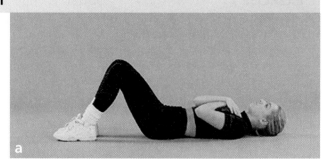

a

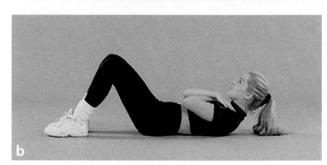

b

EXERCISE 10   Spine Extension (Isometric Exercises)

Instructions: Begin on all fours with your knees below your hips and your hands below your shoulders.

Unilateral spine extension:

(a) Extend your right leg to the rear and reach forward with your right arm. Keep your spine neutral and your raised arm and leg in line with your torso. Don't arch your back or let your hip or shoulder sag. Hold this position for 10–30 seconds. Repeat with your left leg and left arm.

Bilateral spine extension:

(b) Extend your left leg to the rear and reach forward with your right arm. Keep your spine neutral and your raised arm and leg in line with your torso. Don't arch your back or let your hip or shoulder sag. Hold this position for 10–30 seconds. Repeat with your right leg and left arm.

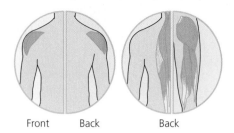

Front   Back   Back

Muscles developed: Erector spinae, gluteus maximus, hamstrings, deltoids

You can make this exercise more difficult by making box patterns with your arms and legs.

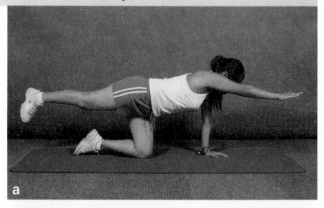

a

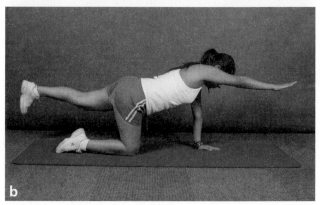

b

EXERCISE 11   Isometric Side Bridge

Instructions: Lie on the floor on your side with your knees bent and your top arm lying alongside your body. Lift your hips so that your weight is supported by your forearm and knee. Hold this position for 3–10 seconds, breathing normally. Repeat on the other side. Perform 3–10 repetitions on each side.

Variation: You can make the exercise more difficult by keeping your legs straight and supporting yourself with your feet and forearm (see Lab 5.3) or with your feet and hand (with elbow straight). You can also do this exercise on an exercise ball.

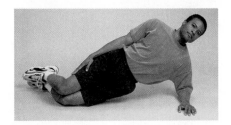

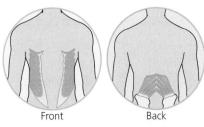

Front   Back

Muscles developed:
Obiques, quadratus, lumborum

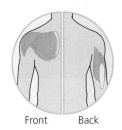

WEIGHT TRAINING EXERCISES: Weight Machines

EXERCISE 1   Bench Press (Chest or Vertical Press)

Instructions: Sit or lie on the seat or bench, depending on the type of machine and the manufacturer's instructions. Your back, hips, and buttocks should be pressed against the machine pads. Place your feet on the floor or the foot supports.

Muscles developed:
Pectoralis major, anterior deltoids, triceps

Front   Back

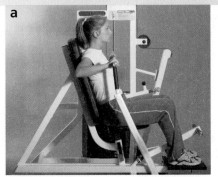

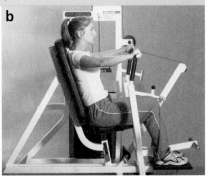

(a) Grasp the handles with your palms facing away from you; the handles should be aligned with your armpits.

(b) Push the bars until your arms are fully extended, but don't lock your elbows. Return to the starting position.

EXERCISE 2   Lat Pull

Instructions: Begin in a seated or kneeling position, depending on the type of lat machine and the manufacturer's instructions.
(a) Grasp the bar of the machine with arms fully extended.
(b) Slowly pull the weight down until it reaches the top of your chest. Slowly return to the starting position.

Muscles developed:
Latissimus dorsi, biceps

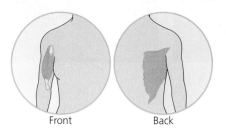

Front   Back

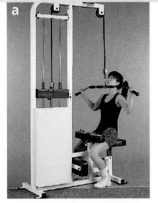

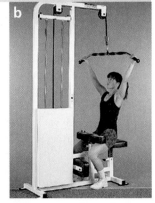

Note: *This exercise focuses on the same major muscles as the assisted pull-up (Exercise 3); choose an appropriate exercise for your program based on your preferences and equipment availability.*

EXERCISE 3 — Assisted Pull-Up

Instructions: Set the weight according to the amount of assistance you need to complete a set of pull-ups—the heavier the weight, the more assistance provided.

(a) Stand or kneel on the assist platform, and grasp the pull-up bar with your elbows fully extended and your palms facing away.

(b) Pull up until your chin goes above the bar and then return to the starting position.

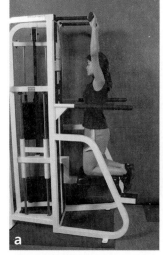
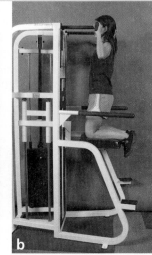

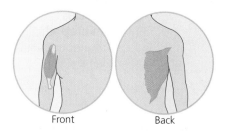

Front   Back

Muscles developed:
Latissimus dorsi, bicep

EXERCISE 4 — Overhead Press (Shoulder Press)

Instructions: Adjust the seat so that your feet are flat on the ground and the hand grips are slightly above your shoulders.

(a) Sit down, facing away from the machine, and grasp the hand grips with your palms facing forward.

(b) Press the weight upward until your arms are extended. Return to the starting position.

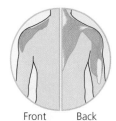

Front   Back

Muscles developed:
Deltoids, trapezius, triceps

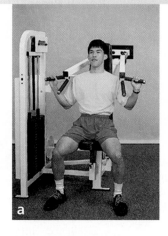
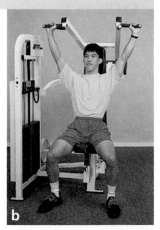

EXERCISE 5 — Biceps Curl

Instructions:

(a) Adjust the seat so that your back is straight and your arms rest comfortably against the top and side pads. Place your arms on the support cushions and grasp the hand grips with your palms facing up.

(b) Keeping your upper body still, flex (bend) your elbows until the hand grips almost reach your collarbone. Return to the starting position.

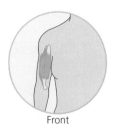

Front

Muscles developed:
Biceps, brachialis

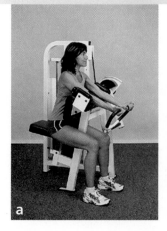
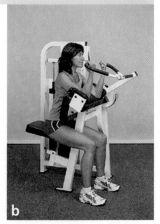

EXERCISE 6   Pullover

Instructions: Adjust the seat so your shoulders are aligned with the cams. Push down on the foot pads with your feet to bring the bar forward until you can place your elbows on the pads. Rest your hands lightly on the bar. If possible, place your feet flat on the floor.

(a) To get into the starting position, let your arms go backward as far as possible.

(b) Pull your elbows forward until the bar almost touches your abdomen. Return to the starting position.

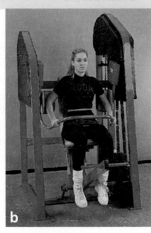
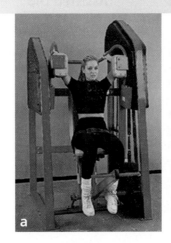

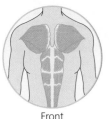
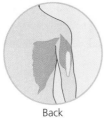

Front   Back

Muscles developed: Latissimus dorsi, pectoralis major and minor, triceps, abdominals

EXERCISE 7   Lateral Raise

Instructions:

(a) Adjust the seat so the pads rest just above your elbows when your upper arms are at your sides, your elbows are bent, and your forearms are parallel to the floor. Lightly grasp the handles.

(b) Push outward and up with your arms until the pads are at shoulder height. Lead with your elbows rather than trying to lift the bars with your hands. Return to the starting position.

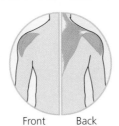

Front   Back

Muscles developed: Deltoids, trapezius

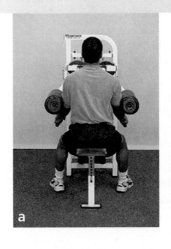
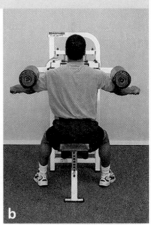

EXERCISE 8   Triceps Extension

Note: *This exercise focuses on some of the same muscles as the assisted dip (Exercise 9); choose an appropriate exercise for your program based on your preferences and equipment availability.*

Instructions:

(a) Adjust the seat so that your back is straight and your arms rest comfortably against the top and side pads. Place your arms on the support cushions and grasp the hand grips with palms facing inward.

(b) Keeping your upper body still, extend your elbows as much as possible. Return to the starting position.

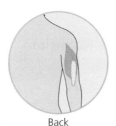

Back

Muscles developed: Triceps

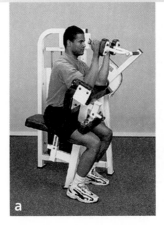
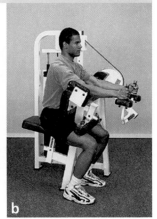

EXERCISE 9   Assisted Dip

Instructions: Set the weight according to the amount of assistance you need to complete a set of dips—the heavier the weight, the more assistance provided.

(a) Stand or kneel on the assist platform with your body between the dip bar. With your elbows fully extended and palms facing your body, support your weight on your hands.

(b) Lower your body until your upper arms are approximately parallel with the bars. Then push up until you reach the starting position.

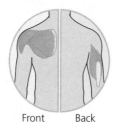

Front   Back

Muscles developed:

Triceps, deltoids, pectoralis major

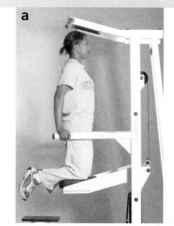

a

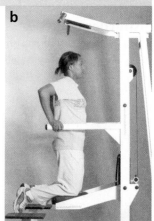

b

EXERCISE 10   Leg Press

Instructions: Sit or lie on the seat or bench, depending on the type of machine and the manufacturer's instructions. Your head, back, hips, and buttocks should be pressed against the machine pads. Loosely grasp the handles at the side of the machine.

(a) Begin with your feet flat on the foot platform about shoulder-width apart. Extend your legs but do not forcefully lock your knees.

(b) Slowly lower the weight by bending your knees and flexing your hips until your knees are bent at about a 90-degree angle or your heels start to lift off the foot platform. Keep your lower back flat against the support pad. Then extend your knees and return to the starting position.

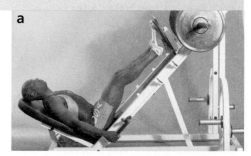

a

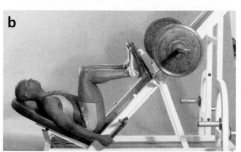

b

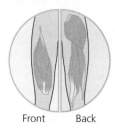

Muscles developed:

Gluteus maximus, quadriceps, hamstrings

Front   Back

EXERCISE 11   Leg Extension (Knee Extension)

Instructions:

(a) Adjust the seat so that the pads rest comfortably on top of your lower shins. Loosely grasp the handles.

(b) Extend your knees until they are almost straight. Return to the starting position.

Knee extensions cause kneecap pain in some people. If you have kneecap pain during this exercise, check with an orthopedic specialist before repeating it.

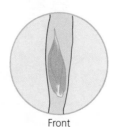

Front

Muscles developed:

Quadriceps

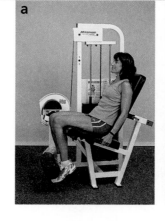

a

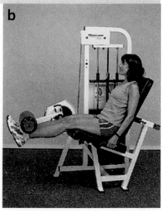

b

EXERCISE 12   Seated Leg Curl

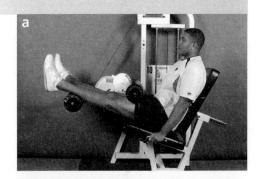

Instructions:

(a) Sit on the seat with your back against the back pad and the leg pad below your calf muscles.

(b) Flex your knees until your lower and upper legs form a 90 degree angle. Return to the starting position.

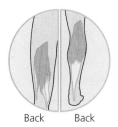

Back   Back

Muscles developed:
Hamstrings, gastrocnemius

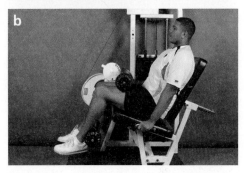

EXERCISE 13   Heel Raise

Instructions:

(a) Stand with your head between the pads and one pad on each shoulder. The balls of your feet should be on the platform. Lightly grasp the handles.

(b) Press down with your toes while lifting your heels. Return to the starting position. Changing the direction your feet are pointing (straight ahead, inward, and outward) will work different portions of your calf muscles.

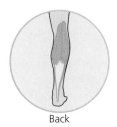

Back

Muscles developed:
Gastrocnemius, soleus

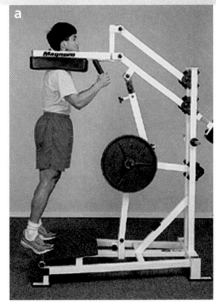

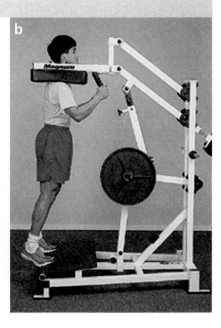

Note: *Abdominal machines and low-back machines are not recommended because of injury risk. Refer to the Free Weights exercise section for appropriate exercises to strengthen the abdominal and low-back muscles. For the rectus abdominus, obliques, and transvere abdominus, perform curl-ups (Exercise 9 in the Free Weights section), and for the erector spinae and quadratus lumborum, perform the spine extension and the isometric side bridge (Exercises 10 and 11 in the Free Weights section).*

Will I gain weight if I do resistance exercises?

Your weight probably will not change significantly as a result of a general fitness program: 1 set of 8–12 repetitions of 8–10 exercises. You will tend to increase muscle mass and lose body fat, so your weight will stay about the same. You may notice a change in how your clothes fit, however, because muscle is more dense than fat. Increased muscle mass will help you control body fat. Muscle increases your metabolism, which means you burn more calories every day. If you combine resistance exercises with cardiovascular (endurance) exercises, you will be on your way to developing a healthier body composition. Concentrate on fat loss rather than weight loss.

Do I need more protein in my diet when I train with weights?

No. Although there is some evidence that power athletes involved in heavy training have a higher-than-normal protein requirement, there is no reason for most people to consume extra protein. Most Canadians take in more protein than they need, so even if there is an increased protein need during heavy training, it is probably supplied by the average diet. (See Chapter 7 for more on dietary needs of athletes and specific recommendations for protein intake.)

What causes muscle soreness the day or two following a weight training workout?

The muscle pain you feel a day or two after a heavy weight training workout is caused by injury to the muscle fibres and surrounding connective tissue. Contrary to popular belief, delayed-onset muscle soreness is not caused by lactic acid buildup. Scientists believe that injury to muscle fibres causes inflammation, which in turn causes the release of chemicals that break down part of the muscle tissue and cause

pain. After a bout of intense exercise that causes muscle injury and delayed-onset muscle soreness, the muscles produce protective proteins that prevent soreness during future workouts. If you don't work out regularly, you lose these protective proteins and become susceptible to muscle soreness again.

Will strength training improve my sports performance?

Strength developed in the weight room does not automatically increase your power in sports such as skiing, tennis, or cycling. Hitting a forehand in tennis and making a turn on skis are precise skills that require coordination between your nervous system and muscles. In skilled people, movements become reflex; you don't think about them when you do them. Increasing strength can disturb this coordination. Only by simultaneously practising a sport and improving fitness can you expect to become more powerful in the skill. Practice helps you integrate your new strength with your skills, which makes you more powerful. Consequently, you can hit the ball harder in tennis or make more graceful turns on the ski slopes. (Refer to Chapter 2 for more on the concept of specificity of physical training.)

Will I improve faster if I train every day?

No. Your muscles need time to recover between training sessions. Doing resistance exercises every day will cause you to become overtrained, which will increase your chance of injury and impede your progress. If your strength training program has reached a plateau, try one of these strategies:

- Vary the number of sets. If you have been performing 1 set of each exercise, add sets.

- Train less frequently. If you are currently training the same muscle groups three or more times per week, you may not be allowing

your muscles to fully recover from intense workouts.

- Change exercises. Using different exercises for a particular muscle group may stimulate further strength development.

- Vary the load and number of repetitions. Try increasing or decreasing the loads you are using and changing the number of repetitions accordingly.

- If you are training alone, find a motivated training partner. A partner can encourage you and assist you with difficult lifts, forcing you to work harder.

If I stop weight training, will my muscles turn to fat?

No. Fat and muscle are two different kinds of tissue, and one cannot turn into the other. Muscles that aren't used become smaller (atrophy), and body fat may increase if caloric intake exceeds calories burned. Although the result of inactivity may be smaller muscles and more fat, the change is caused by two separate processes.

Should I wear a weight belt when I lift?

Until recently, most experts advised people to wear weight belts. However, several studies have shown that weight belts do not prevent back injuries and may, in fact, increase the risk of injury by encouraging people to lift more weight than they are capable of lifting with good form. Although wearing a belt may allow you to lift more weight in some lifts, you may not get the full benefit of your program because use of a weight belt reduces the effectiveness of the workout on the muscles that help support your spine.

Do abdominal machines advertised on television really work?

Studies comparing major types of abdominal exercises have found that "ab" machines are less effective than curl-ups and sit-ups for developing the abdominal muscles. There is no advantage to using an abdominal machine as compared to performing crunches—and a machine may cost $50 or more. A 2004 review of abdominal machines by *Consumer Reports* concluded that no infomercial machine was worth the money and suggested that consumers stick to crunches, possibly with an exercise ball for added difficulty.

Can activities such as yoga and tai chi chuan be used to build muscular strength and endurance?

Each of these forms of exercise involve carefully controlled body movements and precise body positions, so they can help build muscular strength and endurance—although probably not to the degree of traditional weight training exercises.

- Yoga involves a series of physical postures that stretch, strengthen, and relax different parts of the body. Some forms of yoga are much more vigorous than others but most emphasize breathing, stretching, body awareness, and balance.

- Taijíquan (pronounced tie jee choo-en), commonly referred to as "tai chi chuan" or simply "tai chi," is a martial art consisting of a series of slow, fluid, elegant movements that promote relaxation and concentration as well as the development of body awareness, balance, and muscular strength.

To obtain the greatest benefit from these techniques with the least risk of injury, it's best to begin by finding a qualified instructor. See Chapter 10 for more on the use of yoga and tai chi specifically for stress management.

What is circuit training?

Circuit training is a system of organizing a series of exercises that are performed consecutively. Exercises for different muscle groups follow each other, providing a well-rounded workout and helping to delay the onset of fatigue. By moving directly from one exercise to the next, you can keep your heart rate in your training zone and so train both your muscles and your cardiorespiratory system.

Circuit training can be done at home using calisthenic exercises and/or exercises with free weights, or circuits can be put together at a fitness centre. A circuit may include just strength training exercises or may alternate between weight training machines and cardiorespiratory endurance stations. For example, you may perform a set of bench presses followed by 3 minutes on a treadmill and then a set of shoulder presses. Circuit training can be an effective method for building cardiorespiratory endurance and muscular strength during the same workout. It is important to warm up thoroughly before a circuit training workout and to cool down after. Other safety tips include maintaining proper form for each exercise (not rushing), not lifting beyond the limits of your strength, and keeping your heart rate within your target zone.

SUMMARY

- Hypertrophy, or increased muscle fibre size, occurs when weight training causes the number of myofibrils to increase; total muscle size thereby increases. Strength also increases through muscle learning. Most women do not develop large muscles from weight training.

- Improvements in muscular strength and endurance lead to enhanced physical performance, protection against injury, improved body composition, better self-image, improved muscle and bone health with aging, reduced risk of chronic disease, and decreased risk of premature death.

- Muscular strength can be assessed by determining the amount of weight that can be lifted in one repetition of an exercise; muscular endurance can be assessed by determining the number of repetitions of a particular exercise that can be performed.

- Static (isometric) exercises involve contraction without movement. They are most useful when a person is recovering from an injury or surgery or needs to overcome weak points in a range of motion.

- Dynamic (isotonic) exercises involve contraction that results in movement. The two most common types are constant resistance (free weights) and variable resistance (many weight machines).

- Free weights and weight machines have pluses and minuses for developing fitness, although machines tend to be safer.

- Lifting heavy weights for only a few repetitions helps develop strength. Lifting lighter weights for more repetitions helps develop muscular endurance.
- A strength training program for general fitness includes at least 1 set of 8–12 repetitions (enough to cause fatigue) of 8–10 exercises, along with warm-up and cool-down periods; the program should be carried out 2–3 nonconsecutive times a week.
- Safety guidelines for strength training include using proper technique, using spotters and collars when necessary, and taking care of injuries.
- Natural Health Products or drugs that are promoted as instant or quick "cures" usually don't work and are either dangerous or expensive or both.

FOR FURTHER EXPLORATION

Organizations and Websites

Canada's Physical Activity Guide. Offers many suggestions for incorporating physical activity into everyday life; also includes the Physical Activity Readiness Questionnaire (PAR-Q).
> http://www.phac-aspc.gc.ca/pau-uap/paguide/

Exercise: A Guide from the National Institute on Aging. Provides practical advice on fitness for seniors; includes animated instructions for specific weight training exercises.
> http://www.nia.nih.gov/HealthInformation/Publications/ExerciseGuide/

Georgia State University: Strength Training. Provides information about the benefits of strength training and how to develop a safe and effective program; also includes illustrations of a variety of exercises.
> http://www.gsu.edu/~wwwfit/strength.html

Human Anatomy Online. Provides text, illustrations, and animation about the muscular system, nerve-muscle connections, muscular contraction, and other topics.
> http://www.innerbody.com/htm/body.html

National Strength and Conditioning Association. Professional organization that focuses on strength development for fitness and athletic performance.
> http://www.nsca-lift.org

Pilates Association of Canada. Provides information about Pilates and about instructor certification. Can direct you to a certfied Pilates instructor in your area.
> http://www.pilatesassociationofcanada.ca/

University of California, San Diego/Muscle Physiology Home Page. Provides an introduction to muscle physiology, including information about types of muscle fibres and energy cycles.
> http://muscle.ucsd.edu

University of Michigan/Muscles in Action. Interactive descriptions of muscle movements.
> http://www.med.umich.edu/lrc/Hypermuscle/Hyper.html

See also the listings in Chapter 2.

LAB 4.1 Assessing Your Current Level of Muscular Strength

connect ACTIVITY DO IT ONLINE

To assess your strength level and track the progress of your strength training program, you can use data from your weight training workouts to calculate 1-RM. On your workout card, record the amount of weight you lift and the number of repetitions you can complete using that weight. Perform as many repetitions that you can using correct form for each exercise. Use the table below to determine the 1-RM that corresponds to the amount of weight and number of repetitions you lifted. Fill in the following chart to use this method to track your strength gains in major muscle groups as your strength training program progresses. Fill in additional exercises as needed.

Exercise	Date_____ Weight	Reps	1-RM	Date_____ Weight	Reps	1-RM	Date_____ Weight	Reps	1-RM
Bench press									
Overhead press									
Lat pull									
Biceps curl									
Leg press									
Leg extension									

To use the following table to determine 1-RM, find the weight you lifted in the left column and move across the row until you reach the column for the number of repetitions you performed; the number in the corresponding row and column is your 1-RM for that exercise.

Repetitions

Wt (lb)	1	2	3	4	5	6	7	8	9	10	11	12
20	20	21	21	22	23	23	24	25	26	27	28	29
25	25	26	26	27	28	29	30	31	32	33	35	36
30	30	31	32	33	34	35	36	37	39	40	42	43
35	35	36	37	38	39	41	42	43	45	47	48	50
40	40	41	42	44	45	46	48	50	51	53	55	58
45	45	46	48	49	51	52	54	56	58	60	62	65
50	50	51	53	55	56	58	60	62	64	67	69	72
55	55	57	58	60	62	64	66	68	71	73	76	79
60	60	62	64	65	68	70	72	74	77	80	83	86
65	65	67	69	71	73	75	78	81	84	87	90	94
70	70	72	74	76	79	81	84	87	90	93	97	101
75	75	77	79	82	84	87	90	93	96	100	104	108
80	80	82	85	87	90	93	96	99	103	107	111	115
85	85	87	90	93	96	99	102	106	109	113	118	122
90	90	93	95	98	101	105	108	112	116	120	125	130
100	95	98	101	104	107	110	114	118	122	127	132	137

(Continued)

100	100	103	106	109	113	116	120	124	129	133	139	144
105	105	108	111	115	118	122	126	130	135	140	145	151
110	110	113	116	120	124	128	132	137	141	147	152	158
115	115	118	122	125	129	134	138	143	148	153	159	166
120	120	123	127	131	135	139	144	149	154	160	166	173
125	125	129	132	136	141	145	150	155	161	167	173	180
130	130	134	138	142	146	151	156	161	167	173	180	187
135	135	139	143	147	152	157	162	168	174	180	187	194
140	140	144	148	153	158	163	168	174	180	187	194	202
145	145	149	154	158	163	168	174	180	186	193	201	209
150	150	154	159	164	169	174	180	186	193	200	208	216
155	155	159	164	169	174	180	186	192	199	207	215	223
160	160	165	169	175	180	186	192	199	206	213	222	230
165	165	170	175	180	186	192	198	205	212	220	229	238
170	170	175	180	185	191	197	204	211	219	227	235	245
175	175	180	185	191	197	203	210	217	225	233	242	252
180	180	185	191	196	203	209	216	223	231	240	249	259
185	185	190	196	202	208	215	222	230	238	247	256	266
190	190	195	201	207	214	221	228	236	244	253	263	274
195	195	201	206	213	219	226	234	242	251	260	270	281
200	200	206	212	218	225	232	240	248	257	267	277	288
205	205	211	217	224	231	238	246	255	264	273	284	295
210	210	216	222	229	236	244	252	261	270	280	291	303
215	215	221	228	235	242	250	258	267	276	287	298	310
220	220	226	233	240	248	256	264	273	283	293	305	317
225	225	231	238	245	253	261	270	279	289	300	312	324
230	230	237	244	251	259	267	276	286	296	307	319	331
235	235	242	249	256	264	273	282	292	302	313	325	339
240	240	247	254	262	270	279	288	298	309	320	332	346
245	245	252	259	267	276	285	294	304	315	327	339	353
250	250	257	265	273	281	290	300	310	322	333	346	360
255	255	262	270	278	287	296	306	317	328	340	353	367
260	260	267	275	284	293	302	312	323	334	347	360	375
265	265	273	281	289	298	308	318	329	341	353	367	382
270	270	278	286	295	304	314	324	335	347	360	374	389
275	275	283	291	300	309	319	330	341	354	367	381	396
280	280	288	296	305	315	325	336	348	360	373	388	403
285	285	293	302	311	321	331	342	354	367	380	395	411
290	290	298	307	316	326	337	348	360	373	387	402	418
295	295	303	312	322	332	343	354	366	379	393	409	425
300	300	309	318	327	338	348	360	372	386	400	416	432

Table generated using the Brzycki equation: $1\text{-RM} = \text{weight (kg)}/(1.0278 - (0.0278 \times \text{repetitions}))$.

SOURCES: Brzycki, M. 1993. Strength testing. Predicting a one-rep max from a reps-to-fatigue. *Journal of Physical Education,* Recreation, and Dance 64: 88–90, January 1993, a publication of the American Alliance for Health, Physical Education, Recreation, and Dance, http://www.aahperd.org. Reprinted with permission.

CSEP Adapted Prediction of 1 RM

Earlier in the chapter the CSEP Adapted Prediction of 1 RM was discussed as a method by which your 1 RM may be estimated. If you are creating or maintaining a muscle fitness training program, you may be able to more quickly assess your progress by using this table. For example, if you complete 6 repetitions, you can estimate the weight at which you completed the 6 repetitions to be 85% of your repetitions maximum, i.e., 6 reps at 70kg = 70×0.85 = an estimated RM of 59.5kg.

Repetitions Completed	% 1 RM
1	100
2	95
3	93
4	90
5	87
6	85
7	83
8	80
9	77
10	75

The Maximum Bench Press Test

Equipment

If free weights are used, the following equipment is needed:

1. Flat bench (with or without racks)
2. Barbell
3. Assorted weight plates, with collars to hold them in place
4. One or two spotters
5. Weight scale

If a weight machine is preferred, use the following equipment:
1. Universal Gym Dynamic Variable Resistance machine
2. Weight scale.

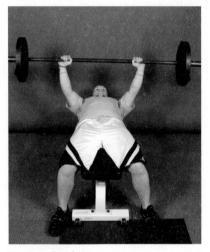

Maximum bench press test.

Preparation

Try a few bench presses with a small amount of weight so you can practise your technique, warm up your muscles, and, if you use free weights, coordinate your movements with those of your spotters. Weigh yourself and record the results.

Body weight: _____ lb

Instructions

1. Use a weight that is lower than the amount you believe you can lift. For free weights, men should begin with a weight about 2/3 of their body weight; women should begin with the weight of just the bar (45 lb).

2. Lie on the bench with your feet firmly on the floor. If you are using a weight machine, grasp the handles with palms away from you; the tops of the handles should be aligned with the tops of your armpits.
   If you are using free weights, grasp the bar slightly wider than shoulder width with your palms away from you. If you have one spotter, she or he should stand directly behind the bench; if you have two spotters, they should stand to the side, one at each end of the barbell. Signal to the spotter when you are ready to begin the test by saying "1, 2, 3." On "3," the spotter should help you lift the weight to a point over your midchest (nipple line).

3. Push the handles or barbell until your arms are fully extended. Exhale as you lift. If you are using free weights, the weight moves from a low point at the chest straight up. Keep your feet firmly on the floor, don't arch your back, and push the weight evenly with your right and left arms. Don't bounce the weight on your chest.

4. Rest for several minutes, then repeat the lift with a heavier weight. It will probably take several attempts to determine the maximum amount of weight you can lift (1 RM).

1 RM: _____ lb Check one: _____ Universal _____ Free weights _____ Other

5. If you used free weights, convert your free weights bench press score to an estimated value for 1 RM on the Universal bench press using the appropriate formula:

Males: Estimated Universal 1 RM = (1.016 × free weights 1 RM _____lb) + 18.41 = _____lb

Females: Estimated Universal 1 RM = (0.848 × free weights 1 RM _____lb) + 21.37 = _____lb

Rating Your Bench Press Result

1. Divide your Universal 1 RM value by your body weight.

1 RM _____ lb ÷ body weight _____ lb = _____

2. Find this ratio in the table below to determine your bench press strength rating. Record the rating here and in the chart at the end of this lab.

Bench press strength rating: _____

Strength Ratings for the Maximum Bench Press Test

	Pounds Lifted/Body Weight (lb)					
Men	*Very Poor*	*Poor*	*Fair*	*Good*	*Excellent*	*Superior*
Age: Under 20	Below 0.89	0.89–1.05	1.06–1.18	1.19–1.33	1.34–1.75	Above 1.75
20–29	Below 0.88	0.88–0.98	0.99–1.13	1.14–1.31	1.32–1.62	Above 1.62
30–39	Below 0.78	0.78–0.87	0.88–0.97	0.98–1.11	1.12–1.34	Above 1.34
40–49	Below 0.72	0.72–0.79	0.80–0.87	0.88–0.99	1.00–1.19	Above 1.19
50–59	Below 0.63	0.63–0.70	0.71–0.78	0.79–0.89	0.90–1.04	Above 1.04
60 and over	Below 0.57	0.57–0.65	0.66–0.71	0.72–0.81	0.82–0.93	Above 0.93
Women						
Age: Under 20	Below 0.53	0.53–0.57	0.58–0.64	0.65–0.76	0.77–0.87	Above 0.87
20–29	Below 0.51	0.51–0.58	0.59–0.69	0.70–0.79	0.80–1.00	Above 1.00
30–39	Below 0.47	0.47–0.52	0.53–0.59	0.60–0.69	0.70–0.81	Above 0.81
40–49	Below 0.43	0.43–0.49	0.50–0.53	0.54–0.61	0.62–0.76	Above 0.76
50–59	Below 0.39	0.39–0.43	0.44–0.47	0.48–0.54	0.55–0.67	Above 0.67
60 and over	Below 0.38	0.38–0.42	0.43–0.46	0.47–0.53	0.54–0.71	Above 0.71

SOURCE: Based on norms from the Cooper Institute for Aerobics Research, Dallas, Texas; from *The Physical Fitness Specialist Manual*, Revised 2002. Used with permission.

Functional Leg Strength Tests

The following tests assess functional leg strength using squats. Most people do squats improperly, increasing their risk of knee and back pain. Before you add weight-bearing squats to your weight training program, you should determine your functional leg strength, check your ability to squat properly, and give yourself a chance to master squatting movements. The following leg strength tests will help you in each of these areas.

These tests are progressively more difficult, so do not move to the next test until you have scored at least a 3 on the current test. On each test, give yourself a rating of 0, 1, 3, or 5, as described in the instructions that follow the fifth test.

1. Chair Squat

Instructions

1. Sit up straight in a chair with your back resting against the backrest and your arms at your sides. Your feet should be placed more than shoulder-width apart so that you can get them under the body.

2. Begin the motion of rising out of the chair by flexing (bending) at the hips—not the back. Then squat up using a hip hinge movement (no spine movement). Stand without rocking forward, bending your back, or using external support, and keep your head in a neutral position.

3. Return to the sitting position while maintaining a straight back and keeping your weight centred over your feet. Your thighs should abduct (spread) as you sit back in the chair. Use your rear hip and thigh muscles as much as possible as you sit.

Do five repetitions.

Your rating: _____ (See rating instructions that follow.)

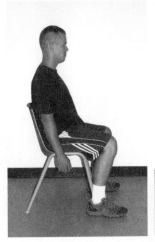
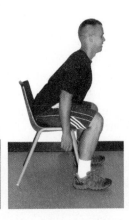
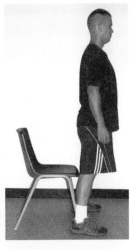

2. Single-Leg Step-Up

Instructions

1. Stand facing a bench, with your right foot placed on the middle of the bench, right knee bent at 90 degrees, and arms at your sides.

2. Step up on the bench until your right leg is straight, maximizing the use of the hip muscles.

3. Return to the starting position. Keep your hips stable, back straight, chest up, shoulders back, and head neutral during the entire movement.

Do five repetitions for each leg.

Your rating: _____ (See rating instructions that follow.)

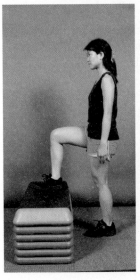
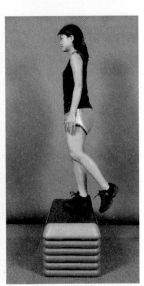

3. Unweighted Squat

Instructions

1. Stand with your feet placed slightly more than shoulder-width apart, toes pointed out slightly, hands on hips or across your chest, head neutral, and back straight. Centre your weight over your arches or slightly behind.

2. Squat down, keeping your weight centred over your arches and actively flexing (bending) your hips until your legs break parallel. During the movement, keep your back straight, shoulders back, and chest out, and let your thighs part to the side so that you are "squatting between your legs."

3. Push back up to the starting position, hinging at the hips and not with the spine, maximizing the use of the rear hip and thigh muscles, and maintaining a straight back and neutral head position.

Do five repetitions.

Your rating: _____ (See rating instructions that follow.)

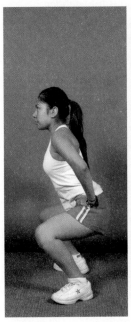
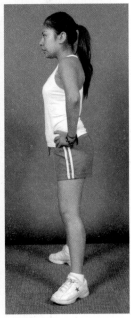

4. Single-Leg Lunge-Squat with Rear-Foot Support

Instructions

1. Stand about 90 cm or 3 feet in front of a bench (with your back to the bench).
2. Place the instep of your left foot on the bench, and put most of your weight on your right leg (your left leg should be bent), with your hands at your sides.
3. Squat on your right leg until your thigh is parallel with the floor. Keep your back straight, chest up, shoulders back, and head neutral.
4. Return to the starting position.

   Do three repetitions for each leg.

   Your rating: _____ (See rating instructions that follow.)

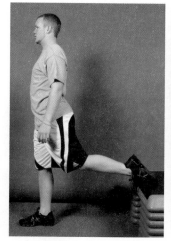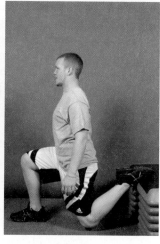

5. Single-Leg Squat from a Bench Preparation

This exercise is the most difficult of the functional leg tests. Use spotters if you haven't done this exercise before or if you do not have the leg strength to perform three repetitions easily.

Instructions

1. Stand on the middle of a bench with your weight on your right leg and your arms extended in front of you. During the test, maintain a straight back and keep your weight over the arches of your feet.
2. Squat down on your right leg until your thigh is parallel with the ground, maximizing the use of your rear hip and thigh muscles. Do not rock forward on your toes or bend at the waist, and maintain a neutral head position.
3. Return to the starting position (stand up) by straightening your right hip and knee, maximizing the use of your rear hip and thigh muscles.

   Perform three repetitions for each leg.

   Your rating: _____ (See rating instructions that follow.)

Rating Your Functional Leg Strength Test Results

5 points: Performed the exercise properly with good back and thigh position, weight centred over the middle or rear of the foot, chest out, and shoulders back; good use of hip muscles on the way down and on the way up, with head in a neutral position throughout the movement; maintained good form during all repetitions; abducted (spread) the thighs on the way down during chair squats and double-leg squats; for single-leg exercises, showed good strength on both sides; for single-leg lunge-squat with rear-foot support, maintained straight back, and knees stayed behind toes.

3 points: Weight was forward on the toes, with some rounding of the back; used thigh muscles excessively, with little use of hip muscles; head and chest were too far forward; showed little abduction of the thighs during double-leg squats; when going down for single-leg exercises, one side was stronger than the other; form deteriorated with repetitions; for single-leg lunge-squat with rear-foot support and single-leg squat from a bench, could not reach parallel (thigh parallel with floor).

1 point: Had difficulty performing the movement, rocking forward and rounding back badly; used thigh muscles excessively, with little use of hip muscles on the way up or on the way down; chest and head were forward; on unweighted squats, had difficulty reaching parallel; and showed little abduction of the thighs; on single-leg exercises, one leg was markedly stronger than the other; could not perform multiple repetitions.

0 points: Could not perform the exercise.

Hand Grip Strength Test

Equipment

Grip strength dynamometer

Preparation

If necessary, adjust the hand grip size on the dynamometer into a position that is comfortable for you; then lock the grip in place. The second joint of your fingers should fit snugly under the handle of the dynamometer.

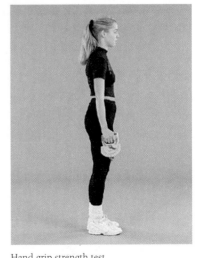

Hand grip strength test.

Instructions

1. Stand with the hand to be tested first at your side, away from your body. The dynamometer should be in line with your forearm and held at the level of your thigh. Squeeze the dynamometer as hard as possible without moving your arm; exhale as you squeeze. During the test, don't let the dynamometer touch your body or any other object.

2. Perform two trials with each hand. Rest for about a minute between trials. Record the scores for each hand to the nearest kilogram.

Right hand: Trial 1: _____ kg   Trial 2: _____ kg   Right hand best trial _____ kg

Left hand: Trial 1: _____ kg   Trial 2: _____ kg   Left hand best trial _____ kg

Rating Your Hand Grip Strength

Refer to the table for a rating of your grip strength. Record the rating below and in the chart at the end of this lab. Total score (sum of the best trial for each hand) _____   Rating for hand grip strength: _____

		Grip Strength* (kg)			
Men	Needs Improvement	Fair	Good	Very Good	Excellent
Age: 15–19	≤ 78	79–89	90–97	98–107	≥ 108
20–29	≤ 83	84–94	95–103	104–114	≥ 115
30–39	≤ 83	84–94	95–103	104–114	≥ 115
40–49	≤ 79	80–87	88–96	97–107	≥ 108
50–59	≤ 75	76–83	84–91	92–100	≥ 101
60–69	≤ 72	73–83	84–90	91–99	≥ 100
Women					
Age: 15–19	≤ 47	48–52	53–59	60–67	≥ 68
20–29	≤ 51	52–57	58–62	63–69	≥ 70
30–39	≤ 50	51–57	58–62	63–70	≥ 71
40–49	≤ 48	49–53	54–60	61–68	≥ 69
50–59	≤ 44	45–48	49–53	54–60	≥ 61
60–69	≤ 40	41–44	45–47	48–53	≥ 54

*Combined right and left hand grip strength.

SOURCE: *Canadian Physical Activity, Fitness & Lifestyle Approach: CSEP—Health & Fitness Program's Appraisal and Counselling Strategy*, 3rd edition. © 2003. Reprinted with permission from the Canadian Society for Exercise Physiology.

Summary of Results

Maximum bench press test from either the 1 RM test or the multiple-repetition test:

Weight pressed: _____ kg   Rating: _____

Functional leg strength tests (0–5): Chair squat: _____ Single-leg step-up: _____ Unweighted squat: _____

Single-leg lunge-squat with rear-foot support: _____ Single-leg squat from a bench: _____

Hand grip strength test: Total score: _____ kg   Rating: _____

Remember that muscular strength is specific: Your ratings may vary considerably for different parts of your body.

Using Your Results

How did you score? Are you at all surprised by your rating for muscular strength? Are you satisfied with your current rating? When examining your ratings, CSEP suggests you consider the ratings to indicate:

"needs improvement" means health risks are present

"fair" means some health benefits are obtained in addition to health risks being present

"good" indicates that some health benefits are obtained

"very good" means that considerable health benefits are seen

"excellent" means optimal health benefits are obtained

If you're not satisfied, set a realistic goal for improvement: _____

Are you satisfied with your current level of muscular strength as evidenced in your daily life—for example, your ability to lift objects, climb stairs, and engage in sports and recreational activities?

If you're not satisfied, set some realistic goals for improvement:

What should you do next? Enter the results of this lab in the Preprogram Assessment column in Appendix C. If you've set goals for improvement, begin planning your strength training program by completing the plan in Lab 4.3. After several weeks of your program, complete this lab again and enter the results in the Postprogram Assessment column of Appendix C. How do the results compare?

Name _____   Section _____   Date _____

LAB 4.2   Assessing Your Current Level of Muscular Endurance

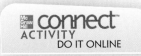

For best results, don't do any strenuous weight training within 48 hours of any test. To assess endurance of the abdominal muscles, perform the partial curl-up test. To assess endurance of muscles in the upper body, perform the push-up test. To assess endurance of the muscles in the lower body, perform the squat endurance test.

The Partial Curl-Up Test

Equipment

1. Four 15-cm strips of self-stick Velcro or heavy tape
2. Ruler
3. Metronome
4. Partner
5. Mat (optional)

Preparation

Affix the strips of Velcro or long strips of tape on the mat or testing surface. Place the strips 10 centimetres apart.

Instructions

1. Start by lying on your back on the floor or mat, arms straight and by your sides, shoulders relaxed, palms down and on the floor, and fingers straight. Adjust your position so that the longest fingertip of each hand touches the end of the near strip of Velcro or tape. Your knees should be bent about 90 degrees, with your feet about 30–45 centimetres from your buttocks.

2. Set the cadence of the metronome to 50 beats per minute. To perform a curl-up, flex your spine while sliding your fingers across the floor until the fingertips of each hand reach the second strip of Velcro or tape. Then, return to the starting position; the shoulders must be returned to touch the mat between curl-ups, but the head need not touch. Shoulders must remain relaxed throughout the curl-up, and feet and buttocks must stay on the floor. Breathe easily, exhaling during the lift phase of the curl-up; do not hold your breath.

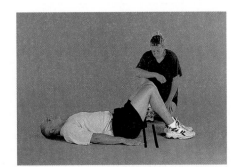

Curl-up test: (a) Starting position.

3. The palms of the hands and the heels must remain in contact with the mat throughout the test. You are not permitted to anchor your feet during the test.

4. Once your partner says "go," perform as many partial curl-ups as you can at the metronome pace with correct form. Your partner counts the curl-ups you perform and calls a stop to the test if she or he notices any incorrect form such as the heels or palms lifting off the floor, or if you are unable to stay on pace with the metronome, or are experiencing discomfort.

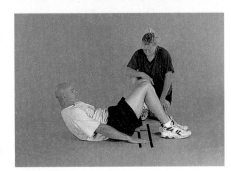

(b) Curl-up.

5. You are to perform as many consecutive partial curl-ups to the metronome cadence as possible in a one-minute period. A maximum of 25 partial curl-ups can be completed in one minute.

   Number of partial curl-ups: _____

Rating Your Partial Curl-Up Test Result

Your score is the number of completed partial curl-ups. Refer to the appropriate portion of the following table for a rating of your abdominal muscular endurance. Record your rating below and in the chart at the end of this lab.

Rating: _____

Ratings for the Partial Curl-Up Test

		Number of Partial Curl-Ups				
Men		*Needs Improvement*	*Fair*	*Good*	*Very Good*	*Excellent*
Age:	15–19	≤ 15	16–20	21–22	23–24	≥ 25
	20–29	≤ 10	11–15	16–20	21–24	≥ 25
	30–39	≤ 10	11–14	15–17	18–24	≥ 25
	40–49	≤ 5	6–12	13–17	18–24	≥ 25
	50–59	≤ 7	8–10	11–16	17–24	≥ 25
	60–69	≤ 5	6–10	11–15	16–24	≥ 25
Women						
Age:	15–19	≤ 11	12–16	17–21	22–24	≥ 25
	20–29	≤ 4	5–13	14–17	18–24	≥ 25
	30–39	≤ 5	6–9	10–18	19–24	≥ 25
	40–49	≤ 3	4–10	11–18	19–24	≥ 25
	50–59	≤ 5	6–9	10–18	19–24	≥ 25
	60–69	≤ 2	3–7	8–16	17–24	≥ 25

SOURCE: *Canadian Physical Activity, Fitness & Lifestyle Approach: CSEP—Health & Fitness Program's Appraisal and Counselling Strategy*, 3rd edition. © 2003. Reprinted with permission from the Canadian Society for Exercise Physiology.

The Push-Up Test

Equipment:

Mat or towel (optional)

Preparation

In this test, you will perform either standard push-ups or modified push-ups, in which you support yourself with your knees. The modified technique reduces the need for upper-body strength in a test of muscular endurance. Therefore, for an accurate assessment of upper-body endurance, men should perform standard push-ups and women should perform modified push-ups. (However, in using push-ups as part of a strength training program, individuals should choose the technique most appropriate for increasing their level of strength and endurance—regardless of gender.)

Instructions

1. *For push-ups:* Start in the push-up position with your body supported by your hands and feet. *For modified push-ups:* Start in the modified push-up position with your body supported by your hands and knees. *For both positions,* your arms and your back should be straight and your fingers pointed forward.

2. Lower your chest to the floor with your back straight, and then return to the starting position.

3. Perform as many push-ups or modified push-ups as you can without stopping.

   Number of push-ups: _____ or number of modified push-ups: _____

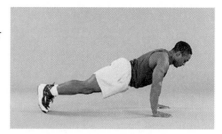

(a) Push-up.

Rating Your Push-Up Test Result

Your score is the number of completed push-ups or modified push-ups. Refer to the appropriate portion of the table below for a rating of your upper-body endurance. Record your rating below and in the chart at the end of this lab.

Rating: _____

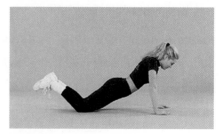

(b) Modified push-up.

Ratings for the Push-Up and Modified Push-Up Tests

Number of Push-Ups

Men		Needs Improvement	Fair	Good	Very Good	Excellent
Age:	15–19	≤ 17	18–22	23–28	29–38	≥ 39
	20–29	≤ 16	17–21	22–28	29–35	≥ 36
	30–39	≤ 11	12–16	17–21	22–29	≥ 30
	40–49	≤ 9	10–12	13–16	17–24	≥ 25
	50–59	≤ 6	7–9	10–12	13–20	≥ 21
	60–69	≤ 4	5–7	8–10	11–17	≥ 18

Number of Modified Push-Ups

Women		Needs Improvement	Fair	Good	Very Good	Excellent
Age:	15–19	≤ 11	12–17	18–24	25–32	≥ 33
	20–29	≤ 9	10–14	15–20	21–29	≥ 30
	30–39	≤ 7	8–12	13–19	20–26	≥ 27
	40–49	≤ 4	5–10	11–14	15–23	≥ 24
	50–59	≤ 1	2–6	7–10	11–20	≥ 21
	60–69	≤ 1	2–4	5–11	12–16	≥ 17

SOURCE: *The Canadian Physical Activity, Fitness and Lifestyle Approach: CSEP—Health & Fitness Program's Health-Related Appraisal & Counselling Strategy*, 3d ed., © 2003. Reprinted with permission from the Canadian Society for Exercise Physiology.

The Squat Endurance Test

Instructions

1. Stand with your feet placed slightly more than shoulder width apart, toes pointed out slightly, hands on hips or across your chest, head neutral, and back straight. Centre your weight over your arches or slightly behind.

2. Squat down, keeping your weight centred over your arches, until your thighs are parallel with the floor. Push back up to the starting position, maintaining a straight back and neutral head position.

3. Perform as many squats as you can without stopping.

   Number of squats: _____

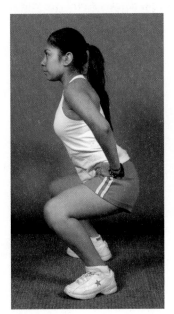

Rating Your Squat Endurance Test Result

Your score is the number of completed squats. Refer to the appropriate portion of the table for a rating of your leg muscular endurance. Record your rating below and in the summary at the end of this lab.

Rating: _____

Ratings for the Squat Endurance Test

Number of Squats Performed

Men		Very Poor	Poor	Below Average	Average	Above Average	Good	Excellent
Age:	18–25	< 25	25–30	31–34	35–38	39–43	44–49	> 49
	26–35	< 22	22–28	29–30	31–34	35–39	40–45	> 45
	36–45	< 17	17–22	23–26	27–29	30–34	35–41	> 41
	46–55	< 9	13–17	18–21	22–24	25–38	29–35	> 35
	56–65	< 9	9–12	13–16	17–20	21–24	25–31	> 31
	65+	< 7	7–10	11–14	15–18	19–21	22–28	> 28

(Continued)

Women	Very Poor	Poor	Below Average	Average	Above Average	Good	Excellent
Age: 18–25	< 18	18–24	25–28	29–32	33–36	37–43	> 43
26–35	< 20	13–20	21–24	25–28	29–32	33–39	> 39
36–45	< 7	7–14	15–18	19–22	23–26	27–33	> 33
46–55	< 5	5–9	10–13	14–17	18–21	22–27	> 27
56–65	< 3	3–6	7–9	10–12	13–17	18–24	> 24
65+	< 2	2–4	5–10	11–13	14–16	17–23	> 23

SOURCE: http://www.topendsports.com/testing/tests/home-squat.htm.

Summary of Results

Curl-up test: Number of curl-ups: _____ Rating: _____

Push-up test: Number of push-ups/modifies push-ups: _____ Rating: _____

Squat endurance test: Number of squats: _____ Rating: _____

Remember that muscular endurance is specific: Your ratings may vary considerably for different parts of your body.

Using Your Results

How did you score? Are you at all surprised by your ratings for muscular endurance? Are you satisfied with your current ratings?

If you're not satisfied, set realistic goals for improvement:

Are you satisfied with your current level of muscular endurance as evidenced in your daily life—for example, your ability to carry groceries or your books, hike, and do yardwork?

If you're not satisfied, set some realistic goals for improvement:

What should you do next? Enter the results of this lab in the Preprogram Assessment column in Appendix C. If you've set goals for improvement, begin planning your strength training program by completing the plan in Lab 4.3. After several weeks of your program, complete this lab again and enter the results in the Postprogram Assessment column of Appendix C. How do the results compare?

Name _____ Section _____ Date _____

LAB 4.3 Designing and Monitoring a Strength Training Program

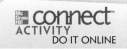

1. *Set goals.* List goals for your strength training program. Your goals can be specific or general, short or long term. In the first section, include specific, measurable goals that you can use to track the progress of your fitness program. These goals might be things like raising your upper body muscular strength rating from fair to good or being able to complete 10 repetitions of a lat pull with 50 kg of resistance. In the second section, include long-term and more qualitative goals, such as improving self-confidence and reducing your risk for back pain.

Specific Goals: Current Status   Final Goal

_____   _____
_____   _____
_____   _____

Other goals: _____
_____
_____

2. *Choose exercises.* Based on your goals, choose 8–10 exercises to perform during each weight training session. If your goal is general training for wellness, use one of the sample programs in Figure 4.2. List your exercises and the muscles they develop in the program plan below.

3. *Frequency: Choose the number of training sessions per week.* Work out at least 2 nonconsecutive days per week. Indicate the days you will train on your program plan; be sure to include days of rest to allow your body to recover.

4. *Intensity: Choose starting weights.* Experiment with different amounts of weight until you settle on a good starting weight, one that you can lift easily for 10–12 repetitions. As you progress in your program, you can add more weight. Fill in the starting weight for each exercise on the program plan.

5. *Time: Choose a starting number of sets and repetitions.* Include at least 1 set of 8–12 repetitions of each exercise. (When you add weight, you may have to decrease the number of repetitions slightly until your muscles adapt to the heavier load.) If your program is focusing on strength alone, your sets can contain fewer repetitions using a heavier load. If you are over approximately 50–60 years of age, your sets should contain more repetitions (10–15) using a lighter load. Fill in the starting number of sets and repetitions of each exercise on the program plan.

6. *Monitor your progress.* Use the workout card on the next page to monitor your progress and keep track of exercises, weights, sets, and repetitions.

Program Plan for Weight Training

Exercise	Muscle(s) Developed	Frequency (check ✓)							Intensity: Weight (lb)	Time	
		M	Tu	W	Th	F	Sa	Su		Repetitions	Sets

WORKOUT CARD FOR _____

Exercise/Date	Wt	Sets	Reps	Wt	Sets	Reps	Wt	Sets	Reps	Wt	Sets	Reps	Wt	Sets	Reps	Wt	Sets	Reps	Wt	Sets	Reps	Wt	Sets	Reps	Wt	Sets	Reps	Wt	Sets	Reps	Wt	Sets	Reps	Wt	Sets	Reps	Wt	Sets	Reps

CHAPTER 5

FLEXIBILITY AND LOW-BACK HEALTH

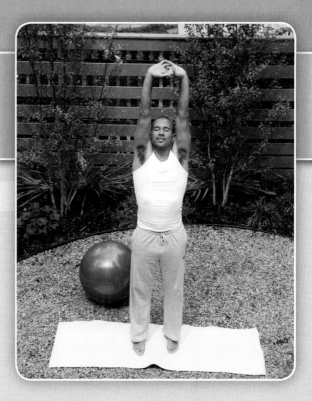

LEARNING OBJECTIVES

After reading this chapter, you should be able to

LO1 List the factors that affect a joint's flexibility

LO2 Identify the potential benefits of flexibility and stretching exercises

LO3 Describe the intensity, duration, and frequency of stretching exercises that will develop the most flexibility with the lowest risk of injury

LO4 Describe the different types of stretching exercises and how they affect muscles

LO5 List safe stretching exercises for major joints

LO6 Explain how low-back pain can be prevented and managed

TEST YOUR KNOWLEDGE

1. **Stretching exercises should be performed**

   a. at the start of a warm-up.
   b. following the active part of a warm-up.
   c. after endurance exercise or strength training.

2. **If you injure your back, it's usually best to rest in bed until the pain is completely gone.**

   True or false?

3. **It is better to hold a stretch for a short time than to "bounce" while stretching.**

   True or false?

ANSWERS

1. **B AND/OR C**. It's best to do stretching exercises when your muscles are warm, after either the active part of a warm-up (5–10 minutes of an activity such as walking or easy jogging) or an endurance or strength training workout. If a high-performance workout is your goal, it is best to stretch after exercise because stretching muscles may temporarily reduce their explosive strength.

2. **FALSE.** Prolonged bed rest may actually worsen back pain. Limit bed rest to a day or less, treat pain and inflammation with cold and then heat, and begin moderate physical activity as soon as possible.

3. **TRUE.** "Bouncing" during stretching can damage your muscles. This type of stretching, called ballistic stretching, should be used only by well-conditioned athletes for specific purposes. A person of average fitness should stretch slowly, holding each stretch for 15–30 seconds.

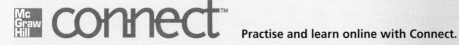

Practise and learn online with Connect.

Flexibility—the ability of a joint to move through its full **range of motion**—is important for general fitness and wellness. Flexibility is a highly adaptable physical fitness component. It increases in response to a regular program of stretching exercises and decreases with inactivity. Flexibility is also specific: Good flexibility in one joint doesn't necessarily mean good flexibility in another. You can increase your flexibility by doing regular stretching exercises for all major joints.

This chapter describes the factors that affect flexibility and the benefits of maintaining good flexibility. It provides guidelines for assessing your current level of flexibility and putting together a successful stretching program. It also examines the common problem of low-back pain.

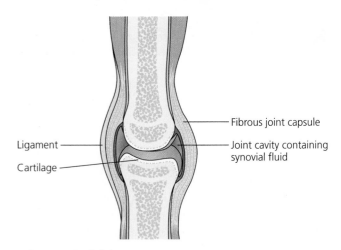

FIGURE 5.1   Basic joint structure.

5.1 TYPES OF FLEXIBILITY

There are two basic types of flexibility:

- *Static flexibility* refers to the ability to hold an extended position at one end or point in a joint's range of motion. For example, static flexibility determines how far you could extend your arm across the front of your body or out to the side. Static flexibility depends on your ability to tolerate stretched muscles, the structure of a joint, and the tightness of muscles, tendons, and ligaments.

- *Dynamic flexibility* is the ability to move a joint through its range of motion with little resistance. For example, dynamic flexibility affects your ability to pitch a ball, swing a golf club. Dynamic flexibility depends on static flexibility, but it also involves strength, coordination, and resistance to movement.

Dynamic flexibility is important for daily activities and sports. Because static flexibility is easier to measure and better researched, however, most assessment tests and stretching programs target that type of flexibility.

LO1   5.2 WHAT DETERMINES FLEXIBILITY?

The flexibility of a joint is affected by its structure, by muscle elasticity and length, and by nervous system regulation. Some factors such as joint structure, can't be changed. Other factors, such as the length of resting muscle fibres, can be changed through exercise; these factors should be the focus of a program to develop flexibility.

Joint Structure

The amount of flexibility in a joint is determined in part by the nature and structure of the joint (Figure 5.1). *Hinge* joints such as those in your fingers and knees allow only limited forward and backward movement; they lock

when fully extended. *Ball-and-socket* joints like the hip enable movement in many different directions and have a greater range of motion. Major joints are surrounded by **joint capsules**, semielastic structures that give joints strength and stability but limit movement. The bone surfaces within the joint are lined with cartilage and separated by synovial fluid to cushion the bones and reduce friction as the joint moves. Ligaments can be found both inside and outside the joint capsule and serve to strengthen and reinforce the joint.

Heredity also plays a part in joint structure and flexibility; for example, although everyone has a broad range of motion in the ball-and-socket hip joint, not everyone can do a split. Gender may also play a role. Some studies have found that women on average have greater flexibility in certain joints.[1]

Muscle Elasticity and Length

Soft tissues, including skin, muscles, tendons, and ligaments, also limit the flexibility of a joint. Muscle tissue is the key to developing flexibility because it can be lengthened if it is regularly stretched. The most important component of muscle tissue related to flexibility is the connective tissue that surrounds and envelops every part of muscle tissue, from individual muscle fibres to entire muscles. Connective tissue provides structure, elasticity, and bulk and makes up about 30% of muscle mass. Two principal types of connective tissue are **collagen,** white fibres that provide structure and support, and **elastin,** yellow fibres that are elastic and flexible.

WELLNESS TIP

Muscles shrink after injury or surgery. Rehabilitation exercises can help muscles grow again. One caution: Overuse of drugs like ibuprofen can slow the regrowth process. Use such drugs only as prescribed by your doctor.

Muscles contain both collagen and elastin, closely intertwined, so muscle tissue exhibits the properties of both types of fibres. A recently discovered structural protein in muscles called *titin* also has elastic properties and contributes to flexibility.

When a muscle is stretched, the wavelike elastin fibres straighten; when the stretch is relieved, they rapidly snap back to their resting position. This temporary lengthening is called **elastic elongation.** If gently and regularly stretched, connective tissues may lengthen and flexibility may improve. This long-term lengthening is called **plastic elongation.** Without regular stretching, the process reverses: These tissues shorten, resulting in decreased flexibility. Regular stretching may contribute to flexibility by lengthening muscle fibres through the addition of contractile units called *sarcomeres.*

The amount of stretch a muscle will tolerate is limited, and as the limits of its flexibility are reached, connective tissue becomes more brittle and may rupture if overstretched. A safe and effective program stretches muscles enough to slightly elongate the tissues but not so much that they are damaged. Research has shown that flexibility is improved best by stretching when muscles are warm[2] (following exercise or the application of heat) and the stretch is applied gradually and conservatively. Sudden, high-stress stretching is less effective and can lead to muscle damage.

Nervous System Regulation

Proprioceptors are nerves that send information about the muscular and skeletal systems to the nervous system. When these nerves detect any change in the position or force of muscles and joints, they send signals to the spine and brain, which in turn send signals back to the muscles to coordinate muscle action in a way that protect muscles and tendons from injury. They help control the speed, strength, and coordination of muscle contractions.

When a muscle is stretched (lengthened), proprioceptors detect the amount and rate of the change in muscle length. The nerves send a signal to the spinal cord, which then sends a signal back to the same muscle, triggering a muscle contraction that resists the change in muscle length. Another signal is sent to the antagonist muscle, causing it to relax, which further facilitates contraction of the stretched muscle. These reflexes occur frequently in active muscles and allow for fine control of muscle length and movement.

Small movements that only slightly stimulate these receptors cause small reflex actions. Rapid, powerful, and sudden movements that strongly stimulate the receptors cause large, powerful reflex muscle contractions. Thus stretches that involve rapid, bouncy movements can be dangerous and cause injury because each bounce causes a reflex contraction and so a muscle might be stretching at the same time it is contracting. Performing a gradual stretch and then holding it allows the proprioceptors to adjust to the new muscle length and to reduce the signals it sends to the spine, thereby allowing muscles to lengthen and, over time, improving flexibility.

The stretching technique called *proprioceptive neuromuscular facilitation (PNF)* takes advantage of nerve activity to improve flexibility. The nervous system reacts to a strong contraction by sending signals to the muscle to promote relaxation. For example, contracting a muscle prior to stretching it can help allow the muscle to stretch farther. The advanced strength training technique called *plyometrics* (see Chapter 4) takes advantage of the nervous system action in stretching and contracting muscles.

Modifying nervous control through movement and specific exercises is the best way to improve the functional range of motion. Regular stretching trains all the proprioceptors to allow greater lengthening of the muscles. Proprioceptors adapt very quickly to stretching (or lack of stretching), so frequent training is beneficial for developing flexibility. Stretching before exercising, however, can disturb proprioceptors and interfere with motor control during exercise. This is another good reason to stretch after exercising.

LO2 5.3 BENEFITS OF FLEXIBILITY

Good flexibility provides benefits for the entire musculoskeletal system; it may also prevent injuries and soreness and improve performance in all physical activities.

Joint Health

Good flexibility is essential to good joint health. When the muscles and other tissues that support a joint are tight, the joint is subject to abnormal stresses that can cause joint deterioration. For example, tight thigh muscles cause excessive pressure on the kneecap, leading to pain in the knee joint. Poor joint flexibility can also cause abnormalities in joint lubrication, leading to deterioration of the sensitive cartilage cells lining the joint; pain and further joint injury can result.

range of motion   The full motion possible in a joint.

joint capsules   Semielastic structures, composed primarily of connective tissue, that surround major joints.

soft tissues   Tissues of the human body that include skin, fat, linings of internal organs and blood vessels, connective tissues, tendons, ligaments, muscles, and nerves.

collagen   White fibres that provide structure and support in connective tissue.

elastin   Yellow fibres that make connective tissue flexible.

elastic elongation   Temporary change in the length of muscles, tendons, and supporting connective tissues.

plastic elongation   Long-term change in the length of muscles, tendons, and supporting connective tissues.

proprioceptor   A nerve that sends information about the muscular and skeletal systems to the nervous system.

TERMS

Does Physical Activity Increase or Decrease the Risk of Bone and Joint Disease?

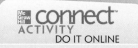
THE EVIDENCE FOR EXERCISE

Most college and university students don't worry much about developing fall-related fractures or chronic bone-related illnesses such as osteoporosis—loss of bone mass—or osteoarthritis—degeneration of the cartilage lining the bones inside joints. Even so, bone health should be a concern throughout life. This is because people begin losing bone mass around age 30; for many, bone loss is accelerated by poor diet and lack of exercise. According to the National Osteoporosis Foundation, 1 in 4 women and at least 1 in 8 men over the age of 50 have osteoporosis and it is estimated that as many as 2 million Canadians may be at risk of osteoporotic fractures during their lifetime.

In addition to getting enough nutrients that are important for bone health (see Chapter 8), there is mounting evidence that exercise can preserve or improve bone health. Even though the relationship between muscle mass and strength and bone health is unclear, experts routinely recommend resistance or weight-bearing exercise as a way to strengthen bones.

For example, several studies have shown an inverse relationship between physical activity and the risk for bone fractures. That is, the more you exercise, the less likely you are to suffer fractures, especially of the upper leg and hip. Research has not determined conclusively how much exercise is required to reduce fracture risk, but reduced risk seems to become apparent when people walk at least 4 hours per week and devote at least 1 hour per week to other forms of physical activity. These findings seem to be consistent for women and men, but some studies disagree on this point, meaning that further research is needed on the sex-related response to exercise as it relates to bone fractures.

Both men and women can prevent fractures and osteoporosis by maintaining or increasing their bone mineral density throughout life, and physical activity plays a significant role in this. One way exercise helps is by increasing the mineral density of bones, or at least by decreasing the loss of mineral density over time. Several 1-year-long studies found that exercise can increase bone mineral density by 1–2% per year, which is significant—especially considering that the same amount of bone mineral density can be lost every 1 to 4 years in older persons. Currently, Heath Canada and the Canadian Society for Exercise Physiology recommend that adults perform weight-bearing

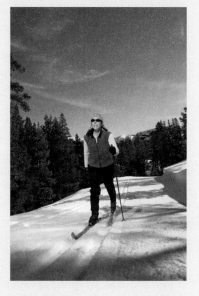

physical activities (such as walking) 3 to 5 days per week and strength training exercises 2 to 4 days per week to increase bone mass or avoid loss of mineral density.

When it comes to exercise and osteoarthritis, the evidence is less conclusive but still fairly positive. All experts agree that regular, moderate-intensity exercise is necessary for joint health. However, they also warn that vigorous or too-frequent exercise may contribute to joint damage and encourage the onset of osteoarthritis. For this reason, experts try to strike a balance in their exercise recommendations, especially for persons with a family history of osteoarthritis. Research seems to support this cautionary approach. Some studies have found that regular physical activity (as recommended for general health) does not increase osteoarthritis risk. Other studies show that moderate activity may provide some protection against the disease, but this evidence is limited.

A few studies also reveal that the type of exercise you do may increase your risk. For example, competitive or strenuous sports such as ballet, orienteering, football, basketball, soccer, and tennis have been associated with the disease, whereas sports such as cross-country skiing, running, swimming, biking, and walking have not.

The bottom line is that the earlier in life you become physically active, the greater your protection against bone loss and bone-related diseases. However, if you have a family history of osteoporosis or osteoarthritis, or if you have already developed symptoms of one of these ailments, be sure to talk to your physician before beginning an exercise program.

SOURCES: American College of Sports Medicine. 2004. ACSM position stand: Physical activity and bone health. *Medicine and Science in Sports and Exercise* 36 (11): 1985–1996; Osteoporosis Canada. 2008. *Breaking Barriers Not Bones: 2008 National Report Card on Osteoporosis Care* (http://www.osteoporosis.ca/; retrieved December 7, 2011); and Canadian Society for Exercise Physiology 2003. *The Canadian Physical Activity, Fitness & Lifestyle Approach,* 3rd ed. Ontario, Canada: CSEP.

Improved flexibility can greatly improve your quality of life, particularly as you get older. People tend to exercise less as they age, leading to loss of joint mobility and increased incidence of joint pain. Aging also decreases the natural elasticity of muscles, tendons, and joints, resulting in stiffness. The problem is often compounded by arthritis (see the box "Does Physical Activity Increase or Decrease the Risk of Bone and Joint Disease?"). Good joint flexibility may prevent arthritis, and stretching may lessen pain in people who have the condition. Another

benefit of good flexibility for older adults is that it increases balance and stability.

Prevention of Low-Back Pain and Injuries

Low-back pain can be related to poor spinal stability, which puts pressure on the nerves leading out from the spinal column. It is estimated that over 80% of Canadians will suffer from low-back pain at some point in their lifespan.[3]

Strength and flexibility in the back, pelvis, and thighs may help prevent this type of back pain but may or may not improve back health or reduce the risk of injury. Good hip and knee flexibility do protect the spine from excessive motion during the tasks of daily living.

Although scientific evidence is limited, people with either high or low flexibility seem to have an increased risk for injury.[4] Extreme flexibility reduces joint stability, and poor flexibility limits a joint's range of motion. Persons of average fitness should try to attain normal flexibility in joints throughout the body, meaning each joint can move through its normal range of motion with no difficulty. Stretching programs are particularly important for older adults, people involved in high-power sports involving rapid changes in direction (such as football and tennis), workers involved in brief bouts of intense exertion (such as police officers and firefighters), and people who sit for prolonged periods (such as office workers and students).

However, stretching before a high-intensity activity (such as sprinting or basketball) may increase the risk of injury by interfering with neuromuscular control and reducing muscles' natural ability to stretch and contract. When injuries do occur, flexibility exercises can be used in treatment: They reduce symptoms and help restore normal range of motion in affected joints.

Additional Potential Benefits

- *Relief of aches and pains* Studying or working in one place for a long time can make your muscles tense. Stretching helps relieve tension, so you can go back to work refreshed and effective.
- *Relief of muscle cramps* Recent research suggests that exercise-related muscle cramps are caused by increased electrical activity within the affected muscle. The best treatment for muscle cramps is gentle stretching, which reduces the electrical activity and allows the muscle to relax.
- *Improved body position and strength for sports (and life)* Good flexibility lets a person assume more efficient body positions and exert force through a greater range of motion. For example, swimmers with more flexible shoulders have stronger strokes because they can pull their arms through the water in the optimal position. Some studies suggest that flexibility training enhances strength development. Do not use stretching however, to enable yourself to exercise excessively.
- *Maintenance of good posture and balance* Good flexibility also contributes to body symmetry and good posture. Bad posture can gradually change your body structures. Sitting in a slumped position, for example, can lead to tightness in the muscles in the front of your chest and overstretching and looseness in the upper spine, causing a rounding of the upper back. This condition, called *kyphosis,*

is common in older people. It may be prevented by stretching regularly.
- *Relaxation* Flexibility exercises reduce mental tension, slow your breathing rate, and reduce blood pressure.
- *Improving impaired mobility* Stretching often decreases pain and improves functional capacity in people with arthritis, stroke, or muscle and nerve diseases and in people who are recovering from surgery or injury.

Assessing Flexibility

Because flexibility is specific to each joint, there are no tests of general flexibility. The most commonly used flexibility test is the sit-and-reach test, which rates the flexibility of the muscles in the lower back and hamstrings. To assess your flexibility and identify inflexible joints, complete Lab 5.1.

LO3 5.4 CREATING A SUCCESSFUL PROGRAM TO DEVELOP FLEXIBILITY

A successful program for developing flexibility contains safe exercises executed with the most effective techniques. Your goal should be to at least attain normal flexibility in the major joints. Balanced flexibility (not too much or too little) provides joint stability and facilitates smooth, economical movement patterns. You can achieve balanced flexibility by performing stretching exercises regularly and by using a variety of stretches and stretching techniques.

Applying the FITT Principle

As with the programs described for developing other health-related components of fitness, the acronym FITT can be used to remember key components of a stretching program: Frequency, Intensity, Time, and Type of exercise.

FREQUENCY Health Canada recommends that stretching exercises be performed a minimum of 2–3 days a week, and ideally 4–7 days a week. Doing these exercises often will provide the most benefits. It's best to stretch when your muscles are warm, so try incorporating your stretching program into your cool-down after cardiorespiratory endurance exercise or weight training.

Never stretch when your muscles are cold; doing so can increase your risk of injury as well as limit the amount of flexibility you can develop. Although stretching before exercise is a time-honoured ritual practised by athletes in many sports, several studies have found that preexercise stretching decreases muscle strength and performance and disturbs neuromuscular control.

If your workout involves participation in a sport or high-performance activity, you may be better off stretching after your workout. For moderate-intensity activities like walking or cycling, stretching before your workout is unlikely to affect performance.

INTENSITY AND TIME (DURATION) For each exercise, slowly stretch your muscles to the point of slight tension or mild discomfort. Hold the stretch for 15–30 seconds. As you hold the stretch, the feeling of slight tension should slowly subside; at that point, try to stretch a bit farther. Throughout the stretch, try to relax and breathe easily. Rest for about 30–60 seconds between each stretch, and do 2–4 repetitions of each stretch. A complete flexibility workout usually takes about 10–30 minutes (Figure 5.2).

LO4 **TYPES OF STRETCHING TECHNIQUES** Stretching techniques vary from simply stretching the muscles during the course of normal activities to sophisticated methods based on patterns of muscle reflexes. Improper stretching can do more harm than good, so it's important to understand the different types of stretching exercises and how they affect the muscles. (See the box "Safe Stretching" for guidelines on creating a safe and effective stretching program.) Four common techniques are static stretches, ballistic stretches, dynamic stretches, and PNF. These techniques can be performed passively or actively.

Warm-up 5–10 minutes or following an endurance or strength training workout	Stretching exercises for major joints **Sample program**	
	Exercise	*Areas stretched*
	Head turns and tilts	Neck
	Towel stretch	Triceps, shoulders, chest
	Across-the-body and overhead stretches	Shoulders, upper back, back of arm
	Upper-back stretch	Upper back
	Lateral stretch	Trunk muscles
	Step stretch	Hip, front of thigh
	Side lunge	Inner thigh, hip, calf
	Inner-thigh stretch	Inner thigh, hip
	Hip and trunk stretch	Trunk, outer thigh, hip, buttocks, lower back
	Modified hurdler stretch	Back of thigh, lower back
	Alternate leg stretcher	Back of thigh, hip, knee, ankle, buttocks
	Lower-leg stretch	Calf, soleus, Achilles tendon

Frequency: 2–3 days per week (minimum); 5–7 days per week (ideal)

Intensity: Stretch to the point of mild discomfort, not pain

Time (duration): All stretches should be held for 15–30 seconds and performed 2–4 times

Type of activity: Stretching exercises that focus on major joints

FIGURE 5.2 A flexibility workout.

Static Stretching In **static stretching**, each muscle is gradually stretched, and the stretch is held for 15–30 seconds. A slow stretch prompts less reaction from proprioceptors, and the muscles can safely stretch farther than usual. Static stretching is the type most often recommended by fitness experts because it's safe and effective. The key to this technique is to stretch the muscles and joints to the point where a pull is felt, but not to the point of pain. (One note of caution: Excess static stretching can decrease joint stability and increase the risk of injury. This may be a particular concern for women, who naturally have joints that are less stable and more flexible than men.) The sample stretching program presented later in this chapter features static stretching exercises.

Ballistic Stretching In **ballistic stretching**, the muscles are stretched suddenly in a forceful bouncing movement. For example, touching the toes repeatedly in rapid succession is a ballistic stretch for the hamstrings. A problem with this technique is that the heightened activity of proprioceptors caused by the rapid stretches can continue for some time, possibly causing injuries during any physical activities that follow. Another concern is that triggering strong responses from the nerves can cause a reflex muscle contraction that makes it harder to stretch. For these reasons, ballistic stretching is usually not recommended for people of average fitness.

Ballistic stretching trains the muscle dynamically, so it can be an appropriate stretching technique for some well-trained athletes. For example, tennis players stretch their hamstrings and quadriceps ballistically when they lunge for a ball during a tennis match. Because this movement is part of their sport, they might benefit from ballistic training of these muscle groups.

Dynamic (Functional) Stretching The emphasis in **dynamic stretching** is on functionally based movements. Dynamic stretching is similar to ballistic stretching in that it includes movement, but it differs in that it does not involve rapid bouncing. Instead, dynamic stretching involves moving the joints through the range of motion used in a specific exercise or sport in an exaggerated but slow and controlled manner; movements are fluid rather than jerky. An example of a dynamic stretch is the lunge walk, in which a person takes slow steps with an exaggerated stride length and reaches a lunge stretch position with each step.

Slow dynamic stretches can lengthen the muscles in many directions without developing high tension in the tissues. These stretches elongate the tissues and train the neuromuscular system. Because dynamic stretches are based on sports movements or movements used in daily life, they develop functional flexibility that translates well into activities.

Dynamic stretches are more challenging than static stretches because they require balance and coordination and may carry a greater risk of muscle soreness and injury. People just beginning a flexibility program might want to start off with static stretches and try dynamic stretches only after they are comfortable with static stretching techniques and have improved their flexibility. It is also a good idea to seek expert advice on dynamic stretching technique and program development.

Serious athletes may use dynamic stretches as part of their warm-up before a competitive event or a high-intensity training session in order to move their joints through the range of motion required for the activity. Functional flexibility training can also be combined with functional strength training. For example, lunge curls, which combine dynamic lunges with free weights biceps curls, stretch the hip, thigh, and calf muscles; stabilize the core muscles in the trunk; and build strength in the arm muscles. Many activities build functional flexibility and strength at the same time, including yoga, Pilates, taijiquan, Olympic weight lifting, plyometrics, stability training (including Swiss and Bosu ball exercises), medicine ball exercises, and functional training machines (for example, Life Fitness and Cybex).

Proprioceptive Neuromuscular Facilitation (PNF)
PNF techniques use reflexes initiated by both muscle and joint receptors to cause greater training effects. The most popular PNF stretching technique is the *contract-relax* stretching method, in which a muscle is contracted before it is stretched. The contraction activates proprioceptors, causing relaxation in the muscle about to be stretched. For example, in a seated stretch of calf muscles, the first step in PNF is to contract the calf muscles. The individual or a partner can provide resistance for an isometric contraction. Following a brief period of relaxation, the next step is to stretch the calf muscles by pulling the tops of the feet toward the body. A duration of 6 seconds for the contraction and 15–30 seconds for the stretch is recommended. PNF appears to be most effective if the individual pushes hard during the isometric contraction.

Another example of a PNF stretch is the *contract-relax-contract pattern*. In this technique, begin by contracting the muscle to be stretched and then relaxing it. Next, contract the opposing muscle (the antagonist). Finally, stretch the first muscle. For example, using this technique to stretch the hamstrings (the muscles in the back of the thigh) would require the following steps: contract the hamstrings, relax the hamstrings, contract the quadriceps (the muscles in the front of the thigh), stretch the hamstrings.

PNF appears to allow more effective stretching, and greater immediate increases in flexibility than static stretching.[5] It also usually requires a partner and takes more time.

Passive versus Active Stretching Stretches can be done either passively or actively. In **passive stretching,**

an outside force or resistance provided by yourself, a partner, gravity, or a weight helps your joints move through their range of motion. For example, a seated stretch of the hamstring and back muscles can be done by reaching the hands toward the feet until a pull is felt in those muscles. You can achieve a greater range of motion (a more intense stretch) using passive stretching. However, because the stretch is not controlled by the muscles themselves, there is a greater risk of injury. Communication between partners in passive stretching is very important to ensure that joints aren't forced outside their normal functional range of motion.

In **active stretching,** a muscle is stretched by a contraction of the opposing muscle (the muscle on the opposite side of the limb). For example, an active seated stretch of the calf muscles occurs when a person actively contracts the muscles on the top of the shin. The contraction of this opposing muscle produces a reflex that relaxes the muscles to be stretched. The muscle can be stretched farther with a low risk of injury.

The only disadvantage of active stretching is that a person may not be able to produce enough stress (enough stretch) to increase flexibility using only the contraction of opposing muscle groups. The safest and most convenient technique is active static stretching, with an occasional passive assist. For example, you might stretch your calves both by contracting the muscles on the top of your shin and by pulling your feet toward you. This way you combine the advantages of active stretching—safety and the relaxation reflex—with those of passive stretching—greater range of motion. People who are just beginning flexibility training may be better off doing active rather than passive stretches. For PNF techniques, it is particularly important to have a knowledgeable partner.

TERMS

static stretching A technique in which a muscle is slowly and gently stretched and then held in the stretched position.

ballistic stretching A technique in which muscles are stretched by the force generated as a body part is repeatedly bounced, swung, or jerked.

dynamic stretching A technique in which muscles are stretched by moving joints slowly and fluidly through their range of motion in a controlled manner; also called *functional stretching*.

passive stretching A technique in which muscles are stretched by force applied by an outside force.

active stretching A technique in which muscles are stretched by the contraction of the opposing muscles.

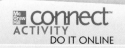
TAKE CHARGE

Safe Stretching

- Do stretching exercises statically. Stretch to the point of mild discomfort, hold the position for 15–30 seconds, rest for 30–60 seconds, and repeat, trying to stretch a bit farther.

- Do not stretch to the point of pain. Any soreness after a stretching workout should be mild and last no more than 24 hours. If you are sore for a longer period, you stretched too intensely.

- Relax and breathe easily as you stretch. Inhale through the nose and exhale through pursed lips during the stretch. Try to relax the muscles being stretched.

- Perform all exercises on both sides of your body.

- Increase intensity and duration gradually over time. Improved flexibility takes many months to develop.

- Stretch when your muscles are warm. Do gentle warm-up exercises such as easy jogging or calisthenics before doing a pre-exercise stretching routine.

- There are large individual differences in joint flexibility. Don't feel you have to compete with others during stretching workouts.

- Engage in a variety of physical activities to help you develop well-rounded functional physical fitness and allow you to perform all types of training more safely and effectively.

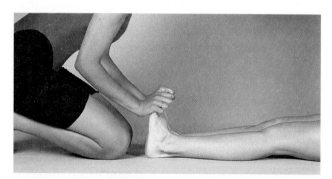

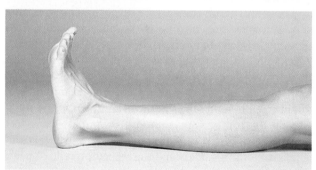

In passive stretching (top), an outside force—such as pressure exerted by another person—helps move the joint and stretch the muscles. In active stretching (bottom), the force to move the joint and stretch the muscles is provided by a contraction of the opposing muscles.

CAREER OPTIONS IN . . .

Flexibility

INSTRUCTING: yoga, tai chi, sport-related coaching.

REHABILITATION: therapeutic assistant, kinesiologist, recreation therapy.

SELF-EMPLOYED: flexibility workshop presenter, life balance trainer.

SOURCE: Physical and Health Education Canada (http://www.phecanada.ca).

Making Progress

As with any type of training, you will make progress and improve your flexibility if you stick with your program. Judge your progress by simply noting your body position while stretching. For example, note how far you can lean forward during a modified hurdler stretch. Repeat the assessment tests that appear in Lab 5.1 periodically and be sure to take the test at the same time of day each time. You will likely notice some improvement after only 2–3 weeks of stretching, but you may need at least 2 months to attain significant improvements. By then, you can expect flexibility increases of about 10–20% in many joints.

LO5 Exercises to Improve Flexibility: A Sample Program

There are hundreds of exercises that can improve flexibility. Your program should include exercises that work all the major joints of the body by stretching their associated muscles (refer back to Figure 4.4). The exercises illustrated here are simple to do and pose a minimum risk of injury. Use these exercises to create a well-rounded program for developing flexibility. Be sure to perform each stretch using the proper technique. Hold each position for 15–30 seconds and perform 2–4 repetitions of each exercise. Avoid exercises that put excessive pressure on your joints (see the box "Stretches to Avoid"). Complete Lab 5.2 when you are ready to start your program.

FITNESS TIP

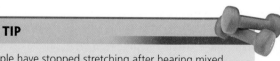

Many people have stopped stretching after hearing mixed results from research studies. This may be a mistake. Stretching after an intense workout can relieve soreness, in addition to providing all the other benefits listed here.

EXERCISE 1 — Head Turns and Tilts

Areas stretched: Neck

Instructions

Head turns: Turn your head to the right and hold the stretch. Repeat to the left.

Head tilts: Tilt your head to the left and hold the stretch. Repeat to the right.

Variation: Place your right palm on your right cheek; try to turn your head to the right as you resist with your hand. Repeat on the left side.

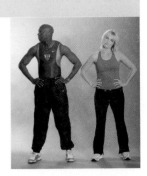

EXERCISE 2 — Towel Stretch

Areas stretched: Triceps, shoulders and chest

Instructions: Roll up a towel and grasp it with both hands, palms down. With your arms straight, slowly lift it back over your head as far as possible. The closer together your hands are, the greater the stretch.

Variation: Repeat the stretch with your arms down and the towel behind your back. Grasp the towel with your palms forward and thumbs pointing out. Gently raise your arms behind your back. This exercise can also be done without a towel.

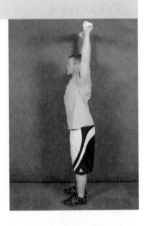

EXERCISE 3 — Across-The-Body and Overhead Stretches

Areas stretched: Shoulders, upper back, back of the arm (triceps)

Instructions:

(a) Keeping your back straight, cross your right arm in front of your body and grasp it with your left hand. Stretch your arm, shoulders, and back by gently pulling your arm as close to your body as possible. Hold.
(b) Bend your right arm over your head, placing your right elbow as close to your right ear as possible. Grasp your right elbow with your left hand over your head. Stretch the back of your arm by gently pulling your right elbow back and toward your head. Hold. Repeat both stretches on your left side.

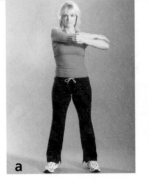
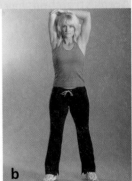

a

b

EXERCISE 4 — Upper-Back Stretch

Areas stretched: Upper back

Instructions: Stand with your feet shoulder-width apart, knees slightly bent, and pelvis tucked under. Lace your fingers in front of your body and press your palms forward.

Variation: In the same position, wrap your arms around your body as if you were giving yourself a hug.

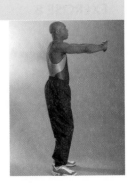

EXERCISE 5   Lateral Stretch

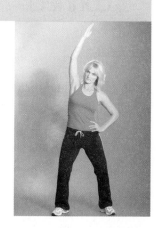

Areas stretched: Trunk muscles

Instructions: Stand with your feet shoulder-width apart, knees slightly bent, and pelvis tucked under. Raise one arm over your head and bend sideways from the waist. Support your trunk by placing the hand or forearm of your other arm on your thigh or hip for support. Be sure you bend directly sideways and don't move your body below the waist. Repeat on the other side.

Variation: Perform the same exercise in a seated position.

EXERCISE 6   Step Stretch

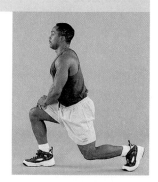

Areas stretched: Hip, front of thigh (quadriceps)

Instructions: Step forward and flex your forward knee, keeping your knee directly above your ankle. Stretch your other leg back so that it is parallel to the floor. Press your hips forward and down to stretch. Your arms can be at your sides, on top of your knee, or on the ground for balance. Repeat on the other side.

EXERCISE 7   Side Lunge

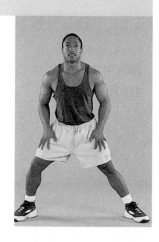

Areas stretched: Inner thigh, hip, calf

Instructions: Stand in a wide straddle with your legs turned out from your hip joints and your hands on your thighs. Lunge to one side by bending one knee and keeping the other leg straight. Keep your knee directly over your ankle; do not bend it more than 90 degrees. Repeat on the other side.

Variation: In the same position, lift the heel of the bent knee to provide additional stretch. The exercise may also be performed with your hands on the floor for balance.

EXERCISE 8   Inner Thigh Stretch

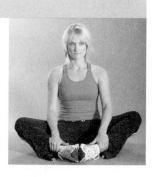

Areas stretched: Inner thigh, hip

Instructions: Sit with the soles of your feet together. Push your knees toward the floor using your hands or forearms.

Variation: When you first begin to push your knees toward the floor, use your legs to resist the movement. Then, relax and press your knees down as far as they will go.

EXERCISE 9   Hip And Trunk Stretch

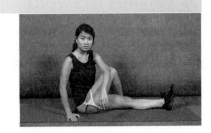

Areas stretched: Trunk, outer thigh and hip, buttocks, lower back

Instructions: Sit with your left leg straight, right leg bent and crossed over the left knee, and right hand on the floor next to your right hip. Turn your trunk as far as possible to the right by pushing against your right leg with your left forearm or elbow. Keep your right foot on the floor. Repeat on the other side.

EXERCISE 10   Modified Hurdler Stretch (Seated Single-Leg Hamstring)

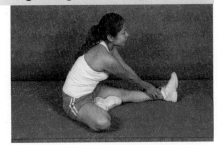

Areas stretched: Back of the thigh (hamstring), lower back

Instructions: Sit with your left leg straight and your right leg tucked close to your body. Reach toward your left foot as far as possible. Repeat for the other leg.

Variation: As you stretch forward, alternately flex and point the foot of your extended leg.

EXERCISE 11   Alternate Leg Stretcher

Areas stretched: Back of the thigh (hamstring), hip, knee, ankle, buttocks

Instructions: Lie flat on your back with both legs straight.

(a) Grasp your left leg behind the thigh, and pull in to your chest.
(b) Hold this position, and then extend your left leg toward the ceiling.
(c) Hold this position, and then bring your left knee back to your chest and pull your toes toward your shin with your left hand. Stretch the back of the leg by attempting to straighten your knee. Repeat for the other leg.

Variation: Perform the stretch on both legs at the same time.

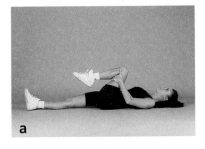

EXERCISE 12   Lower-Leg Stretch

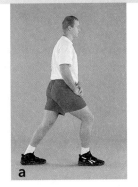
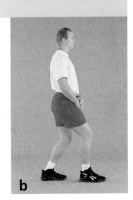

Areas stretched: Back of the lower leg (calf, soleus, Achilles tendon)

Instructions: Stand with one foot about 30–50 centimetres in front of the other, with both feet pointing forward.
(a) Keeping your back leg straight, lunge forward by bending your front knee and pushing your rear heel backward. Hold.
(b) Then, pull your back foot in slightly, and bend your back knee. Shift your weight to your back leg. Hold. Repeat on the other side.

Variation: Place your hands on a wall and extend one foot back, pressing your heel down to stretch; or stand with the balls of your feet on a step or bench and allow your heels to drop below the level of your toes.

Stretches to Avoid

The safe alternatives listed here are described and illustrated in the *Flexibility Exercises* section as part of the complete program of safe flexibility exercises presented in this chapter.

Standing Toe Touch

Problem: Puts excessive strain on the spine.

Alternatives: Modified hurdler stretch (Exercise 10), alternate leg stretcher (Exercise 11), and lower- leg stretch (Exercise 12).

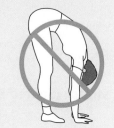

Standing Ankle-to-Buttocks Quadriceps Stretch

Problem: Puts excessive strain on the ligaments of the knee.

Alternative: Step stretch (Exercise 6).

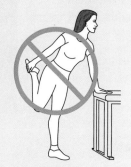

Full Squat with Bent Back

Problem: Puts excessive strain on the ankles, knees, and spine.

Alternatives: Alternate leg stretcher (Exercise 11) and lower-leg stretch (Exercise 12).

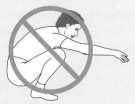

Prone Arch

Problem: Puts excessive strain on the spine, knees, and shoulders.

Alternatives: Towel stretch (Exercise 2) and step stretch (Exercise 6).

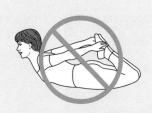

Standing Hamstring Stretch

Problem: Puts excessive strain on the knee and lower back.

Alternatives: Modified hurdler stretch (Exercise 10) and alternate leg stretcher (Exercise 11).

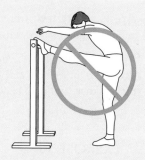

Yoga Plow

Problem: Puts excessive strain on the neck, shoulders and back.

Alternatives: Head turns and tilts (Exercise 1), across the-body and overhead stretches (Exercise 3), and upper-back stretch (Exercise 4).

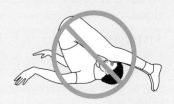

Hurdler Stretch

Problem: Turning out the bent leg can put excessive strain on the ligaments of the knee.

Alternatives: Modified hurdler stretch (Exercise 10).

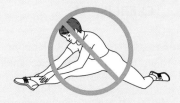

Neck Circles

Problem: Puts excessive strain on the neck and cervical disks.

Alternatives: Head turns and tilts (Exercise 1).

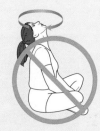

LO6 5.5 PREVENTING AND MANAGING LOW-BACK PAIN

Approximately two-thirds of Canadians experienced back pain in the last year alone and of those who were working, 15% reported that they lost time off work as a result of their back pain. Low-back pain is estimated to cost as much as $12 billion a year in Canada in direct costs such as treatment and rehabilitation alone.[6]

Back pain should be diagnosed by a trained professional and while it can result from sudden traumatic injuries, it is more often the long-term result of weak and inflexible muscles, poor posture, or poor body mechanics during activities like lifting and carrying. Any abnormal strain on the back can result in pain. Most cases of low-back pain clear up within a few weeks or months, but some people have recurrences or suffer from chronic pain.

Function and Structure of the Spine

The spinal column performs many important functions in the body.

- It provides structural support for the body, especially the thorax (upper-body cavity).
- It surrounds and protects the spinal cord.
- It supports much of the body's weight and transmits it to the lower body.

- It serves as an attachment site for a large number of muscles, tendons, and ligaments.
- It allows movement of the neck and back in all directions.

The spinal column is made up of bones called **vertebrae** (Figure 5.3). The spine consists of 7 cervical vertebrae in the neck, 12 thoracic vertebrae in the upper back, and 5 lumbar vertebrae in the lower back. The 9 vertebrae at the base of the spine are fused into two sections and form the sacrum and the coccyx (tailbone). The spine has four curves: the cervical, thoracic, lumbar, and sacral curves. These curves help bring the body weight supported by the spine in line with the axis of the body.

Although the structure of vertebrae depends on their location on the spine, the different types of vertebrae share common characteristics. Each consists of a body, an arch, and several bony processes (Figure 5.4). The vertebral body is cylindrical, with flattened surfaces where **intervertebral disks** are attached. The vertebral body is

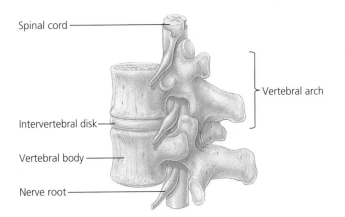

FIGURE 5.4   Vertebrae and an intervertebral disk.

designed to carry the stress of body weight and physical activity. The vertebral arch surrounds and protects the spinal cord. The bony processes serve as joints for adjacent vertebrae and attachment sites for muscles and ligaments. **Nerve roots** from the spinal cord pass through notches in the vertebral arch.

Intervertebral disks, which absorb and disperse the stresses placed on the spine, separate vertebrae from each other. Disks are made up of a gel- and water-filled nucleus surrounded by a series of fibrous rings. The liquid nucleus can change shape when it is compressed, allowing the disk to absorb shock. The intervertebral disks also help maintain the spaces between vertebrae where the spinal nerve roots are located.

Core Muscle Fitness

The **core muscles** include those in the abdomen, pelvic floor, sides of the trunk, back, buttocks, hip, and pelvis (Figure 5.5). There are 29 of these muscles, attaching to the ribs, hips, spinal column, and other bones in the trunk of the body. As described in Chapter 4, the

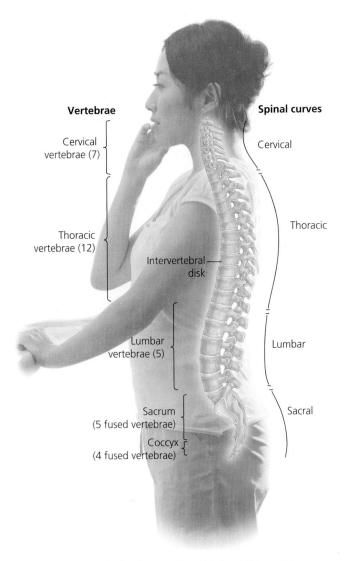

Vertebrae

Cervical vertebrae (7)

Thoracic vertebrae (12)

Intervertebral disk

Lumbar vertebrae (5)

Sacrum (5 fused vertebrae)

Coccyx (4 fused vertebrae)

Spinal curves

Cervical

Thoracic

Lumbar

Sacral

FIGURE 5.3   The spinal column.   The spine is made up of five separate regions and has four distinct curves. An intervertebral disk is located between adjoining vertebrae.

vertebrae   Bony segments composing the spinal column that provide structural support for the body and protect the spinal cord.

intervertebral disk   An elastic disk located between adjoining vertebrae, consisting of a gel- and water-filled nucleus surrounded by fibrous rings; serves as a shock absorber for the spinal column.

nerve root   The base of each of the 31 pairs of spinal nerves that branch off the spinal cord through spaces between vertebrae.

core muscles   The trunk muscles extending from the hips to the upper back.

TERMS

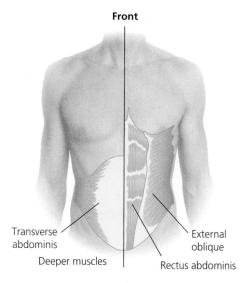

Front

Transverse
abdominis

Deeper muscles

External
oblique

Rectus abdominis

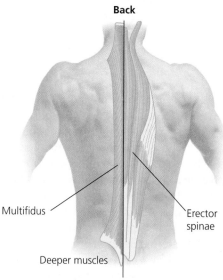

Back

Multifidus

Erector
spinae

Deeper muscles

FIGURE 5.5 Major core muscles.

core muscles stabilize the spine and help transfer force between the upper body and lower body. They stabilize the midsection when you sit, stand, reach, walk, jump, twist, squat, throw, or bend. The muscles on the front, back, and sides of your trunk support your spine when you sit in a chair and fix your midsection as you use your legs to stand up. When hitting a forehand in tennis or batting a softball, most of the force is transferred from the legs and hips, across the core muscles, to the arms. Strong core muscles make movements more forceful and help prevent back pain.

During any dynamic movement, the core muscles work together; some shorten to cause movement, while others contract and hold to provide stability, lengthen to brake the movement, or send signals to the brain about the movements and positions of the muscles and bones (proprioception). When specific core muscles are weak or tired, the nervous system steps in and uses other muscles.

This substitution causes abnormal stresses on the joints, decreases power, and increases the risk of injury.

The best exercises for low-back health are whole-body exercises that force the core muscles to stabilize the spine in many different directions. The low-back exercises presented later in this chapter include several exercises that focus on the core muscles, including the step stretch (lunge), side bridges, and spine extensions. These exercises are generally safe for beginning exercisers and, with physician approval, people with some back pain. More challenging core exercises utilize stability balls or free weights. Stability ball exercises require the core muscles to stabilize the ball (and the body) while performing nearly any type of exercise. Many traditional exercises with free weights can strengthen the core muscles if you do them in a standing position. Weight machines train muscles in isolation, while exercises with free weights done while standing help train the body for real-world movements—an essential principle of core training.

Causes of Back Pain

Back pain can occur at any point along your spine. The lumbar area, because it bears the majority of your weight, is the most common site. Any movement that causes excessive stress on the spinal column can cause injury and pain. The spine is well equipped to bear body weight and the force or stress of body movements along its long axis. However it is less capable of bearing loads at an angle to its long axis or when the trunk is flexed (bent). You do not have to carry a heavy load or participate in a vigorous contact sport to injure your back. Picking a pencil up from the floor using poor body mechanics—reaching too far out in front of you or bending over with your knees straight, for example—can also result in back pain.

Risk factors associated with low-back pain include:

- age greater than 34 years
- degenerative diseases such as arthritis or osteoporosis
- a family or personal history of back pain or trauma, a sedentary lifestyle, low job satisfaction
- low socioeconomic status[7]
- smoking increases risk because smoking appears to increase degenerative changes in the spine
- excess body weight also increases strain on the back
- psychological stress or depression can cause muscle tension and back pain
- occupations and activities associated with low-back pain are those involving physically hard work, such as frequent lifting, twisting, bending, standing up, or straining in forced positions; those requiring high concentration demands (such as computer programming); and those involving vibrations affecting the entire body (such as truck driving).

About 80% of Canadians suffer from back pain at some point in their lives. Back pain can be annoying and even disabling, and every day, many Canadians miss school and work because of their pain. Luckily, you can minimize the risk of back problems by doing a few simple exercises every day. Keep a personal back pain prevention journal and do the following exercises on as many days of the week as possible.

Exercise	Mon.	Tues.	Wed.	Thur.	Fri.	Sat.	Sun.
Curl-ups: 1 set of 10 reps	✓		✓		✓		✓
Side bridge: 5 sets, 3-second hold, each side	✓		✓		✓		✓
Bird dog: 5 sets, 3-second hold, each side	✓		✓		✓		✓
Walking: 15–60 minutes		✓	✓		✓		✓
Kettlebell swings: 1 set of 20 reps	✓				✓	✓	✓

Make a chart like the one shown above, and place a new copy in your training log each week. Enter a check mark every time you do the exercise. Try to enter a check mark for each exercise as often as you can during the week. In this one-week example, the person didn't do all the exercises every day, but she tried to do something on as many days a week as she could. Regularity is the key; if you miss a day, try not to miss the next one.

Underlying causes of back pain include poor muscle endurance and strength in the muscles of the abdomen, back, hips, and legs; excess body weight; poor posture or body position when standing, sitting, or sleeping; and poor body mechanics when performing actions like lifting and carrying, or sports movements. Abnormal spinal loading resulting from any of these causes can have short-term or long-term direct and indirect effects on the spine. Strained muscles, tendons, or ligaments can cause pain and can, over time, lead to injuries to vertebrae or the intervertebral disks.

Stress can cause disks to break down and lose some of their ability to absorb shock. A damaged disk may bulge out between vertebrae and put pressure on a nerve root, a condition commonly referred to as a *slipped or herniated disk*. Painful pressure on nerves can also occur if damage to a disk narrows the space between two vertebrae. With age, you lose fluid from the disks, making them more likely to bulge and put pressure on nerve roots. Depending on the amount of pressure on a nerve, symptoms may include numbness in the back, hip, leg, or foot; radiating pain; loss of muscle function; depressed reflexes; and muscle spasm. If the pressure is severe enough, loss of function can be permanent.

Preventing Low-Back Pain

Incorrect posture is responsible for many back injuries. Strategies for maintaining good posture during daily activities are presented in the box "Good Posture and Low-Back Health." Follow the same guidelines for posture and movement when you engage in sports or recreational activities. Control your movements and warm up thoroughly before you exercise. Take special care when lifting weights.

The role of exercise in preventing and treating back pain is still being investigated. However, many experts do recommend exercise, especially for people who have already experienced an episode of low-back pain. Regular exercise aimed at increasing muscle endurance and strength in the back and abdomen is often recommended to prevent back pain, as is lifestyle physical activity such as walking. Movement helps lubricate your spinal disks and increases muscle fitness in your trunk and legs. Other lifestyle recommendations for preventing back pain include:

- Maintain a healthy weight. Excess fat contributes to poor posture, which can place harmful stress on the spine.
- Stop smoking, and reduce stress.
- Avoid sitting, standing, or working in the same position for too long. Stand up every hour or half-hour and move around.
- Use a supportive seat and a medium-firm mattress. Use lumbar support when driving, particularly for long distances, to prevent back muscle fatigue and pain.
- Warm up thoroughly before exercising.
- Progress gradually when attempting to improve strength or fitness.
- Ensure that you are using proper form and technique when performing any activities, i.e., work, leisure activities, exercising, sports.

Managing Acute Back Pain

Sudden (acute) ack pain usually involves tissue injury. Symptoms may include pain, muscles spasms, stiffness, and inflammation. Many cases of acute back pain go

TAKE CHARGE

Good Posture and Low-Back Health

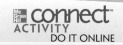

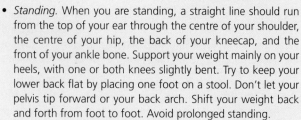

Changes in everyday posture and behaviour can help prevent and alleviate low-back pain.

- *Lying down.* When resting or sleeping, lie on your side with your knees and hips bent. If you lie on your back place a pillow under your knees. Don't lie on your stomach. Use a medium-firm mattress.

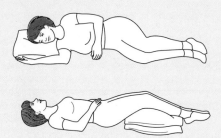

- *Sitting at a computer.* Sit in a slightly reclined position of 100–110 degrees, not an upright 90-degree position. Adjust your chair so your knees are slightly lower than your hips. If your back flattens as you sit, try using a lumbar roll to maintain your back's natural curvature. Place your feet flat on the floor or on a footrest. Place the monitor directly in front of you and adjust it so your eyes are level with the top of the screen; you should be looking slightly downward at the middle of the screen. Adjust the keyboard and mouse so your forearms and wrists are in a neutral position, parallel with the floor.

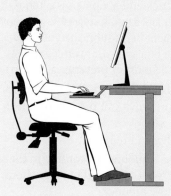

- *Lifting.* If you need to lower yourself to grasp an object, bend at the knees and hips rather than at the waist. Your feet should be about shoulder-width apart. Lift gradually, keeping your arms straight, by standing up or by pushing with your leg muscles. Keep the object close to your body. Don't twist, if you have to turn with the object, change the position of your feet.

- *Standing.* When you are standing, a straight line should run from the top of your ear through the centre of your shoulder, the centre of your hip, the back of your kneecap, and the front of your ankle bone. Support your weight mainly on your heels, with one or both knees slightly bent. Try to keep your lower back flat by placing one foot on a stool. Don't let your pelvis tip forward or your back arch. Shift your weight back and forth from foot to foot. Avoid prolonged standing.

  To check your posture, stand in a normal way with your back to a wall. Your upper back and buttocks should touch the wall; your heels may be a few inches away. Slide one hand into the space between your lower back and the wall. It should slide in easily but should almost touch both your back and the wall. Adjust your posture as needed, and try to hold this position as you walk away from the wall.

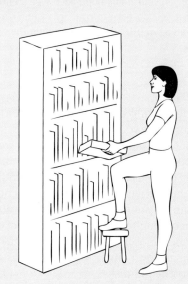

- *Walking.* Walk with your toes pointed straight ahead. Keep your back flat, head up and centred over your body, and chin in. Swing your arms freely. Don't wear high-heeled shoes. Walking briskly is better for back health than walking slowly.

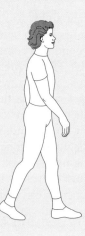

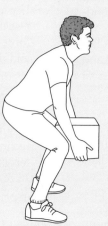

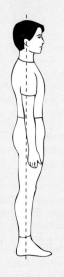

Yoga for Relaxation and Pain Relief

Certain types of exercise can provide relief from back pain, depending on the pain's underlying cause. Effective exercises stretch the muscles and connective tissue in the hips, stabilize the spine, and strengthen and build endurance in the core muscles of the back and abdomen.

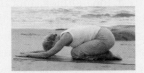

Yoga may be an option for many back pain sufferers because it offers a variety of exercises that target the spine and the core muscles. Yoga is an ancient practice involving slow, gentle movements performed with controlled breathing and focused attention. Yoga practitioners slowly move into a specific posture (called an asana) and hold the posture for up to 60 seconds. There are hundreds of asanas, many of which are easy to do and provide good stretches.

Yoga also involves simple breathing exercises that gently stretch the muscles of the upper back while helping the practitioner focus. Yoga experts say that breathing exercises not only encourage relaxation but also clear the mind and can help

relieve mild to moderate pain. Yoga enthusiasts end their workouts energized and refreshed but calm and relaxed.

Many medical professionals now recommend yoga for patients with back pain, particularly postures that involve arching and gently stretching the back, such as the cat pose (similar to the cat stretch shown in the *Low-Back Exercises* section of this chapter). These are basic asanas that most people can perform repeatedly and hold for a relatively long time.

Because asanas must be performed correctly to be beneficial, qualified instruction is recommended. For those with back pain, physicians advise choosing an instructor who is not only accomplished in yoga but also knowledgeable about back pain and its causes. Such instructors can steer students away from exercises that do more harm than good. It is especially important to choose postures that will benefit the back without worsening the underlying problem. Some asanas can aggravate an injured or painful back if they are performed incorrectly or too aggressively. In fact, a few yoga postures should not be done at all by people with back pain.

If you have back pain, see your physician to determine its cause before beginning any type of exercise program. Even gentle exercise or stretching can be bad for an already injured back, especially if the spinal disks or nerves are involved. For some back conditions, rest or therapy may be better options than exercise, at least in the short term.

---

away by themselves within a few days or weeks. In some cases you may have to actively treat the symptoms with one or more of the following receeommendations.

- You may be able to reduce pain and inflammation by applying cold and then heat. Begin with a cold treatment: Apply ice several times a day; once inflammation and spasms subside, you can apply heat using a heating pad or a warm bath.
- If the pain is bothersome, an over-the-counter, non-steroidal anti-inflammatory medication such as ibuprofen or naproxen may be helpful; stronger pain medications and muscle relaxants are available by prescription.
- Bed rest immediately following the onset of back pain may make you feel better, but it should be of very short duration. Prolonged bed rest—5 days or more—was once thought to be an effective treatment for back pain, but most physicians now advise against it because it may weaken muscles and actually worsen pain. Limit bed rest to one day and begin moderate physical activity as soon as possible.
- Exercise can increase muscular endurance and flexibility and protect your disks from loss of fluid. Three of the back exercises discussed later in the chapter may be particularly helpful following an episode of acute back pain: curl-ups, side bridges, and back extensions.

See your physician if acute back pain doesn't resolve within a short time. Other warning signals of a more severe problem that requires a professional evaluation include the following: severe pain, numbness, pain that radiates down one or both legs, problems with bladder or bowel control, fever, or rapid weight loss.

Managing Chronic Back Pain

Low-back pain is considered chronic if it persists for more than 3 months. Symptoms vary—some people experience stabbing or shooting pain, others a steady ache accompanied by stiffness. Sometimes pain is localized; in other cases, it radiates to another part of the body. Underlying causes of chronic back pain include injuries, infection, muscle or ligament strains, and disk herniations.

Because symptoms and causes are so varied, different people benefit from different treatment strategies, and researchers have found that many treatments have only limited benefits. Potential treatments may include over-the-counter or prescription medications; exercise; physical therapy, massage, or chiropractic care; acupuncture; percutaneous electrical nerve stimulation (PENS), in which acupuncture-like needles are used to deliver an electrical current; education and advice about posture, exercise, and body mechanics; and surgery (see the box "Yoga for Relaxation and Pain Relief").

Psychological therapy may also be beneficial in some cases. Reducing emotional stress that causes muscle tension can provide direct benefits, and other therapies can help people deal better with chronic pain and its effects on their daily lives. Support groups and expressive writing are beneficial for people with chronic pain and other conditions.

Exercises for the Prevention and Management of Low-Back Pain

The tests in Labs 5.3 and 5.4 can help you assess low-back muscular endurance and posture. The exercises that follow are designed to help you maintain a healthy back by stretching and strengthening the major muscle groups that affect the back—the abdominal muscles, the muscles along your spine and sides, and the muscles of your hips and thighs. If you have back problems, check with your physician before beginning any exercise program. Perform the exercises slowly and progress very gradually. Stop and consult your physician if any exercise causes back pain. General guidelines for back exercise programs include the following:

- Do low-back exercises at least 3 days per week; many experts recommend daily back exercises.
- Emphasize muscular endurance rather than muscular strength—endurance is more protective.
- Don't do spine exercises involving a full range of motion early in the morning. Your disks have a high fluid content early in the day and injuries may result.
- Engage in regular endurance exercise such as cycling or walking in addition to performing exercises that specifically build muscular endurance and flexibility. Brisk walking with a vigorous arm swing may help relieve back pain. Start with fast walking if your core muscles are weak or you have back pain.
- Be patient and stick with your program. Increased back fitness and pain relief may require as long as 3 months of regular exercise.
- The adage "no pain, no gain" does not apply to back exercises. Always use good form and stop if you feel pain.

LOW-BACK EXERCISES

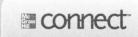

| EXERCISE 1 | Cat Stretch |

Target: Improved flexibility, relaxation, and reduced stiffness in the spine

Instructions: Begin on all fours with your knees below your hips and your hands below your shoulders. Slowly and deliberately move through a cycle of extension and flexion of your spine.
(a) Begin by slowly pushing your back up and dropping your head slightly until your spine is extended (rounded).
(b) Then, slowly lower your back and lift your chin slightly until your spine is flexed (relaxed and slightly arched). *Do not press at the ends of the range of motion.* Stop if you feel pain. Do 10 slow, continuous cycles of the movement.

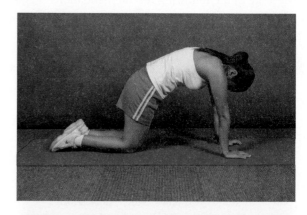

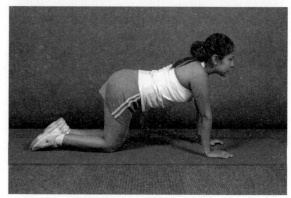

EXERCISE 2   Step Stretch   *(see Exercise 6 in the flexibility program)*

Target: Improved flexibility, strength, and endurance in the muscles of the hip and the front of the thigh

Instructions: Hold each stretch for 10–30 seconds and do at least 4 repetitions on each side.

EXERCISE 3   Alternate Leg Stretcher   *(see Exercise 11 in the flexibility program)*

Target: Improved flexibility in the back of the thigh, hip, knee, and buttocks

Instructions: Hold each stretch for 10–30 seconds and do at least 4 repetitions on each side.

EXERCISE 4   Trunk Twist

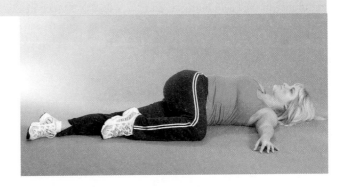

Target: Improved flexibility in the lower back and sides

Instructions: Lie on your side with top knee bent, lower leg straight, lower arm extended out in front of you on the floor, and upper arm at your side. Push down with your upper knee while you twist your trunk backward. Try to get your shoulders and upper body flat on the floor, turning your head as well. Return to the starting position, and then repeat on the other side. Hold the stretch for 10–30 seconds and do at least 4 repetitions on each side.

EXERCISE 5   Curl-Up

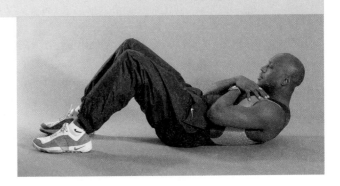

Target: Improved strength and endurance in the abdomen

Instructions: Lie on your back with one or two knees bent and arms crossed on your chest or hands under your lower back. Maintain a neutral spine. Tuck your chin in and slowly curl up, one vertebra at a time, as you use your abdominal muscles to lift your head first and then your shoulders. Stop when you can see your knees and hold for 5–10 seconds before returning to the starting position. Do 10 or more repetitions.

Variation: Add a twist to develop other abdominal muscles. When you have curled up so that your shoulder blades are off the floor, twist your upper body so that one shoulder is higher than the other; reach past your knee with your upper arm. Hold and then return to the starting position. Repeat on the opposite side. Curl-ups can also be done using an exercise ball.

EXERCISE 6 — Isometric Side Bridge *(see Exercise 11 in the free weights program in Chapter 4)*

Target: Increased strength and endurance in the muscles along the sides of the abdomen

Instructions: Hold the bridge position for 10 seconds, breathing normally. Work up to a 60-second hold. Perform one or more repetitions on each side.

Variation: You can make the exercise more difficult by keeping your legs straight and supporting yourself with your feet and forearm (see Lab 5.3) or with your feet and hand (with elbow straight).

EXERCISE 7 — Spine Extensions *(see Exercise 10 in the free weights program in Chapter 4)*

Target: Increased strength and endurance in the back, buttocks, and back of the thighs

Instructions: Hold each position for 10–30 seconds. Begin with one repetition on each side and work up to several repetitions.

Variation: If you have experienced back pain in the past or if this exercise is very difficult for you, do the exercise with both hands on the ground rather than with one arm lifted. You can make this exercise more difficult by doing it balancing on an exercise ball. Find a balance point on your chest while lying face down on the ball with one arm and the opposite leg on the ground. Tense your abdominal muscles while reaching and extending with one arm and reaching and extending with the opposite leg. Repeat this exercise using the other arm and leg.

EXERCISE 8 — Wall Squat (Phantom Chair)

Target: Increased strength and endurance in the lower back, thighs, and abdomen

Instructions: Lean against a wall and bend your knees as though you are sitting in a chair. Support your weight with your legs. Begin by holding the position for 5–10 seconds. Build up to 1 minute or more. Perform one or more repetitions.

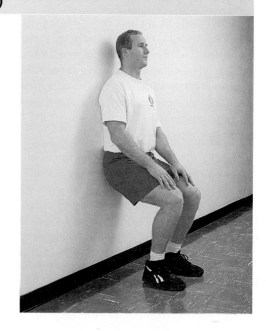

EXERCISE 9   Pelvic Tilt

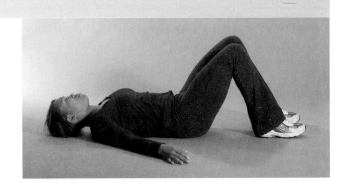

Target: Increased strength and endurance in the abdomen and buttocks

Instructions: Lie on your back with knees bent and arms extended to the side. Tilt your pelvis under and try to flatten your lower back against the floor. Tighten your buttock and abdominal muscles while you hold this position for 5–10 seconds. Don't hold your breath. Work up to 10 repetitions of the exercise. Pelvic tilts can also be done standing or leaning against a wall. (*Note:* Although this is a popular exercise with many therapists, some experts question the safety of pelvic tilts. Stop if you feel pain in your back at any time during the exercise.)

EXERCISE 10   Back Bridge

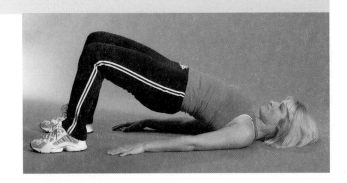

Target: Increased strength and endurance in the hips and buttocks

Instructions: Lie on your back with knees bent and arms extended to the side. Tuck your pelvis under, and then lift your tailbone, buttocks, and lower back from the floor. Hold this position for 5–10 seconds with your weight resting on your feet, arms, and shoulders, and then return to the starting position. Work up to 10 repetitions of the exercise.

✓ TIPS FOR TODAY AND THE FUTURE

To improve and maintain your flexibility, perform stretches that work the major joints at least twice a week.

RIGHT NOW YOU CAN

- Stand up and stretch—do either the upper-back stretch or the across-the-body stretch shown in the chapter.
- Practise the recommended sitting and standing postures suggested in the chapter. If needed, adjust your chair or find something to use as a footrest.

IN THE FUTURE YOU CAN

- Build up your flexibility by incorporating more sophisticated stretching exercises into your routine.
- Increase the frequency of your flexibility workouts to 5 or more days per week.
- Increase the efficiency of your workouts by adding stretching exercises to the cool-down period of your endurance or strength workouts.

Is stretching the same as warming up?

No. They are two distinct activities. A warm-up involves moving the joints through the same motions used during the activity; it increases body temperature so your metabolism works better when you're exercising at high intensity. Stretching increases the movement capability of your joints, so you can move more easily with less risk of injury. Stretching may also induce cellular changes that protect muscles from injury. It is best to stretch at the end of your aerobic or weight training workout, when your muscles are warm. Warmed muscles stretch better than cold ones and are less prone to injury.

How much flexibility do I need?

This question is not always easy to answer. If you're involved in a sport such as gymnastics, figure skating, or ballet, you are often required to reach extreme joint motions to achieve success. However, nonathletes do not need to reach these extreme joint positions. In fact, too much flexibility may, in some cases, increase your risk of injury. As with other types of fitness, moderation is the key. You should regularly stretch your major joints and muscle groups but not aspire to reach extreme flexibility.

Can I stretch too far?

Yes. As muscle tissue is progressively stretched, it reaches a point where it becomes damaged and may rupture.

The greatest danger occurs during passive stretching when a partner is doing the stretching for you. It is critical that your stretching partner not force your joint outside its normal functional range of motion.

Can physical training limit flexibility?

Weight training, jogging, or any physical activity will decrease flexibility if the exercises are not performed through a full range of motion. When done properly, weight training increases flexibility. However, because of the limited range of motion used during the running stride, jogging tends to compromise flexibility. It is important for runners to practice flexibility exercises for the hamstrings and quadriceps regularly.

Does stretching affect muscular strength?

Flexibility training increases muscle strength over time, but preexercise stretching can cause short-term decreases in strength and power. Several recent studies have found that stretching decreases strength, power, and motor control following the stretch. This is one reason some experts suggest that people not stretch as part of their exercise warm-up. It is important to warm up before any workout by engaging in 5–10 minutes of light exercise such as walking or slow jogging.

Can a workout with an exercise ball be useful in preventing and managing low-back pain?

Yes. The exercise or stability ball is an extra-large inflatable ball. It was originally developed for use in physical therapy but has recently become a popular piece of exercise equipment for use in the home or gym. The exercise ball is particularly effective for working the so-called stability muscles in the abdomen, chest, and back—muscles that are important for preventing back problems. The ball's instability forces an exerciser to use the stability muscles to balance the body. Moves such as crunches have been found to be more effective when they are performed with an exercise ball. Beginners should use caution (and choose a larger-sized ball) until they feel comfortable with the movements.

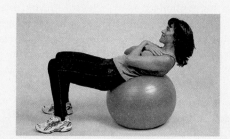

Using an exercise ball for curl-ups works the muscles in the chest, back, buttocks, and legs in addition to those in the abdomen.

SUMMARY

- Flexibility, the ability of joints to move through their full range of motion, is highly adaptable and specific to each joint.
- Range of motion can be limited by joint structure, muscle inelasticity, and stretch receptor activity.
- Developing flexibility depends on stretching the elastic tissues within muscles regularly and gently

until they lengthen. Overstretching can make connective tissue brittle and lead to rupture.
- Signals sent between proprioceptors and the spinal cord can enhance flexibility.
- The benefits of flexibility include preventing abnormal stresses that lead to joint deterioration and possibly reducing the risk of injuries and low-back pain.

- Stretches should be held for 10–30 seconds; perform 2–4 repetitions. Flexibility training should be done a minimum of 2–3 days a week (ideally, 4–7 days per week), preferably following activity, when muscles are warm.

- Static stretching is done slowly and held to the point of mild tension; ballistic stretching consists of bouncing stretches and can lead to injury. Proprioceptive neuromuscular facilitation uses muscle receptors in contracting and relaxing a muscle.

- Passive stretching, using an outside force in moving muscles and joints, achieves a greater range of motion (and has a higher injury risk) than active stretching, which uses opposing muscles to initiate a stretch.

- The spinal column consists of vertebrae separated by intervertebral disks. It provides structure and support for the body and protects the spinal cord. The core muscles stabilize the spine and transfer force between the upper and lower body.

- Acute back pain can be treated as a soft tissue injury, with cold treatment followed by application of heat (once swelling subsides); prolonged bed rest is not recommended. A variety of treatments have been suggested for chronic back pain, including regular exercise, physical therapy, acupuncture, education, and psychological therapy.

- In addition to good posture, proper body mechanics, and regular physical activity, a program for preventing low-back pain includes exercises that stretch and strengthen major muscle groups that affect the lower back.

FOR FURTHER EXPLORATION

Organizations and Websites

The Arthritis Society. Includes general information about the role of exercise in those with various forms of arthritis. Also contains an open forum to ask questions of physicians.
http://www.arthritis.ca

Back Fit Pro. A website maintained by Dr. Stuart McGill, a professor of spine biomechanics at the University of Waterloo, which provides evidence-based information on preventing and treating back pain.
http://www.backfitpro.com

Bone and Joint Decade Canada. Designed to promote the preservation of bone and joint health and improve the health-related quality of life for those with musculo-skeletal disorders.
http://bjdcanada.org/

The Canadian Academy of Sports Medicine. Non-profit group of physicians devoted to the practice of medicine as it applies to all areas of physical activity.
http://www.casm-acms.org/

Canadian Chiropractic Association. Includes information to create awareness about back pain and the role of chiropractors in its treatment. Also provides a questionnaire to assess your risk for suffering low back pain.
http://ccachiro.org

Canadian Orthopaedic Association. Brings together information from physicians promoting orthopaedic care in Canada.
http://www.coa-aco.org/Frameset.html

The Canadian Orthopaedic Foundation. An information source in research, education, and care of those with bone and joint disorders.
http://www.canorth.org

Canadian Physiotherapy Association. Provides SMART stretching tips for a variety of activities.
http://www.physiotherapy.ca/

Exercise: A Guide from the National Institute on Aging. Practical advice on fitness for seniors; includes animated instructions for specific flexibility exercises.
http://www.nia.nih.gov/HealthInformation/Publications/ExerciseGuide/

Georgia State University: Flexibility. Provides information about the benefits of stretching and how to develop a safe and effective program; includes illustrations of stretches.
http://www.gsu.edu/~wwwfit/flexibility.html

MedlinePlus Back Pain Tutorial. An interactive, illustrated tutorial of the causes and prevention of back pain.
http://www.nlm.nih.gov/medlineplus/tutorials/backpain.html

NIH Back Pain Fact Sheet. Basic information on the prevention and treatment of back pain.
http://www.ninds.nih.gov/health_and_medical/disorders/backpain_doc.htm

Stretching and Flexibility. Provides information about the physiology of stretching and different types of stretching exercises.
http://www.ifafitness.com/stretch/index.html

See also the listings for Chapters 2 and 4.

LAB 5.1 Assessing Your Current Level of Flexibility

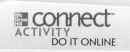

Part I Sit-and-Reach Test

Equipment

Use a modified Wells and Dillon flexometer or construct your own measuring device using a firm box or two pieces of wood about 30 centimetres high attached at right angles to each other. Attach a metric ruler to measure the extent of reach. With the low numbers of the ruler toward the person being tested, set the 26-centimetre mark of the ruler at the footline of the box. (Individuals who cannot reach as far as the footline will have scores below 26 centimetres; those who can reach past their feet will have scores above 26 centimetres.) Most studies show no relationship between performance on the sit-and-reach test and the incidence of back pain.

Preparation

Warm up your muscles with a low-intensity activity such as walking or easy jogging. Then perform slow stretching movements.

Instructions

1. Remove your shoes and sit facing the flexibility measuring device with your knees fully extended and your feet flat against the device about 10 centimetres apart.

2. On an exhale, reach as far forward as you can, with palms down, arms evenly stretched, and knees fully extended; hold the position of maximum reach for about 2 seconds.

3. Perform the stretch 2 times, recording the distance of maximum reach to the nearest 0.5 centimetres: _____ cm

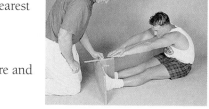

Rating Your Flexibility

Find the score in the table below to determine your flexibility rating. Record it here and on the final page of this lab.

Rating: _____

Ratings for Sit-and-Reach Test

		Rating/Score (cm)*			
Men	Needs Improvement	Fair	Good	Very Good	Excellent
Age: 15–19	≤ 23	24–28	29–33	34–38	≤ 39
20–29	≤ 24	25–29	30–33	34–39	≤ 40
30–39	≤ 22	23–27	28–32	33–37	≤ 38
40–49	≤ 17	18–23	24–28	29–34	≤ 35
50–59	≤ 15	16–23	24–27	28–34	≤ 35
60–69	≤ 14	15–19	20–24	25–32	≤ 33
Women					
Age: 15–19	≤ 28	29–33	34–37	38–42	≤ 43
20–29	≤ 27	28–32	33–36	37–40	≤ 41
30–39	≤ 26	27–31	32–35	36–40	≤ 41
40–49	≤ 24	25–29	30–33	34–37	≤ 38
50–59	≤ 24	25–29	30–32	33–38	≤ 39
60–69	≤ 22	23–26	27–30	31–34	≤ 35

*Footline is set at 26 cm.

SOURCE: *Canadian Physical Activity, Fitness and Lifestyle Approach: CSEP's Health & Fitness Program's Health-Related Appraisal & Counselling Strategy,* Third Edition © 2003. Reprinted with permission from the Canadian Society for Exercise Physiology.

Part II Range-of-Motion Assessment

This portion of the lab can be completed by doing visual comparisons or by measuring joint range of motion with a goniometer or other instrument.

Equipment

1. A partner to do visual comparisons or to measure the range of motion of your joints. (You can also use a mirror to perform your own visual comparisons.)
2. For the measurement method, you need a goniometer, flexometer, or other instrument to measure range of motion.

Preparation

Warm up your muscles with some low-intensity activity such as walking or easy jogging.

Instructions

On the following pages, the average range of motion is illustrated and listed quantitatively for some of the major joints. Visually assess the range of motion in your joints and compare it to that shown in the illustrations. For each joint, note (with a check mark) whether your range of motion is above average, average, or below average and in need of improvement. Average values for range of motion are given in degrees for each joint in the assessment. You can also complete the assessment by measuring your range of motion with a goniometer, flexometer, or other instrument. If you are using this measurement method, identify your rating (above average, average, or below average) and record your range of motion in degrees next to the appropriate category. Although the measurement method is more time-consuming, it allows you to track the progress of your stretching program more precisely and to note changes within the broader ratings categories (below average, above average).

Record your ratings on the following pages and on the chart on the final page of this lab. (Ratings were derived from several published sources.)

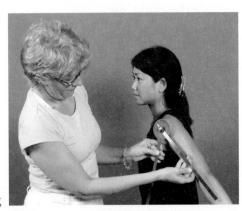

Assessment of range of motion using a goniometer

1. Shoulder Abduction and Adduction

For each position and arm, check one of the following; also fill in degrees if using the measurement method.

Shoulder abduction—raise arm up to the side

Right | Left
_____ | _____ Below average/needs improvement
_____ | _____ Average (92–95°)
_____ | _____ Above average

Shoulder adduction—move arm down and in front of body

Right | Left
_____ | _____ Below average/needs improvement
_____ | _____ Average (124–127°)
_____ | _____ Above average

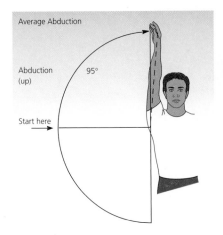

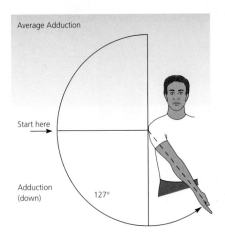

2. Shoulder Flexion and Extension

For each position and arm, check one of the following; also fill in degrees if using the measurement method.

Shoulder flexion—raise arm up in front of the body

Right   Left

_____ _____ Below average/needs improvement

_____ _____ Average (92–95°)

_____ _____ Above average

Shoulder extension—move arm down and behind the body

Right   Left

_____ _____ Below average/needs improvement

_____ _____ Average (145–150°)

_____ _____ Above average

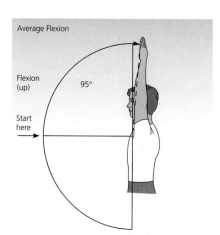

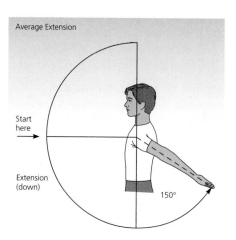

3. Trunk/Low Back Lateral Flexion

Bend directly sideways at your waist. To prevent injury, keep your knees slightly bent, and support your trunk by placing your hand or forearm on your thigh. Check one of the following for each side; fill in degrees if using the measurement method.

Right   Left

_____ _____ Below average/needs improvement

_____ _____ Average (36–40°)

_____ _____ Above average

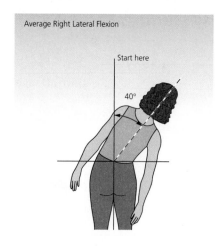

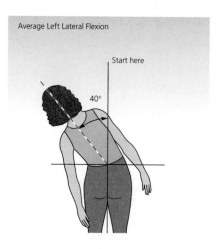

4. Hip Abduction

Raise your leg to the side at the hip. Check one of the following for each leg; fill in degrees if using the measurement meth

Right   Left

_____   _____   Below average/needs improvement

_____   _____   Average (40–45°)

_____   _____   Above average

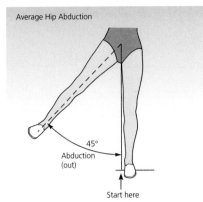

5. Hip Flexion (Bent Knee)

With one leg flat on the floor, bend the other knee and lift the leg up at the hip. Check one of the following for each leg; fill in degrees if using the measurement method.

Right   Left

_____   _____   Below average/needs improvement

_____   _____   Average (121–125°)

_____   _____   Above average

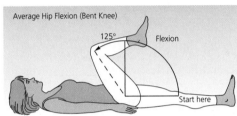

6. Hip Flexion (Straight Leg)

With one leg flat on the floor, raise the other leg at the hip, keeping both legs straight. Take care not to put excess strain on your back. Check one of the following for each leg; fill in degrees if using the measurement method.

Right   Left

_____   _____   Below average/needs improvement

_____   _____   Average (79–81°)

_____   _____   Above average

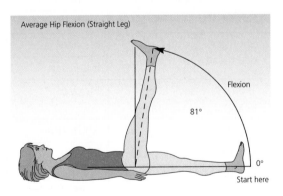

7. Ankle Dorsiflexion and Plantar Flexion

For each position and foot, check one of the following; also fill in degrees if using the measurement method.

Ankle dorsiflexion—pull your toes toward your shin

Right   Left

_____   _____   Below average/needs improvement

_____   _____   Average (9–13°)

_____   _____   Above average

Plantar flexion—point your toes

Right   Left

_____   _____   Below average/needs improvement

_____   _____   Average (50–55°)

_____   _____   Above average

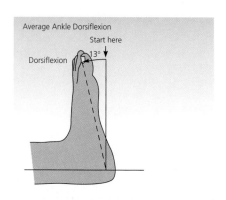

Average Ankle Dorsiflexion

Start here

Dorsiflexion   13°

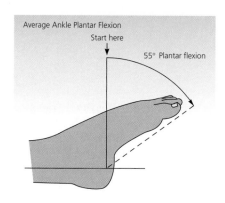

Average Ankle Plantar Flexion

Start here

55° Plantar flexion

Rating Your Flexibility

Sit-and-Reach Test: Score: _____ cm. Rating: _____

Range-of-Motion Assessment

Identify your rating for each joint on each side of the body. If you used the comparison method, put check marks in the appropriate categories; if you measured range of motion, enter the degrees for each joint in the appropriate category.

Joint/Assessment		Right			Left		
		Below Average	*Average*	*Above Average*	*Below Average*	*Average*	*Above Average*
1. Shoulder abduction and adduction	Abduction						
	Adduction						
2. Shoulder flexion and extension	Flexion						
	Extension						
3. Trunk/low-back lateral flexion	Flexion						
4. Hip abduction	Abduction						
5. Hip flexion (bent knee)	Flexion						
6. Hip flexion (straight leg)	Flexion						
7. Ankle dorsiflexion and plantar flexion	Dorsiflexion						
	Plantar flexion						

Using Your Results

How did you score? Are you at all surprised by your ratings for flexibility? Are you satisfied with your current ratings?

If you're not satisfied, set a realistic goal for improvement:

Are you satisfied with your current level of flexibility as expressed in your daily life—for example, your ability to maintain good posture and move easily and without pain?

If you're not satisfied, set some realistic goals for improvement:

What should you do next? Enter the results of this lab in the Preprogram Assessment column in Appendix C. If you've set goals for improvement, begin planning your flexibility program by completing the plan in Lab 5.2. After several weeks of your program, complete this lab again and enter the results in the Postprogram Assessment column of Appendix C. How do the results compare?

Name _____ Section _____ Date _____

LAB 5.2 Creating a Personalized Program for Developing Flexibility

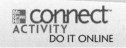

Goals: List goals for your flexibility program. On the left, include specific, measurable goals that you can use to track the progress of your fitness program. These goals might be things like raising your sit-and-reach score from fair to good or your bent-leg hip flexion rating from below average to average. On the right, include long-term and more qualitative goals, such as reducing your risk for back pain.

Specific Goals: Current Status   *Final Goals*

_____   _____

_____   _____

_____   _____

Other goals: _____

_____

Exercises: The exercises in the program plan below are from the general stretching program presented in Chapter 5. You can add or delete exercises depending on your needs, goals, and preferences. For any exercises you add, fill in the areas of the body affected.

Frequency: A minimum frequency of 2–3 days per week is recommended; 4–7 days per week is ideal. You may want to do your stretching exercises the same days you plan to do cardiorespiratory endurance exercise or weight training, because muscles stretch better following exercise, when they are warm.

Intensity: All stretches should be done to the point of mild discomfort, not pain.

Time/duration: All stretches should be held for 10–30 seconds. (PNF techniques should include a 6-second contraction followed by a 10–30-second assisted stretch.) All stretches should be performed 2–4 times.

Program Plan for Flexibility

Exercise	Areas Stretched	M	Tu	W	Th	F	Sa	Su
					Frequency (check ✓)			
Head turns and tilts	Neck							
Towel stretch	Triceps, shoulders, chest							
Across-the-body and overhead stretches	Shoulders, upper back, back of the arm							
Upper-back stretch	Upper back							
Lateral stretch	Trunk muscles							
Step stretch	Hip, front of thigh							
Side lunge	Inner thigh, hip, calf							
Inner-thigh stretch	Inner thigh, hip							
Trunk rotation	Trunk, outer thigh and hip, lower back							
Modified hurdler stretch	Back of the thigh, lower back							
Alternate leg stretcher	Back of the thigh, hip, knee, ankle, buttocks							
Lower-leg stretch	Back of the lower leg							

You can monitor your program using a chart like the following flexibility program chart.

Flexibility Program Chart

Fill in the dates (Frequency) you perform each stretch (Type), the number of seconds (Time) you hold each stretch (should be 15–30 seconds), and the number of repetitions of each (should be 2–4). For an easy check on the duration of your stretches, count "one thousand one, one thousand two," and so on. You will probably find that over time you'll be able to hold each stretch longer (in addition to being able to stretch farther). Recall that your intensity is based on stretching to the point of mild discomfort, not pain.

Exercise/Date																						
	Duration																					
	Reps																					
	Duration																					
	Reps																					
	Duration																					
	Reps																					
	Duration																					
	Reps																					
	Duration																					
	Reps																					
	Duration																					
	Reps																					
	Duration																					
	Reps																					
	Duration																					
	Reps																					
	Duration																					
	Reps																					
	Duration																					
	Reps																					
	Duration																					
	Reps																					
	Duration																					
	Reps																					
	Duration																					
	Reps																					
	Duration																					
	Reps																					
	Duration																					
	Reps																					
	Duration																					
	Reps																					

LAB 5.3 **Assessing Muscular Endurance for Low-Back Health**

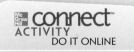

The three tests in this lab evaluate the muscular endurance of major spine stabilizing muscles.

Side Bridge Endurance Test

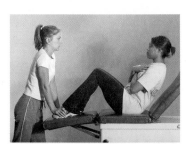

Equipment

1. Stopwatch or clock with a second hand
2. Exercise mat
3. Partner

Preparation

Warm up your muscles with some low-intensity activity such as walking or easy jogging. Practise assuming the side bridge position described below.

Instructions

1. Lie on the mat on your side with your legs extended. Place your top foot in front of your lower foot for support. Lift your hips off the mat so that you are supporting yourself on one elbow and your feet (see photo). Your body should maintain a straight line. Breathe normally; don't hold your breath.

2. Hold the position as long as possible. Your partner should keep track of the time and make sure that you maintain the correct position. Your final score is the total time you are able to hold the side bridge with correct form—from the time you lift your hips until your hips return to the mat.

3. Rest for 5 minutes and then repeat the test on the other side. Record your times here and on the chart at the end of the lab. Right side bridge time: _____ sec. Left side bridge time: _____ sec.

Trunk Flexors Endurance Test

Equipment

1. Stopwatch or clock with a second hand
2. Exercise mat or padded exercise table
3. Two helpers
4. Jig angled at 60° from the floor or padded bench (optional)

Preparation

Warm up with some low-intensity activity such as walking or easy jogging.

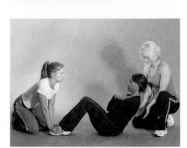

Instructions

1. To start, assume a sit-up posture with your back supported at an angle of 60° from the floor; support can be provided by a jig, a padded bench, or a spotter (see photos). Your knees and hips should both be flexed at 90°, and your arms should be folded across your chest with your hands placed on the opposite shoulders. Your toes should be secured under a toe strap or held by a partner.

2. Your goal is to hold the starting position (isometric contraction) as long as possible after the support is pulled away. To begin the test, a helper should pull the jig or other support back about 10 cm. A helper should keep track of the time; if a spotter is acting as your support, she or he should be ready to support your weight as soon as your torso begins to move back. Your final score is the total time you are able to hold the contraction—from the time the support is removed until any part of your back touches the support. Remember to breathe normally throughout the test.

3. Record your time here and on the chart at the end of the lab. Trunk flexors endurance time: _____ sec.

Back Extensors Endurance Test

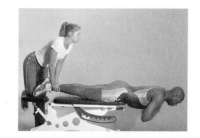

Equipment

1. Stopwatch or clock with a second hand
2. Extension bench with padded ankle support or any padded bench
3. Partner

Preparation

Warm up with some low-intensity activity such as walking or easy jogging.

Instructions

1. Lie face down on the test bench with the upper body extending out over the end of the bench and the pelvis, hips, and knees flat on the bench. Your arms should be folded across your chest with your hands placed on the opposite shoulders. Your feet should be secured under a padded strap or held by a partner.

2. Your goal is to hold your upper body in a straight horizontal line with your lower body as long as possible. Keep your neck straight and neutral; don't raise your head and don't arch your back. Breathe normally. Your partner should keep track of the time and watch your form. Your final score is the total time you are able to hold the horizontal position—from the time you assume the position until your upper body drops from the horizontal position.

3. Record your time here and on the chart below. Back extensors endurance time: _____ sec.

Rating Your Test Results for Muscular Endurance for Low-Back Health

The table below shows mean endurance test times for healthy young college/university students with a mean age of 21 years. Compare your scores with the times shown in the table. (If you are older or have suffered from low-back pain in the past, these ratings are less accurate; however, your time scores can be used as a point of comparison.)

	Right side bridge	Left side bridge	Trunk flexors	Back extensors
	Mean Endurance Times (sec)			
Men	95	99	136	161
Women	75	78	134	185

SOURCE: From S. M. McGill, 2007, *Low Back Disorders: Evidence Based Prevention and Rehabilitation,* 2nd ed., page 211. Reprinted with permission from Human Kinetics (Champaign, IL).

Right side bridge: _____ sec   Rating (above mean, at mean, below mean): _____

Left side bridge: _____ sec   Rating (above mean, at mean, below mean): _____

Trunk flexors: _____ sec   Rating (above mean, at mean, below mean): _____

Back extensors: _____ sec   Rating (above mean, at mean, below mean): _____

Using Your Results

How did you score? Are you at all surprised by your scores for the low-back tests? Are you satisfied with your current ratings?

If you're not satisfied, set a realistic goal for improvement. The norms in this lab are based on healthy young adults, so a score above the mean may or may not be realistic for you. Instead, you may want to set a specific goal based on time rather than rating; for example, set a goal of improving your time by 10%. Imbalances in muscular endurance have been linked with back problems, so if your rating is significantly lower for one of the three tests, you should focus particular attention on that area of the body.

Goal: _____

What should you do next? Enter the results of this lab in the Preprogram Assessment column in Appendix C. If you've set a goal for improvement, begin a program of low-back exercises such as that suggested in this chapter. After several weeks of your program, complete this lab again and enter the results in the Postprogram Assessment column of Appendix C. How do the results compare?

SOURCE: Adapted with permission from S. McGill, 2007, *Low Back Disorders: Evidence-Based Prevention and Rehabilitation,* 2nd edition. (Champaign, IL: Human Kinetics). p. 211.

Name _____ Section _____ Date _____

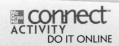

LAB 5.4 Posture Evaluation

For each row, have a partner record the point total that corresponds to the illustration that most closely matches your posture.

5 points	3 points	1 point	Your Score

Head erect (gravity line passes directly through centre) — Head twisted or turned to one side slightly — Head twisted or turned to one side markedly

_____

Shoulders level (horizontally) — One shoulder slightly higher than other — One shoulder markedly higher than other

_____

Spine straight — Spine slightly curved laterally — Spine markedly curved laterally

_____

Hips level (horizontally) — One hip slightly higher — One hip markedly higher

_____

Feet pointed straight ahead — Feet pointed out — Feet pointed out markedly; ankles sag in (pronation)

_____

Arches high — Arches lower, feet slightly flat — Arches low; feet markedly flat

_____

5 points	3 points	1 point	Your Score

 Neck erect, chin in, head in balance directly above shoulders
 Neck slightly forward, chin slightly out
 Neck markedly forward, chin markedly out
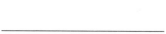

 Chest elevated (breast-bone farthest forward part of body)
 Chest slightly depressed
 Chest markedly depressed (flat)
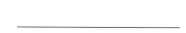

 Shoulders centred
 Shoulders slightly forward
 Shoulders markedly forward (shoulder blades protruding in rear)
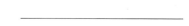

 Upper back normally rounded
 Upper back slightly more rounded
 Upper back markedly rounded
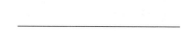

 Trunk erect
 Trunk inclined to rear slightly
 Trunk inclined to rear markedly

 Abdomen flat
 Abdomen protruding
 Abdomen protruding and sagging

 Lower back normally curved
 Lower back slightly hollow
Lower back markedly hollow

Total Score (from both pages) (Scores should be between 13 and 65.) _____

If your posture needs improvement, review the information in the "Yoga for Relaxation and Pain Relief" box presented earlier in the chapter. If you scored 1 point for any item in the evaluation, you may want to consider seeing a physician; professional advice, physical therapy, orthotic devices, or other therapies may help you improve your posture.

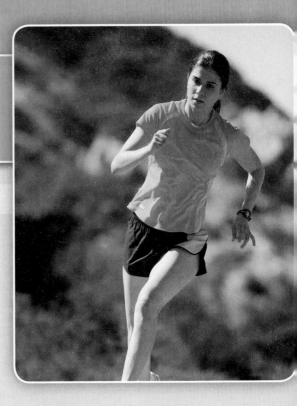

CHAPTER 6

BODY COMPOSITION

LEARNING OBJECTIVES

After reading this chapter, you should be able to

LO1 Define fat-free mass, essential fat, and nonessential fat and describe their functions in the body

LO2 Explain how body composition affects overall health and wellness

LO3 Describe how body mass index, body composition, and body fat distribution are measured and assessed

LO4 Explain how to determine recommended body weight and body fat distribution

TEST YOUR KNOWLEDGE

1. **Exercise helps reduce the risks associated with overweight and obesity even if it doesn't result in improvements in body composition.**

   True or false?

2. **Which of the following is the most significant risk factor for the most common type of diabetes (type 2 diabetes)?**

   a. smoking
   b. low-fibre diet
   c. overweight or obesity
   d. inactivity

3. **In women, excessive exercise and low energy (calorie) intake can cause which of the following?**

   a. unhealthy reduction in body fat levels
   b. amenorrhea (absent menstruation)
   c. bone density loss and osteoporosis
   d. muscle wasting and fatigue

ANSWERS

1. **TRUE.** Regular physical activity provides protection against the health risks of overweight and obesity. People who are fit and obese live longer, healthier lives than normal weight people who are sedentary. However, it is best to both be active and maintain a healthy weight.

2. **C.** All four are risk factors for diabetes, but overweight/obesity is the most significant. It's estimated that 90% of cases of type 2 diabetes could be prevented if people adopted healthy lifestyle behaviours.

3. **ALL FOUR.** Very low levels of body fat, and the behaviours used to achieve them, have serious health consequences for both men and women.

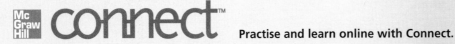

Practise and learn online with Connect.

Body composition, the body's relative amount of fat and fat-free mass, is an important component of fitness for health and wellness. People whose body composition is optimal tend to be healthier, to move more efficiently, and to feel better about themselves. They also have a lower risk of many chronic diseases.

Many people, however, don't succeed in their efforts to obtain a fit and healthy body because they set unrealistic goals and emphasize short-term weight loss rather than the permanent changes in lifestyle that lead to fat loss and a healthy body composition. Successful management of body composition requires the long-term, consistent coordination of many aspects of a wellness program. Even in the absence of changes in body composition, an active lifestyle improves wellness and decreases the risk of disease and premature death (see the box "Why Is Physical Activity Important Even If Body Composition Doesn't Change?").

This chapter focuses on defining and measuring body composition. The aspects of lifestyle that affect body composition are discussed in detail in other chapters: physical activity and exercise in Chapters 2–5, sound nutritional habits in Chapter 7, specific strategies for weight management in Chapter 8, and healthy techniques for managing stress in Chapter 10.

LO1 6.1 WHAT IS BODY COMPOSITION, AND WHY IS IT IMPORTANT?

The human body can be divided into fat-free mass and body fat. As defined in Chapter 2, fat-free mass is composed of all the body's nonfat tissues: bone, water, muscle, connective tissue, organ tissues, and teeth.

A certain amount of body fat is necessary for the body to function. Fat is incorporated into the nerves, brain, heart, lungs, liver, mammary glands, and other body organs and tissues. It is the main source of stored energy in the body; it also cushions body organs and helps regulate body temperature. This **essential fat** makes up about 3–5% of total body weight in men and 8–12% in women (Figure 6.1). The percentage is higher in women due to fat deposits in the breasts, uterus, and other gender-specific sites.

Most of the fat in the body is stored in fat cells, or **adipose tissue**, located under the skin (**subcutaneous fat**) and around major organs (**visceral** or **intra-abdominal fat**). These stored sources of fat are often referred to as **nonessential fat**. People have a genetically determined number of fat cells, but these cells can increase or decrease in size depending on how much fat is being stored. The amount of stored fat depends on several factors, including age, sex, metabolism, diet, and activity level. The primary source of excess body fat is excess calories consumed in the diet—that is, calories consumed in excess of calories expended in metabolism, physical activity, and exercise. A pound of body fat is equal to 3500 calories, so an intake of just 100 calories a day in excess of calories expended will

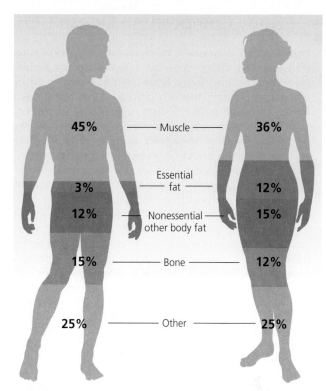

FIGURE 6.1 Body composition of a typical man and woman, 20–24 years old.

SOURCE: Adapted from Brooks, G. A., et al. 2005. *Exercise Physiology: Human Bioenergetics and Its Applications,* 4th ed. New York: McGraw-Hill.

result in a 10-pound weight gain over the course of a year. Excess stored body fat is associated with increased risk of chronic diseases like diabetes and cardiovascular disease, as described later in this chapter.

Overweight and Obesity Defined

Some of the most commonly used methods of assessing and classifying body composition are described later in this chapter. Some methods are based on body fat, and others on total body weight. Methods based on total body weight are less accurate than those based on body fat, but they are commonly used because body weight is easier to measure than body fat.

In the past, many people relied on height/weight tables (which were based on insurance company mortality statistics) to determine whether they were at a healthy weight. Such tables, however, can be highly inaccurate for some people. Because muscle tissue is denser and

essential fat Fat incorporated in various tissues of the body; critical for normal body functioning.

adipose tissue Connective tissue in which fat is stored.

subcutaneous fat Fat located under the skin.

visceral fat Fat located around major organs; also called *intra-abdominal fat*.

nonessential (storage) fat Extra fat or fat reserves stored in the body.

TERMS

Why Is Physical Activity Important Even If Body Composition Doesn't Change?

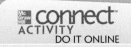
ACTIVITY DO IT ONLINE

Physical activity is important for health even if it produces no changes in body composition—that is, even if a person remains overweight or obese. Physical activity confers benefits no matter how much you weigh; conversely, physical inactivity operates as a risk factor for health problems independently of body composition.

Regular physical activity and exercise block many of the destructive effects of obesity. For example, physical activity improves blood pressure, blood glucose levels, cholesterol levels, and body fat distribution. It also lowers the risk of cardiovascular disease, diabetes, and premature death. Although physical activity and exercise produce these improvements quickly in some people and slowly in others, due to genetic differences, the improvements do occur. Physical activity is particularly important for the many people who have metabolic syndrome or pre-diabetes, both of which are characterized by insulin resistance. Exercise encourages the body's cells to take up and use insulin efficiently for converting nutrients into usable energy.

Although being physically active and not being sedentary may sound identical, experts describe them as different dimensions of the same health issue. Data suggest that it is important not only to be physically active but also to avoid prolonged sitting. In one study, people who watched TV or used a computer 4 or more hours a day had twice the risk of having metabolic syndrome as those who spent less than 1 hour a day in these activities; other studies reported similar results. Thus, in addition to increasing physical activity, avoiding or reducing sedentary behaviour is an important—and challenging—health goal.

Although physical activity is important even if it doesn't change body composition, at a certain level, physical activity and exercise do improve body composition (meaning less fat and more lean muscle mass). Evidence supports a dose-response relation between exercise and fat loss—that is, the more you exercise, the more fat you will lose. This includes

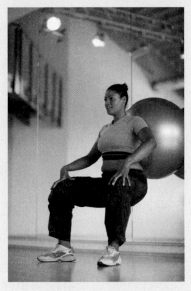

both total body fat and abdominal fat. Additionally, the more body fat a person has, the greater is the loss of abdominal fat with exercise. Studies show that, even without calorie reduction, walking 150 minutes per week at a pace of 4 miles per hour, or jogging 75 minutes a week at 6 miles per hour, produces a decrease in total fat and abdominal fat that is associated with improved metabolic health.

Studies also show, however, that combining exercise with an appropriate reduction in calories is an even better way to reduce levels of body fat and increase lean muscle mass. The results of combining exercise and calorie reduction may not show up as expected on the scale, because the weight of body fat lost is partially offset by the weight of muscle mass gained. Still, your body composition, physical fitness, and overall health have improved.

The question is sometimes asked, Which is more important in combating the adverse health effects of obesity—physical activity or physical fitness? Many studies suggest that both are important; the more active and fit you are, the lower your risk of having health problems and dying prematurely. Of the two, however, physical activity appears to be more important for health than physical fitness.

SOURCES: Baer, H. J., et al. 2011. Risk factors for mortality in the nurses' health study: A competing risks analysis. *American Journal of Epidemiology* 173(3): 319–329; Farrell, S. W. 2010. Cardiorespiratory fitness, adiposity, and all-cause mortality in women. *Medicine and Science in Sports and Exercise* 42(11): 2006–2012; Physical Activity Guidelines Advisory Committee. 2008. *Physical Activity Guidelines Advisory Committee Report, 2008*. Washington, D.C.: U.S. Department of Health and Human Services; and Stephens, B. R., et al. 2011. Effects of 1 day of inactivity on insulin action in healthy men and women: interaction with energy intake. *Metabolism Clinical and Experimental*. 60: 941–949.

heavier than fat, a fit person can easily weigh more than the recommended weight on a height/weight table. For the same reason, an unfit person may weigh less than the table's recommended weight.

When looking at body composition, the most important consideration is the proportion of the body's total weight that is fat—the **percent body fat.** For example, two women may both be 165 centimetres and weigh 60 kilograms. But one woman, a runner, may have only 20% of her body weight as fat, whereas the second, sedentary woman could have 34% body fat. Although neither woman is overweight by most standards, the second woman is overfat. Too much body fat (not total weight) has a negative effect on health and well-being. Just as the amount of body fat is important, so is its location on your body. Visceral fat is more harmful to health than subcutaneous fat.

Overweight is usually defined as total body weight above the recommended range for good health (as determined by large-scale population surveys). **Obesity** is defined as a more serious degree of overweight; the cutoff point for obesity may be set in terms of percent body fat or in terms of some measure of total body weight.

WELLNESS TIP

Sleep problems increase the risk of obesity, especially in children and young adults. Sleep loss increases production of the hormone ghrelin, which boosts appetite and slows metabolic rate. Fatigue can also make it hard to live a healthy lifestyle and maintain a healthy weight.

As obesity rates have increased, so have rates of infertility. Obese men and women are both at greater risk of infertility because obesity interferes with normal hormone levels and functions.

Prevalence of Overweight and Obesity Among Canadians

By any measure, North Americans are getting fatter. In Canada, the prevalence of obesity has increased from 13.8% in 1978/79 to 24.1% in 2009, and more than 34% of Canadian adults are now overweight.[1] Comparatively, approximately 34% of Americans are obese and about 67% are considered overweight.[2] Possible explanations for this increase include more time spent in sedentary work and leisure activities, fewer short trips on foot and more by automobile, fewer daily gym classes for students, more meals eaten outside the home, greater consumption of fast food, increased portion sizes, and increased consumption of soft drinks and convenience foods. In addition, fewer than half of North Americans meet the minimum recommendation of 30 minutes per day of moderate physical activity, and the U.S. Centers for Disease Control and Prevention has estimated that caloric intake has increased by 100–300 calories a day during the past decade[3] and that nearly 40% of adult Americans are physically inactive and get no exercise at all.

LO2 Excess Body Fat and Wellness

As rates of overweight and obesity increase, so do the problems associated with them. The direct financial cost of obesity in Canada alone is reported to be close to $2 billion[4] ($117 billion in the United States[5]) and obesity is now the second-leading preventable cause of death after cigarette smoking. Excess body fat can impact overall wellness through its effects on chronic disease risk, ability to perform physical activities, and body image.

RISK OF CHRONIC DISEASE AND PREMATURE DEATH

Canadians who are obese are 50–100% more likely to die prematurely and even those classified as mildly to moderately overweight will be susceptible to a substantial increase in the risk for premature death. Statistics Canada estimates that obese Canadians are:

- three times more likely to suffer from high blood pressure,
- four times more likely to be diabetic, and
- over 50% more likely to suffer from heart disease than those in healthy weight ranges.

Many overweight and obese people—especially those who are sedentary and eat a poor diet—suffer from a group of symptoms called **metabolic syndrome** (or insulin resistance syndrome). Symptoms include a resistance

to the effects of insulin, high blood pressure, high blood glucose levels, abnormal blood fat levels (high triglycerides and low HDLs, or "good" cholesterol), and fat deposits in the abdominal region. Metabolic syndrome increases the risk of heart disease up to three times in men and six times in women.[6]

Obesity is also associated with an increased risk of death from many types of cancer (e.g., breast, colorectal, endometrial). Other health problems associated with obesity include impaired immune function, gallbladder and kidney disease, skin problems, sleep and breathing disorders, impotence, back pain, arthritis, and other bone and joint disorders.

Even mild to moderate overweight is associated with a substantial increase in the risk of type 2 diabetes. Obese people are more than three times as likely as nonobese people to develop type 2 diabetes, and the incidence of this disease among North Americans has increased dramatically as the rate of obesity has climbed (see the box "Diabetes").

Being obese in itself does not imply that the risk for chronic disease and premature death will be equal. In fact, Statistics Canada has identified differing levels of risk depending upon the status or level of obesity that Canadians suffer from (Figure 6.2 demonstrates the population

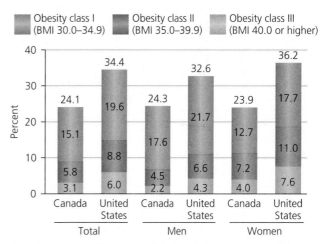

FIGURE 6.2 Prevalence of obesity in adults aged 20 to 79, by sex: Canada, 2007 to 2009 and United States, 2007 to 2008.

SOURCE: Adult obesity prevalence in Canada and the United States, http://www.statcan.gc.ca/pub/82-625-x/2011001/article/11411-e.

Diabetes

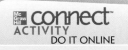

Connect ACTIVITY DO IT ONLINE

Diabetes mellitus is a disease that causes a disruption of normal metabolism. The pancreas normally secretes the hormone insulin, which stimulates cells to take up glucose (blood sugar) to produce energy. Diabetes disrupts this process, causing a buildup of glucose in the bloodstream. Diabetes is associated with kidney failure, nerve damage, circulation problems, retinal damage and blindness, and increased rates of heart attack, stroke, and hypertension. The incidence of diabetes among Canadians has increased dramatically as the rate of obesity has climbed. Diabetes is currently the seventh leading cause of death in Canada.

Types of Diabetes

More than 9 million Canadians live with either diabetes or pre-diabetes. There are two major forms of diabetes. About 10% of people with diabetes have the more serious form, known as *type 1 diabetes*. In this type of diabetes, the pancreas produces little or no insulin, so daily doses of insulin are required. (Without insulin, a person with type 1 diabetes can lapse into a coma.) Type 1 diabetes is usually diagnosed before age 30.

The remaining 90% of Canadians with diabetes have *type 2 diabetes*. This condition can develop slowly, and about 25% of affected individuals are unaware of their condition. In type 2 diabetes, the pancreas doesn't produce enough insulin, cells are resistant to insulin, or both. This condition is usually diagnosed in people over age 40, although there has been a tenfold increase in type 2 diabetes in children in the past two decades. About one-third of people with type 2 diabetes must take insulin; others may take medications that increase insulin production or stimulate cells to take up glucose.

A third type of diabetes occurs in about 2–4% of women during pregnancy. *Gestational diabetes* usually disappears after pregnancy, but does involve an increased risk of both mother and child developing type 2 diabetes.

The term *pre-diabetes* describes blood glucose levels that are higher than normal but not high enough for a diagnosis of type 2 diabetes. Although not everyone with prediabetes will develop type 2 diabetes, many will unless they adopt preventive lifestyle measures.

The major factors involved in the development of diabetes are age, obesity, physical inactivity, a family history of diabetes, and lifestyle. Excess body fat reduces cell sensitivity to insulin, and insulin resistance is usually a precursor of type 2 diabetes. Ethnicity also plays a role. According to the Canadian Diabetes Association, Canadians who are of Aboriginal, Hispanic, Asian, South Asian, or African descent are of greatest risk for being diagnosed with type 2 diabetes.

Treatment

There is no cure for diabetes, but it can be managed successfully by keeping blood sugar levels within safe limits through diet, exercise, and, if necessary, medication. Blood sugar levels can be monitored using a home test, and close control of glucose levels can significantly reduce the rate of serious complications.

The majority of people with type 2 diabetes are overweight when diagnosed, including many who are obese. An important step in treatment is to lose weight. Even a small amount of exercise and weight loss can be beneficial. The Canadian Diabetes Association reports that in one study, people at risk of type 2 diabetes were able to reduce their risk by 58% by exercising moderately for 30 minutes a day and by losing 5 to 7% of their body weight. In people age 60 and older, the risk was cut by almost 71%. Regular exercise and a healthy diet are often sufficient to control type 2 diabetes.

Prevention

It is estimated that 90% of cases of type 2 diabetes could be prevented if people adopted healthy lifestyle behaviours, including regular physical activity, a moderate diet, and modest weight loss. For people with pre-diabetes, lifestyle measures are more effective than medication for delaying or preventing the development of diabetes. Studies of people with pre-diabetes show that a 5–7% weight loss can lower diabetes onset by nearly 60%. Exercise (endurance and/or strength training) makes cells more sensitive to insulin and helps stabilize blood glucose levels; it also helps keep body fat at healthy levels.

A moderate diet to control body fat is perhaps the most important dietary recommendation for the prevention of diabetes. However, the composition of the diet may also be important. Studies have linked diets low in fibre and high in sugar, refined carbohydrates, saturated fat, red meat, and high-fat dairy products to increased risk of diabetes; diets rich in whole grains, fruits, vegetables, legumes, fish, and poultry may be protective. Specific foods linked to higher diabetes risk include soft drinks, white bread, white rice, french fries, processed meats, and sugary desserts.

Warning Signs and Testing

Be alert for the warning signs of diabetes:

- Frequent urination
- Extreme hunger or thirst
- Unexplained weight loss
- Extreme fatigue
- Blurred vision
- Frequent infections
- Cuts and bruises that are slow to heal
- Tingling or numbness in the hands or feet
- Generalized itching with no rash

The best way to avoid complications is to recognize these symptoms and get early diagnosis and treatment. Type 2 diabetes is often asymptomatic in the early stages, however, and major health organizations now recommend routine screening for people over age 45 and anyone younger who is at high risk, including anyone who is obese.

Screening involves a blood test to check glucose levels after either a period of fasting or the administration of a set dose of glucose. A fasting glucose level of 7 mmol/L or higher indicates diabetes; a level of 5.6 mmol/L indicates pre-diabetes. If you are concerned about your risk for diabetes, talk with your physician about being tested.

Exercise, Body Image, and Self-Esteem

If you gaze into the mirror and wish you could change the way your body looks, consider getting some exercise—not to reshape your contours but to firm up your body image and enhance your self-esteem. In a recent study, 82 adults completed a 12-week aerobic exercise program (using cycle ergometry) and had 12 months of follow-up. Compared with the control group, the participants improved their fitness and also benefited psychologically in tests of mood, anxiety, and self-concept. These same physical and psychological benefits were still significant at the 1-year follow-up.

One reason for the findings may be that people who exercise regularly often gain a sense of mastery and competence that enhances their self-esteem and body image. In addition, exercise contributes to a more toned look, which many adults prefer. Research suggests that physically active people are more comfortable with their bodies and their image than sedentary people are. In one workplace study, 60 employees were asked

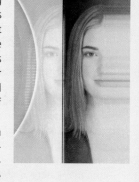

to complete a 36-session stretching program whose main purpose was to prevent muscle strains at work. At the end of the program, besides the significant increase by all participants in measurements of flexibility, their perceptions of their bodies improved and so did their overall sense of self-worth.

Similar results were obtained in a Norwegian study, in which 219 middle-aged people at risk for heart disease were randomly assigned to one of four groups: diet, diet plus exercise, exercise, and no intervention. The greater the participation of individuals in the exercise component of the program, the higher were their scores in perceived competence/self-esteem and coping.

SOURCES: DiLorenzo, T. M., et al. 1999. Long-term effects of aerobic exercise on psychological outcomes. *Preventive Medicine* 28(1): 75–85. Sorensen, M., et al. 1999. The effect of exercise and diet on mental health and quality of life in middle-aged individuals with elevated risk factors for cardiovascular disease. *Journal of Sports Science* 17(5): 369–377; and Moore, T. M. 1998. A workplace stretching program. *AAOHN Journal* 46(12): 563–568.

of Canadians exposed to differing risks as a result of their obesity status). As obese Canadians move from Class I obesity (BMI = 30) to Class III obesity (BMI = 40), there will be an escalation in their health risk. In 2009, obese Canadians were represented by 15.1% in Class I, 5.8% in Class II, and 3.1% in Class III.

BODY FAT DISTRIBUTION AND HEALTH The distribution of fat is also an important indicator of future health. Men and postmenopausal women tend to store fat in the upper regions of their bodies, particularly in the abdominal area (the "apple shape"). Premenopausal women usually store fat in the hips, buttocks, and thighs (the "pear shape"). Excess fat in the abdominal area increases risk of several diseases, including high blood pressure, diabetes, early-onset heart disease, stroke, certain cancers, and mortality. The reason for this increased risk is not entirely clear, but it appears that fat in the abdomen is more easily mobilized and sent into the bloodstream, increasing disease-related blood fat levels.

The risks from body fat distribution are usually assessed by measuring waist circumference. A total waist measurement of more than 102 cm for men and more than 88 cm for women is associated with a significantly increased risk of disease. Waist circumference tends to be higher in taller people, so waist-to-height ratio is a more accurate measure than waist circumference alone. Your waist measurement should be less than half your height. Using this index, a person who is 5 feet 8 inches (173 cm) tall should have a waist circumference of less than 34 inches (86.5 cm). A person who is 6 feet 4 inches (193 cm) tall should have a waist circumferences of less than 38 inches (96.5 cm).

PERFORMANCE OF PHYSICAL ACTIVITIES Too much body fat makes all types of physical activity more difficult because just moving the body through everyday activities means working harder and using more energy. In general, overfat people are less fit than others and don't have the muscular strength, endurance, and flexibility that make normal activity easy. Because exercise is more difficult, they do less of it, depriving themselves of an effective way to improve body composition.

EMOTIONAL WELLNESS AND SELF-IMAGE Obesity can affect psychological as well as physical wellness. Being perceived as fat can be a source of ridicule, ostracism, and sometimes discrimination from others; it can contribute to psychological problems such as depression, anxiety, and low self-esteem.

The popular image of the "ideal" body has changed dramatically in the past 50 years, evolving from slightly plump to unhealthy thin. The ideal body—as presented by the media—is an unrealistic goal for most Canadians. This is because one's ability to change body composition depends on heredity as well as diet and exercise (see the box "Exercise, Body Image, and Self-Esteem"). Body image, problems with body image, and unhealthy ways of dealing with a negative body image are all discussed in Chapter 7.

Problems Associated with Very Low Levels of Body Fat

Though not as prevalent a problem as overweight or obesity, having too little body fat is also dangerous. Essential fat is necessary for the functioning of the body, and

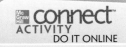

The Female Athlete Triad

While obesity is at epidemic levels in North America, many girls and women strive for unrealistic thinness in response to pressure from peers and a society obsessed with appearance. This quest for thinness has led to an increasingly common, underreported condition called the **female athlete triad.**

The triad consists of three interrelated disorders: abnormal eating patterns (and excessive exercising), followed by lack of menstrual periods **(amenorrhea),** followed by decreased bone density (premature osteoporosis). Left untreated, the triad can lead to decreased physical performance, increased incidence of bone fractures, disturbances of heart rhythm and metabolism, and even death.

Abnormal eating is the event from which the other two components of the triad flow. Abnormal eating ranges from moderately restricting food intake, to binge eating and purging (bulimia), to severely restricting food intake (anorexia nervosa). Whether serious or relatively mild, eating disorders prevent women from consuming enough calories to meet their bodies' needs.

Disordered eating, combined with intense exercise and emotional stress, can suppress the hormones that control the menstrual cycle. If the menstrual cycle stops for three consecutive months, the condition is called amenorrhea. Prolonged amenorrhea can lead to osteoporosis; bone density may erode to the point that a woman in her 20s will have the bone density of a woman in her 60s. Women with osteoporosis have fragile, easily fractured bones. Some researchers have found that even a few missed menstrual periods can decrease bone density.

All physically active women and girls have the potential to develop one or more components of the female athlete triad; for example, it is estimated that 5–20% of women who exercise regularly and vigorously may develop amenorrhea. But the triad is most prevalent among athletes who participate in certain sports: those in which appearance is highly important, those that emphasize a prepubertal body shape, those that require contour-revealing clothing for competition, those that

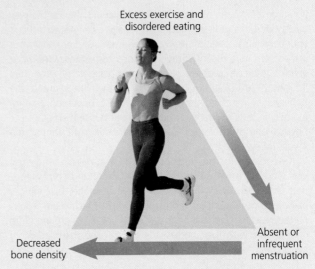

require endurance, and those that use weight categories for participation. Such sports include gymnastics, figure skating, swimming, distance running, cycling, cross-country skiing, track, volleyball, rowing, horse racing, and cheerleading.

The female athlete triad can be life-threatening, and health professionals are taking it seriously. Typical signs of the eating disorders that trigger the condition are extreme weight loss, dry skin, loss of hair, brittle fingernails, cold hands and feet, low blood pressure and heart rate, swelling around the ankles and hands, and weakening of the bones. Female athletes who have repeated stress fractures may be suffering from the condition.

Early intervention is the key to stopping this series of interrelated conditions. Unfortunately, once the condition has progressed, long-term consequences, especially bone loss, are unavoidable. Teenagers may need only to learn about good eating habits; university-age women with a long-standing problem may require intense psychological counselling.

SOURCES: Ackerman, K. E., et al. 2011. Bone health and the female athlete triad in adolescent athletes. *Physician Sportsmedicine* 39(1): 131–141; Nattiv, A., et al. 2007. American College of Sports Medicine position stand: The female athlete triad. *Medicine and Science in Sports and Exercise* 39(10): 1867–1882; Witkop, C. T., et al. 2010. Understanding the spectrum of the female athlete triad. *Obstetrics and Gynecology* 116(6): 1444–1448.

health experts generally view too little body fat—less than about 8–12% for women and 3–5% for men—as a threat to health and well-being. Extreme leanness is linked with reproductive, circulatory, and immune system disorders. Extremely lean people may experience muscle wasting and fatigue. They are also more likely to suffer from dangerous eating disorders, which are described in more detail in Chapter 7. For women, an extremely low percentage of body fat is associated with **amenorrhea** and loss of bone mass (see the box "The Female Athlete Triad").

Of recent concern have been issues of body composition related to low body fat in men. In particular, men who set unrealistic goals for training for strength and size in muscles. In these cases, obsessive-like behaviours may become problematic and place individuals in unhealthy lifestyles.[7]

LO3 6.2 ASSESSING BODY MASS INDEX, BODY COMPOSITION, AND BODY FAT DISTRIBUTION

Although a scale can tell your total weight, it can't reveal whether a fluctuation in weight is due to a change in muscle, body water, or fat. Most importantly, a scale can't differentiate between overweight and overfat.

There are a number of simple, inexpensive ways to estimate healthy body weight and healthy body composition that are more accurate than the bathroom scale. These assessments can provide you with information about the health risks associated with your current body weight and body composition. They can also help

TABLE 6.1   Body Mass Index (BMI) Classification and Disease Risk

Classification	BMI (kg/m^2)	Obesity Class	Disease Risk Relative to Normal Weight and Waist Circumference[a] Men ≤ 102 cm Women ≤ 88 cm	>102 cm >88 cm
Underweight[b]	<18.5		—	—
Normal[c]	18.5–24.9		—	—
Overweight	25.0–29.9		Increased	High
Obesity	30.0–34.9	I	High	Very high
	35.0–39.9	II	Very high	Very high
	≥40.0	III	Extremely high	Extremely high

[a]Disease risk for type 2 diabetes, hypertension, and cardiovascular disease. The waist circumference cutoff points for increased risk are 102 cm for men and 88 cm for women.

[b]Research suggests that a low BMI can be healthy in some cases, as long as it is not the result of smoking, an eating disorder, or an underlying disease process. A BMI of 17.5 or less is sometimes used as a diagnostic criterion for the eating disorder anorexia nervosa.

[c]Increased waist circumference can also be a marker for increased risk, even in persons of normal weight.

SOURCE: Adapted from Health Canada and the National Heart, Lung, and Blood Institute. 1998. *Clinical Guidelines on the Identification, Evaluation, and Treatment of Overweight and Obesity in Adults: The Evidence Report.* Bethesda, Md.: National Institutes of Health.

you establish reasonable goals and set a starting point for current and future decisions about weight loss and weight gain.

Calculating Body Mass Index

Body mass index (BMI) is a measure of body weight that is useful for classifying the health risks of body weight if you don't have access to more sophisticated methods. Though more accurate than height-weight tables, body mass index is also based on the concept that a person's weight should be proportional to their height. BMI is a fairly accurate measure of the health risks of body weight for average people, and it is easy to calculate and rate. Researchers frequently use BMI in studies that examine the health risks associated with body weight.

Because BMI doesn't distinguish between fat weight and fat-free weight, however, it is inaccurate for some groups. For example, athletes who weight train have more muscle mass than average people and may be classified as overweight by the BMI scale; because their "excess" weight is in the form of muscle, however, it is healthy. Further, BMI is not particularly useful for tracking changes in body composition—gains in muscle mass and losses of fat. Women are likely to have more body fat for a given BMI than men. BMI measurements have also over- and under-estimated the prevalence of obesity in several ethnic groups. If you are an athlete, a serious weight trainer, or a person of short stature, do not use BMI as your primary means of assessing whether your current weight is healthy; instead, try one of the methods described in the next section for estimating percent body fat.

BMI is calculated by dividing your body weight (expressed in kilograms) by the square of your height (expressed in metres). The formula appears below. Space for your own calculations can be found in Lab 6.1, and a complete BMI chart appears in Lab 6.2.

1. Multiply your height in metres by itself to obtain the square of the height measurement.

2. Divide your weight in kilograms by the result of step 1 to obtain your BMI.

For example, a person who weighs 59.1 kg and is 1.6 metres tall has a BMI of 59.1 kg ÷ (1.6 m)^2, or 23 kg/m^2.

Under federal guidelines from Health Canada, a BMI between 18.5 and 24.9 is considered healthy. A person is classified as overweight if he or she has a BMI of 25 or above and obese if he or she has a BMI of 30 or above (Table 6.1). A person with a BMI below 18.5 is classified as underweight, although low BMI values may be healthy in some cases if they are not the result of smoking, an eating disorder, or an underlying disease. A BMI of 17.5

female athlete triad   A condition consisting of three interrelated disorders: abnormal eating patterns (and excessive exercising) followed by lack of menstrual periods (amenorrhea) and decreased bone density (premature osteoporosis).

amenorrhea   Absent or infrequent menstruation, sometimes related to low levels of body fat and excessive quantity or intensity of exercise.

body mass index (BMI)   A measure of relative body weight correlating highly with more direct measures of body fat, calculated by dividing total body weight (in kilograms) by the square of body height (in metres).

TERMS

or less is sometimes used as a diagnostic criterion for the eating disorder anorexia nervosa (Chapter 8).

In classifying the health risks associated with overweight and obesity, the Health Canada guidelines consider body fat distribution and other disease risk factors in addition to BMI. As described earlier, excess fat in the abdomen is of greater concern than excess fat in other areas. Methods of assessing body fat distribution are discussed later in the chapter; the Health Canada guidelines use measurement of waist circumference (see Table 6.1). At a given level of overweight, people with a large waist circumference and/or additional disease risk factors are at greater risk for health problems. For example, a man with a BMI of 27, a waist circumference of more than 82 cm, and high blood pressure is at greater risk for health problems than another man who has a BMI of 27 but has a smaller waist circumference and no other risk factors.

Thus, optimal BMI for good health depends on many factors; if your BMI is 25 or above, consult a physician for help in determining a healthy BMI for you. (Weight loss recommendations based on Canadian Society for Exercise Physiology (CSEP) guidelines are discussed further in Chapter 8.)

Estimating Percent Body Fat

Assessing body composition involves estimating percent body fat. The only method for directly measuring the percentage body weight that is fat is autopsy—the dissection and chemical analysis of the body after death. However, there are other indirect techniques that can provide an estimate of percent body fat. One of the most accurate is underwater weighing. Other techniques include skinfold measurements, the Bod Pod, bioelectrical impedance analysis, and dual-energy X-ray absorptiometry.

All of these methods have a margin of error, so it is important not to focus too much on precise values. For example, underwater weighing has an error of about ±3%, meaning that if a person's percent body fat is actually 17%, the test result may be between 14% and 20%; skinfold measurements have an error rate of about ±6%. The results of different methods may also vary, so if you plan to track changes in body composition over time, be sure to use the same method each time to perform the assessment. Table 6.2 provides estimated ranges for healthy percent body fat. As with BMI, the percent body fat ratings indicate cutoff points for health risks associated with underweight and obesity.

UNDERWATER WEIGHING In hydrostatic (underwater) weighing, an individual is weighed under water and on land. The percentages of fat and fat-free weight are then calculated from body density. Muscle has a higher density and fat a lower density than water (1.1 grams per cubic centimetre for fat-free mass; 0.91 gram per cubic

| TABLE 6.2 | Percent Body Fat Classification (when measured or estimated correctly) |

	Percent Body Fat (%)		
	20–39 years	40–59 years	60–79 years
Women			
Essential[a]	8–12	8–12	8–12
Low/athletic[b]	13–20	13–22	13–23
Recommended	21–32	23–33	24–35
Overfat[c]	33–38	34–39	36–41
Obese[c]	⩾39	⩾40	⩾42
Men			
Essential[a]	3–5	3–5	3–5
Low/athletic[b]	6–7	6–10	6–12
Recommended	8–19	11–21	13–24
Overfat[c]	20–24	22–27	25–29
Obese[c]	⩾25	⩾28	⩾30

The cutoffs for recommended, overfat, and obese ranges in this table are based on a study that linked body mass index classifications from the National Institutes of Health with predicted percent body fat (measured using dual energy X-ray absorptiometry).

[a]Essential body fat is necessary for the basic functioning of the body.
[b]Percent body fat in the low/athletic range may be appropriate for some people as long as it is not the result of illness or disordered eating habits.
[c]Health risks increase as percent body fat exceeds the recommended range.

SOURCES: Gallagher, D., et al. 2000. Healthy percentage body fat ranges: An approach for developing guidelines based on body mass index. *American Journal of Clinical Nutrition* 72: 694–701; and American College of Sports Medicine. 2001. *ACSM's Resource Manual for Guidelines for Exercise Testing and Prescription.* 4th ed. Philadelphia: Lippincott, Williams and Wilkins.

centimetre for fat; and 1 gram per cubic centimetre for water). Therefore, fat people tend to float and weigh less under water, and lean people tend to sink and weigh more under water. Most university exercise physiology departments or sports medicine laboratories have an underwater weighing facility. If you want an accurate assessment of your body composition, find a place that does underwater weighing.

SKINFOLD MEASUREMENTS Skinfold measurement is a simple, inexpensive, and practical way to assess body composition. Skinfold measurements can be used to assess body composition because equations can link the thickness of skinfolds at various sites to percent body fat calculations from more precise laboratory techniques.

Skinfold assessment typically involves measuring the thickness of skinfolds at several different sites on the

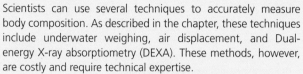
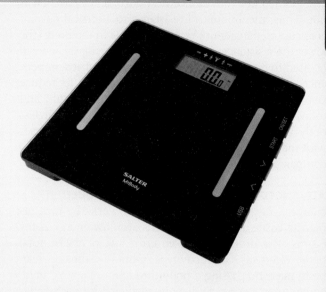

Scientists can use several techniques to accurately measure body composition. As described in the chapter, these techniques include underwater weighing, air displacement, and Dual-energy X-ray absorptiometry (DEXA). These methods, however, are costly and require technical expertise.

You can estimate your body fat and fat-free weight simply and accurately, at home, without the help of a technician. All you need is a digital home scale with a built-in bioelectrical impedance analyzer (BIA). BIA works by measuring the resistance in the body to a small electric current. Electricity flows more slowly through fat tissue than through muscle, so the more fat you have, the more slowly such a current will flow through your body. Conversely, a current will pass through your body more quickly if you have more fat-free (muscle) weight.

To use a BIA scale, just stand on the scale with bare feet. As it checks your weight, the scale sends a low-voltage electrical current through your body and analyzes the speed at which the current travels. Checking your weight and body composition takes no longer than checking your weight alone. Most BIA scales can remember your last weight and body composition measurement, making it easy to compare the measurements from day to day or week to week. Some scales can remember measurements for multiple people, as well.

A study of 22 weight-trained men showed that BIA compared favourably to underwater weighing for measuring body composition. Measurements of fat and lean mass are most valuable for measuring changes in body composition during diet and exercise programs.

Popular BIA scales are manufactured by Taylor, Whynter, Omron, RemedyT, and Tanita. These scales are available in most department stores and online, and cost between $50 and $200 depending on features.

---

body. You can sum up the skinfold values as an indirect measure of body fatness. For example, if you plan to create a fitness (and dietary change) program to improve body composition, you can compare the sum of skinfold values over time as an indicator of your program's progress and of improvements in body composition. You can also plug your skinfold values into equations like those in Lab 6.1 that predict percent body fat. When using these equations, however, it is important to remember that they have a fairly substantial margin of error—(±4% if performed by a skilled technician)—so don't focus too much on specific values. The sum represents only a relative measure of body fatness.

Skinfolds are measured with a device called a **caliper**, which consists of a pair of spring-loaded, calibrated jaws. High-quality calipers are made of metal and have parallel jaw surfaces and constant spring tension. Inexpensive plastic calipers are also available; to ensure accuracy, plastic calipers should be spring-loaded and have metal jaws. Refer to Lab 6.1 for instructions on how to take skinfold measurements. Taking accurate measurements with calipers requires patience, experience, and considerable practice. It's best to take several measurements at each site (or have several different people take each measurement) to help ensure accuracy. Be sure to take the measurements in the exact location called for in the procedure. Because the amount of water in your body changes during the day, skinfold measurements taken in the morning and evening often differ. If you repeat the measurements in the future to track changes in your body composition, measure skinfolds at approximately the same time of day.

AIR DISPLACEMENT (I.E., THE BOD POD) The Bod Pod is a small chamber containing computerized sensors that measures body composition by air displacement. The technique's technical name is *plethysmography*. It determines the percentage of fat by calculating how much air is displaced by the person sitting inside the chamber. The Bod Pod has an error rate of ±2–4% in determining percent body fat.

BIOELECTRICAL IMPEDANCE ANALYSIS (BIA) The BIA technique works by sending a small electrical current through the body and measuring the body's resistance to it. Fat-free tissues, where most body water is located, are good conductors of electrical current, whereas fat is not. Thus, the amount of resistance to electrical current is related to the amount of fat-free tissue in the body (the lower the resistance, the greater the fat-free mass) and can be used to estimate percent body fat. Bioelectrical impedance analysis has an error rate of ±4–5%. To reduce error, follow the manufacturer's instructions carefully and to avoid overhydration or underhydration (more or less body water than normal). Because measurement varies with the type of BIA analyzer, use the same instrument to compare measurements over time.

ADVANCED TECHNIQUES: DEXA AND TOBEC Dual-energy X-ray absorptiometry (DEXA) works by measuring the tissue absorption of high- and low-energy X-ray beams. The procedure has an error rate of ±2%. Total body electrical conductivity (TOBEC) estimates lean body mass by passing a body through a magnetic field. Some fitness centres and sports medicine research facilities offer these body composition assessment techniques.

Assessing Body Fat Distribution

Researchers have studied many different methods for determining the risk associated with body fat distribution. Two of the simplest to perform are waist circumference measurement and waist-to-hip ratio calculation. In the first method, you measure your waist circumference; in the second, you divide your waist circumference by your hip circumference. Waist circumference has been found to be a better indicator of abdominal fat than waist-to-hip ratio. More research is needed to determine the precise degree of risk associated with specific values for these two assessments of body fat distribution.

However, as noted earlier, a total waist measurement of more than 102 cm for men and 88 cm for women and a waist-to-hip ratio above 0.94 for young men and 0.82 for young women are associated with a significantly increased risk of heart disease and diabetes. Lab 6.1 shows you how to measure your body fat distribution.

LO4 6.3 SETTING BODY COMPOSITION GOALS

If assessment tests indicate that fat loss would be beneficial for your health, your first step is to establish a goal. You can use the ratings in Table 6.1 or Table 6.2 to choose a target value for BMI or percent body fat (depending on which assessment you completed).

Make sure your goal is realistic and will ensure good health. Genetics limits your capacity to change your body composition, and few people can expect to develop the body of a fashion model or competitive bodybuilder. However, you can improve your body composition through a program of regular exercise and a healthy diet. If your body composition is in or close to the recommended range, you may want to set a lifestyle goal rather

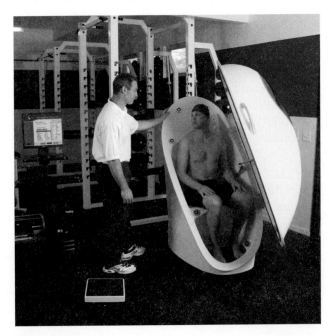

The Bod Pod

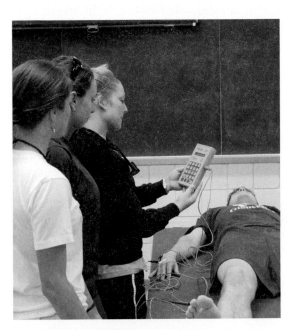

Using bioelectrical impedance analysis to estimate percent body fat

Some studies have found that recording body weight every day helps keep you accountable to your weight-loss program and helps you make faster progress. An easy way to track your weight daily is to write it down in a table like the following:

1. _____	11. _____	21. _____
2. _____	12. _____	22. _____
3. _____	13. _____	23. _____
4. _____	14. _____	24. _____
5. _____	15. _____	25. _____
6. _____	16. _____	26. _____
7. _____	17. _____	27. _____
8. _____	18. _____	28. _____
9. _____	19. _____	29. _____
10. _____	20. _____	30. _____

To make things more interesting, track your weight like this for a few weeks, and then convert the information into a line chart. A chart can help you visualize the data and make it easier for you to gauge your progress. You can easily track daily weights and convert them into charts in a spreadsheet program.

than a specific percent body fat or BMI goal. For example, you might set a goal of increasing your daily physical activity from 20 to 60 minutes or beginning a program of weight training, and then let any improvements in body composition occur as a secondary result of your primary target (physical activity). Remember, a lifestyle that includes regular exercise may be more important for health than trying to reach any ideal weight.

If you are significantly overfat or if you have known risk factors for disease (such as high blood pressure or high cholesterol), consult your physician to determine a body composition goal for your individual risk profile. For people who are obese, small losses of body weight (5–15%) over a 6–12 month period can result in significant health improvements.

Once you've established a body composition goal, you can then set a target range for body weight. Although body weight is not an accurate method of assessing body composition, it's a useful method for tracking progress in a program to change body composition. If you're losing a small or moderate amount of weight and exercising, you're probably losing fat while building muscle mass. Lab 6.2 will help you determine a range for recommended body weight.

Using percent body fat or BMI will generate a fairly accurate target body weight for most people. However, it's best not to stick rigidly to a recommended body weight calculated from any formula; individual genetic, cultural, and lifestyle factors are also important. Decide whether the body weight that the formulas generate for you is realistic, meets all your goals, is healthy, *and* is reasonable for you to maintain.

6.4 MAKING CHANGES IN BODY COMPOSITION

Chapter 8 includes specific strategies for losing or gaining weight and improving body composition. In general, lifestyle should be your focus—regular physical activity, endurance exercise, strength training, and a moderate energy intake. Making significant cuts in food intake in order to lose weight and body fat is a difficult strategy to maintain; focusing on increased physical activity is a better approach for many people. In studies of people who have lost weight and maintained the loss, physical activity was the key to long-term success.

You can track your progress toward your target body composition by checking your body weight periodically. Also, focus on how much energy you have and how your clothes fit.

To get a more accurate idea of your progress, you should directly reassess your body composition occasionally during your program: Body composition changes as weight changes. Losing a lot of weight usually includes losing some muscle mass no matter how hard a person exercises, partly because carrying less weight requires the muscular system to bear a smaller burden. Conversely, a large gain in weight without exercise still causes some gain in muscle mass because muscles are working harder to carry the extra weight.

After you complete your assessments on body composition in this chapter, use Chapter 9 to put together your overall program. This program should include cardiovascular, flexibility, and muscle training. All three areas will assist you in reaching your body composition goals.

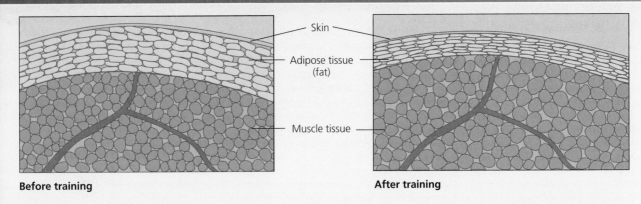

Before training

After training

Effects of exercise on body composition. Endurance exercise and strength training both reduce body fat and increase muscle mass.

Is spot reducing effective?

Spot reducing refers to attempts to lose body fat in specific parts of the body by doing exercises for those parts. Danish researchers have shown that fat use increases in adipose tissue surrounding active muscle, but it is not known if short-term fat use helps reduce fat in specific sites. Most studies show that spot-reducing exercises contribute to fat loss only to the extent that they burn calories. The best way to reduce fat in any specific area is to create an overall negative energy balance: Take in less energy (food) than you use up through exercise and metabolism.

How does exercise affect body composition?

Cardiorespiratory endurance exercise burns calories, thereby helping create a negative energy balance. Weight training does not use many calories and therefore is of little use in creating a negative energy balance. However, weight training increases muscle mass, which maintains a high metabolic rate (the body's energy level) and helps improve body composition. To minimize body fat and increase muscle mass, thereby improving body composition, combine cardiorespiratory

endurance exercise and weight training (see figure).

Are people who have a desirable body composition physically fit?

Having a healthy body composition is not necessarily associated with overall fitness. For example, many bodybuilders have very little body fat but have poor cardiorespiratory capacity and flexibility. Some athletes, such as NFL linemen, weigh 300 pounds or more; they have to lose the weight when they retire if they don't want to jeopardize their health. To be fit, you must rate high on all the components of fitness.

What is liposuction, and will it help me lose body fat?

Suction lipectomy, popularly known as liposuction, is not as commonly performed in Canada as it is in the United States, where it has become the most commonly performed cosmetic procedure. The procedure involves removing limited amounts of fat from specific areas. Typically, no more than 2.5 kg of adipose tissue is removed at a time. The procedure is usually successful if the amount of excess fat is limited

and skin elasticity is good. The procedure is most effective if integrated into a program of dietary restriction and exercise. Side effects include infection, dimpling, and wavy skin contours. Liposuction has a death rate of 1 in 5000 patients, primarily from pulmonary thromboembolism (a blood clot in the lungs) or fat embolism (circulatory blockage caused by a dislodged piece of fat). Other serious complications include shock, bleeding, and impaired blood flow to vital organs.

What is cellulite, and how do I get rid of it?

Cellulite is the name commonly given to ripply, wavy fat deposits that collect just under the skin. The "cottage cheese" appearance stems from the breakdown of tissues supporting the fat. These rippling fat deposits are really the same as fat deposited anywhere else in the body. The only way to control them is to create a negative energy balance—burn up more calories than are taken in. There are no creams or lotions that will rub away surface (subcutaneous) fat deposits, and spot reducing is also ineffective. The solution is sensible eating habits and exercise.

TIPS FOR TODAY AND THE FUTURE

A wellness lifestyle can lead naturally to a body composition that is healthy and appropriate for you.

RIGHT NOW YOU CAN

- Find out what types of body composition assessment techniques are available at facilities on your campus or in your community.
- Do 15 minutes of physical activity—walk, jog, bike, swim, or climb stairs.
- Drink a glass of water instead of a carbonated beverage, and include a high-fibre food such as whole-grain bread or cereal, popcorn, apples, berries, or beans in your next snack or meal.

IN THE FUTURE YOU CAN

- Think about your image of the ideal body type for your sex. Consider where your idea comes from, whether you use this image to judge your own body, and whether it is a realistic goal for you. Write down five positive things about your body.
- Be aware of media messages (especially visual images) that make you feel embarrassed or insecure about your body. Remind yourself that these messages are usually designed to sell a product; they should not form the basis of your body image.

SUMMARY

- The human body is composed of fat-free mass (which includes bone, muscle, organ tissues, and connective tissues) and body fat (essential and nonessential).
- Having too much body fat has negative health consequences, especially in terms of cardiovascular disease and diabetes. Distribution of fat is also a significant factor in health.
- A fit and healthy-looking body, with the right body composition for a particular person, develops from habits of proper nutrition and exercise.
- Measuring body weight is not an accurate way to assess body composition because it does not differentiate between muscle weight and fat weight.

- Body mass index (calculated from weight and height measurements) can help classify the health risks associated with overweight.
- Techniques for estimating percent body fat include underwater weighing, skinfold measurements, the Bod Pod, bioelectrical impedance analysis, DEXA, and TOBEC.
- Body fat distribution can be assessed through the total waist measurement or the waist-to-hip ratio.
- Recommended body composition and weight can be determined by choosing a target BMI or target body fat percentage. Keep heredity in mind when setting a goal, and focus on positive changes in lifestyle.

FOR FURTHER EXPLORATION

Organizations and Websites

Canadian Diabetes Association. Provides numerous resources on diabetes including local resources.
http://www.diabetes.ca/

Canadian Obesity Network. Provides research information on obesity.
http://www.obesitynetwork.ca/

Health Canada. Office of Nutrition Policy and Promotion provides information on Canada's Food Guide and making healthy food choices.
http://www.hc-sc.gc.ca/ahc-asc/branch-dirgen/hpfb-dgpsa/onpp-bppn/index-eng.php

Heart and Stroke Foundation of Canada. Includes a BMI calculator and other information on healthy living.
http://www.heartandstroke.ca/

National Heart, Lung, and Blood Institute. Provides information on the latest federal obesity standards and a BMI calculator.
http://www.nhlbi.nih.gov/guidelines/obesity/ob_home.htm

Public Health Agency of Canada.
http://www.phac-aspc.gc.ca/chn-rcs/index-eng.php

See also the listings for Chapters 2, 7, and 8.

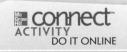

LAB 6.1   Assessing Anthropometric Health Risk

This lab will gather three anthropometric measures (Body Mass Index, Skinfolds, and Waist Circumference) and predict your health risk based on those measurements. Skinfold measurements can be used to determine your Health Benefit Score or to calculate your estimated body fat percentage.

Body Mass Index

Equipment

1. Weight scale
2. Tape measure or other means of measuring height

Instructions

Measure your height and weight, and record the results. Be sure to record the unit of measurement.

Height: _____   Weight: _____

Calculating BMI (see also the shortcut chart of BMI values in Lab 6.2)

1. Square your height measurement.

   Height _____ m × height _____ m = height _____ m^2
2. BMI equals body weight in kilograms divided by height in metres squared (kg/m^2).

   Body weight _____ kg ÷ height _____ m^2 = BMI _____ kg/m^2

             (from step 1)   (from step 3)

Rating Your BMI

Refer to the table for a rating of your BMI. Record the results below and on the final page of this lab.

Classification	BMI (kg/m^2)
Underweight	<18.5
Normal	18.5 – 24.9
Overweight	25.0 – 29.9
Obesity (I)	30.0 – 34.9
Obesity (II)	35.0 – 39.9
Extreme obesity (III)	≥40.0

(Refer to Table 6.1 for additional information.)

BMI _____ kg/m^2

Classification (from table) _____

Skinfold Measurements—Health Benefit Score

Equipment

1. Skinfold calipers
2. Partner to take measurements
3. Marking pen (optional)

Instructions

1. *Select and locate the correct sites for measurement.* All measurements should be taken on the right side of the body with the subject standing. Skinfolds are normally measured on the natural fold line of the skin, either vertically or at a slight angle. The skinfold measurement sites are triceps, biceps, subscapular, iliac crest, and medial calf.

If the person taking skinfold measurements is inexperienced, it may be helpful to mark the correct sites with a marking pen.

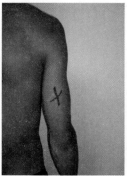 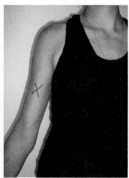 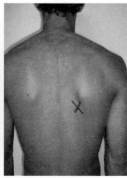 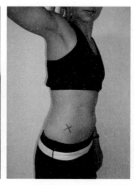 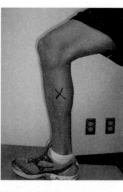

(a) Triceps   (b) Biceps   (c) Subscapular   (d) Iliac Crest   (e) Medial Calf

(a) *Triceps.* Pinch a vertical skinfold on the back of the right arm midway between the shoulder and elbow. To locate the site, place the forearm at 90° with the palm facing up. Locate the site and straighten the arm to 180° before measuring.

(b) *Biceps.* On the front of the arm at the same level as the triceps measurement, pinch a vertical fold along the midline of the front of the arm. The arm should be at the side of the body with the palm facing forward.

(c) *Subscapular.* Pinch a 45° angle fold along the inferior angle of the scapula. Shoulders should be relaxed with the arms by the sides.

(d) *Iliac Crest.* At a site approximately 3 cm above the crest of the ilium, pinch a forward, yet slightly downward fold. The arm of the skinfold side should be raised (such that the upper arm is parallel to the floor) with the hand placed on the same-side shoulder.

(e) *Medial Calf.* The relaxed skinfold foot should be placed on a step with the knee at a 90° angle. Pinch a vertical fold on the medial (inside) calf at the level of the maximum calf girth.

2. *Measuring the appropriate skinfolds.* Pinch a fold of skin between your thumb and forefinger. Pull the fold up so that no muscular tissue is included; don't pinch the skinfold too hard. Hold the calipers perpendicular to the fold and measure the skinfold about 1.0 cm away from your fingers. Allow the tips of the calipers to close on the skinfold and let the reading settle before marking it down. Take two readings at each site with readings measured to the nearest half-millimetre. Measure all five skinfolds before repeating measurements. If the difference between the first two measurements at one site is greater than 0.4 mm, a third measurement is taken. When two measurements are taken, use the average of those two as your final value. When three measurements are taken, the median value is the final value.

3. *Record your measurements.* Record your individual scores and final values in the chart below. Indicate your scores for the sum of skinfold measurements (SO5S) in the chart in the *Assessing Your Health Risk* section of this lab.

Site:	#1	#2	#3	Average/Median
Triceps				
Biceps				
Subscapular				
Illiac Crest				
Medial Calf				

Waist Circumference and Waist-to-Hip Ratio

Equipment

1. Tape measure
2. Partner to take measurements

Preparation

Wear clothes that will not add significantly to your measurements.

Instructions

Stand with your feet together and your arms at your sides. Raise your arms only high enough to allow for taking the measurements. Your partner should make sure the tape is horizontal around the entire circumference and pulled snugly against your skin. The tape shouldn't be pulled so tight that it causes indentations in your skin. Record measurements to the nearest 0.5 cm.

Waist. Measure just above the superior (top) aspect of the iliac crest. To find your iliac crest, feel for the top edge of the supraillium (see Skinfold Measurement below).

See Table 6.1 for a reference to risk associated with your waist-hip-ratio score.

Record your measurement in the chart in the *Assessing Your Health Risk* section

Assessing Your Health Risk

Measurements

Sum of 5 skinfolds (SO5S) _____ mm

Waist circumference: _____ mm

Use the charts on the following pages (one for males and one for females) to calculate your health risk based on body composition scores.

- Start by figuring out which ROW you will score from by comparing your BMI score.
- Move across that row and determine the points your WC converts to—WCP.
- Continue across that row to discover the SO5S points—SO5SP.
- Place these numbers in the formula below to arrive at a Health Benefit Score.

Health Benefit Score $= \dfrac{(\text{WCP} \times 1.5) + \text{SO5SP}}{2.5}$

- Use your Health Benefit Score to gather a Health Benefit Rating and Health Benefit Zone from the following chart:

Scoring of Body Composition: Males

BMI (kg/m²)	Points Column A	WC (cm)	Points Column B	SO5S (mm)	Points Column C
18.5	3	All girths	3	25	3
				25–54	4
				55–79	**3**
				>79	2
18.5–24.9	4	<94	4	<54	4
		94–101	2	54–77	3
		>101	0	>77	2
25–29.9	3	<94	4	<54	4
		94–101	3	54–77	3
		<101	1	>77	2
30.0–32.4	2	<94	4	<54	4
		94–101	2	54–77	3
		>101	0	>77	2

continued

BMI (kg/m²)	Points Column A	WC (cm)	Points Column B	SO5S (mm)	Points Column C
32.5–35.0	1	<94	4	<54	4
		94–101	2	54–77	2
		>101	0	>77	0
>35.0	0	<94	4	<54	4
		94–101	2	54–77	2
		>101	0	>77	0

SOURCE: *Canadian Physical Activity, Fitness & Lifestyle Approach: CSEP—Health & Fitness Program's Appraisal and Counselling Strategy,* 3rd edition. © 2003. Reprinted with permission from the Canadian Society for Exercise Physiology.

Scoring of Body Composition: Females

BMI (kg/m²)	Points Column A	WC (cm)	Points Column B	SO5S (mm)	Points Column C
<18	3	All girths	3	<46	3
				46–83	**4**
				84–113	3
				>113	2
18.5–24.9	4	<80	4	<83	4
		80–87	3	83–113	3
		>87	1	>113	2
25.0–29.9	3	<80	4	<83	4
		80–87	3	83–113	3
		>87	1	>113	2
30.0–32.4	2	<80	4	<83	4
		80–87	2	83–113	3
		>87	0	>113	2
32.5–35.0	1	<80	4	<83	4
		80–87	2	83–113	2
		>87	0	<83	1
>35.0	0	<80	4	<83	4
		80–87	2	83–113	2
		>87	0	>113	0

SOURCE: *Canadian Physical Activity, Fitness & Lifestyle Approach: CSEP—Health & Fitness Program's Appraisal and Counselling Strategy,* 3rd edition. © 2003. Reprinted with permission from the Canadian Society for Exercise Physiology.

Conversion Between Health Benefit Ratings and Scores

Health Benefit Rating	Symbol	Score
Excellent	E	4
Very Good	VG	3
Good	G	2
Fair	F	1
Needs Improvement	NI	0

Health Benefit Zone	
Excellent	Your body composition falls within a range that is generally associated with optimal health benefits.
Very good	Your body composition falls within a range that is generally associated with considerable health benefits.
Good	Your body composition falls within a range that is generally associated with many health benefits.
Fair	Your body composition falls within a range that is generally associated with some health risk. *Continuing to progress from here into the GOOD zone will further increase the health benefits associated with your body composition.*
Needs Improvement	Your body composition falls within a range that is generally associated with considerable health risk. *Try to achieve and maintain a healthy body composition by enjoying regular physical activity and healthy eating. Progressing from here into the FAIR zone is a very significant step to increasing the health benefits associated with your body composition.*

SOURCE: *Canadian Physical Activity, Fitness & Lifestyle Approach: CSEP—Health & Fitness Program's Appraisal and Counselling Strategy,* 3rd edition. © 2003. Reprinted with permission from the Canadian Society for Exercise Physiology.

Skinfold Measurements—Estimated Body Fat Percentage

Equipment

1. Skinfold calipers
2. Partner to take measurements
3. Marking pen (optional)

Instructions

1. Select and locate the correct sites for measurement. All measurements should be taken on the right side of the body with the subject standing. Skinfolds are normally measured on the natural fold line of the skin, either vertically or at a slight angle. The skinfold measurement sites for males are chest, abdomen, and thigh; for females, triceps, suprailium, and thigh. If the person taking skinfold measurements is inexperienced, it may be helpful to mark the correct sites with a marking pen.

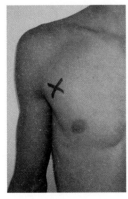

(a) Chest

(b) Abdomen

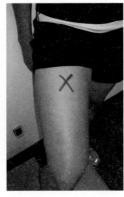

(c) Thigh

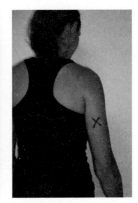

(d) Triceps

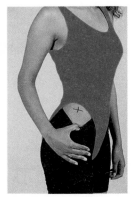

(e) Suprailium

(a) *Chest.* Pinch a diagonal fold halfway between the nipple and the shoulder crease.

(b) *Abdomen.* Pinch a vertical fold about 2 cm to the right of the umbilicus (navel).

(c) *Thigh.* Pinch a vertical fold midway between the top of the hipbone and the kneecap.

(d) *Triceps.* Pinch a vertical skinfold on the back of the right arm midway between the shoulder and elbow. The arm should be straight and should hang naturally.

(e) *Suprailium.* Pinch a fold at the top front of the right hipbone. The skinfold here is taken slightly diagonally according to the natural fold tendency of the skin.

2. *Measure the appropriate skinfolds.* Pinch a fold of skin between your thumb and forefinger. Pull the fold up so that no muscular tissue is included; don't pinch the skinfold too hard. Hold the calipers perpendicular to the fold and measure the skinfold about 0.5 cm away from your fingers. Allow the tips of the calipers to close on the skinfold and let the reading settle before marking it down. Take readings to the nearest half-millimetre. Continue to repeat the measurements until two consecutive measurements match, releasing and repinching the skinfold between each measurement. Make a note of the final measurement for each site.

Time of day of measurements:

Men		*Women*	
Chest: _____ mm		Triceps: _____ mm	
Abdomen: _____ mm		Suprailium: _____ mm	
Thigh: _____ mm		Thigh: _____ mm	

Determining Percent Body Fat

Add the measurements of your three skinfolds. Use this sum as a point of comparison for future assessments and/or find the percent body fat that corresponds to your total in the appropriate table. For example, a 19-year-old female with measurements of 16 mm, 19 mm, and 22 mm would have a skinfold sum of 57 mm; according to the following table, her percent body fat is 22.7.

Sum of three skinfolds: _____ mm Percent body fat: _____%

Percent Body Fat Estimate for Women: Sum of Triceps, Suprailium, and Thigh Skinfolds

Sum of Skinfolds (mm)	Age								
	Under 22	23–27	28–32	33–37	38–42	43–47	48–52	53–57	Over 57
23–25	9.7	9.9	10.2	10.4	10.7	10.9	11.2	11.4	11.7
26–28	11.0	11.2	11.5	11.7	12.0	12.3	12.5	12.7	13.0
29–31	12.3	12.5	12.8	13.0	13.3	13.5	13.8	14.0	14.3
32–34	13.6	13.8	14.0	14.3	14.5	14.8	15.0	15.3	15.5
35–37	14.8	15.0	15.3	15.5	15.8	16.0	16.3	16.5	16.8
38–40	16.0	16.3	16.5	16.7	17.0	17.2	17.5	17.7	18.0
41–43	17.2	17.4	17.7	17.9	18.2	18.4	18.7	18.9	19.2
44–46	18.3	18.6	18.8	19.1	19.3	19.6	19.8	20.1	20.3
47–49	19.5	19.7	20.0	20.2	20.5	20.7	21.0	21.2	21.5
50–52	20.6	20.8	21.1	21.3	21.6	21.8	22.1	22.3	22.6
53–55	21.7	21.9	22.1	22.4	22.6	22.9	23.1	23.4	23.6
56–58	22.7	23.0	23.2	23.4	23.7	23.9	24.2	24.4	24.7
59–61	23.7	24.0	24.2	24.5	24.7	25.0	25.2	25.5	25.7
62–64	24.7	25.0	25.2	25.5	25.7	26.0	26.7	26.4	26.7
65–67	25.7	25.9	26.2	26.4	26.7	26.9	27.2	27.4	27.7
68–70	26.6	26.9	27.1	27.4	27.6	27.9	28.1	28.4	28.6
71–73	27.5	27.8	28.0	28.3	28.5	28.8	29.0	29.3	29.5
74–76	28.4	28.7	28.9	29.2	29.4	29.7	29.9	30.2	30.4
77–79	29.3	29.5	29.8	30.0	30.3	30.5	30.8	31.0	31.3
80–82	30.1	30.4	30.6	30.9	31.1	31.4	31.6	31.9	32.1
83–85	30.9	31.2	31.4	31.7	31.9	32.2	32.4	32.7	32.9
86–88	31.7	32.0	32.2	32.5	32.7	32.9	33.2	33.4	33.7
89–91	32.5	32.7	33.0	33.2	33.5	33.7	33.9	34.2	34.4
92–94	33.2	33.4	33.7	33.9	34.2	34.4	34.7	34.9	35.2
95–97	33.9	34.1	34.4	34.6	34.9	35.1	35.4	35.6	35.9
98–100	34.6	34.8	35.1	35.3	35.5	35.8	36.0	36.3	36.5
101–103	35.3	35.4	35.7	35.9	36.2	36.4	36.7	36.9	37.2
104–106	35.8	36.1	36.3	36.6	36.8	37.1	37.3	37.5	37.8
107–109	36.4	36.7	36.9	37.1	37.4	37.6	37.9	38.1	38.4
110–112	37.0	37.2	37.5	37.7	38.0	38.2	38.5	38.7	38.9
113–115	37.5	37.8	38.0	38.2	38.5	38.7	39.0	39.2	39.5
116–118	38.0	38.3	38.5	38.8	39.0	39.3	39.5	39.7	40.0
119–121	38.5	38.7	39.0	39.2	39.5	39.7	40.0	40.2	40.5
122–124	39.0	39.2	39.4	39.7	39.9	40.2	40.4	40.7	40.9
125–127	39.4	39.6	39.9	40.1	40.4	40.6	40.9	41.1	41.4
128–130	39.8	40.0	40.3	40.5	40.8	41.0	41.3	41.5	41.8

SOURCE: Jackson, A. S., and M. L. Pollock. 1985. Practical assessment of body composition. *Physician and Sportsmedicine* 13(5): 76–90. Reproduced by permission of The McGraw-Hill Companies.

Percent Body Fat Estimate for Men: Sum of Chest, Abdomen, and Thigh Skinfolds

Sum of Skinfolds (mm)	Age								
	Under 22	23–27	28–32	33–37	38–42	43–47	48–52	53–57	Over 57
8–10	1.3	1.8	2.3	2.9	3.4	3.9	4.5	5.0	5.5
11–13	2.2	2.8	3.3	3.9	4.4	4.9	5.5	6.0	6.5
14–16	3.2	3.8	4.3	4.8	5.4	5.9	6.4	7.0	7.5
17–19	4.2	4.7	5.3	5.8	6.3	6.9	7.4	8.0	8.5
20–22	5.1	5.7	6.2	6.8	7.3	7.9	8.4	8.9	9.5
23–25	6.1	6.6	7.2	7.7	8.3	8.8	9.4	9.9	10.5
26–28	7.0	7.6	8.1	8.7	9.2	9.8	10.3	10.9	11.4
29–31	8.0	8.5	9.1	9.6	10.2	10.7	11.3	11.8	12.4
32–34	8.9	9.4	10.0	10.5	11.1	11.6	12.2	12.8	13.3
35–37	9.8	10.4	10.9	11.5	12.0	12.6	13.1	13.7	14.3
38–40	10.7	11.3	11.8	12.4	12.9	13.5	14.1	14.6	15.2
41–43	11.6	12.2	12.7	13.3	13.8	14.4	15.0	15.5	16.1
44–46	12.5	13.1	13.6	14.2	14.7	15.3	15.9	16.4	17.0
47–49	13.4	13.9	14.5	15.1	15.6	16.2	16.8	17.3	17.9
50–52	14.3	14.8	15.4	15.9	16.5	17.1	17.6	18.2	18.8
53–55	15.1	15.7	16.2	16.8	17.4	17.9	18.5	19.1	19.7
56–58	16.0	16.5	17.1	17.7	18.2	18.8	19.4	20.0	20.5
59–61	16.9	17.4	17.9	18.5	19.1	19.7	20.2	20.8	21.4
62–64	17.6	18.2	18.8	19.4	19.9	20.5	21.1	21.7	22.2
65–67	18.5	19.0	19.6	20.2	20.8	21.3	21.9	22.5	23.1
68–70	19.3	19.9	20.4	21.0	21.6	22.2	22.7	23.3	23.9
71–73	20.1	20.7	21.2	21.8	22.4	23.0	23.6	24.1	24.7
74–76	20.9	21.5	22.0	22.6	23.2	23.8	24.4	25.0	25.5
77–79	21.7	22.2	22.8	23.4	24.0	24.6	25.2	25.8	26.3
80–82	22.4	23.0	23.6	24.2	24.8	25.4	25.9	26.5	27.1
83–85	23.2	23.8	24.4	25.0	25.5	26.1	26.7	27.3	27.9
86–88	24.0	24.5	25.1	25.7	26.3	26.9	27.5	28.1	28.7
89–91	24.7	25.3	25.9	26.5	27.1	27.6	28.2	28.8	29.4
92–94	25.4	26.0	26.6	27.2	27.8	28.4	29.0	29.6	30.2
95–97	26.1	26.7	27.3	27.9	28.5	29.1	29.7	30.3	30.9
98–100	26.9	27.4	28.0	28.6	29.2	29.8	30.4	31.0	31.6
101–103	27.5	28.1	28.7	29.3	29.9	30.5	31.1	31.7	32.3
104–106	28.2	28.8	29.4	30.0	30.6	31.2	31.8	32.4	33.0
107–109	28.9	29.5	30.1	30.7	31.3	31.9	32.5	33.1	33.7
110–112	29.6	30.2	30.8	31.4	32.0	32.6	33.2	33.8	34.4
113–115	30.2	30.8	31.4	32.0	32.6	33.2	33.8	34.5	35.1
116–118	30.9	31.5	32.1	32.7	33.3	33.9	34.5	35.1	35.7
119–121	31.5	32.1	32.7	33.3	33.9	34.5	35.1	35.7	36.4
122–124	32.1	32.7	33.3	33.9	34.5	35.1	35.8	36.4	37.0
125–127	32.7	33.3	33.9	34.5	35.1	35.8	36.4	37.0	37.6

SOURCE: Jackson, A. S., and M. L. Pollock. 1985. Practical assessment of body composition. *Physician and Sportsmedicine* 13(5): 76–90. Reproduced by permission of The McGraw-Hill Companies.

Rating Your Body Composition

Refer to Table 6.2 to rate your percent body fat. Record it below:

Rating: _____

Using Your Results

How did you score? Are you at all surprised by your ratings for health risk? Are your current ratings in the range for good health? Are you satisfied with your current body composition? Why or why not?

If you're not satisfied, set a realistic goal for improvement:

What should you do next? Enter the results of this lab in the Preprogram Assessment column in Appendix C. If you've determined that you need to change your body composition, plan your program using the labs in Chapters 7 and 9 and the weight management section of the Daily Fitness and Nutrition Journal. After several weeks or months of an exercise and/or dietary change program, complete this lab again and enter the results in the Postprogram Assessment column of Appendix C.

Name _____   Section _____   Date _____

LAB 6.2 Setting Goals for Target Body Weight

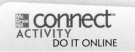

This lab is designed to help you set body weight goals based on a target BMI or percent body fat. If the results of Lab 6.1 indicate that a change in body composition would be beneficial for your health, you may want to complete this lab to help you set goals. Remember, though, that a wellness lifestyle—including a balanced diet and regular exercise—is more important for your health than achieving any specific body weight, BMI, or percent body fat. You may want to set goals for improving your diet and increasing physical activity and let your body composition change as a result. If so, use the labs in Chapters 3, 4, 7, and 8 as your guides.

Equipment

Calculator (or pencil and paper for calculations).

Preparation

Determine percent body fat and/or calculate BMI as described in Lab 6.1. Keep track of height and weight as measured for these calculations.

Height: _____ Weight: _____

Instructions: Target Body Weight from Target BMI

Use the chart below to find the target body weight that corresponds to your target BMI. Find your height in the left column, and then move across the appropriate row until you find the weight that corresponds to your target BMI. Remember, BMI is only an indirect measurement of body composition. It is possible to improve body composition without any significant change in weight. For example, a weight training program may result in increased muscle mass and decreased fat mass without any change in overall weight. For this reason, you may want to set alternative or additional goals, such as improving the fit of your clothes or decreasing your waist measurement.

	<18.5		18.5–24.9						25–29.9					30–34.9					35–39.9					≥40
	Underweight		Normal						Overweight					Obesity (Class I)					Obesity (Class II)					Extreme Obesity
BMI	17	18	19	20	21	22	23	24	25	26	27	28	29	30	31	32	33	34	35	36	37	38	39	40
Height													Body Weight (pounds)											
4'10"	81	86	91	96	101	105	110	115	120	124	129	134	139	144	148	153	158	163	168	172	177	182	187	192
4'11"	84	89	94	99	104	109	114	119	124	129	134	139	144	149	154	159	163	168	173	178	183	188	193	198
5'	87	92	97	102	108	113	118	123	128	133	138	143	149	154	159	164	169	174	179	184	190	195	200	205
5'1"	90	95	101	106	111	117	122	127	132	138	143	148	154	159	164	169	175	180	185	191	196	201	207	212
5'2"	93	98	104	109	115	120	126	131	137	142	148	153	159	164	170	175	181	186	191	197	202	208	213	219
5'3"	96	102	107	113	119	124	130	136	141	147	153	158	164	169	175	181	186	192	198	203	209	215	220	226
5'4"	99	105	111	117	122	128	134	140	146	152	157	163	169	175	181	187	192	198	204	210	216	222	227	233
5'5"	102	108	114	120	126	132	138	144	150	156	162	168	174	180	186	192	198	204	210	216	222	229	235	241
5'6"	105	112	118	124	130	136	143	149	155	161	167	174	180	186	192	198	205	211	217	223	229	236	242	248
5'7"	109	115	121	128	134	141	147	153	160	166	173	179	185	192	198	204	211	217	224	230	236	243	249	256
5'8"	112	118	125	132	138	145	151	158	165	171	178	184	191	197	204	211	217	224	230	237	244	250	257	263
5'9"	115	122	129	136	142	149	156	163	169	176	183	190	197	203	210	217	224	230	237	244	251	258	264	271
5'10"	119	126	133	139	146	153	160	167	174	181	188	195	202	209	216	223	230	237	244	251	258	265	272	279
5'11"	122	129	136	143	151	158	165	172	179	187	194	201	208	215	222	230	237	244	251	258	265	273	280	287
6'	125	133	140	148	155	162	170	177	184	192	199	207	214	221	229	236	243	251	258	266	273	280	288	295
6'1"	129	137	144	152	159	167	174	182	190	197	205	212	220	228	235	243	250	258	265	273	281	288	296	303
6'2"	132	140	148	156	164	171	179	187	195	203	210	218	226	234	242	249	257	265	273	281	288	296	304	312
6'3"	136	144	152	160	168	176	184	192	200	208	216	224	232	240	248	256	264	272	280	288	296	304	312	320
6'4"	140	148	156	164	173	181	189	197	206	214	222	230	238	247	255	263	271	280	288	296	304	312	321	329

SOURCE: Ratings from the National Heart, Lung, and Blood Institute. 1998. *Clinical Guidelines on the Identification, Evaluation, and Treatment of Overweight and Obesity in Adults.* Bethesda, Md.: National Institutes of Health.

Current BMI: _____ Target BMI: _____ Target body weight (from chart): _____

Alternative/additional goals: _____

_____

Note: You can calculate target body weight from target BMI more precisely by using the following formula: (1) convert your height measurement to metres, (2) square your height measurement, (3) multiply this number by your target BMI to get your target weight in kilograms:

1. Height _____ in. $\times$ 0.0254 m/in. = height _____ m

2. Height _____ m $\times$ height _____ m = _____ m^2

3. Target BMI _____ $\times$ height _____ m^2 = target weight _____ kg

Note: If you are more comfortable referring to your weight in pounds, multiply your weight in kg by 2.2 to estimate your weight in pounds.

Setting a Goal

Based on these calculations and other factors (including heredity, individual preference, and current health status), select a target weight or range of weights for yourself.

Target body weight: _____

CHAPTER 7

NUTRITION

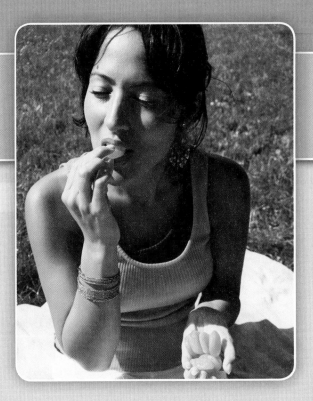

LEARNING OBJECTIVES

After reading this chapter, you should be able to

LO1 List the essential nutrients and describe the functions they perform in the body

LO2 Describe the guidelines that have been developed to help people choose a healthy diet, avoid nutritional deficiencies, and protect themselves from diet-related chronic diseases

LO3 Discuss nutritional guidelines for vegetarians and for special population groups

LO4 Explain how to use food labels and other consumer tools to make informed choices about foods

LO5 Put together a personal nutrition plan based on affordable foods that you enjoy and that will promote wellness, today and in the future

TEST YOUR KNOWLEDGE

1. **Three ounces of chicken or meat, the amount considered to be one serving, is approximately the size of which of the following?**

   a. a domino
   b. a deck of cards
   c. a small paperback book

2. **Candy is the leading source of added sugars in the North American diet.**

   True or false?

3. **Which of the following is NOT a whole grain?**

   a. brown rice
   b. wheat flour
   c. popcorn

ANSWERS

1. **B.** Many people underestimate the size of the servings they eat, leading to overconsumption of calories and fat.

2. **FALSE.** Regular (nondiet) carbonated beverages are the leading source, with an average of 99.7 litres consumed per person per year in Canada. Each 360 ml beverage supplies about 10 teaspoons of sugar, the total recommended daily limit for a 2000-calorie diet.

3. **B.** Unless labelled "whole wheat," wheat flour is processed to remove the bran and germ and is not a whole grain.

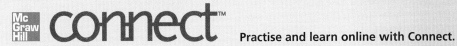

Practise and learn online with Connect.

In your lifetime, you'll spend about 6 years eating—about 70 000 meals and 60 tonnes of food. What you eat affects your energy level, well-being, and overall health (see the box "Eating Habits and Total Wellness"). Your nutritional habits help determine your risk of the major chronic diseases, including heart disease, cancer, stroke, and diabetes. Choosing foods that provide adequate amounts of the nutrients you need while limiting the substances linked to disease should be an important part of your daily life.

Choosing a healthy diet is a two-part project. First, you have to know which nutrients are necessary and in what amounts. Second, you have to translate those requirements into a diet consisting of foods you like to eat that are both available and affordable. Once you have an idea of what constitutes a healthy diet for you, you may also have to make adjustments in your current diet to bring it into line with your goals.

This chapter provides the basic principles of **nutrition.** It introduces the six classes of essential nutrients, explaining their role in the functioning of the body. It also provides different sets of guidelines that you can use to design a healthy diet plan. Finally, it offers practical tools and advice to help you apply the guidelines to your own life. Diet is an area of your life in which you have almost total control.

LO1 7.1 NUTRITIONAL REQUIREMENTS: COMPONENTS OF A HEALTHY DIET

You probably think about your diet in terms of the foods you like to eat. What's important for your health, though, are the nutrients contained in those foods. Your body requires proteins, fats, carbohydrates, vitamins, minerals,

and water—about 45 **essential nutrients.** The word essential in this context means that you must get these substances from food because your body is unable to manufacture them at all, or at least not fast enough to meet your physiological needs. The six classes of nutrients, along with their functions and major sources, are listed in Table 7.1.

The body needs some essential nutrients in relatively large amounts. These **macronutrients** include protein, fat, and carbohydrate. **Micronutrients,** such as vitamins and minerals, are required in much smaller amounts. Your body obtains nutrients through the process of **digestion,** which breaks down food into compounds that the gastrointestinal tract can absorb and the body can use (see Figure 7.1). A diet that provides enough essential nutrients is vital because they provide energy, help build and maintain body tissues, and help regulate body functions.

Calories

The energy in foods is expressed as **kilocalories.** One kilocalorie represents the amount of heat it takes to raise the temperature of 1 litre of water 1°C. A person needs about 2000 kilocalories a day to meet energy needs. In common usage, people usually refer to kilocalories as calories, which is a much smaller energy unit: 1 kilocalorie contains 1000 calories. This text uses the familiar word calorie to stand for the larger energy unit; you'll also find calorie used on food labels.

Of the six classes of essential nutrients, three supply energy:

- Fat = 9 calories per gram
- Protein = 4 calories per gram
- Carbohydrate = 4 calories per gram

Alcohol, although it is not an essential nutrient, also supplies energy, providing 7 calories per gram. (One gram

---

TABLE 7.1 The Six Classes of Essential Nutrients

Nutrient	Function	Major Sources
Proteins (4 calories/gram)	Form important parts of muscles, bone, blood, enzymes, some hormones, and cell membranes; repair tissue; regulate water and acid-base balance; help in growth; supply energy	Meat, fish, poultry, eggs, milk products, legumes, nuts
Carbohydrates (4 calories/gram)	Supply energy to cells in brain, nervous system, and blood; supply energy to muscles during exercise	Grains (breads and cereals), fruits, vegetables, milk
Fats (9 calories/gram)	Supply energy; insulate, support, and cushion organs; provide medium for absorption of fat-soluble vitamins	Animal foods, grains, nuts, seeds, fish, vegetables
Vitamins	Promote (initiate or speed up) specific chemical reactions within cells	Abundant in fruits, vegetables, and grains; also found in meat and dairy products
Minerals	Help regulate body functions; aid in the growth and maintenance of body tissues; act as catalysts for the release of energy	Found in most food groups
Water	Makes up 50–60% of body weight; provides a medium for chemical reactions; transports chemicals; regulates temperature; removes waste products	Fruits, vegetables, and liquids

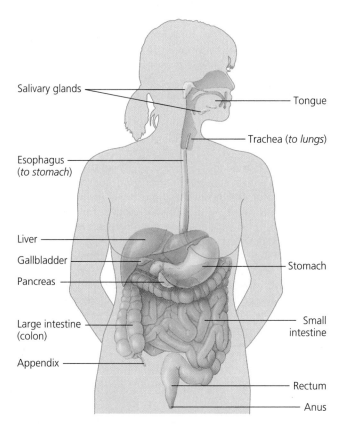

FIGURE 7.1 The digestive system. Food is partially broken down by being chewed and mixed with saliva in the mouth. As food moves through the digestive tract, it is mixed by muscular contractions and broken down by chemicals. After travelling to the stomach via the esophagus, food is broken down further by stomach acids. Most absorption of nutrients occurs in the small intestine, aided by secretions from the pancreas, gallbladder, and intestinal lining. The large intestine reabsorbs excess water; the remaining solid wastes are collected in the rectum and excreted through the anus.

equals a little less than 0.04 ounce.) The high caloric content of fat is one reason experts often advise against high fat consumption; most of us do not need the extra calories to meet energy needs. Regardless of their source, calories consumed in excess of energy needs can be converted to fat and stored in the body.

But just meeting energy needs is not enough. Our bodies need enough of all the essential nutrients to grow and function properly. Practically all foods contain mixtures of nutrients, although foods are commonly classified according to their predominant nutrients. For example, spaghetti is considered a carbohydrate food although it contains small amounts of other nutrients. Let's take a closer look at the functions and sources of the six classes of nutrients.

Proteins—The Basis of Body Structure

Proteins form important parts of the body's main structural components: muscles and bones. Proteins also form important parts of blood, enzymes, cell membranes, and

some hormones. As mentioned above, protein also provide energy (4 calories per gram) for the body.

AMINO ACIDS The building blocks of proteins are called **amino acids.** Twenty common amino acids are found in food; nine of these are essential: histidine, isoleucine, leucine, lysine, methionine, phenylalanine, threonine, tryptophan, and valine. The other 11 amino acids can be produced by the body as long as the necessary components are supplied by foods.

COMPLETE AND INCOMPLETE PROTEINS Individual protein sources are considered "complete" if they supply all the essential amino acids in adequate amounts and "incomplete" if they do not. Meat, fish, poultry, eggs, milk, cheese, and soy provide complete proteins. Incomplete proteins, which come from plant sources such as **legumes** and nuts, are good sources of most essential amino acids, but are usually low in one or two.

Combining two vegetable proteins, such as wheat and peanuts in a peanut butter sandwich, allows each vegetable protein to make up for the amino acids missing in the other protein. The combination yields a complete protein. It was once believed that vegetarians had to "complement" their proteins at each meal in order to receive the benefit of a complete protein. It is now known, however, that proteins consumed throughout

TERMS

nutrition The science of food and how the body uses it in health and disease.

essential nutrients Substances the body must get from food because it cannot manufacture them at all or fast enough to meet its needs. These nutrients include proteins, fats, carbohydrates, vitamins, minerals, and water.

macronutrients Essential nutrients required by the body in relatively large amounts.

micronutrients Essential nutrients required by the body in minute amounts.

digestion The process of breaking down foods in the gastrointestinal tract into compounds the body can absorb.

kilocalorie A measure of energy content in food; 1 kilocalorie represents the amount of heat needed to raise the temperature of 1 litre of water 1°C; commonly referred to as a calorie.

protein An essential nutrient that form important parts of the body's main structures (muscle and bones) as well as blood, enzymes, hormones, and cell membranes; also provides energy.

amino acids The building blocks of proteins.

legumes Vegetables such as peas and beans that are high in fibre and are also important sources of protein.

Eating Habits and Total Wellness

Healthy eating does more than nourish your body—it enhances your ability to enjoy life to the fullest by improving overall wellness, both physical and mental. A recent study examined a group of adults who followed a healthy eating plan for four years. At the end of this period, the study subjects were more confident with their food choices and more satisfied with their lives in general than their peers who did not make any dietary changes. The reverse is also true—when people overeat they often have feelings of guilt, anger, discouragement, and even self-loathing. Out-of-control eating can erode self-confidence and lead to depression.

Can individual foods affect the way we feel? Limited scientific evidence points to some correlation between certain foods and one's mood. Many people, especially women, seem to crave chocolate when they are "blue." Studies show that chocolate, in small quantities, may indeed give you a lift. Sugary foods tend to temporarily raise serotonin levels in the brain, which can improve mood (serotonin is a neurotransmitter associated with a calm, relaxed state). The fat found in chocolate acts to increase endorphins, brain chemicals that reduce pain and increase feelings of well-being. Chocolate also contains caffeine,

theobromine, phenylethylamine, and a variety of other less studied chemicals that may have a positive impact on mood.

Some recent research shows that eating certain carbohydrate-rich foods, such as a plain baked potato or a bagel with jelly, can have a temporary calming effect. This effect is most pronounced when rapidly digestible carbohydrates are consumed alone, with no fats or protein in the meal. The practical implications of this research are uncertain.

If you are looking for a mental boost, some scientists think that eating a meal consisting primarily of protein-rich foods may be helpful. The theory is that proteins contain the amino acid tyrosine, which is used by the body to manufacture the neurotransmitters dopamine and norepinephrine. Some researchers postulate that eating protein-containing foods could increase the synthesis of these neurotransmitters, which can speed reaction time and increase alertness. Whether this really works, especially in well-nourished individuals who have not been lacking these nutrients to begin with, remains to be seen. In the meantime, it wouldn't hurt, and might even help, to include some protein in the meal you eat prior to your next big exam.

---

the course of the day can complement each other to form a pool of amino acids from which the body can draw to produce the necessary proteins. Vegetarians should include a variety of vegetable protein sources in their diets to make sure they get all the essential amino acids in adequate amounts. (Healthy vegetarian diets are discussed later in the chapter.)

RECOMMENDED PROTEIN INTAKE Adequate daily intake of protein for adults is 0.8 gram per kilogram of body weight, or about 50 grams of protein per day for someone who weighs 64 kg (140 pounds) and 65 grams of protein for someone who weighs 82 kg (180 pounds). Table 7.2 lists some popular food items and the amount of protein each provides.

WELLNESS TIP

Research shows that some protein-rich foods can give you a quick mental boost, which can be helpful before an exam.

The majority of Canadians consume acceptable levels of protein required for adequate nutrition.[1] Protein consumed beyond what the body needs is synthesized into fat for energy storage or burned for energy requirements. A little extra protein is not harmful, but it can contribute fat to the diet because protein-rich foods are often fat-rich as well. A very high protein intake can also strain the kidneys.

A fairly broad range of protein intake is associated with good health, and Health Canada recommends that the amount adults eat should fall within the range of 10–30% of the total daily calorie intake. The average Canadian adult diet includes about 16% of total daily calories as protein.[2] (See Chapter 8 for more information about high-protein diets advocated for weight loss.)

Fats—Essential in Small Amounts

Fats, also known as *lipids*, are the most concentrated source of energy, at 9 calories per gram. The fats stored in your body represent usable energy, help insulate your body, and support and cushion your organs. Fats in the diet help your body absorb fat-soluble vitamins and add flavour and texture to foods. Fats are the major fuel for the body during periods of rest and light activity. Two fats—linoleic acid and alpha-linolenic acid—are essential

TABLE 7.2	Protein Content of Common Food Items
Item	**Protein (grams)**
3 ounces lean meat, poultry, or fish	20–25
½ cup tofu	20–25
1 cup dried beans	15–20
1 cup milk, yogurt	8–12
1½ ounces cheese	8–12
1 serving of cereals, grains, nuts, vegetables	2–4

How much junk food do you eat on any given day? Let's find out. Write down all the different kinds of junk food you eat during the day today:

_____

_____

_____

_____

_____

_____

_____

Now, write down your reason for eating each of those items:

_____

_____

_____

_____

_____

Whether you eat junk for pleasure or to help cope with stress, it pays to be mindful of your eating habits. Consider your reasons for eating junk food, and try to catch yourself the next time you're tempted to reach for some. If you're able to stop yourself, you can make healthier choices.

to the diet; they are key regulators of such body functions as the maintenance of blood pressure and the progress of a healthy pregnancy.

TYPES AND SOURCES OF FATS Most of the fats in food are fairly similar in composition, generally including a molecule of glycerol (an alcohol) plus three fatty acid chains attached to it. The resulting structure is called a triglyceride. Animal fat, for example, is primarily made of triglycerides.

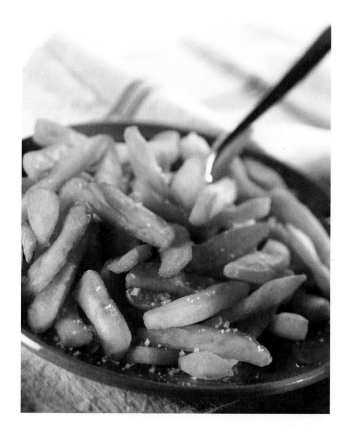

Within a triglyceride, differences in the fatty acid structure result in different types of fats. Depending on this structure, a fat may be unsaturated, monounsaturated, polyunsaturated, or saturated. (The essential fatty acids—linoleic and alpha-linolenic acids—are both polyunsaturated.) The different types of fatty acids have different characteristics and different effects on your health.

Food fats are often composed of both saturated and unsaturated fatty acids; the dominant type of fatty acid determines the fat's characteristics. Food fats containing large amounts of saturated fatty acids are usually solid at room temperature; they are generally found naturally in animal products. The leading sources of saturated fat in the Canadian diet are red meats (hamburger, steak, roasts), whole milk, cheese, hot dogs, and lunch meats. Food fats containing large amounts of monounsaturated and polyunsaturated fatty acids are usually from plant sources and are liquid at room temperature. Olive, canola, safflower, and peanut oils contain mostly monounsaturated fatty acids. Corn, soybean, and cottonseed oils contain mostly polyunsaturated fatty acids.

HYDROGENATION There are notable exceptions to these generalizations. When unsaturated vegetable oils undergo the process of **hydrogenation,** a mixture of saturated and unsaturated fatty acids is produced, creating a more solid fat from a liquid oil. Hydrogenation

hydrogenation A process by which hydrogens are added to unsaturated fats, increasing the degree of saturation and turning liquid oils into solid fats. Hydrogenation produces a mixture of saturated fatty acids and standard and trans forms of unsaturated fatty acids.

TERMS

also changes some unsaturated fatty acids into **trans fatty acids (trans fats)**, unsaturated fatty acids with an atypical shape that affects their behaviour in the body. Food manufacturers use hydrogenation to increase the stability of an oil so it can be reused for deep frying; to improve the texture of certain foods (to make pastries and pie crusts flakier, for example); and to extend the shelf life of foods made with oil. Hydrogenation is also used to transform liquid vegetable oils into margarine or shortening.

Many baked and fried foods are prepared with hydrogenated vegetable oils, so they can be relatively high in saturated and trans fatty acids. Leading sources of trans fats in the Canadian diet are deep-fried fast foods such as french fries and fried chicken (typically fried in vegetable shortening rather than oil); baked and snack foods such as pot pies, cakes, cookies, pastries, doughnuts, and chips; and stick margarine.

In general, the more solid a hydrogenated oil is, the more saturated and trans fats it contains. For example, stick margarines typically contain more saturated and trans fats than do tub or squeeze margarines. Small amounts of trans fatty acids are also found naturally in meat and milk.

Hydrogenated vegetable oils are not the only plant fats that contain saturated fats. Palm and coconut oils, although derived from plants, are also highly saturated. Yet fish oils, derived from an animal source, are rich in polyunsaturated fats.

FATS AND HEALTH　Different types of fats have very different effects on health. Many studies have examined the effects of dietary fat intake on blood **cholesterol** levels and the risk of heart disease. Saturated and trans fatty acids raise blood levels of **low-density lipoprotein (LDL)**, or "bad" cholesterol, thereby increasing a person's risk of heart disease. Unsaturated fatty acids, with the exception of trans fatty acids, lower LDL. Monounsaturated fatty acids, such as those found in olive and canola oils, may also increase levels of **high-density lipoproteins (HDL)**, or "good" cholesterol, providing even greater benefits for heart health. Saturated fats have been found to impair the ability of HDLs to prevent inflammation of the blood vessels, one of the key factors in vascular disease; they have

also been found to reduce the ability of the blood vessels to react normally to stress. Thus, to reduce the risk of heart disease, it is important to choose unsaturated fats instead of saturated and trans fats. (See Chapter 11 for more on cholesterol and a heart-healthy diet.)

Canadians were once the largest consumers of trans fats in the world. Thankfully, Canadian consumption of trans fats has declined by about 40% over the last decade (8.3 to 4.9 g per day).[3] However, health experts are particularly concerned about trans fats because of their double negative effect on heart health—they both raise LDL and lower HDL—and because there is less public awareness of trans fats. In January 2003 Canada became the first country to require the inclusion of trans fatty acid content on food labels. Recently a task force combining the House of Commons, Health Canada, and the Heart and Stroke Foundation of Canada was formed in an effort to further develop strategies for lowering processed trans fat levels in foods.

For heart health, it's important to limit your consumption of both saturated and trans fats. The best way to reduce saturated fat in your diet is to lower your intake of meat and full-fat dairy products (whole milk, cream, butter, cheese, ice cream). To lower trans fats, decrease your intake of deep-fried foods and baked goods made with hydrogenated vegetable oils; use liquid oils rather than margarine or shortening for cooking; and favour tub or squeeze margarines or those labelled low-trans or trans-free over standard stick margarines. Remember, the softer or more liquid a fat is, the less saturated and trans fat it is likely to contain.

Although saturated and trans fats pose health hazards, other fats are beneficial. Monounsaturated fatty acids, as found in avocados, most nuts, and olive, canola, peanut, and safflower oils, improve cholesterol levels and may help protect against some cancers. **Omega-3 fatty acids**, a form of polyunsaturated fat found primarily in fish, may be even more healthful. Omega-3s and the compounds the body makes from them have a number of heart-healthy effects: They reduce the tendency of blood to clot, inhibit inflammation and abnormal heart rhythms, and reduce blood pressure and risk of heart attack and stroke in some people. Because of these benefits, nutritionists recommend that Canadians increase the proportion of omega-3s in their diet by eating fish two or more times a week. Salmon, tuna, trout, mackerel, herring, sardines, and anchovies are all good sources of omega-3s; lesser amounts are found in plant sources, including dark-green leafy vegetables; walnuts; flaxseeds; and canola, walnut, and flaxseed oils.

Most of the polyunsaturated fats currently consumed by North Americans are omega-6s, primarily from corn oil and soybean oil. Foods rich in omega-6s are important because they contain the essential nutrient linoleic acid. However, some nutritionists recommend that people reduce the proportion of omega-6s they consume in favour of omega-3s. To make this adjustment, use canola

TERMS

trans fatty acid (trans fat)　A type of unsaturated fatty acid produced during the process of hydrogenation; trans fats have an atypical shape that affects their chemical activity.

cholesterol　A waxy substance found in the blood and cells and needed for cell membranes, vitamin D, and hormone synthesis.

low-density lipoprotein (LDL)　Blood fat that transports cholesterol to organs and tissues; excess amounts result in the accumulation of fatty deposits on artery walls.

high-density lipoprotein (HDL)　Blood fat that helps transport cholesterol out of the arteries, thereby protecting against heart disease.

omega-3 fatty acids　Polyunsaturated fatty acids commonly found in fish oils that are beneficial to cardiovascular health.

oil rather than corn oil in cooking, and check for corn, soybean, or cottonseed oil in products such as mayonnaise, margarine, and salad dressing.

In addition to its effects on heart disease risk, dietary fat can affect health in other ways. Diets high in fatty red meat are associated with an increased risk of certain forms of cancer, especially colon cancer. A high-fat diet can also make weight management more difficult. Because fat is a concentrated source of calories (9 calories per gram versus 4 calories per gram for protein and carbohydrate), a high-fat diet is often a high-calorie diet that can lead to weight gain. In addition, there is some evidence that calories from fat are more easily converted to body fat than calories from protein or carbohydrate.

Although more research is needed on the precise effects of different types and amounts of fat on overall health, a great deal of evidence points to the fact that most people benefit from lowering their overall fat intake to recommended levels and choosing unsaturated fats instead of saturated and trans fats. The types of fatty acids and their effects on health are summarized in Figure 7.2.

RECOMMENDED FAT INTAKE To meet the body's need for essential fats, adult men need about 17 grams per day of linoleic acid and 1.6 grams per day of alpha-linolenic acid; for women, the daily need is 12 grams of linoleic acid and 1.1 grams of alpha-linolenic acid. About 3–4 teaspoons (15–20 grams) of vegetable oil per day incorporated into your diet will supply the essential fats. Most Canadians consume sufficient amounts of the essential fats, and limiting unhealthy fats is a much greater health concern.

Limits for total, saturated, and trans fat intake have been set by a number of government and research organizations. In 2002, the Food and Nutrition Board in conjunction with Health Canada released recommendations for the balance of energy sources in a healthful diet. These recommendations, called Acceptable Macronutrient Distribution Ranges (AMDRs), are based on ensuring adequate intake of essential nutrients while also reducing the risk of chronic diseases like heart disease and cancer. As with protein, a range of levels of fat intake is associated with good health; the AMDR for total fat is 20–35% of total calories. Although

	Type of Fatty Acid	Found In[a]	Possible Effects on Health
Keep Intake Low	SATURATED	Animal fats (especially fatty meats and poultry fat and skin) Butter, cheese, and other high-fat dairy products Palm and coconut oils	Raises total cholesterol and "bad" (LDL) cholesterol levels Increases risk of heart disease May increase risk of colon and prostate cancers
	TRANS	French fries and other deep-fried fast foods Stick margarines, shortening Packaged cookies and crackers Processed snacks and sweets	Raises total cholesterol and "bad" (LDL) cholesterol levels Lowers "good" (HDL) cholesterol levels May increase risk of heart disease and breast cancer
Choose Moderate Amounts	MONOUNSATURATED	Olive, canola, and safflower oils Avocados, olives Peanut butter (without added fat) Many nuts, including almonds, cashews, pecans, pistachios	Lowers total cholesterol and "bad" (LDL) cholesterol levels May reduce blood pressure and lower triglyceride levels (a risk factor for CVD) May reduce risk of heart disease, stroke, and some cancers
	POLYUNSATURATED (two groups)[b]		
	Omega-3 fatty acids 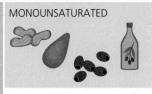	Fatty fish, including salmon, white albacore tuna, mackerel, anchovies, and sardines Lesser amounts in walnut, flaxseed, canola, and soybean oils; tofu; walnuts; flaxseeds; and dark-green, leafy vegetables	Reduces blood clotting and inflammation and inhibits abnormal heart rhythms Lowers triglyceride levels (a risk factor for CVD) May lower blood pressure in some people May reduce risk of fatal heart attack, stroke, and some cancer
	Omega-6 fatty acids 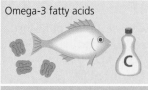	Corn, soybean, and cottonseed oils (often used in margarine, mayonnaise, and salad dressing)	Lowers total cholesterol and "bad" (LDL) cholesterol levels May lower "good" (HDL) cholesterol levels May reduce risk of heart disease May slightly increase risk of cancer if omega-6 intake is high and omega-3 intake is low

[a] Food fats contain a combination of types of fatty acids in various proportions; for example, canola oil is composed mainly of monounsaturated fatty acids (62%) but also contains polyunsaturated (32%) and saturated (6%) fatty acids. Food fats are categorized here according to their predominant fatty acid.

[b] The essential fatty acids are polyunsaturated: Linoleic acid is an omega-6 fatty acid and alpha-linolenic acid is an omega-3 fatty acid.

FIGURE 7.2 Types of fatty acids and their possible effects on health. The health effects of dietary fats are still being investigated. In general, nutritionists recommend that we consume a diet moderate in overall fat and that we substitute unsaturated fats for saturated and trans fats. Monounsaturated fats and omega-3 polyunsaturated fats may be particularly good choices for promoting health. Eating lots of fat of any type can provide excess calories because all types of fats are rich sources of energy (9 calories per gram).

Setting Intake Goals for Protein, Fat, and Carbohydrates

Goals have been established by the Food and Nutrition Board and Health Canada to help ensure adequate intake of the essential amino acids, fatty acids, and carbohydrates. The daily goals for adequate intake for adults are as follows:

	Men	Women
Protein	56 grams	46 grams
Fat: Linoleic acid	17 grams	12 grams
Alpha-linolenic acid	1.6 gram	1.1 grams
Carbohydrate	130 grams	130 grams

Protein intake goals can be calculated more specifically by multiplying your body weight in kilograms by 0.8. (Refer to the Nutrition Resources section at the end of the chapter for information for specific age groups and life stages.)

To meet your daily energy needs, you need to consume more than the minimally adequate amounts of the energy-providing nutrients listed above, which alone supply only about 800–900 calories. The Food and Nutrition Board provides additional guidance in the form of Acceptable Macronutrient Distribution Ranges (AMDRs). The ranges can help you balance your intake of the energy-providing nutrients in ways that ensure adequate intake while reducing the risk of chronic disease. The AMDRs for protein, total fat, and carbohydrate are as follows:

Protein	10–30% of total daily calories
Total fat	20–35% of total daily calories
Carbohydrate	45–65% of total daily calories

To set individual goals, begin by estimating your total daily energy (calorie) needs; if your weight is stable, your current energy intake is the number of calories you need to maintain your weight at your current activity level. Next, select percentage goals for protein, fat, and carbohydrate. You can allocate your total daily calories among the three classes of macronutrients to suit your preferences; just make sure that the three percentage values you select total 100% and that you meet the minimum intake goals listed. Two samples reflecting different total energy intake and nutrient intake goals are shown in the table below.

To translate your own percentage goals into daily intake goals expressed in calories and grams, multiply the appropriate percentages by total calorie intake and then divide the results by the corresponding calories per gram. For example, a fat limit of 35% applied to a 2200-calorie diet would be calculated as follows: 0.35 × 2200 = 770 calories of total fat; 770 ÷ 9 calories per gram = 86 grams of total fat. (Remember that fat has 9 calories per gram and that protein and carbohydrate have 4 calories per gram.)

Two Sample Macronutrient Distributions

Nutrient	AMDR	Sample 1 Individual Goals	Sample 1 Amounts for a 1600-calorie diet	Sample 2 Individual Goals	Sample 2 Amounts for a 2800-calorie diet
Protein	10–30%	15%	240 calories = 60 grams	20%	560 calories = 140 grams
Fat	20–35%	30%	480 calories = 53 grams	20%	560 calories = 62 grams
Carbohydrate	45–65%	55%	880 calories = 220 grams	60%	1680 calories = 420 grams

SOURCE: Food and Nutrition Board, Institute of Medicine, National Academies. 2002. *Dietary Reference Intakes: Energy, Carbohydrate, Fibre, Fat, Fatty Acids, Cholesterol, Protein, and Amino Acids.* Washington, D.C.: National Academy Press. Reprinted with permission from *Dietary Reference Intakes: Applications in Dietary Planning.* Copyright © 2003 by the National Academy of Sciences. Courtesy of the National Academies Press, Washington, D.C.

more difficult for consumers to monitor, AMDRs have also been set for omega-6 fatty acids (5–10%) and omega-3 fatty acids (0.6–1.2%) as part of total fat intake. Because any amount of saturated and trans fat increases the risk of heart disease, saturated and trans fat intake should be kept as low as possible and most fat in a healthy diet should be unsaturated. Canadian adults currently consume about 31% of total calories as fat.

For advice on setting individual intake goals, see the box, "Setting Intake Goals for Protein, Fat, and Carbohydrate." To determine how close you are to meeting these intake goals for fat, keep a running total over the course of the day. For prepared foods, food labels list the number of grams of fat, protein, and carbohydrate; the breakdown for many foods and popular fast-food items can be found in Appendices A and B. Nutrition information is also available in many grocery stores, in published nutrition guides, and online (see For Further Exploration at the end of the chapter). By checking these resources, you can keep track of the total grams of fat, protein, and carbohydrate you eat and assess how close your current diet is to the recommended intake goals.

In reducing fat intake to recommended levels, the emphasis should be on lowering saturated and trans fats (see Figure 7.2). You can still eat high-fat foods, but it makes good sense to limit the size of your portions and to balance your intake with low-fat foods. For example, peanut butter is high in fat, with 8 grams (72 calories) of fat in each 90-calorie tablespoon. Two tablespoons of peanut butter eaten on whole-wheat bread and served with a banana, carrot sticks, and a glass of nonfat milk makes a nutritious lunch—high in protein and carbohydrate, relatively low in total and saturated fat (500 calories, 18 grams of total fat, 4 grams of saturated fat). Four tablespoons of peanut butter on high-fat crackers with potato chips, cookies, and whole milk is a less healthy combination (1000 calories, 62 grams of total fat, 15 grams of saturated fat). So although it's important to evaluate individual food items for their fat content, it is more important to look at them in the context of your overall diet.

Carbohydrates—An Ideal Source of Energy

Carbohydrates are needed in the diet primarily to supply energy to body cells. Some cells, such as those in the brain and other parts of the nervous system and in the blood, use only carbohydrates for fuel. During high-intensity exercise, muscles also get most of their energy from carbohydrates.

SIMPLE AND COMPLEX CARBOHYDRATES Carbohydrates are classified into two groups: simple and complex. *Simple carbohydrates* include sucrose (table sugar), fructose (fruit sugar, honey), maltose (malt sugar), and lactose (milk sugar). Simple carbohydrates provide much of the sweetness in foods. They are found naturally in fruits and milk and are added to soft drinks, fruit drinks, candy, and sweet desserts. There is no evidence that any type of simple sugar is more nutritious than any other.

Complex carbohydrates include starches and most types of dietary fibre. Starches are found in a variety of plants, especially grains (wheat, rye, rice, oats, barley, millet), legumes, and tubers (potatoes and yams). Most other vegetables contain a mix of starches and simple carbohydrates. Fibre is found in fruits, vegetables, and grains.

During digestion in the mouth and small intestine, your body breaks down carbohydrates into simple sugar molecules, such as **glucose,** for absorption. Once the glucose is in the bloodstream, the pancreas releases insulin, which allows cells to take up glucose and use it for energy. The liver and muscles also take up glucose and store it in the form of a starch called **glycogen.** The muscles use glucose from glycogen as fuel during endurance events or long workouts. Carbohydrates consumed in excess of the body's energy needs can be changed into fat and stored. Whenever calorie intake exceeds calorie expenditure, fat storage can lead to weight gain. This is true whether the excess calories come from carbohydrates, proteins, fat, or alcohol.

REFINED CARBOHYDRATES VERSUS WHOLE GRAINS Complex carbohydrates can be further divided between refined, or processed, carbohydrates and unrefined carbohydrates, or whole grains. Before they are processed, all grains are **whole grains,** consisting of an inner layer of germ, a middle layer called the endosperm, and an outer layer of bran (Figure 7.3). During processing, the

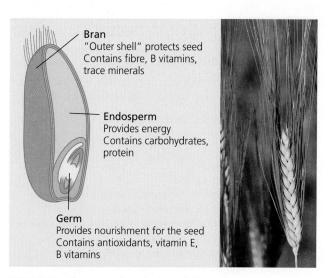

FIGURE 7.3 The parts of a whole grain kernel.

germ and bran are often removed, leaving just the starchy endosperm. The refinement of whole grains transforms whole-wheat flour to white flour, brown rice to white rice, and so on.

Refined carbohydrates usually retain all the calories of their unrefined counterparts, but they tend to be much lower in fibre, vitamins, minerals, and other beneficial compounds. Many refined grain products are enriched or fortified with vitamins and minerals, but often the nutrients lost in processing are not replaced.

Unrefined carbohydrates tend to take longer to chew and digest than refined ones; they also enter the bloodstream more slowly. This slower digestive pace tends to make people feel full sooner and for a longer period, lessening the chance that they will overeat. Also, a slower rise in blood glucose levels following consumption of complex carbohydrates may help in the prevention and management of diabetes. Whole grains are also high in dietary fibre (discussed later). Consumption of whole grains has been linked to reduced risk for heart disease, diabetes, high blood pressure, stroke, and certain forms of cancer. For all these reasons, whole grains are recommended over those that have been refined. This does not mean that you should never eat refined carbohydrates such as white bread or white rice, simply that whole-wheat bread, brown rice, and other whole grains are healthier choices. See the box "Choosing More Whole-Grain Foods" for tips on increasing your intake of whole grains.

carbohydrate An essential nutrient; sugars, starches, and dietary fibre are all carbohydrates.

glucose A simple sugar that is the body's basic fuel.

glycogen An animal starch stored in the liver and muscles.

whole grain The entire edible portion of a grain such as wheat, rice, or oats, including the germ, endosperm, and bran. During milling or processing, parts of the grain are removed, often leaving just the endosperm.

TERMS

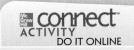

TAKE CHARGE

Choosing More Whole-Grain Foods

What Are Whole Grains?

The first step in increasing your intake of whole grains is to correctly identify them. The following are whole grains:

whole wheat	whole-grain corn
whole rye	popcorn
whole oats	brown rice
oatmeal	barley

Other choices include bulgur (cracked wheat), millet, kasha (roasted buckwheat kernels), quinoa, teff, wheat and rye berries, amaranth, graham flour, whole-grain kamut, whole-grain spelt, and whole-grain triticale.

Wheat flour, unbleached flour, enriched flour, and degerminated corn meal are not whole grains. Wheat germ and wheat bran are also not whole grains, but they are the constituents of wheat typically left out when wheat is processed and so are healthier choices than regular wheat flour, which typically contains just the endosperm.

Reading Food Packages to Find Whole Grains

To find packaged foods rich in whole grains, read the list of ingredients. The first item on the list of ingredients should be one of the whole grains listed above. In addition, the Health Canada has recently suggested that Canadian manufacturers follow new US Food and Drug Administration guidelines. These include special health claims for foods that contain 51% or more whole-grain ingredients. Such products may contain a statement such as the following on their packaging: "Rich in whole grain," "Made with 100% whole grain," or "Diets rich in whole-grain foods may help reduce the risk of heart disease and certain cancers." While potentially helpful, many whole-grain products will not be able to meet the criteria necessary to carry such claims.

Incorporating Whole Grains into Your Daily Diet

- Bread: Look for sandwich breads, bagels, English muffins, buns, and pita breads with a whole grain listed as the first ingredient.

- Breakfast cereals: Whole-grain choices include oatmeal, muesli, shredded wheat, and some types of raisin bran, bran flakes, wheat flakes, toasted oats, and granola.

- Rice: Choose brown rice or rice blends that include brown rice.

- Pasta: Look for whole-wheat, whole-grain kamut, or whole-grain spelt pasta.

- Tortillas: Choose whole-wheat or whole-corn tortillas.

- Crackers and snacks: Some varieties of crackers are made from whole grains, including some flatbreads or crisp-breads, woven wheat crackers, and rye crackers. Other whole-grain snack possibilities include popcorn, popcorn cakes, brown rice cakes, whole-corn tortilla chips, and whole-wheat fig cookies. Be sure to check food labels for fat content, as many popular snacks are also high in fat.

- Mixed-grain dishes: Combine whole grains with other foods to create healthy mixed dishes such as tabouli; soups made with hulled barley or wheat berries; and pilafs, casseroles, and salads made with brown rice, whole-wheat couscous, kasha, millet, wheat bulgur, and quinoa.

If your grocery store doesn't carry these items, try your local health food store.

GLYCEMIC INDEX AND GLYCEMIC RESPONSE Insulin and glucose levels rise and fall following a meal or snack containing any type of carbohydrate. Some foods cause a quick and dramatic rise in glucose and insulin levels; others have a slower, more moderate effect. A food that has a strong effect on blood glucose levels is said to have a high **glycemic index.** Research findings have been mixed, but some studies have found that a meal containing high glycemic index foods may increase appetite. Over the long term, diets rich in these foods may increase the risk of diabetes and heart disease in some people. High glycemic index foods do not, as some popular diets claim, directly cause weight gain beyond the calories they contain.

Attempting to base food choices on glycemic index is a difficult task, however. Although unrefined complex carbohydrates and high-fibre foods tend to have a low glycemic index, patterns are less clear for other types of foods and do not follow a simple distinction such as that of simple versus complex carbohydrates. For example, some fruits with fairly high levels of simple carbohydrates have only a moderate effect on blood glucose levels, while white rice, potatoes, and white bread, which are rich in complex carbohydrates, have a high glycemic index. Watermelon has a glycemic index more than twice that of strawberries, and the glycemic index of a banana changes dramatically as it ripens. Spaghetti has a glycemic index half that of white bread, even when the two items are made from the same ingredients. The acid and

TERMS

glycemic index (GI) A measure of how high and how fast a particular food raises blood glucose levels.

WELLNESS TIP

Certain carbohydrate-rich foods, such as a bagel or a plain baked potato, can have a temporary calming effect on some people during stressful situations.

fat content of a food also affect glycemic index—the more acidic and higher in fat a food is, the lower its effect on glucose levels.

This complexity is one reason why major health organizations have not issued specific guidelines for glycemic index. For people with particular health concerns, glycemic index may be an important consideration, but it should not be the sole criterion for food choices. For example, ice cream and chocolate have much lower glycemic index values than brown rice and carrots—but that doesn't make them healthier choices overall. Remember that most unrefined grains, fruits, vegetables, and legumes are rich in nutrients and have a low-to-moderate glycemic index. Choose a variety of vegetables daily, and avoid heavy consumption of white potatoes. Limit foods that are high in added sugars but provide few other nutrients. Some studies have singled out regular soda, with its large dose of rapidly absorbable sugar, as specifically linked to increased diabetes risk.

RECOMMENDED CARBOHYDRATE INTAKE On average, Canadians consume 358 grams of carbohydrate per day, well above the 130 grams needed to meet the body's requirement for essential carbohydrate.[4] A range of intakes is associated with good health, and experts recommend that adults consume 45–65% of total daily calories as carbohydrate, about 225–325 grams of carbohydrate for someone consuming 2000 calories per day. The focus should be on consuming a variety of foods rich in complex carbohydrates, especially whole grains.

Health experts offer separate guidelines for intake of added sugars as part of total carbohydrate consumption. The Food and Nutrition Board and Health Canada set an AMDR for added sugars of 25% or less of total daily calories, but many health experts recommend a substantially lower intake. Guidelines released by the World Health Organization in 2003 suggested a limit of 10% of total daily calories from added sugars. Foods high in added sugar are generally high in calories and low in nutrients and fibre, thus providing "empty" calories. To reduce your intake of added sugars, limit soft drinks, candy, sweet desserts, and sweetened fruit drinks. The simple carbohydrates in your diet should come from food sources in which they are found naturally—including fruits, which are excellent sources of vitamins and minerals, and from milk, which is high in protein and calcium.

Athletes in training can especially benefit from high carbohydrate diets (60–70% of total daily calories), which enhance the amount of carbohydrates stored in their muscles (as glycogen) and therefore provide more carbohydrate fuel for use during endurance events or long workouts. In addition, carbohydrates consumed during prolonged athletic events can help fuel muscles and extend the availability of the glycogen stored in muscles. Caution is in order, however, because overconsumption of carbohydrates can lead to feelings of fatigue and underconsumption of other nutrients.

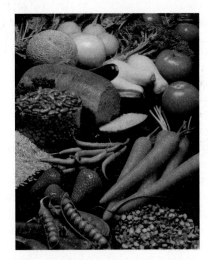

Fruits, vegetables, and whole grains are excellent sources of carbohydrates and fibre.

Fibre—A Closer Look

Fibre is the term given to nondigestible carbohydrates provided mainly by plants. Instead of being digested, like starch, fibre passes through the intestinal tract and provides bulk for feces in the large intestine, which in turn facilitates elimination. In the large intestine, some types of fibre are broken down by bacteria into acids and gases, which explains why consuming too much fibre can lead to intestinal gas. Because humans cannot digest fibre, it is not a source of carbohydrate in the diet; however, the consumption of fibre is necessary for good health.

TYPES OF FIBRE The Food and Nutrition Board and Health Canada have defined two types of fibre:

- **Dietary fibre** refers to nondigestible carbohydrates and lignin that are present naturally in plants such as grains, legumes, and vegetables.
- **Functional fibre** refers to nondigestible carbohydrates that have been either isolated from natural sources or synthesized in a lab and then added to a food product or supplement.
- **Total fibre** is the sum of dietary and functional fibre.

Fibres have different properties that lead to different physiological effects in the body. **Soluble (viscous) fibre** slows the body's absorption of glucose and binds cholesterol-containing compounds in the intestine, lowering

dietary fibre Nondigestible carbohydrates and lignin that are intact in plants.

functional fibre Nondigestible carbohydrates either isolated from natural sources or synthesized; these may be added to foods and dietary supplements.

total fibre The total amount of dietary fibre and functional fibre in the diet.

soluble (viscous) fibre Fibre that dissolves in water or is broken down by bacteria in the large intestine.

TERMS

blood cholesterol levels and reducing the risk of cardio-vascular disease. **Insoluble fibre** binds water, making the feces bulkier and softer so they pass more quickly and easily through the intestines.

Both kinds of fibre contribute to disease prevention; but the evidence is mixed. As an example, a fibre-rich diet was long thought to lower the risk of colon cancer. Although a large-scale European study concluded that fibre can reduce the risk of colon cancer by 40%, American studies showed that fibre has no impact on colon cancer risk. Still, other limited research indicates that a diet high in soluble fibre can help people manage diabetes and high blood cholesterol levels; a diet high in insoluble fibre can help prevent a variety of health problems, including constipation, hemorrhoids, and diverticulitis. Some studies have linked diets high in fibre-rich fruits, vegetables, and grains with a lower risk of some kinds of cancer; however, it is unclear whether fibre or other food components are responsible for this reduction in risk.

SOURCES OF DIETARY FIBRE   All plant foods contain some dietary fibre. Fruits, legumes, oats (especially oat bran), and barley are particularly rich in soluble fibre. Wheat (especially wheat bran), cereals, grains, and vegetables are all good sources of insoluble fibre. Psyllium, which is often added to cereals or used in fibre supplements and laxatives, improves intestinal health and also helps control glucose and cholesterol levels. The processing of packaged foods can remove fibre, so it's important to depend on fresh fruits and vegetables and foods made from whole grains as sources of dietary fibre.

RECOMMENDED INTAKE OF DIETARY FIBRE   To reduce the risk of chronic disease and maintain intestinal health, the Food and Nutrition Board and Health Canada recommend a daily fibre intake of 38 grams for adult men and 25 grams for adult women. Canadians currently consume about 14 grams of fibre.[5] Fibre should come from foods, not supplements, which should be used only under medical supervision.

Vitamins—Organic Micronutrients

Vitamins are organic (carbon-containing) substances required in very small amounts to regulate various processes within living cells (Table 7.3). Humans need 13 vitamins. Four are fat-soluble (A, D, E, and K), and nine are water-soluble (C and the eight B-complex vitamins: thiamin, riboflavin, niacin, vitamin B-6, folate, vitamin B-12, biotin, and pantothenic acid).

Solubility affects how a vitamin is absorbed, transported, and stored in the body. The water-soluble vitamins are absorbed directly into the bloodstream, where they travel freely. Excess water-soluble vitamins are removed by the kidneys and excreted in urine. Fat-soluble vitamins require a more complex absorptive process. They are usually carried in the blood by special proteins and are stored in the body in fat tissues rather than excreted.

FUNCTIONS OF VITAMINS   Many vitamins help chemical reactions take place. They provide no energy to the body directly but help unleash the energy stored in carbohydrates, proteins, and fats. Vitamins are critical in the production of red blood cells and the maintenance of the nervous, skeletal, and immune systems. Some vitamins act as **antioxidants,** which help preserve healthy cells in the body. Key vitamin antioxidants include vitamin E, vitamin C, and the vitamin A precursor beta-carotene. (Antioxidants are described later in the chapter.)

SOURCES OF VITAMINS   The human body does not manufacture most of the vitamins it requires and must obtain them from foods. Vitamins are abundant in fruits, vegetables, and grains. In addition, many processed foods, such as flour and breakfast cereals, contain added vitamins. A few vitamins are made in certain parts of the body: The skin makes vitamin D when it is exposed to sunlight, and intestinal bacteria make vitamin K. Nonetheless, you still need to obtain vitamin D and vitamin K from foods (Table 7.3).

VITAMIN DEFICIENCIES AND EXCESSES   If your diet lacks sufficient amounts of a particular vitamin, characteristic symptoms of deficiency develop (see Table 7.3). For example, vitamin A deficiency can cause blindness, and vitamin B-6 deficiency can cause seizures. Vitamin deficiency diseases are most often seen in developing countries; they are relatively rare in Canada because vitamins are readily available from our food supply. However, intakes below recommended levels can have adverse effects on health even if they are not low enough to cause a deficiency disease. For example, low intake of folate increases a woman's chance of giving birth to a baby with a neural tube defect (a congenital malformation of the central nervous system). Low intake of folate and vitamins B-6 and B-12 has been linked to increased heart disease risk. Many Canadians consume less-than-recommended amounts of vitamins A, C, B-6, and E.

Extra vitamins in the diet can be harmful, especially when taken as supplements. High doses of vitamin A are

TABLE 7.3 Facts About Vitamins

Vitamin	Important Dietary Sources	Major Functions	Signs of Prolonged Deficiency	Toxic Effects of Megadoses
Fat-Soluble				
Vitamin A	Liver, milk, butter, cheese, and fortified margarine; carrots, spinach, and other orange and deep-green vegetables and fruits	Maintenance of vision, skin, linings of the nose, mouth, digestive and urinary tracts, immune function	Night blindness; dry, scaling skin; increased susceptibility to infection; loss of appetite; anemia; kidney stones	Liver damage, miscarriage and birth defects, headache, vomiting and diarrhea, vertigo, double vision, bone abnormalities
Vitamin D	Fortified milk and margarine, fish oils, butter, egg yolks (sunlight on skin also produces vitamin D)	Development and maintenance of bones and teeth, promotion of calcium absorption	Rickets (bone deformities) in children; bone softening, loss, and fractures in adults	Kidney damage, calcium deposits in soft tissues, depression, death
Vitamin E	Vegetable oils, whole grains, nuts and seeds, green leafy vegetables, asparagus, peaches	Protection and maintenance of cellular membranes	Red blood cell breakage and anemia, weakness, neurological problems, muscle cramps	Relatively nontoxic, but may cause excess bleeding or formation of blood clots
Vitamin K	Green leafy vegetables; smaller amounts widespread in other foods	Production of proteins essential for blood clotting and bone metabolism	Hemorrhaging	None reported
Water-Soluble				
Biotin	Cereals, yeast, egg yolks, soy flour, liver; widespread in foods	Synthesis of fat, glycogen, and amino acids	Rash, nausea, vomiting, weight loss, depression, fatigue, hair loss	None reported
Folate	Green leafy vegetables, yeast, oranges, whole grains, legumes, liver	Amino acid metabolism, synthesis of RNA and DNA, new cell synthesis	Anemia, weakness, fatigue, irritability, shortness of breath, swollen tongue	Masking of vitamin B-12 deficiency
Niacin	Eggs, poultry, fish, milk, whole grains, nuts, enriched breads and cereals, meats, legumes	Conversion of carbohydrates, fats, and protein into usable forms of energy	Pellagra (symptoms include diarrhea, dermatitis, inflammation of mucous membranes, dementia)	Flushing of the skin, nausea, vomiting, diarrhea, liver dysfunction, glucose intolerance
Pantothenic acid	Animal foods, whole grains, broccoli, potatoes; widespread in foods	Metabolism of fats, carbohydrates, and proteins	Fatigue, numbness and tingling of hands and feet, gastrointestinal disturbances	None reported
Riboflavin	Dairy products, enriched breads and cereals, lean meats, poultry, fish, green vegetables	Energy metabolism; maintenance of skin, mucous membranes, and nervous system structures	Cracks at corners of mouth, sore throat, skin rash, hypersensitivity to light, purple tongue	None reported
Thiamin	Whole-grain and enriched breads and cereals, organ meats, lean pork, nuts, legumes	Conversion of carbohydrates into usable forms of energy, maintenance of appetite and nervous system function	Beriberi (symptoms include muscle wasting, mental confusion, anorexia, enlarged heart, nerve changes)	None reported
Vitamin B-6	Eggs, poultry, fish, whole grains, nuts, soybeans, liver, kidney, pork	Metabolism of amino acids and glycogen	Anemia, convulsions, cracks at corners of mouth, dermatitis, nausea, confusion	Neurological abnormalities and damage
Vitamin B-12	Meat, fish, poultry, fortified cereals	Synthesis of blood cells; other metabolic reactions	Anemia, fatigue, nervous system damage, sore tongue	None reported
Vitamin C	Peppers, broccoli, brussels sprouts, spinach, citrus fruits, strawberries, tomatoes, potatoes, cabbage, other fruits and vegetables	Maintenance and repair of connective tissue, bones, teeth, and cartilage; promotion of healing; aid in iron absorption	Scurvy, anemia, reduced resistance to infection, loosened teeth, joint pain, poor wound healing, hair loss, poor iron absorption	Urinary stones in some people, acid stomach from ingesting supplements in pill form, nausea, diarrhea, headache, fatigue

SOURCES: Food and Nutrition Board, Institute of Medicine. 2006. *Dietary Reference Intakes: The Essential Guide to Nutrient Requirements.* Washington, D.C.: National Academies Press. The complete Dietary Reference Intake reports are available from the National Academies Press (http://www.nap.edu). Shils, M. E., et al., eds. 2005. *Modern Nutrition in Health and Disease,* 10th ed. Baltimore: Lippincott Williams and Wilkins.

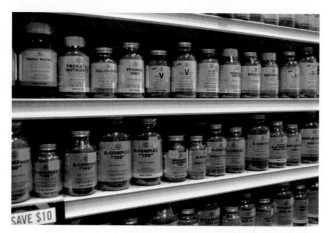

Vitamin and mineral supplements are popular, but they are not usually necessary for healthy people who eat a balanced diet.

toxic and increase the risk of birth defects, for example. Vitamin B-6 can cause irreversible nerve damage when taken in large doses. Megadoses of fat-soluble vitamins are particularly dangerous because the excess will be stored in the body rather than excreted, increasing the risk of toxicity. Even when supplements are not taken in excess, relying on them for an adequate intake of vitamins can be a problem: There are many substances in foods other than vitamins and minerals, and some of these compounds may have important health effects. Later in the chapter we discuss specific recommendations for vitamin intake and when a supplement is advisable. For now, keep in mind that it's best to obtain most of your vitamins from foods rather than supplements.

The vitamins and minerals in foods can be easily lost or destroyed during storage or cooking. To retain their value, eat or process vegetables immediately after buying them. If you can't do this, then store them in a cool place, covered to retain moisture—either in the refrigerator (for a few days) or in the freezer (for a longer term). To reduce nutrient losses during food preparation, minimize the amount of water used and the total cooking time. Develop a taste for a crunchier texture in cooked vegetables. Baking, steaming, broiling, and microwaving are all good methods of preparing vegetables.

Minerals—Inorganic Micronutrients

Minerals are inorganic (non-carbon-containing) elements you need in small amounts to help regulate body functions, aid in the growth and maintenance of body tissues, and help release energy (Table 7.4). There are about 17 essential minerals. The major minerals, those that the body needs in amounts exceeding 100 milligrams per day, include calcium, phosphorus, magnesium, sodium, potassium, and chloride. The essential trace minerals, those that you need in minute amounts, include copper, fluoride, iodine, iron, selenium, and zinc.

Characteristic symptoms develop if an essential mineral is consumed in a quantity too small or too large for good health. The minerals most commonly lacking in the Canadian diet are iron, calcium, magnesium, and potassium.[6] Focus on good food choices for these nutrients (see Table 7.4). Iron-deficiency **anemia** is a problem in some age groups, and researchers fear poor calcium intakes are sowing the seeds for future **osteoporosis,** especially in women. See the box "Eating for Healthy Bones" to learn more.

Water—Vital but Often Ignored

Water is the major component in both foods and the human body: You are composed of about 50–60% water. Your need for other nutrients, in terms of weight, is much less than your need for water. You can live up to 50 days without food but only a few days without water.

Water is distributed all over the body, among lean and other tissues and in urine and other body fluids. Water is used in the digestion and absorption of food and is the medium in which most of the chemical reactions take place within the body. Some water-based fluids like blood transport substances around the body; other fluids serve as lubricants or cushions. Water also helps regulate body temperature.

Water is contained in almost all foods, particularly in liquids, fruits, and vegetables. The foods and fluids you consume provide 80–90% of your daily water intake; the remainder is generated through metabolism. You lose water each day in urine, feces, and sweat and through evaporation in your lungs.

Most people maintain a healthy water balance by consuming beverages at meals and drinking fluids in response to thirst. In 2004, the Food and Nutrition Board and Health Canada set levels of adequate water intake to maintain hydration (Table 7.5); all fluids, including those

CAREER OPTIONS IN . . .

Nutrition

HEALTH CARE: dietician/nutritionist, professor, doctor.

COMMUNITY: life sciences or home economics teacher, wellness coordinator.

INDUSTRY: food scientist, product health claims researcher, food and nutrition admininstration.

SOURCES: Physical and Health Education Canada (http://www.phecanada.ca); Mount Saint Vincent University. Nutrition Related Career Options (http://www.msvu.ca/en/home/programsdepartments/professionalstudies/appliedhumannutrition/becomingadietitiannutritionprofessional/nutritioncareers.aspx).

WELLNESS TIP

If you take a supplement, *never* take more than the recommended dosage unless your doctor tells you to.

TABLE 7.4 Facts About Selected Minerals

Mineral	Important Dietary Sources	Major Functions	Signs of Prolonged Deficiency	Toxic Effects of Megadoses
Calcium	Milk and milk products, tofu, fortified orange juice and bread, green leafy vegetables, bones in fish	Formation of bones and teeth; control of nerve impulses, muscle contraction, blood clotting	Stunted growth in children, bone mineral loss in adults; urinary stones	Kidney stones, calcium deposits in soft tissues, inhibition of mineral absorption, constipation
Fluoride	Fluoridated water, tea, marine fish eaten with bones	Maintenance of tooth and bone structure	Higher frequency of tooth decay	Increased bone density, mottling of teeth, impaired kidney function
Iodine	Iodized salt, seafood, processed foods	Essential part of thyroid hormones, regulation of body metabolism	Goiter (enlarged thyroid), cretinism (birth defect)	Depression of thyroid activity, hyperthyroidism in susceptible people
Iron	Meat and poultry, fortified grain products, dark-green vegetables, dried fruit	Component of hemoglobin, myoglobin, and enzymes	Iron-deficiency anemia, weakness, impaired immune function, gastrointestinal distress	Nausea, diarrhea, liver and kidney damage, joint pains, sterility, disruption of cardiac function, death
Magnesium	Widespread in foods and water (except soft water); especially found in grains, legumes, nuts, seeds, green vegetables, milk	Transmission of nerve impulses, energy transfer, activation of many enzymes	Neurological disturbances, cardiovascular problems, kidney disorders, nausea, growth failure in children	Nausea, vomiting, diarrhea, central nervous system depression, coma; death in people with impaired kidney function
Phosphorus	Present in nearly all foods, especially milk, cereal, peas, eggs, meat	Bone growth and maintenance, energy transfer in cells	Impaired growth, weakness, kidney disorders, cardiorespiratory and nervous system dysfunction	Drop in blood calcium levels, calcium deposits in soft tissues, bone loss
Potassium	Meats, milk, fruits, vegetables, grains, legumes	Nerve function and body water balance	Muscular weakness, nausea, drowsiness, paralysis, confusion, dysruption of cardiac rhythm	Cardiac arrest
Selenium	Seafood, meat, eggs, whole grains	Defense against oxidative stress and regulation of thyroid hormone action	Muscle pain and weakness, heart disorders	Hair and nail brittleness and loss, nausea and vomiting, weakness, irritability
Sodium	Salt, soy sauce, fast food, and processed foods, especially lunch meats, canned soups and vegetables, salty snacks, and processed cheese	Body water balance, acid-base balance, nerve function	Muscle weakness, loss of appetite, nausea, vomiting; deficiency is rarely seen	Edema, hypertension in sensitive people
Zinc	Whole grains, meat, eggs, liver, seafood (especially oysters)	Synthesis of proteins, RNA, and DNA; wound healing; immune response; ability to taste	Growth failure, loss of appetite, impaired taste acuity, skin rash, impaired immune function, poor wound healing	Vomiting, impaired immune function, decline in blood HDL levels, impaired copper absorption

SOURCES: Food and Nutrition Board, Institute of Medicine. 2006. *Dietary Reference Intakes: The Essential Guide to Nutrient Requirements.* Washington, D.C.: National Academies Press. The complete Dietary Reference Intake reports are available from the National Academies Press (http://www.nap.edu). Shils, M. E., et al., eds. 2005. *Modern Nutrition in Health and Disease,* 10th ed. Baltimore: Lippincott Williams and Wilkins.

containing caffeine, can count toward your total daily fluid intake. Men need to consume about 3.7 total litres of water, with 3.0 litres (about 13 cups) coming from beverages; women need 2.7 total litres, with 2.2 litres (about 9 cups) coming from beverages. (See Table 1 in the Nutrition Resources section at the end of the chapter for recommendations for specific age groups.) If you exercise vigorously or live in a hot climate, you need to consume additional fluids to maintain a balance between water consumed and water lost. See the "Do Athletes Need a Different Diet?" box later in the chapter for more on the fluid needs of athletes and active people.

Other Substances in Food

Many substances in food are not essential nutrients but that may influence health.

minerals   Inorganic compounds needed in small amounts for regulation, growth, and maintenance of body tissues and functions.

anemia   A deficiency in the oxygen-carrying material in the red blood cells.

osteoporosis   A condition in which the bones become thin and brittle and break easily.

TERMS

TABLE 7.5 Adequate Daily Water Intake

Life stage		Total water intake from fluids and food	Fluid intake (water and beverages) as part of total water intake
Children	1–3 years	1.3 litres	0.9 litres (about 4 cups)
	4–8 years	1.7 litres	1.2 litres (about 5 cups)
Males	9–13 years	2.4 litres	1.8 litres (about 8 cups)
	14–18 years	3.3 litres	2.6 litres (about 11 cups)
	19 years and older	3.7 litres	3.0 litres (about 13 cups)
Females	9–13 years	2.1 litres	1.6 litres (about 7 cups)
	14–18 years	2.3 litres	1.8 litres (about 8 cups)
	19 years and older	2.7 litres	2.2 litres (about 9 cups)

Infant fluid intake (0.7–0.8 litres/day) is assumed to be from human milk and, for infants 7–12 months, from complementary foods and beverages.

SOURCE: Reprinted with permission from the National Academy of Science. "Dietary Reference Intake: Water, Potassium, Sodium, Chloride, and Sulfate." 2004. Institute of Medicine, National Academies.

ANTIOXIDANTS   When the body uses oxygen or breaks down certain fats or proteins as a normal part of metabolism, it gives rise to substances called **free radicals.** Environmental factors such as cigarette smoke, exhaust fumes, radiation, excessive sunlight, certain drugs, and stress can increase free radical production. A free radical is a chemically unstable molecule that reacts with fats, proteins, and DNA, damaging cell membranes and mutating genes. Free radicals have been implicated in aging, cancer, cardiovascular disease, and other degenerative diseases like arthritis.

Antioxidants found in foods can help protect the body by blocking the formation and action of free radicals and repairing the damage they cause. Some antioxidants, such as vitamin C, vitamin E, and selenium, are also essential nutrients. Others, such as carotenoids, found in yellow, orange, and dark-green leafy vegetables, are not. Researchers recently identified the top antioxidant-containing foods and beverages as blackberries, walnuts, strawberries, artichokes, cranberries, brewed coffee, raspberries, pecans, blueberries, cloves, grape juice, unsweetened baking chocolate, sour cherries, and red wine. Also high in antioxidants are Brussels sprouts, kale, cauliflower, and pomegranates.

PHYTOCHEMICALS   Antioxidants fall into the broader category of **phytochemicals,** substances found in plant foods that may help prevent chronic disease. Researchers have just begun to identify and study all the different compounds found in foods, and many preliminary findings are promising. For example, certain substances found in soy foods may help lower cholesterol levels. Sulforaphane, a compound isolated from broccoli and other **cruciferous vegetables,** may render some carcinogenic compounds harmless. Limited research has shown that you can get the most benefit from cruciferous vegetables by eating them raw. Allyl sulfides, a group of chemicals found in garlic and onions, appear to boost the activity of cancer-fighting immune cells. Further research on phytochemicals may extend the role of nutrition to the prevention and treatment of many chronic diseases.

To increase your intake of phytochemicals, it is best to obtain them by eating a variety of fruits and vegetables rather than relying on supplements. Like many vitamins and minerals, isolated phytochemicals may be harmful if taken in high doses. In addition, it is likely that their health benefits are the result of chemical substances working in combination. The role of phytochemicals in disease prevention is discussed further in Chapters 11 and 12.

LO2 7.2 NUTRITIONAL GUIDELINES: PLANNING YOUR DIET

Various tools have been created by scientific and government groups to help people design healthy diets. The **Dietary Reference Intakes (DRIs)** are standards for nutrient intake designed to prevent nutritional deficiencies and reduce the risk of chronic disease. **Canada's Food Guide** translates these nutrient recommendations into a balanced food-group plan that includes all essential nutrients. Together, the DRIs and the Food Guide make up a complete set of resources for dietary planning.

FITNESS TIP

Drink plenty of water before, during, and after workouts, especially when the weather is warm. Proper hydration helps you avoid cramps and heat-related problems such as heat stroke.

Osteoporosis is a condition in which the bones become dangerously thin and fragile over time. It currently afflicts as many as 2 million Canadians with women over 50 twice as likely to suffer from it as males over 50.

Most bone mass is built by age 18. After bone density peaks between ages 25 and 35, bone mass is lost over time. To prevent osteoporosis, the best strategy is to build as much bone as possible during your youth and do everything you can to maintain it as you age. Up to 50% of bone loss is determined by controllable lifestyle factors such as diet and exercise. Key nutrients for bone health include the following:

Calcium Getting enough calcium is important throughout life to build and maintain bone mass. Health Canada recommends that most adults consume 1000–200mg of calcium per day. Milk, yogurt, canned salmon and sardines with the bones, and calcium-fortified orange juice, bread, and cereals are all good sources.

Vitamin D Vitamin D is necessary for bones to absorb calcium; 600 IU (15 mcg) a day is recommended for children and adults aged 9–70 years. Vitamin D can be obtained from foods and is manufactured by the skin when exposed to sunlight. Because the sun is weaker in northern latitudes, most Canadians are good candidates for vitamin D supplements. People who don't eat many foods rich in vitamin D, such as milk, eggs and oily fish, and those who don't expose their face, arms, and hands to the sun (without sunscreen) for 5–15 minutes a few times each week are at risk.

Vitamin K Vitamin K promotes the synthesis of proteins that help keep bones strong. Broccoli and leafy green vegetables are rich in vitamin K.

Other nutrients Other nutrients that may play an important role in bone health include vitamin C, magnesium, potassium, manganese, zinc, copper, and boron.

On the flip side, there are several dietary substances that may have a negative effect on bone health, especially if consumed in excess, including alcohol, sodium, caffeine, and retinol (a form of vitamin A). Drinking lots of soda, which often replaces milk in the diet and which is high in phosphorus (a mineral that may interfere with calcium absorption), has been shown to increase the risk of bone fracture in teenage girls.

The effect of protein intake on bone mass depends on other nutrients: Protein helps build bone as long as calcium and vitamin D intake are adequate; but if intake of calcium and vitamin D is low, high protein intake can lead to bone loss.

Weight-bearing aerobic activities help maintain bone mass throughout life. In fact, just jumping in place or skipping rope for 2 minutes a day can help maintain bone density. Normal weight-bearing activities of daily living (such as carrying a load of laundry up a flight of stairs) also go a long way to keeping your bones strong. Walking is a great way keep bones strong. Strength training improves bone density, muscle mass, strength, and balance.

SOURCES: Osteoporosis Canada (http:// www.osteoporosis.ca) and Health Canada. 2010. *Food and Nutrition: Vitamin D and Calcium: Updated Dietary Reference Intakes* (http://www.hc-sc.gc.ca/fn-an/nutrition/vitamin/vita-d-eng.php#t5; retrieved December 10, 2011).

Dietary Reference Intakes (DRIs)

How much vitamin C, iron, calcium, and other nutrients do you need to stay healthy? The Food and Nutrition Board of the National Academy of Sciences and Health Canada have partnered to establish dietary standards, or recommended intake levels, for North Americans of all ages. The current set of standards, called Dietary Reference Intakes (DRIs), is relatively new, having been introduced in 1997. An earlier set of standards, called the **Recommended Dietary Allowances (RDAs)**, focused on preventing nutritional deficiency diseases such as anemia; the RDAs were established in 1941 and updated periodically, most recently in 1989. The newer DRIs have a broader focus because recent research has looked not just at the prevention of nutrient deficiencies but also at the role of nutrients in promoting optimal health and preventing chronic diseases such as cancer, osteoporosis, and heart disease.

The DRIs include standards for both recommended intakes and maximum safe intakes. The recommended intake of each nutrient is expressed as either a *Recommended Dietary Allowance (RDA)* or *Adequate Intake (AI)*. An AI is set when there is not enough information available to set an RDA value; regardless of the type of standard used, however, the DRI represents the best available estimate of

intake for optimal health. The *Tolerable Upper Intake Level (UL)* sets the maximum daily intake by a healthy person that is unlikely to cause health problems. For example, the RDA for calcium for an 18-year old female is 1300 mg per day; the UL is 2500 mg per day.

TERMS

free radical An electron-seeking compound that can react with fats, proteins, and DNA, damaging cell membranes and mutating genes in its search for electrons; produced through chemical reactions in the body and by exposure to environmental factors such as sunlight and tobacco smoke.

phytochemical A naturally occurring substance found in plant foods that may help prevent and treat chronic diseases such as heart disease and cancer; phyto means plant.

cruciferous vegetables Vegetables of the cabbage family, including cabbage, broccoli, Brussels sprouts, kale, and cauliflower; the flower petals of these plants form the shape of a cross, hence the name.

Dietary Reference Intakes (DRIs) An umbrella term for four types of nutrient standards: Adequate Intake (AI), Estimated Average Requirement (EAR), and Recommended Dietary Allowance (RDA) set levels of intake considered adequate to prevent nutrient deficiencies and reduce the risk of chronic disease; Tolerable Upper Intake Level (UL) sets the maximum daily intake that is unlikely to cause health problems.

Canada's Food Guide A food-group plan that provides practical advice to ensure a balanced intake of the essential nutrients.

Recommended Dietary Allowances (RDAs) Amounts of certain nutrients considered adequate to prevent deficiencies in most healthy people; will eventually be replaced by the Dietary Reference Intakes (DRIs).

Because of lack of data, ULs have not been set for all nutrients. This does not mean that people can tolerate chronic intakes of these vitamins and minerals above recommended levels. Like all chemical agents, nutrients can produce adverse effects if intakes are excessive. There is no established benefit from consuming nutrients at levels above the RDA or AI. The DRIs can be found in the Nutrition Resources section at the end of the chapter. For more information, visit the website of the National Academies' Food and Nutrition Board (see For Further Exploration at the end of the chapter.)

DAILY VALUES Because the DRIs are far too cumbersome to use as a basis for food labels, the U.S. Food and Drug Administration developed another set of dietary standards, the **Daily Values.** The Daily Values are based on several different sets of guidelines and include standards for fat, cholesterol, carbohydrate, dietary fibre, and selected vitamins and minerals. The Daily Values represent appropriate intake levels for a 2000-calorie diet. The percent Daily Value shown on a food label shows how well that food contributes to your recommended daily intake. Food labels are described in detail later in the chapter.

SHOULD YOU TAKE SUPPLEMENTS? The aim of the DRIs is to guide you in meeting your nutritional needs primarily with food, rather than with vitamin and mineral supplements. Supplements lack potentially beneficial phytochemicals and fibre that are found only in whole foods. Nutrition scientists generally agree that most Canadians can obtain most of the vitamins and minerals they need by consuming a varied, nutritionally balanced diet like the one recommended by Canada's Food Guide.

The question of whether to take supplements is a serious one. Some vitamins and minerals are dangerous when ingested in excess, as described in Tables 7.3 and 7.4. Large doses of particular nutrients can also cause health problems by affecting the absorption of other vitamins and minerals. For all these reasons, you should think carefully about whether to take supplements; consider consulting a physician or registered dietitian.

Over the past two decades, high-dose supplement use has been promoted as a way to prevent or delay the onset of many diseases, including heart disease and several forms of cancer. These claims remain controversial, however, and a growing body of research shows that vitamin or mineral supplements have no significant impact on the risk of developing such illnesses. For example, a 2008 study conducted as part of the Women's Health Initiative showed no differences in the levels of heart disease, cancer, or overall mortality between postmenopausal women who took multivitamin supplements and those who did not. A similar study of adult men indicated that taking vitamins C and E did not reduce the risk of heart disease or certain cancers. According to the experts behind these and other studies, the research provides further proof that a balanced diet of whole foods—not high-dose supplementation—is the best way to promote health and prevent disease.

In setting the DRIs, the Food and Nutrition Board recommended supplements of particular nutrients for the following groups:

- Women who are capable of becoming pregnant should take 400 μg per day of folic acid (the synthetic form of the vitamin folate) from fortified foods and/or supplements in addition to folate from a varied diet. Research indicates that this level of folate intake will reduce the risk of neural tube defects. (This defect occurs early in pregnancy, before most women know they are pregnant; therefore, the recommendation for the folate intake applies to all women of reproductive age rather than only to pregnant women.) Enriched breads, flours, corn meals, rice, noodles, and other grain products have been fortified with small amounts of folic acid. Folate is found naturally in leafy green vegetables, legumes, oranges and orange juice, and strawberries.

- People over age 50 should consume foods fortified with vitamin B-12, B-12 supplements, or both to meet the majority of the DRI of 2.4 mg of B-12 daily. Up to 30% of people over 50 have problems absorbing protein-bound B-12 in foods. Vitamin B-12 in supplements and fortified foods is more readily absorbed and can help prevent a deficiency.

- Because of the oxidative stress caused by smoking, the Food and Nutrition Board and Health Canada also recommend that smokers consume 35 mg more vitamin C per day than the DRI intake level set for their age and sex (for adults, recommended daily vitamin C intakes for nonsmokers are 90 mg for men and 75 mg for women). However, supplements are not usually needed because this extra vitamin C can easily be obtained from foods. For example, one cup of orange juice has about 100 mg of vitamin C.

Supplements may also be recommended in other cases. Women with heavy menstrual flows may need extra iron to compensate for the monthly loss. Older people, people with dark skin, and people exposed to little sunlight may need extra vitamin D. Some vegetarians may need supplemental calcium, iron, zinc, and vitamin B-12, depending on their food choices. Newborns need a single dose of vitamin K, which must be administered under the direction of a physician. People who consume few calories, who have certain diseases, or who take certain medications may need specific vitamin and mineral

TERMS

Daily Values A simplified version of the RDAs used on food labels; also included are values for nutrients with no established RDA.

Studies have shown that most people underestimate the size of their food portions, in many cases by as much as 50%. If you need to retrain your eye, try using measuring cups and spoons and an inexpensive kitchen scale when you eat at home. With a little practice, you'll learn the difference between 3 and 8 ounces of chicken or meat and what a half-cup of rice really looks like. For quick estimates, use these equivalents:

- 1 teaspoon of margarine = one dice

- 30 grams of cheese = your thumb, four dice stacked together, or an ice cube

- 60 grams of chicken or meat = a deck of cards

- ½ cup of rice, past, or potato = an ice cream scoop or ½ a baseball

- 2 tablespoons of peanut butter = a ping-pong ball or large marshmallow

- 1 60-gram bagel = a hockey puck or yo-yo

- 1 60-gram muffin or roll = a plum or a large egg

- 1 medium fruit (apple or orange) = a baseball

- ¼ cup nuts = a golf ball

- small cookie or cracker = a poker chip

---

supplements. Such supplement decisions must be made by a physician because some vitamins and minerals counteract the actions of certain medications.

In deciding whether to take a vitamin and mineral supplement, consider whether you already eat a fortified breakfast cereal every day. Many breakfast cereals contain almost as many nutrients as a vitamin pill! If you do decide to take a supplement, choose a balanced formulation that contains 50–100% of the Daily Value for vitamins and minerals. Avoid supplements containing large doses of particular nutrients.

Canada's Food Guide

The Food Guide (Figure 7.4) is an outline of what to eat each day—not a rigid prescription, but a general guide that lets you choose a healthful diet that's right for you. It calls for eating a variety of foods to get the nutrients you need and at the same time the right amount of calories to maintain a healthy weight. Access the online version of Canada's Food Guide at www.hc-sc.gc.ca/fn-an/food-guide-aliment/index-eng.php and click on "My food guide" to create your own personal Food Guide based on your daily requirements. Your personal food guide will identify how many servings of each food group that YOU should be consuming on a daily basis.

FOOD GUIDE SERVINGS AND THEIR SIZES The number of servings (Figure 7.4) recommended for each group in the Food Guide is based on specific serving sizes that may differ from your own typical portion sizes and the serving sizes listed on food labels. For example, one Food Guide serving of pasta is ½ cup; if your portion at a meal is 1½ cups of pasta, it would count as 3 servings toward your daily total from the Grain Products food group. When evaluating your current diet or planning dietary changes, it is very important to consider the serving sizes given in the Food Guide. If you are one of the many

people who have trouble identifying 30 grams of cereal or a half-cup of rice, see the strategies in the box "Judging Serving Sizes."

GRAIN PRODUCTS (3–8 SERVINGS) Foods from this group are usually low in fat and rich in complex carbohydrates, dietary fibre (if grains are unrefined), and many vitamins and minerals, including thiamin, riboflavin, iron, niacin, folate, and zinc. Although 3–8 servings may seem like a large amount of food, many people eat several servings at a time. A single serving is the equivalent of the following:

- 1 slice of bread or half a hamburger bun, English muffin, or bagel
- 1 small roll, biscuit, or muffin
- 30 g of ready-to-eat cereal
- ½ cup cooked cereal, rice, or pasta
- 5–6 small or 2–3 large crackers
- 1 18-cm corn or flour tortilla

Choose foods that are typically made with little fat or sugar (bread, rice, pasta) over those that are high in fat and sugar (croissants, chips, cookies, doughnuts). For maximum nutrition, choose half of these servings per day from whole grains, such as whole-wheat bread, high-fibre cereal, whole-wheat pasta, and brown rice.

FRUIT AND VEGETABLES (4–10 SERVINGS) Fruit and vegetables are rich in carbohydrates, dietary fibre, vitamin A, vitamin C, folate, magnesium, and other nutrients. They are also naturally low in fat (both) and sodium (fruits). A serving of vegetables is equivalent to the following:

- 1 cup raw leafy vegetables
- 1 medium sized fruit or vegetable
- ½ cup tomato sauce

- ½ cup fruit or vegetable juice
- ½ cup cooked dry beans (legumes)
- 1 cup bean or vegetable soup

Fruits and vegetables vary in the nutrients they provide so it is important to consume a variety of types to obtain maximum nutrition. Many Canadians consume only a few different types of vegetables, with white potatoes (baked or served as french fries) being the most popular. A suggestion would be to try to consume at least one serving from each of the following vegetable groups on most days of the week:

- Dark-green vegetables like spinach, chard, collards, broccoli, romaine, and turnip and mustard greens
- Deep-yellow and orange vegetables like carrots, winter squash, sweet potatoes, and pumpkin
- Legumes like pinto beans, kidney beans, black beans, lentils, chickpeas, and tofu; legumes can be counted as servings of vegetables or as alternatives to meat
- Starchy vegetables like corn, green peas, and white potatoes
- Other vegetables; tomatoes, bell peppers (red, orange, yellow, or green), green beans, and cruciferous vegetables like cauliflower are good choices

Good choices of fruits are citrus fruits and juices, melons, pears, apples, bananas, and berries. Choose whole fruits often—they are higher in fibre and often lower in calories than fruit juices. Fruit juices typically contain more nutrients than fruit drinks. For canned fruits, choose those packed in their own juice rather than in syrup.

MILK AND ALTERNATIVES (2–4 SERVINGS) Foods from this group are high in protein, carbohydrate, calcium, riboflavin, and vitamin D. To limit the fat in your diet, choose servings of low-fat or nonfat items from this group:

- 1 cup milk
- 50 g of block cheese
- 2 slices processed cheese

Cottage cheese is lower in calcium than most other cheeses, and 1 cup of cottage cheese counts as only half a serving for this food group. Ice cream is also lower in calcium than many other dairy products (½ cup is equivalent to 1/3 serving); in addition, it is high in sugar and fat. The number of servings you should consume each day will be dependent upon your age and health status (Figure 7.4).

MEAT AND ALTERNATIVES (2–3 SERVINGS) This food group provides protein, niacin, iron, vitamin B-6, zinc, and thiamin; the animal foods in the group also provide vitamin B-12. The Food Guide recommends 2–3

servings each day of foods from this group. The total amount of these servings should be the equivalent of 150–300 grams of cooked lean meat, poultry, or fish a day. Many people misjudge what makes up a single serving for this food group:

- 50–100 g cooked lean meat, poultry, or fish (an average hamburger or a medium chicken breast half is about 100 g, or ½ cup of drained canned tuna counts as about 75 g)
- The following portions of nonmeat foods are equivalent to 30 grams of lean meat: ½ cup cooked dry beans (if not counted as a vegetable), 1 egg, 2 tablespoons peanut butter, 1/3 cup nuts, ¼ cup seeds, and 1/3 cup tofu

One egg at breakfast, a cup of pinto beans at lunch, and a hamburger at dinner would add up to the equivalent of 225 g of lean meat for the day. To limit your intake of fat and saturated fat, choose lean cuts of meat and skinless poultry, eat nuts and seeds in moderation, and watch your serving sizes carefully. Additionally, you may choose to eat fish such as salmon twice a week to increase your consumption of healthier fats. Choose at least one serving of such plant proteins as black beans, lentils, or tofu every day.

Canada's Food Guide also includes a category for Oils and Fats which gives advice on foods such as oils and sugars that are not found on the Food Guide. Health Canada suggests that you consume products found in this group in moderation. Foods in this group tend to be higher in fat and calorie content. See the box "Reducing the Saturated and Trans Fats in Your Diet," for ways to reduce their intake. In addition, a new section on Beverages helps us to identify healthier selections of beverages that may even be counted towards other food groups on the guide.

Canada's Food Guide to Healthy Eating is a general guide to what you should eat every day. By eating a balanced variety of foods from each of the four food groups and including some plant proteins, you can ensure that your daily diet is adequate in all nutrients. A diet using low-fat food choices contains only about 1800 calories but meets all known nutritional needs, except possibly for iron in some women who have heavy menstrual periods. For these women, foods fortified in iron, such as breakfast cereals, can make up the deficit.

COMPLEMENTING CANADA'S FOOD GUIDE Health Canada has recognized that there are groups of Canadians who may consume diets that require the same guidance as the Food Guide but include foods not found in the Food Guide, or include foods required in different ratios. In 2007, the Eating Well With Canada's Food Guide— First Nations, Inuit, and Métis (see Figure 7.5), was published in three languages (Cree, Ojibwe, and Inuktitut).

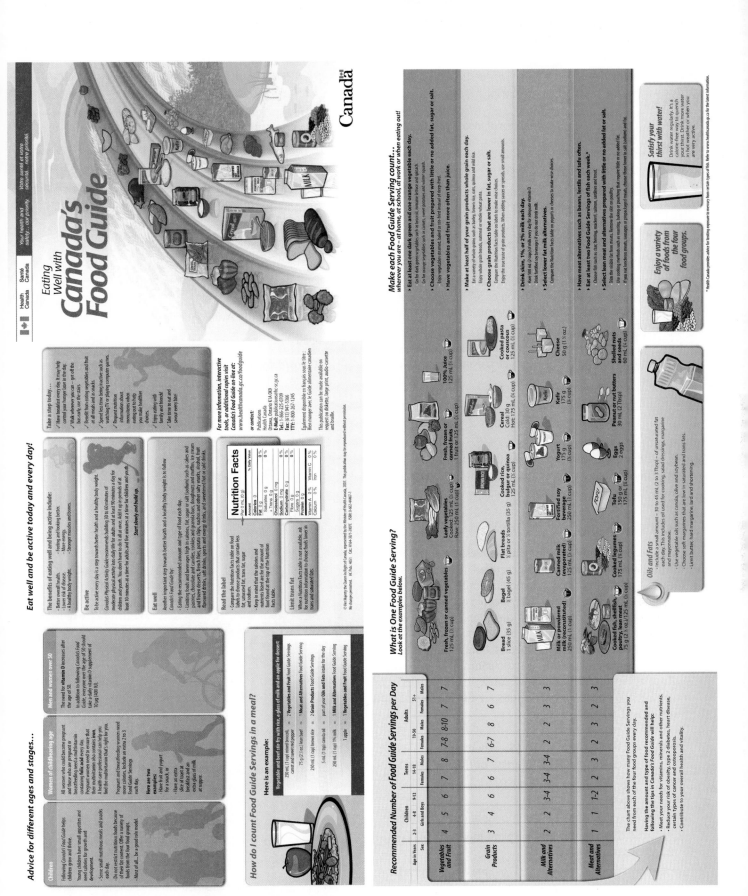

FIGURE 7.4 Canada's Food Guide and recommended servings.

SOURCE: Adapted and reproduced with the permission of the Minister of Public Works and Government Services Canada, 2008.

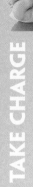

Reducing the Saturated and Trans Fats in Your Diet

Your overall goal is to limit total fat intake to no more than 35% of total calories. Favour unsaturated fats over saturated and trans fats.

- Be moderate in your consumption of foods high in fat, including fast food, commercially prepared baked goods and desserts, deep-fried foods, meat, poultry (with skin), nuts and seeds, and regular dairy products.

- When you do eat high-fat foods, limit your portion sizes, and balance your intake with foods low in fat.

- Choose lean cuts of meat, and trim any visible fat from meat before and after cooking. Remove skin from poultry before or after cooking.

- Drink fat-free or low-fat milk instead of whole milk, and use lower-fat varieties when cooking or baking. Substitute plain low-fat yogurt, low-fat cottage cheese, or buttermilk for sour cream.

- Use vegetable oil instead of butter or margarine. Use tub or squeeze margarine instead of stick margarine. Look for margarines that are free of trans fats. Minimize intake of coconut or palm oil.

- Season vegetables, seafood, and meats with herbs and spices rather than with creamy sauces, butter, or margarine.

- Use olive oil or lemon juice on salad, or use a yogurt-based salad dressing instead of mayonnaise or sour cream dressings.

- Steam, boil, bake, or microwave vegetables, or stir-fry them in a small amount of canola oil.

- Roast, bake, or broil meat, poultry, or fish so that fat drains away as the food cooks.

- Use a nonstick pan for cooking so that added fat will be unnecessary; use a vegetable spray for frying.

- Substitute egg whites for whole eggs when baking; limit the number of egg yolks when scrambling eggs.

- Choose fruits as desserts most often.

- Eat a low-fat vegetarian main dish at least once a week.

In addition, the following pages detail the use of a guide that enables many vegetarians to consume foods that will assist in meeting daily intake values.

LO3 The Vegetarian Alternative

Some people choose a diet with one essential difference from the diets we've already described. That is, this type of diet eliminates or restricts foods of animal origin (meat, poultry, fish, eggs, milk) . Many people choose such diets for health reasons; vegetarian diets tend to be lower in saturated fat, cholesterol, and animal protein and higher in complex carbohydrates, dietary fibre, folate, vitamins C and E, carotenoids, and phytochemicals. Some people adopt a vegetarian diet out of concern for the environment, for financial considerations, or for reasons related to ethics or religion.

TYPES OF VEGETARIAN DIETS   There are various vegetarian styles; the wider the variety of the diet eaten, the easier it is to meet nutritional needs.

- **Vegans** eat only plant foods.
- **Lacto-vegetarians** eat plant foods and dairy products.
- **Lacto-ovo-vegetarians** eat plant foods, dairy products, and eggs.

Others can be categorized as **partial vegetarians, semivegetarians,** or **pescovegetarians.** These people eat plant foods, dairy products, eggs, and usually a small selection of poultry, fish, and other seafood. Many other people choose vegetarian meals frequently but are not

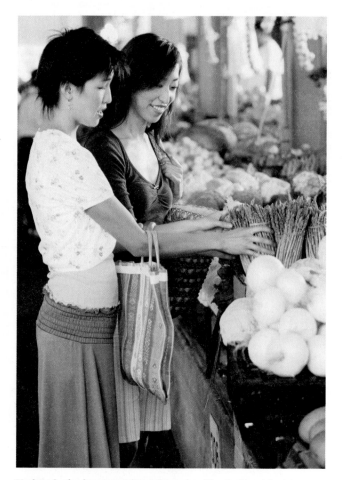

Variety is the key to maintaining a healthy, balanced vegetarian diet.

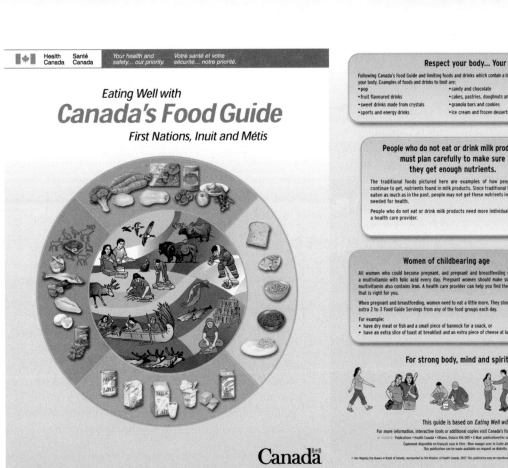

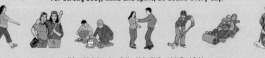

FIGURE 7.5 Eating Well with Canada's Food Guide—First Nations, Métis, and Inuit.

SOURCE: Canada's Food Guide to Healthy Eating, For People Four Years and Over. Health Canada, 2007. Reproduced with permission from the Minister of Health, 2012.

strictly vegetarian. Including some animal protein (such as dairy products) in a vegetarian diet makes planning easier, but it is not necessary.

A FOOD GUIDE FOR VEGETARIANS Health Canada's newest Food Guide is considered to be more "friendly" to vegetarians in that its Meat and Alternatives group places a greater emphasis on the consumption of vegetarian options instead of meat-only products. Although a vegetarian-only version of Canada's Food Guide has not been created, the Dieticians of Canada has released a Public Policy Statement[7] called "A New Food Guide for North American Vegetarians" (see Figure 7.6) that should be considered a complement to Canada's Food Guide.

If you are using the basic Food Guide, it can be adapted for use by vegetarians with only a few key modifications (see Figure 1 in the Nutrition Resources section at the end of the chapter):

- Grain Products group (5–12 servings per day)
- Fruit and Vegetables group (5–10 servings per day)
- Milk and Alternatives group (0–4 servings per day); vegans and other vegetarians who do not consume any dairy products must find other rich sources of calcium (see below)
- Dry Beans, Nuts, Seeds, Eggs, and Meat Substitutes group (2–3 servings per day); this group includes such foods as soy milk, legumes, eggs or egg whites, nuts, seeds, tofu (soybean curd), tempeh (a cultured soy product), and peanut butter

A healthy vegetarian diet emphasizes a wide variety of plant foods. Although plant proteins are generally incomplete, choosing a variety of plant foods will supply all of the essential amino acids. Choosing minimally processed and unrefined foods will maximize nutrient value and provide ample dietary fibre. Daily consumption of a variety of plant foods in amounts that meet total energy needs can provide all needed nutrients, except vitamin B-12 and possibly vitamin D. Strategies for obtaining these and other nutrients of concern include the following:

- Vitamin B-12 is found naturally only in animal foods; if dairy products and eggs are limited or avoided, B-12 can be obtained from fortified foods such as ready-to-eat cereals, soy beverages, meat substitutes, and special yeast products or from supplements.
- Vitamin D can be obtained by spending 5–15 minutes a day out in the sun, by consuming vitamin D-fortified products like ready-to-eat cereals and soy or rice milk, or by taking a supplement.
- Calcium is found in legumes, tofu processed with calcium, dark-green leafy vegetables, nuts, tortillas made from lime-processed corn, and fortified orange juice, soy milk, bread, and other foods.
- Iron is found in whole grains, fortified bread and breakfast cereals, dried fruits, green leafy vegetables, nuts and seeds, legumes, and soy foods. The iron in plant foods is more difficult for the body to absorb than the iron from animal sources; consuming a

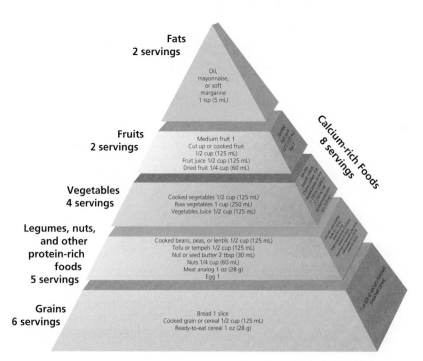

Fats
2 servings
Oil, mayonnaise, or soft margarine 1 tsp (5 mL)

Calcium-rich Foods
8 servings

Fruits
2 servings
Medium fruit 1
Cut up or cooked fruit 1/2 cup (125 mL)
Fruit juice 1/2 cup (125 mL)
Dried fruit 1/4 cup (60 mL)

Vegetables
4 servings
Cooked vegetables 1/2 cup (125 mL)
Raw vegetables 1 cup (250 mL)
Vegetables Juice 1/2 cup (125 mL)

Legumes, nuts, and other protein-rich foods
5 servings
Cooked beans, peas, or lentils 1/2 cup (125 mL)
Tofu or tempeh 1/2 cup (125 mL)
Nut or seed butter 2 tbsp (30 mL)
Nuts 1/4 cup (60 mL)
Meat analog 1 oz (28 g)
Egg 1

Grains
6 servings
Bread 1 slice
Cooked grain or cereal 1/2 cup (125 mL)
Ready-to-eat cereal 1 oz (28 g)

FIGURE 7.6 Vegetarian Food Guide Pyramid.

SOURCE: Reprinted from A new food guide for North American vegetarians, 103, Messina V, Melina V, Mangels AR, Vegetarian Food Guide Pyramid, 771–775., Copyright 2003, with permission from Elsevier.

good source of vitamin C with most meals is helpful because vitamin C improves iron absorption.

- Zinc is found in whole grains, nuts, legumes, and soy foods.

If you are a vegetarian or are considering becoming one, devote some extra time and thought to your diet. It's especially important that you eat as wide a variety of foods as possible to ensure that all your nutritional needs are satisfied. Consulting with a registered dietitian will make your planning even easier. Vegetarian diets for children, teens, and pregnant and lactating women warrant professional guidance.

Dietary Challenges for Special Population Groups

Canada's Food Guide to Healthy Eating provides a basis that everyone can use to create a healthy diet. However, some population groups face special dietary challenges.

CHILDREN AND TEENAGERS Young people often simply need to be encouraged to eat. Perhaps the best thing a parent can do for younger children is provide a variety of foods. For example, parents can add vegetables to casseroles and fruit to cereal, or they can offer fruit and vegetable juices or homemade yogurt or fruit shakes instead of sugary drinks. Allowing children to help prepare meals is another good way to encourage good eating habits.

WOMEN Women tend to be smaller and to weigh less than men, meaning they have lower energy needs and therefore consume fewer calories. Because of this, women have more difficulty getting adequate amounts of all the essential nutrients and need to focus on nutrient-dense foods. Two nutrients of special concern are calcium and iron, minerals for which many women fail to meet the DRIs. Low calcium intake may be linked to the development of osteoporosis in later life. Nonfat and low-fat dairy products and fortified cereal, bread, and orange juice are good choices.

Iron is also a concern: Menstruating women have higher iron requirements than other groups, and a lack of iron in the diet can lead to iron-deficiency anemia. Lean red meat, green leafy vegetables, and fortified breakfast cereals are good sources of iron. As discussed earlier, all women capable of becoming pregnant should consume adequate folic acid from fortified foods and/or supplements.

MEN Men are seldom thought of as having nutritional deficiencies because they generally have high-calorie diets. However, many men have a diet that does not follow the Food Guide and that includes more red meat and fewer fruits, vegetables, and grains than recommended. This dietary pattern is linked to heart disease and some types of cancer. A high intake of calories can lead to weight gain in the long term if a man's activity

---

FITNESS TIP

Consumption of red meats, sweets, eggs, and butter is greatly reduced or eliminated entirely in most forms of the Mediterranean diet.

---

level decreases as he ages. Men should use the Food Guide as a basis for their overall diet and focus on increasing their consumption of fruits, vegetables, and grains to obtain vitamins, minerals, dietary fibre, and phytochemicals.

The "5 to 10 a day" initiative developed in partnership with the Canadian Cancer Society, Heart and Stroke Foundation of Canada, and the Canadian Produce Marketing Association promotes increased intake of fruits and vegetables among Canadians in general. Visit www.5to10aday.com.

UNIVERSITY/COLLEGE STUDENTS Foods that are convenient for university and college students are not always the healthiest choices. However, it is possible to make healthy eating both convenient and affordable. See tips in the box "Eating Strategies for University/College Students."

OLDER ADULTS As people age, they tend to become less active, so they require fewer calories to maintain their weight. At the same time, the absorption of nutrients tends to be lower in older adults because of age-related changes in the digestive tract. Thus, they must consume nutrient-dense foods to meet their nutritional requirements. As discussed earlier, foods fortified with vitamin B-12 and/or B-12 supplements are recommended for people over age 50. Because constipation is a common problem, consuming foods high in dietary fibre and obtaining adequate fluids are important goals.

ATHLETES Key dietary concerns for athletes are meeting increased energy and fluid requirements for training and making healthy food choices throughout the day. For more on this topic, see the box "Do Athletes Need a Different Diet?"

PEOPLE WITH SPECIAL HEALTH CONCERNS Many Canadians have special health concerns that affect their dietary needs. For example, women who are pregnant or breastfeeding require extra calories, vitamins, and

---

TERMS

vegan A vegetarian who eats no animal products at all.

lacto-vegetarian A vegetarian who includes milk and cheese products in the diet.

lacto-ovo-vegetarian A vegetarian who eats no meat, poultry, or fish, but does eat eggs and milk products.

partial vegetarian, semivegetarian, or pescovegetarian A vegetarian who includes eggs, dairy products, and small amounts of poultry and seafood in their diet.

Eating Strategies for University/College Students

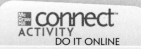

General Guidelines

- Eat slowly and enjoy your food. Set aside a separate time to eat. Don't eat while you study.

- Eat a colourful, varied diet. The more colourful your diet is, the more varied and rich in fruits and vegetables it will be. Many Canadians eat few fruits and vegetables, despite the fact that these foods are typically inexpensive, delicious, rich in nutrients, and low in fat and calories. Don't limit your vegetable choices to french fries, which are typically high in saturated and trans fats.

- Eat breakfast. You'll have more energy in the morning and be less likely to grab an unhealthy snack later on. Whole-grain cereals or whole-grain toast are excellent breakfast choices.

- Choose healthy snacks—fruits, vegetables, grains, and cereals—as often as you can.

- Drink water more often than soft drinks or other sweetened beverages. Rent a mini-refrigerator for your residence room and stock up on healthy beverages.

- Pay attention to portion sizes. Read food labels carefully, and take special note of serving sizes and the total number of servings in the package. You may find that your favourite bottled drinks and packaged snack foods provide multiple servings and that you are consuming more calories, fat, and added sugars than you realize.

- Combine physical activity with healthy eating. You'll look and feel better and have a much lower risk of many chronic diseases. Even a little exercise is better than none.

Eating on Campus

- If menus are posted or distributed, decide what you want to eat before getting in line and stick to your choices. Consider what you plan to do and eat for the rest of the day before making your choices.

- Ask for large servings of vegetables and small servings of meat and other high-fat main dishes. Build your meals around grains and vegetables.

- Choose whole grains.

- Choose leaner poultry, fish, or bean dishes rather than high-fat meats and fried entrées.

- Ask that gravies and sauces be served on the side; limit your intake.

- Choose broth-based or vegetable soups rather than cream soups.

- At the salad bar, load up on leafy greens, beans, and fresh vegetables. Avoid mayonnaise-coated salads (macaroni salad, potato salad), bacon, croutons, and high-fat dressings. Put dressing on the side; dip your fork into it rather than pouring it over the salad.

- Choose fruit for dessert rather than pastries, cookies, or cakes.

Eating in Fast-Food Restaurants

- Most fast-food chains can provide a brochure with a nutritional breakdown of the foods on the menu. Ask for it and identify the healthiest options. (See also the information in Appendix B.)

- Order small single burgers with no cheese instead of double burgers with many toppings.

- Ask for items to be prepared without mayonnaise, tartar sauce, sour cream, or other high-fat sauces. Ketchup, mustard, and fat-free mayonnaise or sour cream are better choices and are available at many fast-food restaurants.

- Choose whole-grain buns or bread for sandwiches.

- Choose chicken items made from chicken breast, not processed chicken.

- Order vegetable pizzas without extra cheese.

- If you order french fries or onion rings, get the smallest size and/or share them with a friend. Better yet, get a salad or fruit cup instead.

  Fast-food meals are a health concern. A large cheeseburger, large order of fries, and large (32 oz) nondiet soft drink may provide about 1600 calories, 75 grams of fat, and 30 teaspoons of added sugars. If you have a fast-food meal, balance it with healthy, nutrient-rich foods during the rest of the day.

Eating on the Run

Are you chronically short of time? The following healthy and filling items can be packed for a quick snack or meal:

- fresh or dried fruit, fruit juices, raw fresh vegetables

- plain bagels, bread sticks, whole-wheat fig bars, low-fat cheese sticks or cubes, lowfat crackers or granola bars

- nonfat or low-fat yogurt, snack-size cereal boxes, pretzels, rice or corn cakes

- plain popcorn, soup (if you have access to a microwave), or water.

minerals. People with diabetes benefit from a well-balanced diet that is low in simple sugars, high in complex carbohydrates, and relatively rich in mono-unsaturated fats. And people with high blood pressure need to limit their sodium consumption and control their weight. If you have a health problem or concern that may require a special diet, discuss your situation with a physician or registered dietitian.

If you exercise vigorously and frequently, or if you are an athlete in training, you likely have increased energy and fluid requirements. Research supports the following recommendations for athletes:

- **Energy intake:** Someone engaged in a vigorous training program may have energy needs as high as 6000 calories per day—far greater than the energy needs of a moderately active person. For athletes, it is recommend to consume a diet with 60–65% of calories coming from carbohydrates, 10–15% from protein, and no more than 30% from fat.

  Athletes who need to maintain low body weight and fat (such as gymnasts, skaters, and wrestlers) need to get enough calories and nutrients while avoiding unhealthy eating patterns such as bulimia. The combination of low body fat, high physical activity, disordered eating habits–and, in women, amenorrhea–is associated with osteoporosis, stress fractures, and other injuries. If keeping your weight and body fat low for athletic reasons is important to you, seek dietary advice from a qualified dietician and make sure your physician is aware of your eating habits.

- **Carbohydrates:** Endurance athletes involved in competitive events lasting longer than 90 minutes may benefit from increasing carbohydrate intake to 65–70% of their total calories. Specifically, the American College of Sports Medicine (ACSM) recommends that athletes consume 2.7–4.5 grams per pound of body weight daily, depending on their weight, sport, and other nutritional needs. This increase should come in the form of complex carbohydrates.

  High carbohydrate intake builds and maintains glycogen stores in the muscles, resulting in greater endurance and delayed fatigue during competitive events. The ACSM recommends that before exercise an active adult or athlete eat a meal or snack that is relatively high in carbohydrates, moderate in protein, and low in fat and fibre. Eating carbohydrates 30 minutes, 2 hours, and 4 hours after exercise can help replenish glycogen stores in the liver and muscles.

- **Fat:** It is recommended that all athletes get 20–35% of calories from fat in their diets. This is in line with the daily intake suggested by Health Canada. Reducing fat intake to less than 20% of daily calories can negatively affect performance and be harmful to health.

- **Protein:** For endurance and strength-trained athletes, the ACSM and the Dieticians of Canada recommend eating

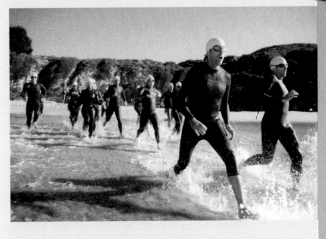

1.2–1.7 gram of protein per kg of body weight each day, which is considerably higher than the standard DRI of 0.8 gram per kg. This level of protein is easily obtainable from foods; in fact, most Canadians eat more protein than they need every day. A balanced, moderate-protein diet can provide the protein most athletes need.

There is no evidence that consuming supplements containing vitamins, minerals, protein, or specific amino acids builds muscle or improves sports performance. Strength and muscle are built with exercise, not extra protein, and carbohydrates provide the fuel needed for muscle-building exercise.

- **Fluids:** If you exercise heavily or live in a hot climate, you should drink extra fluids to maximize performance and prevent heat illness. For a strenuous endurance event, prepare yourself the day before by drinking plenty of fluids. The ACSM and Dieticians of Canada recommend drinking 4–6 millilitres of fluid per kg of body weight about 4 hours before the event. During the event, take in enough fluids to compensate for fluid loss due to sweating; the amount required depends on the individual and his or her sweat rate. Afterward, drink enough to replace lost fluids—about 16–24 ounces for every pound of weight lost.

  Water is a good choice for fluid replacement for events lasting 60–90 minutes. For longer workouts or events, a sports drink can be a good choice. These contain water, electrolytes, and carbohydrates and can provide some extra energy as well as replace electrolytes like sodium lost in sweat.

SOURCE: American College of Sports Medicine. 2009. *American College of Sports Medicine Position Stand: Nutrition and Athletic Performance* (http://www .acsm-msse.org/pt/pt-core/template-journal/msse/media/0309nutrition.pdf; retrived April 23, 2011).

LO4   7.3 NUTRITIONAL PLANNING: MAKING INFORMED CHOICES ABOUT FOOD

Knowing about nutrition is a good start to making sound choices about food. It also helps if you can interpret food labels, understand food additives, and avoid foodborne illnesses.

Reading Food Labels

Consumers can get help in applying the principles of the Food Guide and the DRIs from nutrition labels. Since 2003 nutrition labelling on all pre-packaged foods in Canada has been mandatory. Every nutrition label shows a variety of information such as serving sizes and the amount of fat, saturated fat, cholesterol, protein, dietary fibre, and sodium in each serving. To make intelligent choices about food, learn to read and understand nutrition labels (see the box "Using Nutrition Labels"). Research has shown that people who read nutrition labels eat less fat.

Because most meat, poultry, fish, fruits, and vegetables are not processed, they were not covered by the 2003 law. You can obtain information on the nutrient content of these items from basic nutrition books, registered dietitians, nutrient analysis computer software, the World Wide Web, and the companies that produce or distribute these foods. Also, supermarkets often have large posters or pamphlets listing the nutrient contents of these foods. Lab 7.3 gives you the opportunity to compare foods using the information provided on their labels.

Reading Dietary Supplement Labels

Dietary supplements include vitamins, minerals, amino acids, herbs, enzymes, and other compounds. Although dietary supplements are often thought of as safe and natural, they contain powerful bioactive chemicals that have the potential for harm. About one-quarter of all pharmaceutical drugs are derived from botanical sources, and even essential vitamins and minerals can have toxic effects if consumed in excess.

A 2010 Ipsos-Reid survey shows that 73% of Canadians regularly take natural health products (NHPs) like vitamins and minerals, herbal products, and homeopathic medicines. In Canada, these supplements are regulated by the Natural Health Products Regulations. Before they are approved by Health Canada and put on the market, all supplements undergo assessment to determine if it is safe, effective, and of a high quality. Products are then given a product licence and can be sold in Canada.

Food Additives

Today, some 2800 substances are intentionally added to foods for one or more of the following reasons: (1) to maintain or improve nutritional quality, (2) to maintain freshness, (3) to help in processing or preparation, or (4) to alter taste or appearance. Additives make up less than 1% of our food. The most widely used are sugar, salt, and corn syrup; these three, plus citric acid, baking soda, vegetable colours, mustard, and pepper, account for 98% by weight of all food additives used in North America.

Food additives pose no significant health hazard to most people because the levels used are well below any that could produce toxic effects. Two additives that are occasionally used in higher quantities are sulfites, used to keep vegetables from turning brown, and monosodium glutamate (MSG), used as a flavour enhancer. To protect yourself, eat a variety of foods in moderation. If you have any sensitivity to an additive, check food labels when you shop and ask questions when you eat out.

Foodborne Illness

Many people worry about additives or pesticide residues in their food. However, a greater threat to the safety of the food supply comes from microorganisms that cause foodborne illnesses. Raw or undercooked animal products, such as chicken, hamburger, and oysters, pose the greatest risk for contamination. Health Canada and the Centers for Disease Control in the United States estimate that 2.2 million Canadians and 76 million Americans become sick each year as a result of foodborne illness. In most cases, foodborne illness produces acute gastroenteritis, characterized by diarrhea, vomiting, fever, and weakness. People often mistake foodborne illness for a bout of the flu. Although the effects of foodborne illness are usually not serious, some groups, such as children and older people, are at risk for severe complications, including rheumatic diseases, kidney failure, seizures, blood poisoning, and death.

CAUSES OF FOODBORNE ILLNESSES Most cases of foodborne illness are caused by pathogens, disease-causing microorganisms that contaminate food, usually from improper handling. The threats are numerous and varied; among them are the sometimes deadly Escherichia coli (E. coli) O157:H7 in meat and water; Salmonella in eggs, on vegetables, and on poultry; Vibrio in shellfish; Cyclospora and hepatitis A virus on fruit; Cryptosporidium in drinking water; Campylobacter jejuni in meat and poultry; and Listeria monocytogenes in lunch meats, sausages, and hot dogs.

You can't tell by taste, smell, or sight whether a food is contaminated. Although most pathogens are usually destroyed during cooking, it is important to recognize that your handling of foods before cooking can be critical. In addition, while foodborne illness outbreaks associated with food-processing plants make headlines, most cases of illness trace back to poor food handling in the home or in food-service establishments. The Canadian Partnership for Consumer Food Safety Education is taking steps to bring down levels of contamination by educating Canadians about the importance of food safety in the home. See the box "Safe Food Handling" for more information.

TREATING FOODBORNE ILLNESS If you think you may be having a bout of foodborne illness, drink plenty of clear fluids to prevent dehydration and rest to speed recovery. To prevent further contamination, wash your hands often and always before handling food until you recover. A fever higher than 39°C, blood in the stool, or dehydration deserves a physician's evaluation, especially if the symptoms persist for more than 2–3 days. In cases of suspected botulism—characterized by symptoms such as double vision, paralysis, dizziness, and vomiting— consult a physician immediately.

WELLNESS TIP

To get produce as clean as possible, rub it with a soft brush while holding it under running water.

The key to protecting yourself from foodborne illness is to handle, cook, and store foods in ways that prevent bacteria from spreading and multiplying:

- Don't buy food in containers that leak, bulge, or are severely dented. Refrigerated foods should be cold, and frozen foods should be solid.

- Refrigerate perishable items as soon as possible after purchase. Use or freeze fresh meats within 3–5 days and fresh poultry, fish, and ground meat within 1–2 days.

- Store raw meat, poultry, fish, and shellfish in containers in the refrigerator so that the juices don't drip onto other foods. Keep these items away from other foods, surfaces, utensils, or serving dishes to prevent cross-contamination.

- Thaw frozen food in the refrigerator or in the microwave oven, not on the kitchen counter.

- Thoroughly wash your hands with warm soapy water for 20 seconds before and after handling food, especially raw meat, fish, poultry, or eggs.

- Make sure counters, cutting boards, dishes, and other equipment are thoroughly cleaned before and after use using hot, soapy water. Wash dishcloths and kitchen towels frequently.

- Thoroughly rinse and scrub fruits and vegetables with a brush, if possible, or peel off the skin.

- Cook foods thoroughly, especially beef, poultry, fish, pork, and eggs; cooking kills most micro organisms. Use a food thermometer to ensure that foods are cooked to a safe temperature. Hamburgers should be cooked to 160°F. Turn or stir microwaved food to make sure it is heated evenly throughout. When eating out, order hamburger cooked well-done and make sure foods are served piping hot.

- Cook stuffing separately from poultry; or wash poultry thoroughly, stuff immediately before cooking, and transfer the stuffing to a clean bowl immediately after cooking. The temperature of cooked stuffing should reach 165°F.

- Keep hot foods hot (140°F or above) and cold foods cold (40°F or below); harmful bacteria can grow rapidly between these two temperatures. Refrigerate foods within 2 hours of purchase or preparation, and within 1 hour if the air temperature is above 90°F. Refrigerate foods at or below 5°C and freeze at or below −18°C. Use refrigerated leftovers within 3–4 days.

- Don't eat raw animal products, including raw eggs in homemade hollandaise sauce, eggnog, or cookie dough. Use only pasteurized milk and juice, and look for pasteurized eggs.

- Cook eggs until they're firm and fully cook foods containing eggs. Store eggs in the coldest part of the refrigerator, not on the door, and use them within 3–5 weeks.

- Because of possible contamination with E. coli O157:H7 and Salmonella, avoid raw sprouts. Even sprouts grown under clean conditions in the home can be risky because bacteria may be present in the seeds. Cook sprouts before eating them.

- Read the food label and package information, and follow safety instructions such as "Keep Refrigerated" and the "Safe Handling Instructions."

- "When in doubt, throw it out." Even if a food looks and smells fine, it may not be safe. If you aren't sure that a food has been prepared, served, and stored safely, don't eat it.

Additional precautions are recommended for people at particularly high risk for foodborne illness—pregnant women, young children, older persons, and people with weakened immune systems or certain chronic illnesses. If you are a member of one of these groups, don't eat or drink any of the following products: unpasteurized juices; raw sprouts; unpasteurized (raw) milk and products made from unpasteurized milk; raw or undercooked meat, poultry, eggs, fish, and shellfish; and soft cheeses such as feta, Brie, Camembert, or blue-veined cheeses. To protect against Listeria, it's also important to avoid ready-to-eat foods such as hot dogs, luncheon meats, and cold cuts unless they are reheated until they are steaming hot.

Irradiated Foods—A Technique of Biotechnology

Food irradiation is the treatment of foods with gamma rays, X rays, or high-voltage electrons to kill potentially harmful pathogens, including bacteria, parasites, insects, and fungi that cause foodborne illness. It also reduces spoilage and extends shelf life. Even though irradiation has been generally endorsed by agencies such as the World Health Organization and the Centers for Disease Control and Prevention, few irradiated foods are currently on the market due to consumer resistance and skepticism. Studies haven't conclusively identified any harmful effects of food irradiation, and the newer methods of irradiation involving electricity and X rays do not require the use of any radioactive materials. Studies indicate that

when consumers are given information about the process of irradiation and the benefits of irradiated foods, most want to purchase them.

All primary irradiated foods (meat, vegetables, and so on) are labelled with the flowerlike radura symbol and a brief information label; spices and foods that are merely ingredients do not have to be so labelled. It is important to remember that although irradiation kills most pathogens, it does not

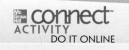

Using Nutrition Labels

Nutrition labels are designed to help consumers make food choices based on the nutrients that are most important to good health. In addition to listing nutrient content by weight, the label puts the information in the context of a daily diet of 2000 calories that includes no more than 65 grams of fat (approximately 30% of total calories). For example, if a serving of a particular product has 13 grams of fat, the label will show that the serving represents 20% of the daily fat allowance. If your daily diet contains fewer or more than 2000 calories, you need to adjust these calculations accordingly.

Nutrition labels contain uniform serving sizes. This means that if you look at different brands of salad dressing, for example, you can compare calories and fat content based on the serving amount. (Nutrition label serving sizes may be larger or smaller than Food Guide serving sizes, however.) Regulations also require that foods meet strict definitions if their packaging includes the terms low-fat, or high in fibre (see below). Health claims such as "good source of dietary fibre" or "low in saturated fat" on packages are signals that those products can wisely be included in your diet. Overall, the food label is an important tool to help you choose a diet that conforms to the Food Guide.

Selected Nutrient Claims and What They Mean

The Canadian Food Inspection Agency has set out guidelines based on which the Nutrition Labels are permitted to include health claims. Listed below are some of the more common health claims you may see on foods. For a full listing of the regulations, please see inspection.gc.ca.

Source of energy Food provides at least 100 calories per serving.

Reduced or fewer At least 25% less of a nutrient than a similar product; can be applied to fat ("reduced fat"), saturated fat, cholesterol, sodium, and calories.

Low calorie 40 calories or less per serving.

Fat-free/non-fat Less than 0.5 g of fat per serving.

Low-fat 3 g or less of fat per serving.

Saturated fatty acids-free Less than 0.2 g of saturated fat and 0.2 g of trans fatty acids per serving.

Low in saturated fatty acids 2 g or less of saturated fatty acids and trans fatty acids combined per serving.

Cholesterol-free Less than 2 mg of cholesterol and 2 g or less of saturated-fat per serving.

Low cholesterol 20 mg or less of cholesterol and 2 g or less of saturated fat per serving.

Sugar keep in mind that sugar does not always appear as 'sugar.' Typically words on the ingredients list ending in 'ose' imply that those sources are in fact, sugar sources.

1. Serving size: Determine how many servings there are in the food package and compare it to how much you actually eat. You may need to adjust the rest of the nutrient values based on your typical serving size.

2. Calories and calories from fat: Note whether a serving is high in calories and fat. The sample food shown here is low in fat, with only 30 of its 235 calories from fat.

3. Daily Values: Based on a 2000-calorie diet, Daily Value percentages tell you whether the nutrients in a serving of food contribute a lot or a little to your total daily diet.

> 5% or less is low
> 20% or more is high

4. Limit these nutrients: Look for foods low in fat, saturated fat, trans fat, cholesterol, and sodium.

5. Get enough of these nutrients: Look for foods high in dietary fibre, vitamin A, vitamin C, calcium, and iron.

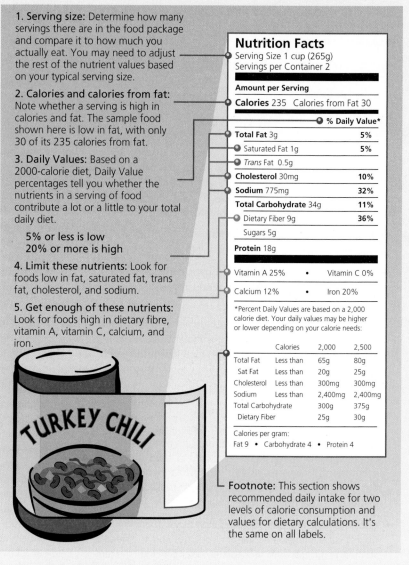

Footnote: This section shows recommended daily intake for two levels of calorie consumption and values for dietary calculations. It's the same on all labels.

Source of fibre 2 g or more fibre per serving.

High in fibre 4 g or more fibre per serving.

Low sodium 140 mg or less of sodium per serving.

Low in protein Contains no more than 1 g of protein per 100 g of the food.

Source of protein Food has a protein rating of 20 or more. Foods such as proteins can be assigned a biological value (BV), or in this case protein rating, identifying an approximate percentage of the nutrient that the body is able to utilize.

High in protein Food has a protein rating of 40 or more.

Lean Meat or poultry that has not been ground, marine or fresh water animals or a product of any of these; and contains 10% or less fat.

Extra-lean Meat or poultry that has not been ground, marine or fresh water animals or a product of any of these; and contains 7.5% or less fat.

completely sterilize foods. Proper handling of irradiated foods is still critical for preventing foodborne illness.

Organic Foods—Stricter Standards for a Booming Industry

Some people who are concerned about pesticides and other environmental contaminants choose to buy foods that are **organic.** Since 2009, the Canadian Organics Products Regulations (OPR), of the Canadian Food Inspection Agency, have been responsible for certifying foods as organic according to strict production, processing, handling, and labelling criteria. Food certified as organic will carry the new Biologique Canada Organic logo below.

 Foods that are organic are not chemical-free, however. They may be contaminated with pesticides used on neighbouring lands or on foods transported in the same train or truck. However, they do tend to have lower levels of pesticide residues than conventionally grown crops. Some experts recommend that consumers who want to buy organic fruits and vegetables spend their money on those that carry lower pesticide residues than their conventional counterparts (the "dirty dozen"): apples, bell peppers, celery, cherries, imported grapes, nectarines, peaches, pears, potatoes, red raspberries, spinach, and strawberries. Experts also recommend buying organic beef, poultry, eggs, dairy products, and baby food. Fruits and vegetables that carry little pesticide residue whether grown conventionally or organically include asparagus, avocadoes, bananas, broccoli, cauliflower, corn, kiwi, mangoes, onions, papaya, pineapples, and peas. All foods are subject to strict pesticide limits; the debate about the health effects of small amounts of residue is ongoing.

Whether organic foods are better for your health, organic farming is better for the environment. It helps maintain biodiversity of crops and replenish the Earth's resources. It is less likely to degrade soil, contaminate water, or expose farm workers to toxic chemicals. As multinational food companies get into the organic food business, however, consumers who want to support environmentally friendly farming methods should look for foods that are not only organic but also locally grown.

LO5 7.4 A PERSONAL PLAN: APPLYING NUTRITIONAL PRINCIPLES

Based on your particular nutrition and health status, there probably is an ideal diet for you, but there is no single type of diet that provides optimal health for everyone. Many cultural dietary patterns can meet people's nutritional requirements (see the box "Ethnic Foods"). Every individual needs to customize a food plan based on age, gender, weight, activity level, medical risk factors—and, of course, personal tastes.

Assessing and Changing Your Diet

The first step in planning a healthy diet is to examine what you currently eat. Labs 7.1 and 7.2 are designed to help you analyze your current diet and compare it with optimal dietary goals. (This analysis can be completed using Appendix A, a nutritional analysis software program, or one of several websites.)

To put your plan into action, use the behavioural self-management techniques and tips described in Chapter 1. If you identify several changes you want to make, focus on one at a time. You might start, for example, by substituting nonfat or low-fat milk for whole milk. When you become used to that, you can try substituting whole-wheat bread for white bread. The information on eating behaviour in Lab 7.1 will help you identify and change unhealthy patterns of eating.

Staying Committed to a Healthy Diet

Beyond knowledge and information, you also need support in difficult situations. Refer back to the Cycle of Behaviour Change presented in Chapter 1 to help you construct a plan that will be easier to maintain. Use the tips below to help keep yourself on track.

- Keeping to your plan is easiest when you choose and prepare your own food at home.
- Consider utilizing a meal plan such as the 100-Mile diet. Based on the efforts of two residents of northern British Columbia who for one year, restricted their diets to only foods grown within 100 miles of their residence. In addition to assisting the local community and helping the environment, the 100-Mile diet is also thought to be safer and more nutritious. For more information on the 100-Mile diet, see www.dietitians.ca/Dietitians-Views/100-Mile-Diet.aspx.
- Advance planning is the key: mapping out meals and shopping appropriately, cooking in advance when possible, and preparing enough food for leftovers later in the week. A tight budget does not necessarily make it more difficult to eat healthy meals. It makes good health sense and good budget sense to use only small amounts of meat and to have a few meatless meals each week.
- In restaurants, keeping to food plan goals becomes somewhat more difficult. Portion sizes in restaurants tend to be larger than serving sizes of the Food Guide, but by remaining focused on your goals, you can eat only part of your meal and take the rest home for a meal later in the week. Don't hesitate to

organic A designation applied to foods grown and produced according to strict guidelines limiting the use of pesticides, nonorganic ingredients, hormones, antibiotics, genetic engineering, irradiation, and other practices.

TERMS

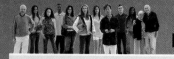

Ethnic Foods

There is no one ethnic diet that clearly surpasses all others in providing people with healthful foods. However, every diet has its advantages and disadvantages and, within each cuisine, some foods are better choices. The dietary guidelines described in this chapter can be applied to any ethnic cuisine. For additional guidance, refer to the table below.

	Choose More Often	Choose Less Often
Chinese	Dishes that are steamed, poached (jum), boiled (chu), roasted (kow), barbecued (shu), or lightly stir-fried Hoisin sauce, oyster sauce, wine sauce, plum sauce, velvet sauce, or hot mustard Fresh fish and seafood, skinless chicken, tofu Mixed vegetables, Chinese greens Steamed rice, steamed spring rolls, soft noodles	Fried wontons or egg rolls Crab rangoon Crispy (Peking) duck or chicken Sweet-and-sour dishes made with breaded and deep-fried meat, poultry, or fish Fried rice Fried or crispy noodles
French	Dishes prepared au vapeur (steamed), en brochette (skewered and broiled), or grillé (grilled) Fresh fish, shrimp, scallops, or mussels or skinless chicken, without sauces Clear soups	Dishes prepared à la crème (in cream sauce), au gratin or gratinée (baked with cream and cheese), or en croûte (in pastry crust) Drawn butter, hollandaise sauce, and remoulade (mayonnaise-based sauce)
Greek	Dishes that are stewed, broiled, or grilled, including shish kabobs (souvlaki) Dolmas (grape leaves) stuffed with rice Tzatziki (yogurt, cucumbers, and garlic) Tabouli (bulgur-based salad) Pita bread, especially whole wheat	Moussaka, saganaki (fried cheese) Vegetable pies such as spanakopita and tyropita Baba ghanoush (eggplant and olive oil) Deep-fried falafel (chickpea patties) Gyros stuffed with ground meat Baklava
Indian	Dishes prepared masala (curry), tandoori (roasted in a clay oven), or tikke (pan roasted); kabobs Raita (yogurt and cucumber salad) and other yogurt-based dishes and sauces Dal (lentils), pullao or pilau (basmati rice) Chapati (baked bread)	Ghee (clarified butter) Korma (meat in cream sauce) Samosas, pakoras (fried dishes) Molee and other coconut milk-based dishes Poori, bhatura, or paratha (fried breads)
Italian	Pasta primavera or pasta, polenta, risotto, or gnocchi with marinara, red or white wine, white or red clam, or light mushroom sauce Dishes that are grilled or prepared cacciatore (tomato-based sauce), marsala (broth and wine sauce), or piccata (lemon sauce) Cioppino (seafood stew) Vegetable soup, minestrone or fagioli (beans)	Antipasto (cheese, smoked meats) Dishes that are prepared alfredo, frito (fried), crema (creamed), alla panna (with cream), or carbonara Veal scaloppini Chicken, veal, or eggplant parmigiana Italian sausage, salami, and prosciutto Buttered garlic bread Cannoli
Japanese	Dishes prepared nabemono (boiled), shabu-shabu (in boiling broth), mushimono (steamed), nimono (simmered), yaki (broiled), or yakimono (grilled) Sushi or domburi (mixed rice dish) Steamed rice or soba (buckwheat), udon (wheat), or rice noodles	Tempura (battered and fried) Agemono (deep fried) Katsu (fried pork cutlet) Sukiyaki Fried tofu
Mexican	Soft corn or wheat tortillas Burritos, fajitas, enchiladas, soft tacos, and tamales filled with beans, vegetables, or lean meats Refried beans, nonfat or low-fat, rice and beans Ceviche (fish marinated in lime juice) Salsa, enchilada sauce, and picante sauce Gazpacho, menudo, or black bean soup Fruit or flan for dessert	Crispy, fried tortillas Dishes that are fried, such as chile relleños, chimichangas, flautas, and tostadas Nachos and cheese, chili con queso, and other dishes made with cheese or cheese sauce Guacamole, sour cream, and extra cheese Refried beans made with lard Fried ice cream
Thai	Dishes that are barbecued, sautéed, broiled, boiled, steamed, braised, or marinated Sàté (skewered and grilled meats) Fish sauce, basil sauce, chili or hot sauces Bean thread noodles, Thai salad	Coconut milk soup Peanut sauce or dishes topped with nuts Mee-krob (crispy noodles) Red, green, and yellow curries, which typically contain coconut milk

SOURCES: National Heart, Lung, and Blood Institute. 2006. Guidelines on Overweight and Obesity: Electronic Textbook (http://www.nhlbi.nih.gov/guidelines/obesity/e_txtbk/appndx/6a3b.htm, retrieved December 10, 2011); and Duyff, R. L. 2006. *The American Dietetic Association's Complete Food and Nutrition Guide,* 2nd ed. Hoboken, N.J.: Wiley.

ask questions when you're eating in a restaurant. Most restaurant personnel are glad to explain how menu selections are prepared and to make small adjustments, such as serving salad dressings and sauces on the side so they can be avoided or used sparingly. To limit your fat intake, order meat or fish broiled or grilled rather than fried or sautéed, choose rice or a plain baked potato over french fries, and select a clear soup rather than a creamy one. Desserts that are irresistible can, at least, be shared.

Strategies like these can be helpful, but small changes cannot change a fundamentally high-fat, high-calorie meal into a moderate, healthful one. Often, the best advice is to bypass a large steak with potatoes au gratin for a flavourful but low-fat entrée. Many of the selections offered in ethnic restaurants are healthy choices (refer to the box on ethnic foods for suggestions).

Knowledge of food and nutrition is essential to the success of your program. The information provided in this chapter should give you the tools you need to design and implement a diet that promotes long-term health and well-being. If you need additional information or have questions about nutrition, be sure the source you consult is reliable.

TIPS FOR TODAY AND THE FUTURE

Opportunities to improve your diet present themselves every day, and small changes add up.

RIGHT NOW YOU CAN

- Substitute a healthy snack—an apple, a banana, or plain popcorn—for a bag of chips or cookies.
- Drink a glass of water and put a bottle of water in your backpack for tomorrow.
- Plan to make healthy selections when you go to dinner, such as a baked potato instead of french fries or salmon instead of steak.

IN THE FUTURE, YOU CAN

- Visit the Canada's Food Guide site at www.hc-sc.gc.ca/fn-an/food-guide-aliment/index-eng.php and use the online tools to create a personalized nutrition plan and begin tracking your eating habits.
- Learn to cook healthier meals. There are hundreds of free websites and low-cost cookbooks that provide recipes for healthy dishes.

SUMMARY

- The six classes of nutrients are carbohydrates, proteins, fats, vitamins, minerals, and water.

- The nutrients essential to humans are released into the body through digestion. Nutrients in foods provide energy, measured in kilocalories (commonly called calories); build and maintain body tissues; and regulate body functions.

- Protein, an important component of body tissue, is composed of amino acids; nine are essential to a diet. Foods from animal sources provide complete proteins; plants provide incomplete proteins.

- Fats, a major source of energy, also insulate the body and cushion the organs; 3–4 teaspoons of vegetable oil per day supplies the essential fats. For most people, dietary fat intake should be 20–35% of total calories, and unsaturated fats should be favoured over saturated and trans fats.

- Carbohydrates provide energy to the brain, nervous system, and blood and to muscles during high-intensity exercise. Naturally occurring simple carbohydrates and unrefined complex carbohydrates should be favoured over added sugars and refined carbohydrates.

- Fibre includes plant substances that are impossible for the human body to digest. It helps reduce cholesterol levels and promotes the passage of wastes through the intestines.

- The 13 essential vitamins are organic substances that promote specific chemical and cell processes and act as antioxidants. The 17 known essential minerals are inorganic substances that regulate body functions, aid in growth and tissue maintenance, and help in the release of energy from food. Deficiencies in vitamins and minerals can cause severe symptoms over time, but excess doses are also dangerous.

- Water aids in digestion and food absorption, allows chemical reactions to take place, serves as a lubricant or cushion, helps regulate body temperature, flushes toxins and eliminates wastes.

- Foods contain other substances, such as phytochemicals, that may not be essential nutrients but that may protect against chronic diseases.

- The Dietary Reference Intakes and Canada's Food Guide for Healthy Eating provide standards and recommendations for getting all essential nutrients from a varied, balanced diet and for eating in ways that protect against chronic disease.

- Basic recommendations for a healthy diet include aiming for a healthy weight through diet and physical activity; building a healthy base for our diets by following the Guide, choosing a variety of plant foods, and handling foods safely; and making sensible choices that consider intake of fat, sugar, salt, and alcohol.

Which should I eat—butter or margarine?

Both butter and margarine are concentrated sources of fat, containing about 11 grams of fat and 100 calories per tablespoon. Butter is higher in saturated fat, which raises levels of artery-clogging LDL ("bad" cholesterol). Each tablespoon of butter has about 8 grams of saturated fat; margarine has about 2. Butter also contains cholesterol, which margarine does not.

Margarine, on the other hand, contains trans fat, which not only raises LDL but lowers HDL ("good" cholesterol). A tablespoon of stick margarine contains about 2 grams of trans fat. Butter contains a small amount of trans fat as well. Although butter has a combined total of saturated and trans fats that is twice that of stick margarine, the trans fat in stick margarine may be worse for you. Clearly, you should avoid both butter and stick margarine. To solve this dilemma, remember that softer is better. The softer or more liquid a margarine or spread is, the less hydrogenated it is and the less trans fat it contains. Tub and squeeze margarines contain less trans fat than stick margarines; some margarines are modified to be low-trans or trans-free and are labelled as such. Vegetable oils are an even better choice for cooking and for table use (such as olive oil for dipping bread) because most are low in saturated fat and completely free of trans fats.

Canada's Food Guide seems to recommend such a large number of servings. How can I possibly follow its recommendations without gaining weight?

First of all, consider how many servings from each food group are appropriate for you. The suggested number of servings is given as a range, 3–8 servings of grain products, 4–10 of fruits and vegetables, and so on. The smaller number of servings is for people who consume about 1800 calories a day, such as many sedentary women. The larger number is for those who consume about 3200 calories a day, such as active men. If the smaller number of servings is appropriate for you, concentrate on choosing nutrient-dense foods—those that are rich in nutrients but relatively low in calories, such as most grains, fruits, and vegetables.

Second, compare the serving sizes of the foods you eat with those used in the Food Guide. Some of the Guide's serving sizes are smaller than what you might typically eat. For example, many people eat a cup or more of pasta or rice in a meal, which would correspond to 2 or more servings from the grain products group. You'll probably find that your current diet already includes the minimum number of servings from most of the food groups. If not, you may find that you are eating too many servings from one group and not enough from another. Make small changes in your eating habits and food choices to bring your diet into line with the recommendations in the Guide, paying particular attention to your consumption of fat and added sugars. The Food Guide is designed to help you balance your food choices to ensure good health. Strategies for successful weight management are described in detail in Chapter 8.

What exactly are genetically modified foods? Are they safe? How can I recognize them on the shelf, and how can I know when I'm eating them?

Genetic engineering involves altering the characteristics of a plant, animal, or microorganism by adding, rearranging, or replacing genes in its DNA; the result is a genetically modified (GM) organism. New DNA may come from related species or organisms or from

- A vegetarian diet requires special planning but can meet all nutritional needs.
- Different population groups, such as university/college students and athletes, face special dietary challenges and should plan their diets to meet their particular needs.
- Consumers can get help applying nutritional principles by reading the standardized labels that appear on all packaged foods and on dietary supplements.
- Although nutritional basics are well established, no single diet provides wellness for everyone. Individuals should focus on their particular needs and adapt general dietary principles to meet them.

FOR FURTHER EXPLORATION

Organizations, Hotlines, and Websites

Mix It Up. Campaign to encourage Canadians of all ages to include more fruits and vegetables as part of a healthy diet.
  http://5to10aday.com

Canadian Food Inspection Agency. Delivers information related to food, animal health, and plant protection. Includes allergy alerts and food releases important to Canadians.
  http://www.inspection.gc.ca

entirely different types of organisms. Many GM crops are already grown in the Canada: About 60% of all processed food in Canada contain some genetic modifications. Products made with GM organisms include juice, carbonated drinks, nuts, tuna, frozen pizza, spaghetti sauce, canola oil, chips, salad dressing, and soup.

The potential benefits of GM foods cited by supporters include improved yields overall and in difficult growing conditions, increased disease resistance, improved nutritional content, lower prices, and less use of pesticides. Critics of biotechnology argue that unexpected effects may occur: Gene manipulation could elevate levels of naturally occurring toxins or allergens, permanently change the gene pool and reduce biodiversity, and produce pesticide-resistant insects through the transfer of genes. In 2000, a form of GM corn approved for use only in animal feed was found to have commingled with other varieties of corn and to have been used in human foods; this mistake sparked fears of allergic reactions and led to recalls. Opposition to GM foods is particularly strong in Europe; in many developing nations that face food shortages, responses to GM crops have tended to be more positive.

There is currently no Canadian legislation governing the labelling of GM foods in Canada, meaning that Canadians will have virtually no knowledge of their consumption of GM foods. The one exception to this rule is when a food's composition has changed significantly and in such a way that a known allergen is introduced. For example, soybeans that contain a gene from a peanut would have to be labelled because peanuts are a common allergen. The only foods guaranteed not to contain GM ingredients are those certified as organic.

How can I tell if I'm allergic to a food?

A true food allergy is a reaction of the body's immune system to a food or food ingredient, usually a protein. This immune reaction can occur within minutes of ingesting the food, resulting in symptoms such as hives, diarrhea, difficulty breathing, or swelling of the lips or tongue. The most severe response is a systemic reaction called anaphylaxis, which involves a potentially life-threatening drop in blood pressure. Food allergies affect only about 2% of the adult population and about 4–6% of infants. Just a few foods account for most of the food allergies in Canada: cow's milk, eggs, peanuts, tree nuts (walnuts, cashews, and so on), soy, wheat, fish, and shellfish.

Many people who believe they have food allergies may actually suffer from a food intolerance, a much more common source of adverse food reactions that typically involves problems with metabolism rather than with the immune system. The body may not be able to adequately digest a food or the body may react to a particular food compound. Food intolerances have been attributed to lactose (milk sugar), gluten (a protein in some grains), tartrazine (yellow food colouring), sulfite (a food additive), MSG, and the sweetener aspartame. Although symptoms of a food intolerance may be similar to those of a food allergy, they are typically more localized and not life-threatening. Many people with food intolerance can safely and comfortably consume small amounts of the food that affects them.

If you suspect you have a food allergy or intolerance, a good first step is to keep a food diary. Note everything you eat or drink, any symptoms you develop, and how long after eating the symptoms appear. Then make an appointment with your physician to go over your diary and determine if any additional tests are needed. People at risk for severe allergic reactions must diligently avoid trigger foods and carry medications to treat anaphylaxis.

Dietitians of Canada. Provides a variety of educational materials and self-awareness activities on nutrition.
   http://dietitians.ca

FDA Center for Food Safety and Applied Nutrition. Offers information about topics such as food labelling, food additives, and foodborne illness.
   http://vm.cfsan.fda.gov

Food Safety Hotlines. Provide information on the safe purchase, handling, cooking, and storage of food.
   888-SAFEFOOD (FDA)
   800-535-4555 (USDA Meat and Poultry Hotline)

Gateways to Government Nutrition Information. Provides access to government resources relating to food safety, including consumer advice and information on specific pathogens.
   http://www.nutrition.gov
   http://www.foodsafety.gov

Harvard School of Public Health: Nutrition Source. Provides advice on interpreting news on nutrition; an overview of the Healthy Eating Pyramid, an alternative to the basic USDA pyramid; and suggestions for building a healthy diet.
   http://www.hsph.harvard.edu/nutritionsource

Health Canada—Food and Nutrition. Site detailing all relevant areas of food and nutrition including labelling, genetically modified foods and Canada's Food Guide to Healthy Eating.
   http://www.hc-sc.gc.ca/fn-an/nutrition/index_e.html

Heart and Stroke Foundation of Canada. Provides information about heart and stroke and healthy living in Canada.
   http://heartandstroke.ca

MedlinePlus: Nutrition. Provides links to information from government agencies and major medical associations on a wide variety of nutrition topics.
   http://www.nlm.nih.gov/medlineplus/nutrition.html

National Academies' Food and Nutrition Board. Provides information about the Dietary Reference Intakes and related guidelines.
http://www.iom.edu/board.asp?id=3788

Osteoporosis Society of Canada. Provides resources and support networks for those suffering from osteoporosis.
http://www.osteoporosis.ca/

USDA Food and Nutrition Information Center. Provides a variety of materials relating to the Dietary Guidelines, food labels, Food Guide Pyramid, and many other topics.
http://www.nal.usda.gov/fnic

Vegetarian Resource Group. Information and links for vegetarians and people interested in learning more about vegetarian diets.
http://www.vrg.org

You can obtain nutrient breakdowns of individual food items from the following sites:

Nutrition Analysis Tools, and System
http://nat.crgq.com

USDA Food and Nutrition Information Center
http://www.ars.usda.gov/ba/bhnrc/ndl

See also the resources listed in Chapters 8, 11, and 12.

Nutrition Resources

TABLE 1 Dietary Reference Intakes (DRIs): Recommended Levels for Individual Intake

Life Stage	Group	Biotin (μg/day)	Choline (mg/day)a	Folate (μg/day)b	Niacin (mg/day)c	Pantothenic Acid (mg/day)	Riboflavin (mg/day)	Thiamin (mg/day)	Vitamin A (μg/day)d	Vitamin B-6 (mg/day)	Vitamin B-12 (μg/day)	Vitamin C (mg/day)e	Vitamin D (μg/day)f	Vitamin E (mg/day)g
Infants	0–6 months	5	125	65	2	1.7	0.3	0.2	400	0.1	0.4	40	5	4
	7–12 months	6	150	80	4	1.8	0.4	0.3	500	0.3	0.5	50	5	5
Children	1–3 years	8	**200**	**150**	**6**	2	**0.5**	**0.5**	**300**	**0.5**	**0.9**	**15**	5	**6**
	4–8 years	12	**250**	**200**	**8**	3	**0.6**	**0.6**	**400**	**0.6**	**1.2**	**25**	5	**7**
Males	9–13 years	20	**375**	**300**	**12**	4	**0.9**	**0.9**	**600**	**1.0**	**1.8**	**45**	5	**11**
	14–18 years	25	**550**	**400**	**16**	5	**1.3**	**1.2**	**900**	**1.3**	**2.4**	**75**	5	**15**
	19–30 years	30	550	400	16	5	1.3	1.2	900	1.3	2.4	90	5	15
	31–50 years	30	550	400	16	5	1.3	1.2	900	1.3	2.4	90	5	15
	51–70 years	30	550	400	16	5	1.3	1.2	900	1.7	2.4h	90	10	15
	>70 years	30	550	400	16	5	1.3	1.2	900	1.7	2.4h	90	15	15
Females	9–13 years	20	**375**	**300**	**12**	4	**0.9**	**0.9**	**600**	**1.0**	**1.8**	**45**	5	**11**
	14–18 years	25	**400**	**400i**	**14**	5	**1.0**	**1.0**	**700**	**1.2**	**2.4**	**65**	5	**15**
	19–30 years	30	425	400i	14	5	1.1	1.1	700	1.3	2.4	75	5	15
	31–50 years	30	425	400i	14	5	1.1	1.1	700	1.3	2.4	75	5	15
	51–70 years	30	425	400i	14	5	1.1	1.1	700	1.5	2.4h	75	10	15
	>70 years	30	425	400	14	5	1.1	1.1	700	1.5	2.4h	75	15	15
Pregnancy	≤18 years	30	450	600i	18	6	1.4	1.4	750	1.9	2.6	80	5	15
	19–30 years	30	450	600i	18	6	1.4	1.4	770	1.9	2.6	85	5	15
	31–50 years	30	450	600i	18	6	1.4	1.4	770	1.9	2.6	85	5	15
Lactation	≤18 years	35	550	500	17	7	1.6	1.4	1200	2.0	2.8	115	5	19
	19–30 years	35	550	500	17	7	1.6	1.4	1300	2.0	2.8	120	5	19
	31–50 years	35	550	500	17	7	1.6	1.4	1300	2.0	2.8	120	5	19
Tolerable Upper Intake Levels for Adults (19–70)			3500	1000k	35k				3000	100		2000	50	1000k

Note: The table includes values for the type of DRI standard—Adequate Intake (AI) or Recommended Dietary Allowance (RDA)—that has been established for that particular nutrient and life stage; RDAs are shown in **bold type.** The final row of the table shows the Tolerable Upper Intake Levels (ULs) for adults; refer to the full DRI report for information on other ages and life stages. A UL is the maximum level of daily nutrient intake that is likely to pose no risk of adverse effects. There is insufficient data to set ULs for all nutrients, but this does not mean that there is no potential for adverse effects; source of intake should be from food only to prevent high levels of intake of nutrients without established ULs. In healthy individuals, there is no established benefit from nutrient intakes above the RDA or AI.

aAlthough AIs have been set for choline, there are few data to assess whether a dietary supply of choline is needed at all stages of the life cycle, and it may be that the choline requirement can be met by endogenous synthesis at some of these stages.

bAs dietary folate equivalents (DFE); 1 DFE = 1 μg food folate = 0.6 μg folate from fortified food or as a supplement consumed with food = 0.5 μg of a supplement taken on an empty stomach.

cAs niacin equivalents (NE): 1 mg niacin = 60 mg tryptophan.

TABLE 1   Dietary Reference Intakes (DRIs): Recommended Levels for Individual Intake (continued)

Life Stage	Group	Vitamin K (μg/day)	Calcium (mg/day)	Chromium (μg/day)	Copper (μg/day)	Fluoride (mg/day)	Iodine (mg/day)	Iron (mg/day)l	Magnesium (mg/day)	Manganese (mg/day)	Molybdenum (μg/day)	Phosphorus (mg/day)	Selenium (μg/day)	Zinc (mg/day)m
Infants	0–6 months	2.0	210	0.2	200	0.01	110	0.27	30	0.003	2	100	15	2
	7–12 months	2.5	270	5.5	220	0.5	130	11	75	0.6	3	275	20	3
Children	1–3 years	30	500	11	340	0.7	90	7	80	1.2	17	460	20	3
	4–8 years	55	800	15	440	1	90	10	130	1.5	22	500	30	5
Males	9–13 years	60	1300	25	700	2	120	8	240	1.9	34	1250	40	8
	14–18 years	75	1300	35	890	3	150	11	410	2.2	43	1250	55	11
	19–30 years	120	1000	35	900	4	150	8	400	2.3	45	700	55	11
	31–50 years	120	1000	35	900	4	150	8	420	2.3	45	700	55	11
	51–70 years	120	1200	30	900	4	150	8	420	2.3	45	700	55	11
	>70 years	120	1200	30	900	4	150	8	420	2.3	45	700	55	11
Females	9–13 years	60	1300	21	700	2	120	8	240	1.6	34	1250	40	8
	14–18 years	75	1300	24	890	3	150	15	360	1.6	43	1250	55	9
	19–30 years	90	1000	25	900	3	150	18	310	1.8	45	700	55	8
	31–50 years	90	1000	25	900	3	150	18	320	1.8	45	700	55	8
	51–70 years	90	1200	20	900	3	150	8	320	1.8	45	700	55	8
	>70 years	90	1200	20	900	3	150	8	320	1.8	45	700	55	8
Pregnancy	≤18 years	75	1300	29	1000	3	220	27	400	2.0	50	1250	60	13
	19–30 years	90	1000	30	1000	3	220	27	350	2.0	50	700	60	11
	31–50 years	90	1000	30	1000	3	220	27	360	2.0	50	700	60	11
Lactation	≤18 years	75	1300	44	1300	3	290	10	360	2.6	50	1250	70	14
	19–30 years	90	1000	45	1300	3	290	9	310	2.6	50	700	70	12
	31–50 years	90	1000	45	1300	3	290	9	320	2.6	50	700	70	12
Tolerable Upper Intake Levels for Adults (19–70)			2500		10,000	10	1100	45	350^k	11	2000	4000	400	40

d As retinol activity equivalents (RAEs): 1 RAE = 1 μg retinol, 12 μg β-carotene, or 24 μg α-carotene or β-cryptoxanthin. Preformed vitamin A (retinol) is abundant in animal-derived foods; provitamin A carotenoids are abundant in some dark yellow, orange, red, and deep-green fruits and vegetables. For preformed vitamin A and for provitamin A carotenoids in supplements, IRE = 1 RAE; for provitamin A carotenoids in foods, divide the REs by 2 to obtain RAEs. The UL applies only to preformed vitamin A.

e Individuals who smoke require an additional 35 mg/day of vitamin C over that needed by nonsmokers; nonsmokers regularly exposed to tobacco smoke should ensure they meet the RDA for vitamin C.

f As cholecalciferol: 1 μg cholecalciferol = 40 IU vitamin D. DRI values are based on the absence of adequate exposure to sunlight.

g As α-tocopherol. Includes naturally occurring RRR- α-tocopherol and the 2R-stereoisomeric forms from supplements; does not include the 2S-stereoisomeric forms from supplements.

h Because 10–30% of older people may malabsorb food-bound B-12, those over age 50 should meet their RDA mainly with supplements or foods fortified with B-12.

i In view of evidence linking folate intake with neural tube defects in the fetus. It is recommended that all women capable of becoming pregnant consume 400 μg of folate from supplements or fortified foods in addition to consuming folate from a varied diet.

j It is assumed that women will continue consuming 400 μg from supplements or fortified food until their pregnancy is confirmed and they enter prenatal care, which ordinarily occurs after the end of the periconceptional period—the critical time for formation of the neural tube.

k The UL applies only to intake from supplements, fortified foods, and/or pharmacological agents and not to intake from foods.

l Because the absorption of iron from plant foods is low compared to that from animal foods, the RDA for strict vegetarians is approximately 1.8 times higher than the values established for omnivores (14 mg/day for adult male vegetarians; 33 mg/day for premenopausal female vegetarians). Oral contraceptives (OCs) reduce menstrual blood losses, so women taking them need less daily iron; the RDA for premenopausal women taking OCs is 10.9 mg/day. For more on iron requirements for other special situations, refer to *Dietary Reference Intakes for Vitamin A, Vitamin K, Arsenic, Boron, Chromium, Copper, Iodine, Iron, Manganese, Molybdenum, Nickel, Silicon, Vanadium, and Zinc* (visit http://www.nap.edu for the complete report).

m Zinc absorption is lower for those consuming vegetarian diets so the zinc requirement for vegetarians is approximately twofold greater than for those consuming a nonvegetarian diet.

TABLE 1 Dietary Reference Intakes (DRIs): Recommended Levels for Individual Intake (*continued*)

Life Stage	Group	Potassium (g/day)	Sodium (g/day)	Chloride (g/day)	Carbohydrate RDA/AI (g/day)	Carbohydrate AMDR[n] (%)	Total Fiber RDA/AI (g/day)	Total Fat AMDR[o] (%)	Linoleic Acid RDA/AI (g/day)	Linoleic Acid AMDR[o] (%)	Alpha-linolenic Acid RDA/AI (g/day)	Alpha-linolenic Acid AMDR[o] (%)	Protein[n] RDA/AI (g/day)	Protein[n] AMDR[o] (%)	Water[p] (L/day)
Infants	0–6 months	0.4	0.12	0.18	60	ND[q]	ND	r	4.4	ND[q]	0.5	ND[q]	9.1	ND[q]	0.7
	7–12 months	0.7	0.37	0.57	95	ND[q]	ND	r	4.6	ND[q]	0.5	ND[q]	13.5	ND[q]	0.8
Children	1–3 years	3.0	1.0	1.5	130	45–65	19	30–40	7	5–10	0.7	0.6–1.2	13	5–20	1.3
	4–8 years	3.8	1.2	1.9	130	45–65	25	25–35	10	5–10	0.9	0.6–1.2	19	10–30	1.7
Males	9–13 years	4.5	1.5	2.3	130	45–65	31	25–35	12	5–10	1.2	0.6–1.2	34	10–30	2.4
	14–18 years	4.7	1.5	2.3	130	45–65	38	25–35	16	5–10	1.6	0.6–1.2	52	10–30	3.3
	19–30 years	4.7	1.5	2.3	130	45–65	38	20–35	17	5–10	1.6	0.6–1.2	56	10–35	3.7
	31–50 years	4.7	1.5	2.3	130	45–65	38	20–35	17	5–10	1.6	0.6–1.2	56	10–35	3.7
	51–70 years	4.7	1.3	2.0	130	45–65	30	20–35	14	5–10	1.6	0.6–1.2	56	10–35	3.7
	>70 years	4.7	1.2	1.8	130	45–65	30	20–35	14	5–10	1.6	0.6–1.2	56	10–35	3.7
Females	9–13 years	4.5	1.5	2.3	130	45–65	26	25–35	10	5–10	1.0	0.6–1.2	34	10–30	2.1
	14–18 years	4.7	1.5	2.3	130	45–65	26	25–35	11	5–10	1.1	0.6–1.2	46	10–30	2.3
	19–30 years	4.7	1.5	2.3	130	45–65	25	20–35	12	5–10	1.1	0.6–1.2	46	10–35	2.7
	31–50 years	4.7	1.5	2.3	130	45–65	25	20–35	12	5–10	1.1	0.6–1.2	46	10–35	2.7
	51–70 years	4.7	1.3	2.0	130	45–65	21	20–35	11	5–10	1.1	0.6–1.2	46	10–35	2.7
	>70 years	4.7	1.2	1.8	130	45–65	21	20–35	11	5–10	1.1	0.6–1.2	46	10–35	2.7
Pregnancy	≤18 years	4.7	1.5	2.3	175	45–65	28	20–35	13	5–10	1.4	0.6–1.2	71	10–35	3.0
	19–30 years	4.7	1.5	2.3	175	45–65	28	20–35	13	5–10	1.4	0.6–1.2	71	10–35	3.0
	31–50 years	4.7	1.5	2.3	175	45–65	28	20–35	13	5–10	1.4	0.6–1.2	71	10–35	3.0
Lactation	≤18 years	5.1	1.5	2.3	210	45–65	29	20–35	13	5–10	1.3	0.6–1.2	71	10–35	3.8
	19–30 years	5.1	1.5	2.3	210	45–65	29	20–35	13	5–10	1.3	0.6–1.2	71	10–35	3.8
	31–50 years	5.1	1.5	2.3	210	45–65	29	20–35	13	5–10	1.3	0.6–1.2	71	10–35	3.8
Tolerable Upper Intake Level for Adults (19–70)			2.3	3.6											

[n]Daily protein recommendations are based on body weight for reference body weights. To calculate for a specific body weight, use the following values: 1.5 g/kg for infants, 1.1 g/kg for 1–3 years, 0.95 g/kg for 4–13 years, 0.85 g/kg for 14–18 years, 0.8 g/kg for adults, and 1.1 g/kg for pregnant (using prepregnancy weight) and lactating women.

[o]Acceptable Macronutrient Distribution Range (AMDR), expressed as a percent of total daily calories, is the range of intake for a particular energy source that is associated with reduced risk of chronic disease while providing intakes of essential nutrients. If an individual consumes in excess of the AMDR, there is a potential for increasing the risk of chronic diseases and/or insufficient intakes of essential nutrients.

[p]Total water intake from fluids and food.

[q]Not determinable due to lack of data of adverse effects in this age group and concern with regard to lack of ability to handle excess amounts. Source of intake should be from food only to prevent high levels of intake.

[r]For infants, Adequate Intake of total fat is 31 grams/day (0–6 months) and 30 grams per day (7–12 months) from breast milk and, for infants 7–12 months, complementary food and beverages.

SOURCE: Food and Nutrition Board, Institute of Medicine, National Academies. 2004. Dietary Reference Intakes Tables. Washington, D.C.: National Academies Press. The complete Dietary Reference Intake reports are available from the National Academy Press (http://www.nap.edu).

*Reprinted with permission from *Dietary Reference Intakes Applications in Dietary Planning*. Copyright © 2004 by the National Academy of Sciences. Reprinted with permission from the National Academies Press, Washington, D.C.

Name _____   Section _____   Date _____

LAB 7.1 Your Daily Diet versus the Food Guide

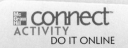

Keep a record of everything you eat for 3 consecutive days. Record all foods and beverages you consume, breaking each food item into its component parts (for example, a turkey sandwich would be listed as 2 slices of bread, 100 grams of turkey, 1 tsp of mayonnaise, and so on) and list them separately in the column labelled 'food'. Complete the first two columns of the chart during the course of the day; fill in the remaining information at the end of the day using Figure 7.4 and the *Canada's Food Guide* section of this chapter.
(Note: This lab can also be completed using nutritional analysis software or websites.)

DAY 1

Food	Your Portion Size	Food Group	Number of Food Guide Servings*

Daily Total

Food Group	Number of Servings
Milk, yogurt, cheese	
Meat, poultry, fish, dry beans, eggs, nuts	
Fruits	
Vegetables	
Breads, cereals, rice, pasta	
Water	
Other foods, i.e., soft drinks, unhealthy snacks	

*Your portion sizes may be smaller or larger than the serving sizes given in the Food Guide, list the actual number of Food Guide servings contained in the foods you eat.

DAY 2

Food	Your Portion Size	Food Group	Number of Food Guide Servings*

Daily Total

Food Group	Number of Servings
Milk, yogurt, cheese	
Meat, poultry, fish, dry beans, eggs, nuts	
Fruits	
Vegetables	
Breads, cereals, rice, pasta	
Water	
Other foods, i.e., soft drinks, unhealthy snacks	

*Your portion sizes may be smaller or larger than the serving sizes given in the Food Guide, list the actual number of Food Guide servings contained in the foods you eat.

DAY 3

Food	Your Portion Size	Food Group	Number of Food Guide Servings*

Daily Total

Food Group	Number of Servings
Milk, yogurt, cheese	
Meat, poultry, fish, dry beans, eggs, nuts	
Fruits	
Vegetables	
Breads, cereals, rice, pasta	
Water	
Other foods, i.e., soft drinks, unhealthy snacks	

*Your portion sizes may be smaller or larger than the serving sizes given in the Food Guide, list the actual number of Food Guide servings contained in the foods you eat.

Next, average your serving totals for the 3 days and enter them in the chart below. Fill in the recommended serving totals that apply to you from Figure 7.4.

Food Group	Recommended Number of Daily Servings	Actual (Average) Number of Daily Servings
Milk, yogurt, cheese		
Meat, poultry, fish, dry beans, eggs, nuts		
Fruits		
Vegetables		
Breads, cereals, rice, pasta		
Water		
Other foods, i.e., soft drinks, unhealthy snacks		

Using Your Results

How did you score? How close is your diet to that recommended by the Food Guide? Are you at all surprised by the actual number of servings you're consuming from each food group?

What should you do next? If the results of the assessment indicate that you could boost your level of wellness by improving your diet, set realistic goals for change. Do you need to increase or decrease your consumption of any food groups? Be sure to use the information on portion sizes in this chapter. List any areas of concern below, along with a goal for change and strategies for achieving the goal you've set. If you see that you are falling short in one food group, such as fruits or vegetables, you might try increasing those servings by consuming an apple, a bunch of grapes, or some baby carrots. Think carefully about the reasons behind your food choices. For example, if you eat doughnuts for breakfast every morning because you feel rushed, make a list of ways to save time to allow for a healthier breakfast.

Problem: _____

Goal: _____

Strategies for change: _____

_____

_____

Problem: _____

Goal: _____

Strategies for change: _____

_____

_____

Problem: _____

Goal: _____

Strategies for change: _____

_____

_____

Enter the results of this lab in the Preprogram Assessment column in Appendix C. If you've set goals and identified strategies for change, begin putting your plan into action. After several weeks of your program, complete this lab again and enter the results in the Postprogram Assessment column of Appendix C. How do the results compare?

Name _____   Section _____   Date _____

LAB 7.2 Dietary Analysis

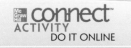

You can complete this activity using either a nutrition analysis software program or the food composition data in Appendix B and the charts printed below. Information about the nutrient content of foods is also available online; see the For Further Exploration section for recommended websites. (This lab asks you to analyze one day's diet. For a more complete and accurate assessment of your diet, analyze the results from several different days, including a weekday and a weekend day.)

DATE _____   DAY: M Tu W Th F Sa Su

Food	Amount	Calories	Protein (g)	Carbohydrate (g)	Dietary fibre (g)	Fat, total (g)	Saturated fat (g)	Cholesterol (mg)	Sodium (mg)	Vitamin A (mg)	Vitamin C (mg)	Calcium (mg)	Iron (mg)
Recommended totals[a]			10–30%	45–65%	25–38 g	20–35%	≤10%	≤300 mg	≤2300 mg	RE	mg	mg	mg
Actual totals[b]		cal	g / %	g / %	g	g / %	g / %	mg	mg	RE	mg	mg	mg

[a]Fill in the appropriate DRI values for vitamin A, vitamin C, calcium, and iron from Table 1 in the Nutrition Resources section.
[b]Total the values in each column. To calculate the percentage of total calories from protein, carbohydrates, fat, and saturated fat, use the formulas from the "Setting Intake Goals for Protein, Fat, and Carbohydrates" box, presented earlier in the chapter. Protein and carbohydrate provide 4 calories per gram; fat provides 9 calories per gram. For example, if you consume a total of 270 grams of carbohydrate and 2000 calories, your percentage of total calories from carbohydrate would be (270 g × 4 cal/g) ÷ 2000 cal = 54%. Do not include data for alcoholic beverages in your calculations. Percentages may not total 100% due to rounding.

Using Your Results

How did you score? How close is your diet to that recommended by the Dietary Reference Intakes, and other guidelines? Are you surprised by any of the results of this assessment?

What should you do next? Enter the results of this lab in the Preprogram Assessment column in Appendix C. If your daily diet meets all the recommended intakes, congratulations—and keep up the good work. If the results of the assessment pinpoint areas of concern, then work with your food record on the previous page to determine what changes you could make to meet all the guidelines. Make changes, additions, and deletions until it conforms to all or most of the guidelines. Or, if you prefer, start from scratch to create a day's diet that meets the guidelines. Use the chart below to experiment and record your final, healthy sample diet for one day. Then put what you learned from this exercise into practice in your daily life. After several weeks of your program, complete this lab again and enter the results in the Postprogram Assessment column of Appendix C. How do the results compare?

DATE _____   DAY: M Tu W Th F Sa Su

Food	Amount	Calories	Protein (g)	Carbohydrate (g)	Dietary fibre (g)	Fat, total (g)	Saturated fat (g)	Cholesterol (mg)	Sodium (mg)	Vitamin A (mg)	Vitamin C (mg)	Calcium (mg)	Iron (mg)
Recommended totals[a]			10–30%	45–65%	25–38 g	20–35%	≤10%	≤300 mg	≤2300 mg	RE	mg	mg	mg
Actual totals[b]		cal	g / %	g / %	g	g / %	g / %	mg	mg	RE	mg	mg	mg

LAB 7.3 Informed Food Choices

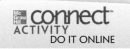

Part I Using Nutrition Labels

Choose three food items to evaluate. You might want to select three similar items, such as regular, low-fat, and non-fat salad dressing, or three very different items. Record the information from their nutrition labels in the table below.

Food Items			
Serving size			
Calories	cal	cal	cal
Total fat—grams	g	g	g
—% Daily Value	%	%	%
Saturated fat—grams	g	g	g
—% Daily Value	%	%	%
Trans fat—grams	g	g	g
Cholesterol—milligrams	mg	mg	mg
Sodium —milligrams	mg	mg	mg
—% Daily Value	%	%	%
Carbohydrates (total)—grams	g	g	g
—% Daily Value	%	%	%
Fibre—grams	g	g	g
—% Daily Value	%	%	%
Sugars—grams	g	g	g
Protein—grams	g	g	g
Vitamin A—% Daily Value	%	%	%
Vitamin C—% Daily Value	%	%	%
Calcium—% Daily Value	%	%	%
Iron—% Daily Value	%	%	%

How do the items you chose compare? You can do a quick nutrient check by totalling the Daily Value percentages for nutrients you should limit (total fat, sodium) and the nutrients you should favour (fibre, vitamin A, vitamin C, calcium, iron) for each food. Which food has the largest percent Daily Value sum for nutrients to limit? For nutrients to favour?

Food Items			
Calories	cal	cal	cal
% Daily Value total for nutrients to limit (total fat, sodium)	%	%	%
% Daily Value total for nutrients to favour (fibre, vitamin A, vitamin C, calcium, iron)	%	%	%

Part II Evaluating Fast Food

Use the information from Appendix B, Nutritional Content of Popular Items from Fast-Food Restaurants, to complete the chart on this page for the last fast-food meal you ate. Add up your totals for the meal. Compare the values for fat, protein, carbohydrate, cholesterol, and sodium content for each food item and for the meal as a whole with the levels suggested by Health Canada and the Food and Nutrition Board. Calculate the percentage of total calories derived from fat, saturated fat, protein, and carbohydrate using the formulas given.

If you haven't recently been to one of the restaurants included in the appendix, fill in the chart for any sample meal you might eat. If some of the food items you selected don't appear in Appendix B, ask for a nutrition information brochure when you visit the restaurant, or check out online fast-food information: Arby's (www.arbysrestaurant.com), Burger King (www.burgerking.com), Domino's Pizza (www.dominos.com), KFC (www.kfc.com), McDonald's (www.mcdonalds.com), Subway (www.subway.com), Taco Bell (www.tacobell.com), Wendy's (www.wendys.com).

FOOD ITEMS

	AMDR							Total[b]
Serving size (g)		g	g	g	g	g	g	g
Calories		cal	cal	cal	cal	cal	cal	cal
Total fat—grams		g	g	g	g	g	g	g
—% calories[a]	20–35%	%	%	%	%	%	%	%
Saturated fat—grams		g	g	g	g	g	g	g
—% calories[a]	≤10%	%	%	%	%	%	%	%
Protein—grams		g	g	g	g	g	g	g
—% calories[a]	10–30%	%	%	%	%	%	%	%
Carbohydrate—grams		g	g	g	g	g	g	g
—% calories[a]	45–65%	%	%	%	%	%	%	%
Cholesterol[c]	100 mg	mg	mg	mg	mg	mg	mg	mg
Sodiumc	800 mg	mg	mg	mg	mg	mg	mg	mg

[a]To calculate the percentage of total calories from each food energy source (fat, carbohydrate, protein), use the following formula:

$$\frac{(\text{number of grams of energy source}) \times (\text{number of calories per gram of energy source})}{(\text{total calories in serving of food item})}$$

(Note: Fat and saturated fat provide 9 calories per gram; protein and carbohydrate provide 4 calories per gram.) For example, the percentage of total calories from protein in a 150-calorie dish containing 10 grams of protein is

$$\frac{(10 \text{ grams of protein}) \times (4 \text{ calories per gram})}{(150 \text{ calories})} = \frac{40}{150} = 0.27, \text{ or } 27\% \text{ of total calories from protein}$$

[b]For the Total column, add up the total grams of fat, carbohydrate, and protein contained in your sample meal and calculate the percentages based on the total calories in the meal. (Percentages may not total 100% due to rounding.) For cholesterol and sodium values, add up the total number of milligrams.

[c]Recommended daily limits of cholesterol and sodium are divided by 3 here to give an approximate recommended limit for a single meal.

Using Your Results

Consider your nutritional intake from fast food and compare it to your intake of a meal that was not fast food. What differences did you notice in the proportion of nutrients that came from each nutrient group?

What changes do you need to make to your fast food intake to enhance your nutritional intake?

CHAPTER 8

WEIGHT MANAGEMENT

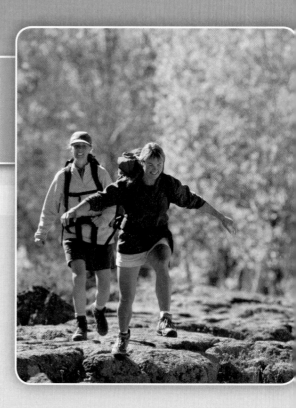

LEARNING OBJECTIVES

After reading this chapter, you should be able to

LO1 Explain the health risks associated with overweight and obesity

LO2 Explain the factors that may contribute to a weight problem, including genetic, physiological, lifestyle, and psychosocial factors

LO3 Describe lifestyle factors that contribute to weight gain and loss, including the role of food choices, exercise, and emotional factors

LO4 Identify and describe the symptoms of eating disorders and the health risks associated with them

LO5 Design a personal plan for successfully managing body weight

TEST YOUR KNOWLEDGE

1. **About what percentage of Canadian adults are overweight?**
   a. 6%
   b. 26%
   c. 36%

2. **Approximately what percentage of those with eating disorders are women?**
   a. 50%
   b. 70%
   c. 90%

3. **The consumption of low-calorie sweeteners has helped Canadians control their weight.**

   True or false?

ANSWERS

1. **C.** About 36% of Canadian adults are overweight, including approximately 26% of adult men and 23% of adult women who are obese.

2. **C.** 90%. Health Canada reports that over 152 000 Canadian women suffer from either anorexia nervosa or bulimia with many developing the disorder between the ages of 14 and 25.

3. **FALSE.** Since the introduction of low-calorie sweeteners, both total calorie intake and total sugar intake have increased, as has the proportion of Canadians who are overweight.

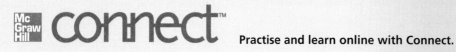

Achieving and maintaining a healthy body weight is a serious public health challenge in Canada and a source of distress for many Canadians. The 2010 Canadian Community Health Survey reported that 34% of Canadians are considered overweight and about 2% underweight. In addition, trends for the past 25 years suggest a 9% increase in the number of Canadian adults reported to be obese.[1] By comparison, Canadian figures now mimic those of the United States in overall numbers of overweight and obese adults. Although overall numbers are similar, distinctions are found in the number of Canadian men (24.3%) and women (23.9.%) who are obese compared to American men (32.6%) and women (36.2%). It is anticipated that if current rates of weight gain continue, all American adults will be overweight by 2030.[2]

Controlling body weight is really a matter of controlling body fat. As explained in Chapter 6, the most important consideration for health is not total weight but body composition—the proportion of fat to fat-free mass. Many people who are "overweight" are also "over-fat," and the health risks they face are due to the latter condition. Although this chapter uses the common terms weight management and weight loss, the goal for wellness is to adopt healthy behaviours and achieve an appropriate body composition, not to conform to rigid standards of total body weight.

Although not completely understood, managing body weight is not a mysterious process. The "secret" is balancing calories consumed with calories expended in daily activities—in other words, eating a moderate diet and participating in regular physical activity.

Body image is a related area of concern. More and more people are becoming unhappy with their bodies and obsessed with their weight. A large number of people seem to contradict what they believe and practise about their body image. Even as the Canadian National Obesity Survey reminded Canadians that those who were overweight and obese were twice as likely as healthy-weight Canadians to suffer from conditions such as high blood pressure and type 2 diabetes, 70% of respondents said that they were satisfied with their weight. It was also slightly perplexing that overweight Canadians were as likely as healthy-weight Canadians to believe that being overweight might lead to a greater risk of suffering from these health conditions.[3] Dissatisfaction with body weight and shape is associated with dangerous eating patterns such as binge eating or self-starvation and with eating disorders.

This chapter explores the factors that contribute to the development of overweight and obesity as well as to eating disorders. It also takes a closer look at weight management through lifestyle and suggests specific strategies for reaching and maintaining a healthy weight. This information is designed to provide the tools necessary for integrating effective weight management into a wellness lifestyle.

LO1 8.1 HEALTH IMPLICATIONS OF OVERWEIGHT AND OBESITY

As rates of overweight and obesity have risen in Canada, so has the prevalence of the health conditions associated with overweight—including a more than 33% rise in the rate of type 2 diabetes in just the past decade. It's estimated that inactivity and overweight account for more than 21,000 premature deaths annually in Canada.[4] About $2 billion per year is spent treating obesity-related health problems.[5] Overweight and obesity are two of the most serious and widespread challenges to wellness.

Obesity is one of six major controllable risk factors for heart disease; it also increases risk for other forms of cardiovascular disease (CVD), hypertension, certain forms of cancer, diabetes, gallbladder disease, respiratory problems, joint diseases, skin problems, impaired immune function, and sleep disorders. Obesity doubles mortality rates from many causes; severe obesity (weighing twice your healthy weight) can reduce life expectancy by 8–10 years. A 2008 study of 46 000 Swedish military recruits showed that people who are obese at age 18 are three times more likely to die prematurely than people who are normal weight at that age.

Gaining weight over the years has also been found to be dangerous; in one study, women who gained more than 22 pounds since they were 18 years old had a sevenfold increase in the risk of heart disease. Many studies have confirmed that obesity and—to a lesser extent—overweight shorten lives.

At the same time, even modest weight loss can have a significant positive impact on health. A weight loss of just 5–10% in obese individuals can reduce the risk of weight-related conditions and increase life expectancy.

Can Someone be Overfat and Fit?

The general answer is yes. Recent research at the Cooper Institute in the United States indicates that those who are fit (based on cardiovascular testing) have a lower mortality risk than those who are unfit, even if overweight or obese. While it is important to focus some attention on increasing obesity rates, many suggest that we then neglect the benefits of exercise and fitness. As a rule, lower body fat levels are preferred but it is possible to have higher, and in some cases overfat or obese levels of fat, and still be considered to be fit.

LO2 8.2 FACTORS CONTRIBUTING TO EXCESS BODY FAT

Several factors determine body weight and composition. These factors can be grouped into genetic, physiological, lifestyle, and psychosocial factors.

Beating the "Freshman 15"

How much weight have you put on since you started going to university/college? It isn't unusual for first-year university/college students to gain some weight (often called the "Freshman 15"), and many students continue gaining weight throughout their university/college years.

If you've gained weight since starting university/college, write down the number of pounds you've gained: _____ pounds

Next, think of five reasons why you have gained this weight, and list them below:

1: _____

2: _____

3: _____

4: _____

5: _____

Now, think of five things you can start doing right now either to stop gaining weight or start losing weight:

1: _____

2: _____

3: _____

4: _____

5: _____

Keep these lists in mind as you work through this chapter, its labs, and the Behaviour Change Workbook at the end of the text. The lists may become the starting point for creating a personal weight-management plan, should you decide you need one.

Genetic Factors

Estimates of the genetic contribution to obesity vary widely, from about 25–40% of an individual's body fat. More than 600 genes have been linked to obesity, but their actions are still under study. Genes can influence body size and shape, body fat distribution, and metabolic rate. Genetic factors may also affect the ease with which weight is gained as a result of overeating and where on the body extra weight is added.

If both parents are overweight, their children have an 80% risk of being obese; children with one obese parent face a 40% risk of becoming obese.[6] In studies that compared adoptees and their biological parents, the weights of the adoptees were found to be more like those of the biological parents than the adoptive parents, again indicating a strong genetic link.

Hereditary influences, however, must be balanced against the contribution of environmental factors. Not all children of obese parents become obese, and normal-weight parents can have overweight children. Environmental factors like diet and exercise are probably responsible for such differences. Thus, the tendency to develop obesity may be inherited, but the expression of this tendency is affected by environmental influences.

Physiological Factors

Metabolism is a key physiological factor in the regulation of body fat and body weight. Hormones also play a role. A few other physiological factors have been proposed as causes for weight gain, such as carbohydrate craving due to low levels of the neurotransmitter serotonin, but research on this and other theories has so far been inconclusive.

METABOLISM AND ENERGY BALANCE Metabolism is the sum of all the vital processes by which food energy and nutrients are made available to and used by the body. The largest component of metabolism, **resting metabolic rate (RMR)**, is the energy required to maintain vital body functions, including respiration, heart rate, body temperature, and blood pressure, while the body is at rest. As shown in Figure 8.1, RMR accounts for 65–70% of daily energy expenditure. The energy required to digest food accounts for an additional ±10% of daily energy expenditure. The remaining 20–30% is expended during physical activity.

Both heredity and behaviour affect metabolic rate. Men, who have a higher proportion of muscle mass than women, have a higher RMR (muscle tissue is more metabolically

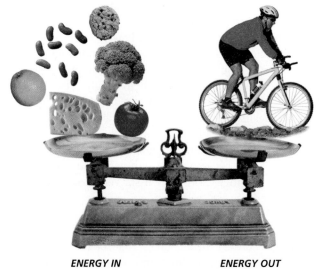

ENERGY IN
Food calories

ENERGY OUT
Physical activity 20–30%
Food digestion ±10%
Resting metabolism 65–70%

FIGURE 8.1 The energy-balance equation.

active than fat). Also, some individuals inherit a higher or lower RMR than others. A higher RMR means that a person burns more calories while at rest and can therefore take in more calories without gaining weight.

Weight loss or gain also affects metabolic rate. When a person loses weight, both RMR and the energy required to perform physical tasks decrease. The reverse occurs when weight is gained. One of the reasons exercise is so important during a weight-loss program is that exercise, especially resistance training, helps maintain muscle mass and metabolic rate.

Exercise has a positive effect on metabolism. When people exercise, they slightly increase their RMR—the number of calories their bodies burn at rest. They also increase their muscle mass, which is associated with a higher metabolic rate. The exercise itself also burns calories, raising total energy expenditure. The higher the energy expenditure, the more the person can eat without gaining weight.

The energy-balance equation is the key to weight management. If you burn the same amount of energy as you take in (a *neutral* [isocaloric] energy balance), your weight remains constant. If you consume more calories than you expend (a *positive* energy balance), your weight increases. If you burn more calories than you consume (a *negative* energy balance), your weight decreases.

To create a negative energy balance and lose weight and body fat, you can increase the amount of energy you burn by increasing your level of physical activity and/or decreasing the amount of energy you take in by consuming fewer calories.

HORMONES Hormones clearly play a role in the accumulation of body fat, especially for females. Hormonal changes at puberty, during pregnancy, and at menopause contribute to the amount and location of fat accumulation. For example, during puberty, hormones cause the development of secondary sex characteristics, including larger breasts, wider hips, and a fat layer under the skin. This addition of body fat at puberty is normal and healthy.

One hormone thought to be linked to obesity is *leptin*. Secreted by the body's fat cells, leptin is carried to the brain, where it appears to let the brain know how big or small the body's fat stores are. With this information, the brain can regulate appetite and metabolic rate accordingly. Researchers hope to use these hormones to develop treatments for obesity based on appetite control. As most of us will admit, however, hunger is often not the primary reason we overeat. Cases of obesity based solely or primarily on hormone abnormalities do exist, but they are rare.

LO3 Lifestyle Factors

Genetic and physiological factors may increase risk for excess body fat, but they are not sufficient to explain the increasingly high rate of obesity seen in Canada. The gene pool has not changed dramatically in the past 40 years, but the rate of obesity among Canadians has nearly tripled. Clearly, other factors are at work—particularly lifestyle factors such as increased energy intake and decreased physical activity.

EATING North Americans generally have access to an abundance of highly palatable and calorie-dense foods, and many have eating habits that contribute to weight gain. Most overweight adults will admit to eating more than they should of high-fat, high-sugar, high-calorie foods. People eat out more frequently now than in the past, and we rely more heavily on fast food and packaged convenience foods. Restaurant and convenience food portion sizes tend to be very large, and the foods themselves are more likely to be high in fat, sugar, and calories and low in nutrients. The Neilsen Company reported that 24% of Canadians eat at a restaurant once or twice a week; 9% of Canadians eat out three to six times a week and 2% of Canadians report that they eat out every day. Interestingly, Canadians report the largest percentage of consumers in the world who choose breakfast as the meal they usually eat out. Studies of adults have also found that the more people eat out, the more calories they consume, especially when they choose a fast-food restaurant.[7]

Research has consistently found that people underestimate portion sizes (i.e., suggest that they are smaller than they actually are) by as much as 25%. When participants in one recent study were asked to report their food intake over the previous 24 hours, the majority underestimated their actual intake by about 600 calories.

According to the Dieticians of Canada, the average calorie intake by Canadians has increased by over 400 calories per day since 1991. Coupled with a decline in the levels of physical activity, the net result has been a substantial increase in the number of Canadians who are overweight. Even small increases in energy intake make a difference. For example, 150 additional calories per day, the amount of calories in one can of pop or beer, can translate into a 7-kilogram weight gain in one year (7700 calories corresponds to one kilogram of body fat). Compared to 1991, Canadians today consume significantly more carbohydrates (about 50 more grams per day), a lot more fat, and about the same amount of protein. The additional carbohydrate calories do not come from the fruits, vegetables, and whole grains recommended by health experts but rather from salty snacks, soft drinks, pizza, and sweet desserts. Other factors contributing to increased calorie intake include increased portion sizes and consumption of more high-calorie meals away from home.

PHYSICAL ACTIVITY Activity levels among Canadians are declining, beginning in childhood and continuing throughout the life cycle. Most adults drive to work, sit

> **resting metabolic rate (RMR)** The energy required (in calories) to maintain vital body functions, including respiration, heart rate, body temperature, and blood pressure, while the body is at rest.

Looking for an easy way to cut calories? Cut down on soda pop or beer. A 12-ounce can of regular soda pop or beer contains about 150 calories. Reduce your consumption by just one can a day, and you can lose about 15 pounds in a year!

all day, and then relax in front of the TV at night. During leisure time, both children and adults surf the Internet, play video games, or watch TV rather than bicycle, participate in sports, or just do yardwork or chores around the house. One study found that 60% of the incidence of overweight can be linked to excessive television viewing. Internet use has fast become the "new" TV. The 2004 Household Internet Use Survery reported that 64% of Canadian households had at least one member who regularly used the Internet. Other modern conveniences such as remote controls, elevators, and power mowers have also reduced daily physical activity. This increase in sedentary lifestyles can also lead to an increased risk for obesity. In fact, the Canadian Community Health Survey (CCHS) reported that 27% of sedentary men were obese compared with only 20% of active men.[8]

PSYCHOSOCIAL FACTORS Many people have learned to use food as a means of coping with stress and negative emotions. Eating can provide a powerful distraction from difficult feelings—loneliness, anger, boredom, anxiety, shame, sadness, inadequacy. It can be used to combat low moods, low energy levels, and low self-esteem. When food and eating become the primary means of regulating emotions, **binge eating** or other unhealthy eating patterns can develop. University/college living often makes it difficult to maintain a healthy weight. Fast foods and sedentary habits can lead to weight problems in both the short and the long term.

Obesity is strongly associated with socioeconomic status. The CCHS found that more women tend to be obese at lower income levels while more men are obese at higher income levels.[9] These differences may reflect the greater sensitivity and concern for a slim physical appearance among upper-income women, as well as greater access to information about nutrition and to low-fat and low-calorie foods. It may also reflect the greater acceptance of obesity among certain ethnic groups, as well as different cultural values related to food choices.

In some families and cultures, food is used as a symbol of love and caring. It is an integral part of social gatherings and celebrations. In such cases, it may be difficult to change established eating patterns because they are linked to cultural and family values.

8.3 ADOPTING A HEALTHY LIFESTYLE FOR SUCCESSFUL WEIGHT MANAGEMENT

When all the research has been assessed, it is clear that most weight problems are lifestyle problems. Even though more and more young people are developing weight problems, most arrive at early adulthood with the advantage of having a normal body weight—neither too fat nor too thin. In fact, many young adults get away with very poor eating and exercise habits and don't develop a weight problem. But as the rapid growth of adolescence slows and family and career obligations increase, maintaining a healthy weight becomes a greater challenge. Slow weight gain is a major cause of overweight and obesity, so weight management is important for everyone, not just for people who are currently overweight. A good time to develop a lifestyle for successful weight management is during early adulthood, when healthy behaviour patterns have a better chance of taking hold.

Permanent weight loss is not something you start and stop. You need to adopt healthy behaviours that you can maintain throughout your life including eating habits, physical activity and exercise, an ability to think positively and manage your emotions effectively, and the coping strategies you use to deal with the stresses and challenges in your life.

Diet and Eating Habits

In contrast to dieting, which involves some form of food restriction, the term *diet* refers to your daily food choices. Quick-fix dieting methods are typically short-term efforts that rarely produce long-term changes in body composition. Everyone has a diet, but not everyone is dieting. It is important to develop a diet that you enjoy and that enables you to maintain a healthy body composition.

Use Canada's Food Guide as the basis for planning a healthy diet (see Chapter 7); choose the healthiest options within each food group. For weight management, you may need to pay special attention to total calories, portion sizes, energy density, fat and carbohydrate intake, and eating habits.

TOTAL CALORIES Canada's Food Guide suggests we consume foods from the food groups that will permit each Canadian to consume calories between

- 1600 calories: Many smaller, sedentary women and some older adults and
- 2800 calories: Teenage boys, many active men, and some very active women

The precise number of calories needed to maintain weight will vary from individual to individual based on heredity, fitness status, level of physical activity, and other factors. It may be more important to focus on individual energy balance than on a general recommendation for daily calorie intake. To maintain your current weight, the total number of calories you eat must equal the number you burn (refer to the energy-balance equation in Figure 8.1). To lose weight, you must decrease your calorie intake and/or increase the number of calories you burn; to gain weight, the reverse is true. To calculate your approximate daily caloric needs, complete the calculations in Lab 8.1.

The best approach for weight loss is combining an increase in physical activity with moderate calorie restriction. Don't go on a crash diet. You need to eat and drink enough to meet your need for essential nutrients. To maintain weight loss, you will probably have to maintain some degree of the calorie restriction you used to lose the weight. Therefore, it is important that you adopt a level of food intake that you can live with over the long term. For most people, maintaining weight loss is more difficult than losing the weight in the first place. To identify weight-loss goals and ways to meet them, complete Lab 8.2.

PORTION SIZES Overconsumption of total calories is closely tied to portion sizes. Many Canadians are unaware that the portion sizes of packaged foods and of foods served at restaurants have increased in size, and most of us significantly underestimate the amount of food we eat. One study found that the larger the meal, the greater the underestimation of calories.[10] Limiting portion sizes

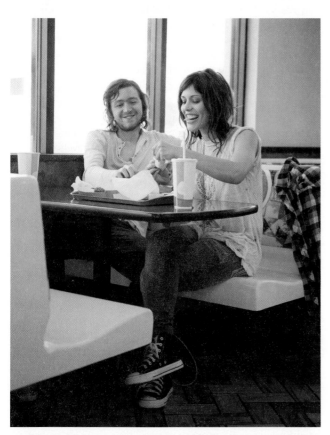

Having a regular schedule of meals and snacks is important for successful weight management. Select the healthiest choices from within the food groups: A breakfast of whole-grain cereal, whole fruit, and juice can help get the day off to a good start.

to those recommended in the Food Guide is critical for weight management. For many people, concentrating on portion sizes is easier than counting calories. See Chapter 7 for more information and hints on choosing appropriate portion sizes.

ENERGY (CALORIE) DENSITY Experts also recommend that you pay attention to *energy density*—the number of calories per ounce or gram of weight in a food. Studies suggest that it isn't consumption of a certain amount of fat or calories in food that reduces hunger and leads to feelings of fullness and satisfaction. Rather, it is consumption of a certain weight of food. Foods that are low in energy density have more volume and bulk—that is, they are relatively heavy but have few calories (Table 8.1). For example, for the same 100 calories, you could eat 20 baby carrots or four pretzel twists; you are more likely to feel full after eating the serving of carrots because it weighs 10 times that of the serving of pretzels (10 ounces versus 1 ounce).

Fresh fruits and vegetables, with their high water and fibre content, are low in energy density, as are whole-grain foods. Fresh fruits contain fewer calories and more fibre than fruit juices or drinks. Meat, ice cream, potato chips, croissants, crackers, and cakes and cookies are examples of foods high in energy density. Strategies for lowering the energy density of your diet include the following:

- Eat fruit with breakfast and for dessert.
- Add extra vegetables to sandwiches, casseroles, stirfry dishes, pizza, pasta dishes, and fajitas.
- Start meals with a bowl of broth-based soup; include a green salad or fruit salad.
- Snack on fresh fruits and vegetables rather than crackers, chips, or other energy-dense snack foods.
- Limit serving sizes of energy-dense foods such as butter, mayonnaise, cheese, chocolate, fatty meats,

TABLE 8.1	Examples of Foods Low in Energy Density	
Food	**Amount**	**Calories**
Carrot, raw	1 medium	25
Popcorn, air popped	2 cups	62
Apple	1 medium	72
Vegetable soup	1 cup	72
Plain instant oatmeal	½ cup	80
Fresh blueberries	1 cup	80
Corn on the cob (plain)	1 ear	80
Cantaloupe	½ melon	95
Light (fat-free) yogurt with fruit	170 ml	100
Unsweetened apple sauce	1 cup	100
Pear	1 medium	100
Corn flakes	1 cup	101
Sweet potato, baked	1 medium	120

Evaluating Fat and Sugar Substitutes

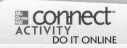

CRITICAL CONSUMER

Foods made with fat and sugar substitutes are often promoted for weight loss. But just what are fat and sugar substitutes? And can they really contribute to weight management?

Fat Substitutes

A variety of substances are used to replace fats in processed foods and other products. Some contribute calories, protein, fibre, and/or other nutrients; others do not. Fat replacers can be classified into three general categories:

- Carbohydrate-based fat replacers include starch, fibres, gums, cellulose, polydextrose, and fruit purees. They are found in dairy and meat products, baked goods, salad dressing, and many other prepared foods. Newer types such as Oatrim, Z-trim, and Nutrim are made from types of dietary fibre that may actually lower cholesterol levels. Carbohydrate-based fat replacers contribute up to 4 calories per gram.

- Protein-based fat replacers are typically made from milk, egg whites, soy, or whey; trade names include Simplesse, Dairy-lo, and Supro. They are used in cheese, sour cream, mayonnaise, margarine spreads, frozen desserts, salad dressings, and baked goods. Protein-based fat replacers typically contribute 1–4 calories per gram.

- Fat-based fat replacers include glycerides, olestra, and other types of fatty acids. Some of these compounds are not absorbed well by the body and so provide fewer calories per gram (5 calories compared with the standard 9 for fats); others are impossible for the body to digest and so contribute no calories at all. In many cases, these fat replacers also act to inhibit the absorption of nutrients that the body needs. Olestra has been banned for use in Canada as a food additive due to the risk of harmful side effects.

Nonnutritive Sweeteners and Sugar Alcohols

Sugar substitutes are often referred to as nonnutritive sweeteners because they provide no calories or essential nutrients. By 2004, five types of nonnutritive sweeteners had been approved for use in Canada: acesulfame-K (Sunett), aspartame (Nutra-Sweet, Equal), saccharin (Sweet 'N Low, Hermesetas), sucralose (Splenda), and cyclamate (Sucaryl, Sugar Twin, Weight Watchers). They are used in beverages, desserts, baked goods, yogurt, chewing gum, and products such as toothpaste, mouthwash, and cough syrup.

Sugar alcohols are made by altering the chemical form of sugars extracted from fruits and other plant sources; they include erythritol, isomalt, lactitol, maltitol, mannitol, sorbitol, and xylitol. Sugar alcohols provide 0.2 to 2.5 calories per gram, compared to 4 calories per gram in standard sugar. They have typically been used to sweeten sugar-free candies but are now being added to many sweet foods (candy, cookies, and so on) promoted as low-carbohydrate products. Sugar alcohols are digested in a way that can create gas, cramps, and diarrhea if they are consumed in large amounts—more than about 10 grams in one meal.

Fat and Sugar Substitutes in Weight Management

Whether fat and sugar substitutes help you achieve and maintain a healthy weight depends on your eating and activity habits. When evaluating foods containing fat and sugar substitutes, consider these issues:

- Is the food lower in calories or just lower in fat? Reduced-fat foods often contain extra sugar to improve the taste and texture lost when fat is removed, so such foods may be as high or even higher in total calories than their fattier counterparts.

- Are you choosing foods with fat and/or sugar substitutes *instead of* foods you typically eat or *in addition* to foods you typically eat? If you consume low-fat, no-sugar-added ice cream instead of regular ice cream, you may save calories. But if you add such ice cream to your daily diet simply because it is lower in fat and sugar, your overall calorie consumption—and your weight—may increase.

- How many foods containing fat and sugar substitutes do you consume each day? Although Health Canada has given at least provisional approval to all the sugar substitutes currently available, health concerns about some of these products linger. One way to limit any potential adverse effects is to read labels and monitor how much of each product you consume.

- Is an even healthier choice available? Many of the foods containing fat and sugar substitutes are low-nutrient snack foods. Fruits, vegetables, and whole grains are healthier snack choices.

---

croissants, and snack foods that are fried or high in added sugars (including reduced-fat products), or contain trans fat.

- Avoid processed foods, which can be high in fat and sodium. Even processed foods labelled "fat-free" or "reduced fat" may be high in calories. Such products may contain sugar and fat substitutes (see the box "Evaluating Fat and Sugar Substitutes").

EATING HABITS Equally important to weight management is eating small, frequent meals—four or five meals per day including breakfast and snacks—on a regular schedule. Skipping meals leads to excessive hunger; feelings of deprivation, and increased vulnerability to binge eating or snacking. Establish a regular pattern of eating, and set some rules governing food choices. Rules governing breakfast might be these, for example: Choose a sugar-free, high-fibre cereal with nonfat milk and fruit most of the time; have a hard-boiled egg no more than three times a week; save pancakes and waffles for special occasions. For effective weight management, it is better to consume the majority of calories during the day rather than in the evening.

Decreeing some foods off-limits generally sets up a rule to be broken. The better principle is "everything in moderation." No foods need to be entirely off-limits, though some should be eaten judiciously.

8.4 PHYSICAL ACTIVITY AND EXERCISE

Regular physical activity is another important lifestyle factor in weight management. Physical activity and exercise burn calories and keep the metabolism geared to using food for energy instead of storing it as fat. Making significant cuts in food intake in order to lose weight is a difficult strategy to maintain; increasing your physical activity is a much better strategy. Regular physical activity also protects against weight gain and is essential for maintaining weight loss.

PHYSICAL ACTIVITY   All physical activity will help you manage your weight. The first step in becoming more active is to incorporate more physical activity into your daily life. If you are currently sedentary, follow the recommendations of Health Canada by accumulating 150 minutes or more of moderate-intensity physical activity—walking, gardening, housework—or 75 minutes of vigorous-intensity physical activity—e.g., jogging, aerobics—or a combination of the two every week. Take the stairs instead of the elevator, walk or bike instead of driving. In the long term, even a small increase in activity level can help maintain your current weight or help you lose a moderate amount of weight (Table 8.2). In fact, research suggests that fidgeting—stretching, squirming, standing up, and so on—may help prevent weight gain in some people. If you simply walked around during TV commercials while watching 2 hours

of prime-time programming, you'd accumulate more than 30 minutes of physical activity. Short bouts of activity (no less than 10 minutes each) spread throughout the day can produce many of the same health benefits as continuous physical activity.

If you are overweight and want to lose weight, or if you are trying to maintain a lower weight following weight loss, a greater amount of physical activity can help. Researchers have found that people who lose weight and don't regain it typically burn about 2800 calories per week in physical activity—the equivalent of about 1 hour of brisk walking per day. The Institute of Medicine and the World Health Organization recommend at least 60 minutes of moderate physical activity per day.

EXERCISE   Once you become more active every day, begin a formal exercise program that includes cardio-respiratory endurance exercise, resistance training, and stretching exercises. (See the box "What Is the Best Way to Exercise for Weight Loss?") Moderate-intensity endurance exercise, if performed frequently for a relatively long duration, can burn a significant number of calories. Endurance training also increases the rate at which your body uses calories after your exercise session is over—burning an additional 5–180 extra calories, depending on the intensity of

---

TABLE 8.2	Calorie Costs of Selected Physical Activities*						

To determine how many calories you burn when you engage in a particular activity, multiply the calorie multiplier given below by your body weight (in pounds) and then by the number of minutes you exercise.

Activity	Cal/lb/min	×	Body Weight	×	Min	=	Total Calories
Cycling (21 km/h)	.071		_____		_____		_____
Dancing (popular)	.049		_____		_____		_____
Digging	.062		_____		_____		_____
Driving a car	.020		_____		_____		_____
Housework	.029		_____		_____		_____
Painting a house	.034		_____		_____		_____
Shovelling snow	.052		_____		_____		_____
Sitting quietly	.009		_____		_____		_____
Sleeping and resting	.008		_____		_____		_____
Standing quietly	.012		_____		_____		_____
Typing or writing	.013		_____		_____		_____
Walking briskly (7 km/h)	.048		_____		_____		_____

*See Chapter 9 for the energy costs of fitness activities.

SOURCE: Adapted from Kusinitz, I. and M. Fine. 1995. *Your Guide to Getting Fit,* 3d ed. Mountain View, Calif.: Mayfield.

What Is the Best Way to Exercise for Weight Loss?

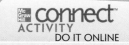
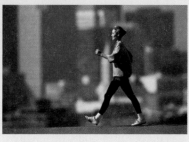

If weight loss is your primary goal, the guidelines for planning a fitness program can vary depending on your weight, body composition, and current level of fitness. For example, there is some dispute among fitness experts about the best target heart rate (THR) zone to use when exercising for weight loss. Some experts recommend exercising at a moderate THR (55–69% of maximum heart rate) because the body burns fat at a slightly more efficient rate at this level of exertion. Others recommend exercising vigorously (70–90% of maximum heart rate) because exercise at this intensity burns more calories overall. According to some estimates, for example, a 30-minute workout at 80–85% of maximum heart rate burns about 30% more calories overall than a 30-minute workout at 60–65% maximum heart rate—but the lower-intensity workout burns roughly 20% more fat calories than the higher-intensity workout.

Regardless, if you are obese or your fitness level is very low, start with a lower-intensity workout (55% of maximum heart rate) and stick with it until your cardiorespiratory fitness level improves enough to support short bouts of higher-intensity exercise. This way, you will burn more fat, reduce the risk of injury and strain on your heart, and improve your chances of staying with your program. Even if your primary goal is to lose weight, you are also improving your cardiorespiratory fitness. Any amount of exercise, even at low to moderate intensity, will help you achieve both goals. But patience is required, especially if you need to lose a great deal of weight.

For weight loss to occur, exercise at lower intensities has to be offset by longer and/or more frequent exercise sessions. As mentioned in this chapter, 60–90 minutes of daily exercise is recommended for anyone who needs to lose weight or maintain weight loss. If you cannot fit such a large block of activity into your daily schedule, break your workouts into short segments—as little as 10–15 minutes each. This approach is probably best for someone who has been sedentary, because it allows the body to become accustomed to exercise at a gradual pace while preventing injury and avoiding strain on the heart.

Many research studies have shown that walking is an ideal form of exercise for losing weight and avoiding weight gain. A landmark 15-year study by the University of North Carolina at Charlotte showed that, over time, people who walked only 30 minutes per day gained 18 pounds less than people who didn't walk. Those who regularly walked farther were better able to lose or maintain weight. Other studies found that people who walked 30 minutes five times per week lost an average of 5 pounds in 6–12 months, without dieting, watching what they ate, or exercising intensely. You can lose even more weight if you eat sensibly and walk farther and faster.

As noted in Chapter 9, a 165-pound adult who walks at a speed of 5 kilometres per hour for 60 minutes a day, 5 days a week, can lose about one-quarter kilogram of body weight per week. Regular walking is the simplest and most effective health habit for controlling body weight and promoting health. Even if you're sedentary, a few months of walking can increase your fitness level to the point where more vigorous types of exercise—and even greater health benefits—are possible.

If you are obese or have never exercised, it may be wise to get a professional assessment of your cardiorespiratory fitness before starting an exercise program. (Refer to Chapter 2 and Lab 2.1 for additional cautions.) Such assessments are available at most exercise physiology labs and at many YMCAs, fitness facilities, and campus wellness centres. By measuring your maximum heart rate and oxygen consumption during exercise, this type of assessment can help you determine a specific THR zone for exercise. If you cannot locate an exercise physiology lab in your area, ask your physician if he or she can provide a referral.

SOURCES: Gordon-Larsen, P., et al. 2009. Fifteen-year longitudinal trends in walking patterns and their impact on weight change. *American Journal of Clinical Nutrition* 89(1): 19–26; Levine, J. A., et al. 2008. The role of free-living daily walking in human weight gain and obesity. *Diabetes* 57(3): 548–554; Nelson, M. E., and S. C. Folta. 2009. Further evidence for the benefits of walking. *American Journal of Clinical Nutrition* 89(1): 15–16; and Physical Activity Guidelines Advisory Committee. 2008. *Physical Activity Guidelines Advisory Committee Report, 2008.* Washington, D.C.: U.S. Department of Health and Human Services.

exercise. Resistance training builds muscle mass, and more muscle translates into a higher metabolic rate. Resistance training can also help you maintain your muscle mass during a period of weight loss, helping you avoid the significant drop in RMR associated with weight loss.

Regular physical activity, maintained throughout life, makes weight management easier. The sooner you establish good habits, the better. The key to success is making exercise an integral part of a lifestyle you can enjoy now and will enjoy in the future.

Thoughts and Emotions

The way you think about yourself and your world influences, and is influenced by, how you feel and how you act. In fact, research on people who have a weight problem indicates that low self-esteem and the negative emotions that accompany it are significant problems. People with low self-esteem mentally compare the actual self to an internally held picture of the "ideal self," an image based on perfectionistic goals and beliefs about how they and others should be. The more these two pictures differ, the larger the impact on self-esteem and the more likely the presence of negative emotions.

Besides the internal picture we carry of ourselves, all of us carry on a internal dialogue about events happening to us and around us. This *self-talk* can be either self-deprecating or positively motivating, depending on our beliefs and attitudes. Having realistic beliefs and goals and engaging in positive self-talk and problem solving support a healthy lifestyle. (Chapter 10 and Activity 11

If you're trying to lose weight or maintain your current weight, it's a good idea to write down everything you eat, including how many calories it contains. Researchers have found that writing down the food choices you make every day increases your commitment and helps you stick to your diet, especially during high-risk times such as holidays, parties, and family gatherings.

Writing every day also serves as a reminder to you that losing weight is important. In a multicentre study conducted over 6 months in 2008, dieters who kept a daily food journal lost twice as much weight as those who didn't track what they ate.

Besides tracking what you eat, keep track of your formal exercise program and other daily physical activities so you can begin increasing either their intensity or duration. People who succeed in their health program expend lots of energy in physical activity—according to one study, an average of 2700 calories a week. Tracking your physical activities and daily exercise routines provides all the same benefits as tracking your eating habits. Your log will help you see your progress, track fitness improvements and weight loss, and maintain a positive perspective on your efforts. All this will help you take your program seriously over the long term.

---

in the Behaviour Change Workbook at the end of the text include strategies for developing realistic self-talk.)

Coping Strategies

Appropriate coping strategies help you deal with the stresses of life; they are also an important lifestyle factor in weight management. Many people use eating as a way to cope. (Others may use drugs, alcohol, smoking, or gambling.) Those who overeat might use food to alleviate loneliness or to serve as a pickup for fatigue, as an antidote to boredom, or as a distraction from problems. Some people even overeat to punish themselves for real or imagined transgressions.

Those who recognize that they are using food in these ways can analyze their eating habits with fresh eyes. They can consciously attempt to find new coping strategies and begin to use food appropriately—to fuel life's activities, to foster growth, and to bring pleasure, not to manage stress. For a summary of the components of weight management through healthy lifestyle choices, see the box "Lifestyle Strategies for Successful Weight Management."

8.5 APPROACHES TO OVERCOMING A WEIGHT PROBLEM

Now you know the factors that contribute to a weight problem, and you understand the importance of diet and physical activity in successful weight management. If you are overweight, you may already be planning how to go about losing weight and keeping it off. You have many options.

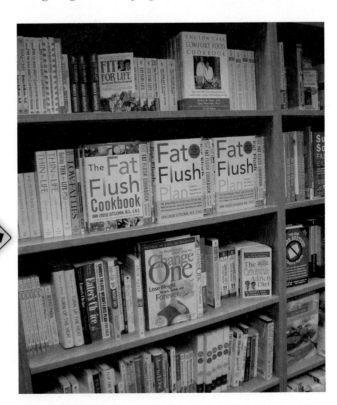

There are many plans and supplements promoted for weight loss, but few have any research supporting their effectiveness for long-term weight management.

CAREER OPTIONS FOR . . .

Weight Management

COMMUNITY: weight loss consultant, lifestyle coach, provincial sport or active living organization, physical activity journalist.

RECREATION AND LEISURE: commercial recreation (e.g., hotel, cruise ship or workplace recreation), youth program manager (e.g., YMCA/YWCA, Boys and Girls Clubs), provincial and federal government (e.g., tourism promotion or national/territorial park employee).

SOURCE: Physical and Health Education Canada (http://www.phecanada.ca).

Lifestyle Strategies for Successful Weight Management

Food Choices

- Follow the recommendations in Canada's Food Guide for eating a moderate, varied diet. Focus on making good choices from within each food group.

- Favour foods with *low* energy density and *high* nutrient density.

- Check food labels for serving sizes, calories, and nutrient levels.

- Watch for hidden calories. Reduced-fat foods often have as many calories as their full-fat versions. Fat-based condiments like butter, margarine, mayonnaise, and salad dressings provide about 100 calories per tablespoon; added sugars such as jams, jellies, and syrup are also packed with calories.

- Drink fewer calories. Many Canadians consume high-calorie beverages such as pop, fruit drinks, sports drinks, alcohol, and specialty coffees and teas.

- For problem foods, try eating small amounts under controlled conditions. Go out for a scoop of ice cream, for example, rather than buying a litre for your freezer.

Planning and Serving

- Keep a log of what you eat. Before you begin your program, your log will provide a realistic picture of your current diet and what changes you can make. Once you start your program, a log will keep you focused on your food choices and portion sizes. Consider tracking the following:

  - food eaten
  - hunger level
  - circumstances (location, other activities)
  - outside influences (environment, other people)
  - thoughts and emotions

- Eat four to five meals a day, including breakfast. In studies, people who eat breakfast consume fewer calories overall over the course of the day. Fix more meals yourself and eat out less often. Keep low-calorie snacks on hand to combat the "munchies." Baby carrots, popcorn, and fresh fruits and vegetables are good choices.

- When shopping for food, make a list and stick to it. Don't shop when you're hungry. Avoid aisles that contain problem foods.

- Consume the majority of your daily calories *during the day*, not in the evening.

- Pay special attention to portion sizes. Use measuring cups and spoons and a food scale to become more familiar with appropriate portion sizes.

- Serve meals on small plates and in small bowls to help you eat smaller portions without feeling deprived.

- Eat only in specifically designated spots. Remove food from other areas of your house or apartment.

- When you eat, just eat—don't do anything else, such as read or watch TV.

- *Avoid late-night eating,* a behaviour specifically associated with weight gain among university/college students.

- Eat slowly. It takes time for your brain to get the message that your stomach is full. Take small bites and chew food thoroughly. Pay attention to every bite, and enjoy your food. Between bites, try putting your fork or spoon down and taking sips of beverage.

- When you've finished eating, remove your plate. Cue yourself that the meal is over—drink a glass of water, suck on a mint, chew gum, or brush your teeth.

Special Occasions

- When you eat out, choose a restaurant where you can make healthy food choices. Ask the server not to put bread and butter on the table before the meal and request that sauces and salad dressings be served on the side. If portion sizes are large, take half your food home for a meal later in the week. Don't choose supersized meals.

- If you cook a large meal for friends, send leftovers home with your guests.

- If you're eating at a friend's, eat a little and leave the rest. Don't eat to be polite; if someone offers you food you don't want, thank the person and decline firmly.

- Take care during the winter holidays. Research indicates that people gain less than they think during the winter holidays (about half a kilogram) but that the weight isn't lost during the rest of the year, leading to slow, steady weight gain.

Physical Activity and Stress Management

- Increase your level of daily physical activity. If you have been sedentary for a long time or are seriously overweight, increase your level of activity slowly. Start by walking 10 minutes at a time, and work toward 30–60 minutes or more of moderate physical activity per day.

- Begin a formal exercise program that includes cardiorespiratory endurance exercise, strength training, and stretching.

- Develop techniques for handling stress—go for a walk or use a relaxation technique. Practise positive self-talk. Get adequate sleep. (See Chapter 10 for more on stress management.)

- Develop strategies for coping with non-hunger cues to eat, such as boredom, sleepiness, or anxiety. Try calling a friend, taking a shower, or reading a magazine.

- Tell family members and friends that you're making some changes in your eating and exercise habits. Ask them to be supportive.

Doing It Yourself

If you need to lose weight, focus on adopting the healthy lifestyle described throughout this book. The "right" weight for you will naturally evolve, and you won't have to diet. Combine modest cuts in energy intake with exercise, and avoid very-low-calorie diets. (In general, a low-calorie diet should provide 1200–1500 calories per day.) By achieving a negative energy balance of 250–1000 calories per day, you'll produce the recommended weight loss of ½–2 pounds per week.

Most low-calorie diets cause a rapid loss of body water at first. When this phase passes, weight loss declines. As a result, people are often misled into believing that their efforts are not working. They give up, not realizing that smaller losses later in the diet are actually better than the initial big losses, because later loss is mostly fat loss, whereas initial loss is primarily fluid. For someone who is overweight, reasonable weight loss is 8–10% of body weight over 6 months.

For many Canadians, maintaining weight loss is a bigger challenge than losing weight. Most weight lost during a period of dieting is regained. When planning a weight management program, you need to include strategies that you can maintain over the long-term, both for food choices and for physical activity. Weight-management is a lifelong project. A registered dietitian or nutritionist can recommend an appropriate plan for you when you want to lose weight on your own. For more tips on losing weight on your own, refer to the section later in the chapter on creating an individual weight-management plan.

Diet Books

Many people who try to lose weight by themselves fall prey to one or more of the dozens of diet books on the market. Although some books contain useful advice and motivational tips, most make empty promises. Here are some guidelines for evaluating and choosing a diet book:

1. Reject books that advocate an unbalanced way of eating, such as a high-carbohydrate-only diet or low-carbohydrate, high-protein diets. Also reject books promoting a single food, such as cabbage or grapefruit.

2. Reject books that claim to be based on a "scientific breakthrough" or to have the "secret" to success.

3. Reject books that use gimmicks, like matching eating to blood type, hyping insulin resistance as the single cause of obesity, combining foods in special ways to achieve weight loss, rotating levels of calories, or purporting that a weight problem is due to food allergies, food sensitivities, yeast infections, or hormone imbalances.

4. Reject books that promise quick weight loss or that limit the selection of foods.

5. Accept books that advocate a balanced approach to diet plus exercise and sound nutrition advice.

Many diets cause weight loss if maintained; the real difficulty is finding a safe and healthy pattern of food choices and physical activity that results in long-term maintenance of a healthy body weight and reduced risk of chronic disease (see the box "Is Any Diet Best for Weight Loss?").

Dietary Supplements and Diet Aids

The number of dietary supplements and other weight-loss aids on the market has also increased in recent years. Promoted in advertisements, magazines, direct mail campaigns, infomercials, and websites, these products typically promise a quick and easy path to weight loss. Most of these products are marketed as dietary supplements and so are subject to fewer regulations than over-the-counter (OTC) medications. A 2002 report from the Federal Trade Commission stated that more than half of the advertisements for weight-loss products made representations that are likely to be false. In addition, use of OTC products doesn't help in the adoption of lifestyle behaviours that can help people achieve and maintain a healthy weight over the long term.

The bottom line on nonprescription diet aids is, *caveat emptor* (Let the buyer beware). There is no quick and easy way to lose weight. The most effective approach is to develop healthy diet and exercise habits and to make them a permanent part of your lifestyle. The following sections describe some commonly marketed OTC products for weight loss.

FORMULA DRINKS AND FOOD BARS Canned diet drinks, powders used to make shakes, and diet food bars and snacks are designed to achieve weight loss by substituting for some or all of a person's daily food intake. However, most people find it difficult to use these products for long periods, and muscle loss and other serious health problems may result if they are used as the sole source of nutrition for an extended period. Use of such products sometimes results in rapid short-term weight loss, but the weight is typically regained because users don't learn to change their eating and lifestyle behaviours.

HERBAL SUPPLEMENTS As described in Chapter 7, herbs are marketed as dietary supplements, so there is little information about effectiveness, proper dosage, drug interactions, and side effects. In addition, labels may not accurately reflect the ingredients and dosages present, and safe manufacturing practices are not guaranteed.

There are currently no guidelines for the sale of herbal supplements for weight loss in Canada. If you are considering using an herbal supplement, check its ingredients carefully and be sure to check with your doctor before starting your supplement regime.

OTHER SUPPLEMENTS Fibre is another common ingredient in OTC diet aids, promoted for appetite control. However, dietary fibre acts as a bulking agent in the large intestine, not the stomach, so it doesn't have a pronounced effect on appetite. In addition, many diet aids

Is Any Diet Best for Weight Loss?

Experts agree that reducing calorie intake promotes weight loss. However, many popular weight-loss plans include a special hook and promote specific food choices and macronutrient (protein, fat, carbohydrate) combinations as best for weight loss. Research findings have been mixed, but two points are clear. Total calorie intake matters, and the best diet is probably the one you can stick with.

Low-Carbohydrate Diets

Some low-carb diets advocate fewer than 10% of total calories from carbohydrates, compared to the 45–65% recommended by Health Canada. Some suggest daily carbohydrate intake below the 130 grams needed to provide essential carbohydrates in the diet. Small studies have found that low-carbohydrate diets can help with short-term weight loss and be safe for relatively short periods of time—although unpleasant effects such as bad breath, constipation, and headache are fairly common.

Some low-carb diets tend to be very high in protein and saturated fat and low in fibre, whole grains, vegetables, and fruits (and thus lack some essential nutrients). Diets high in protein and saturated fat have been linked to an increased risk of heart disease, high blood pressure, and cancer. Other low-carb diets, though still emphasizing protein, limit saturated fats, allow most vegetables after an initial period, and advocate switching to "healthy carbs." These diets are healthier than the more extreme versions.

Low-Fat Diets

Many experts advocate diets that are relatively low in fat, high in carbohydrates, and moderate in protein. Critics of these diets blame them for rising rates of obesity and note that very-low-fat, very-high-carbohydrate diets can increase triglyceride levels and reduce levels of good (HDL) cholesterol in some people. These negative effects can be counteracted with moderate-intensity exercise, however, and low-fat diets combined with physical activity can be safe and effective for many people.

Few experts take the position that low-fat, high-carbohydrate diets, apart from overall diet and activity patterns, are responsible for the increase in obesity among North Americans. However, the debate has highlighted the importance of total calorie intake and the quality of carbohydrate choices. A low-fat diet is not a licence to consume excess calories, even in low-fat foods.

How Do Popular Diets Measure Up?

In one recent study, obese people on a very-low-carbohydrate, high-fat diet lost more weight over a 6-month period than people following a moderate-fat diet. After a year, however, the difference in weight loss between the two groups was no longer significant, and the dropout rate from both groups was high.

A 2005 study followed participants in four popular diets that emphasize different strategies—Weight Watchers (restricted portion sizes and calories), Atkins (low-carbohydrate, high-fat), Zone (relatively high protein, moderate fat and carbohydrate), and Ornish (very low fat). Each of these diets modestly reduced body weight and heart disease risk factors. There was no significant difference in weight loss at 1 year among the diets, and the more closely people adhered to each diet, the more weight they lost. A 2008 study comparing the Atkins Diet, the Mediterranean Diet, and a standard low-fat diet yeilded similar results.

Energy Balance Counts: Healthy Living Unit—Public Health Agency of Canada

Future research may determine that certain macronutrient patterns are somewhat more helpful for disease reduction in people with particular risk profiles. In terms of weight loss, however, such differences among diets are likely overshadowed by the importance of total calorie intake and physical activity. Important lessons about energy balance can be drawn from the Public Health Agency of Canada's Healthy Living Unit (www.phac-aspc.gc.ca/pau-uap/fitness/index.html): Here Canadians can learn about ways to manage their energy balance through the development of proper eating habits and the incorporation of physical activity into their daily routine.

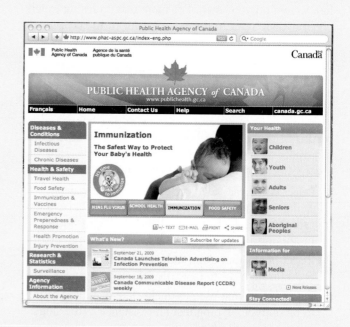

SOURCES: Battle of the diet books II. 2006. *Nutrition Action Healthletter,* July/August; Dansinger, M. L., et al. 2005. Comparison of the Atkins, Ornish, Weight Watchers, and Zone diets for weight loss and heart disease risk reduction. *Journal of the American Medical Association* 293(1): 43–53; Hays, N. P., et al. 2004. Effects of an ad libitum low-fat, high-carbohydrate diet on body weight, body composition, and fat distribution in older men and women. *Archives of Internal Medicine* 164(2): 210–217; Hill, J., and R. Wing. 2003. *Permanente Journal* 7(3): 34–37; Bravata, D. M., et al. 2003. Efficacy and safety of low-carbohydrate diets. *Journal of the American Medical Association* 289: 1837–1850; Foster, G. D., et al. 2003. A randomized trial of low-carbohydrate diet for obesity. *New England Journal of Medicine* 348: 2082–2090; and Shai, I., et al. 2008. Weight Loss with a Low-Carbohydrate, Mediterranean, or Low-Fat Diet. *New England Journal of Medicine* 359(3): 229–241.

contain only 3 or fewer grams of fibre, which does not contribute much toward the recommended daily intake of 25–38 grams. Other popular dietary supplements include conjugated linoleic acid, carnitine, chromium, pyruvate, calcium, B vitamins, chitosan, and a number of products labelled "fat absorbers," "fat blockers," or "starch blockers." Research has not found these products to be effective, and many have potentially adverse side effects.

Weight-Loss Programs

Weight-loss programs come in a variety of types, including noncommercial support organizations, commercial programs, websites, and medically supervised clinical programs.

NONCOMMERCIAL WEIGHT-LOSS PROGRAMS Noncommercial programs such as TOPS (Take Off Pounds Sensibly) and Overeaters Anonymous (OA) mainly provide group support. They do not advocate any particular diet, but they do recommend seeking professional advice for creating an individualized diet and exercise plan. Like Alcoholics Anonymous, OA is a 12-step program with a spiritual orientation that promotes "abstinence" from compulsive overeating. These types of programs are generally free. Your physician or a registered dietitian can also provide information and support for weight loss.

COMMERCIAL WEIGHT-LOSS PROGRAMS Commercial programs such as Weight Watchers and Jenny Craig, typically provide group support, nutrition education, physical activity recommendations, and behaviour modification advice. Some also make available packaged foods to assist in following dietary advice. Many Canadian commercial programs voluntarily belong to the Partnership for Healthy Weight Management established by the United States' Federal Trade Commission in 1999.

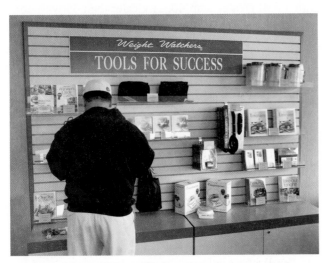

A variety of commercial weight-loss programs are available. These programs yield mixed results, but most provide nutritional counselling and support for people who are serious about losing weight.

By doing so, they agree to provide clients with information on staff training and education, the risks associated with overweight and obesity, the risks associated with each program or product, the costs of the program, and the expected outcomes of the program, including rates of success. A responsible and safe weight-loss program should have the following features:

1. The recommended diet should be safe and balanced, include all the food groups, and meet the DRIs for all nutrients. Physical activity and exercise should be strongly encouraged.

2. The program should promote slow, steady weight loss averaging 0.25–1 kg per week. (There may be rapid weight loss initially due to fluid loss.)

3. If a participant plans to lose more than 10 kilograms, has any health problems, or is taking medication on a regular basis, physician evaluation and monitoring should be recommended. The staff of the program should include qualified counsellors and health professionals.

4. The program should include plans for weight maintenance after the weight-loss phase is over.

5. The program should provide information on all fees and costs, including those of supplements and prepackaged foods, as well as data on risks and expected outcomes of participating in the program.

You should also consider whether a program fits your lifestyle and whether you are truly ready to make a commitment to it. A strong commitment and a plan for maintenance are especially important because only 10–15% of program participants maintain their weight loss; the rest gain back all or more than they had lost. One study of participants found that regular exercise was the best predictor of maintaining weight loss, and frequent television viewing was the best predictor of weight gain.

ONLINE WEIGHT-LOSS PROGRAMS Internet-based weight-loss programs have proliferated over the last decade. Most such websites include a cross between self-help and group support through chat rooms, bulletin boards, and e-newsletters. Many sites offer online self-assessment for diet and physical activity habits as well as a meal plan; some provide access to a staff professional for individualized help. Many are free but some charge a small weekly or monthly fee.

Research suggests that this type of program provides an alternative to in-person diet counselling and can lead to weight loss for some people. Studies found that people who logged on more frequently tended to lose more weight; weekly online contact in terms of behaviour therapy proved most successful for weight loss. The criteria used to evaluate commercial programs can also be applied to Internet-based programs. In addition, make sure a program offers member-to-member support and access to staff professionals.

CLINICAL WEIGHT-LOSS PROGRAMS   Medically supervised clinical programs are usually located in a hospital or other medical setting. Designed to help those who are severely obese, these programs typically involve a closely monitored very-low-calorie diet. The cost of a clinical program is usually high, but insurance often covers part of the fee.

Prescription Drugs

For a medicine to cause weight loss, it must reduce energy consumption, increase energy expenditure, and/or interfere with energy absorption. The medications most often prescribed for weight loss are appetite suppressants that reduce feelings of hunger or increase feelings of fullness. Appetite suppressants usually work by increasing levels of catecholamine or serotonin, two brain chemicals that affect mood and appetite.

While not all prescription weight-loss drugs are legal for use in Canada, they all have potential side effects. Those that affect catecholamine levels, including phentermine (Ionamin, Obenix, Fastin, and Adipex-P), diethylpropion (Tenuate), and mazindol (Sanorex), may cause sleeplessness, nervousness, and euphoria. Sibutramine (legal for use in Canada) acts on both the serotonin and catecholamine systems; it may trigger increases in blood pressure and heart rate. Headaches, constipation or diarrhea, dry mouth, and insomnia are other side effects. Be sure to confirm a drug's legality and safety with Health Canada's website before using weight-loss drugs.

Another Canadian medication approved for long-term use in reducing obesity is orlistat (Xenical), which lowers calorie consumption by blocking fat absorption in the intestines; it prevents about 30% of the fat in food from being digested. Similar to the fat substitute olestra, orlistat reduces the absorption of fat-soluble vitamins and antioxidants. Side effects include diarrhea, cramping, and other gastrointestinal problems if users do not follow a low-fat diet. Orlistat and sibutramine are currently the only two drugs approved for use in weight loss in Canada.

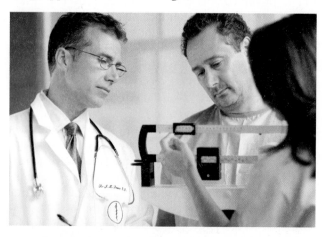

Severely obese people may get the most benefit from a clinical weight-loss program, where diet and activity are monitored closely by health professionals.

A new drug, rimonabant (Acomplia) has been used successfully in Europe and is awaiting Health Canada approval for use in Canada. Rimonabant suppresses appetite by acting on certain brain receptors. Studies show that rimonabant may lead to greater weight loss than other drugs and may help users keep weight off for a longer time. Side effects include mild diarrhea, dizziness, and nausea. Some users also suffer psychological side effects such as depression and suicidal thoughts.

All of these medications work best in conjunction with behaviour modification. Appetite suppressants produce modest weight loss—about 2–10 kg above the loss expected with nondrug obesity treatments. Individuals respond differently, however, and some experience more weight loss than others., Weight loss tends to level off or reverse after 4 to 6 months on a medication, and many people regain the weight they've lost if they stop taking the drugs.

Prescription weight-loss drugs are not for people who want to lose a few kilograms. The latest federal guidelines advise people to try lifestyle modification for at least 6 months before trying drug therapy. Prescription drugs are recommended—in conjunction with lifestyle changes—only in certain cases: for people who have been unable to lose weight with non-drug options and who have a BMI over 30 (or over 27 if two or more additional risk factors such as diabetes and high blood pressure are present).

Surgery

About 3% of Canadians are morbidly obese,[11] meaning they have a BMI of 40 or higher. Morbid obesity is a serious medical condition that is often complicated by other health problems such as diabetes, sleep disorders, heart disease, and arthritis. Surgical intervention may be necessary as a treatment of last resort. According to a National Institutes of Health Consensus Conference, gastric bypass surgery may be recommended for patients with a BMI greater than 40, or greater than 35 with obesity-related illnesses. Due to the increasing prevalence of severe obesity, surgical treatment of obesity is growing worldwide. Obesity-related health conditions, as well as risk of premature death, generally improve after surgical weight loss. Surgery is not without risks, however, and is generally appropriate only for people with severe obesity-related health problems.

Bariatric surgery modifies the gastrointestinal tract by changing either the size of the stomach by partitioning the stomach with staples or a band, or by modifying the way the stomach drains (gastric bypass). In either type of surgical intervention, the goal is to promote weight loss by reducing the amount of food the patient can eat. The two most common surgeries are the Roux-en-Y gastric bypass and the vertical banded gastroplasty (VGB/Lap-Band). Potential complications from surgery include nutritional deficiencies, fat intolerance, nausea, vomiting, and reflux. As many as 10–20% of patients may require follow-up surgery to address complications.

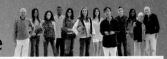
connect
ACTIVITY
DO IT ONLINE

Body Image and Gender

Women are much more likely than men to be dissatisfied with their bodies, often wanting to be thinner than they are. In one study, only 30% of eighth-grade girls reported being content with their bodies, while 70% of their male classmates expressed satisfaction with their looks. Girls and women are much more likely than boys and men to diet and develop eating disorders.

One reason that girls and women are dissatisfied with their bodies is that they are influenced by the media—particularly advertisements and women's fashion magazines. Most teen girls report that the media influence their idea of the perfect body and their decision to diet. In a study of adult women, viewing pictures of thin models in magazines had an immediate negative effect on their mood. In another study, 68% of female university/college students felt worse about their own appearance after looking through women's magazines. Some 75% of normal-weight women think they are overweight.

The image of the "perfect" woman presented in the media is often unrealistic and even unhealthy. In a review of BMI data for Miss America pageant winners since 1922, researchers noted a significant decline in BMI over time, with an increasing number of recent winners having BMIs in the "underweight" category. The average fashion model is 10–18 centimetres taller and 8 kilograms lighter than the average North American woman.

Our culture may be promoting an unattainable masculine ideal as well. Researchers studying male action figures such as GI Joe from the past 40 years noted that they have become increasingly muscular. A recent Batman action figure, if projected onto a man of average height, would result in someone with a 75-cm waist, 142-cm chest, and 67-cm biceps. Such media messages can be demoralizing; and although not as commonly, boys and men also suffer from body image problems.

Body Image and Ethnicity

Although some groups espouse thinness as an ideal body type, others do not. In many traditional African societies, for example, full-figured women's bodies are seen as symbols of health, prosperity, and fertility. African-Canadiann teenage girls have a much more positive body image than white girls; in one survey, two-thirds of them defined beauty as "the right attitude," whereas white girls were more preoccupied with weight and body shape. Nevertheless, recent evidence indicates that African-Canadian women are as likely to engage in disordered eating behaviour, especially binge eating and vomiting, as their First Nations, Métis, Inuit, and white counterparts. This finding underscores the complex nature of eating disorders and body image.

Avoiding Body Image Problems

To minimize your risk of developing a body image problem, keep the following strategies in mind:

- Focus on healthy habits and good physical health.

- Focus on good psychological health and put concerns about physical appearance in perspective. Your worth as a human being does not depend on how you look.

- Practise body acceptance. You can influence your body size and type through lifestyle to some degree, but the basic fact is that some people are genetically designed to be bigger or heavier than others.

- Find things to appreciate in yourself besides an idealized body image. People who can learn to value other aspects of themselves are more accepting of the physical changes that occur naturally with age.

- View eating as a morally neutral activity.—eating dessert isn't "bad" and doesn't make you a bad person. Healthy eating habits is an important part of a wellness lifestyle, but the things you really care about and do are more important in defining who you are.

- See the beauty and fitness industries for what they are. Realize that one of their goals is to prompt dissatisfaction with yourself so that you will buy their products.

Weight loss from surgery generally ranges between 40% and 70% of total body weight over the course of a year. The key to success is to have adequate follow-up and to stay motivated so that life behaviours and eating patterns are changed permanently.

The surgical technique of liposuction involves the removal of small amounts of fat from specific locations. Liposuction is not a method for treating obesity.

Psychological Help

When concern about body weight and shape have developed into an eating disorder, professional help is recommended. A therapist should have experience working with weight management, body image issues, eating disorders, addictions, and abuse issues.

8.6 BODY IMAGE

The collective picture of the body as seen through the mind's eye, **body image** consists of perceptions, images, thoughts, attitudes, and emotions. A negative body image is characterized by dissatisfaction with the body in general or some part of the body in particular. Dissatisfaction with body weight and shape is associated with dangerous eating patterns such as binge eating or self-starvation and with eating disorders.

body image The mental representation a person holds about her or his body at any given moment in time, consisting of perceptions, images, thoughts, attitudes, and emotions about the body.

TERMS

Severe Body Image Problems

Poor body image can cause significant psychological distress. A person can become preoccupied by a perceived defect in appearance, thereby damaging self-esteem and interfering with relationships. Adolescents and adults who have a negative body image are more likely to diet restrictively, eat compulsively, or develop some other form of disordered eating.

When dissatisfaction becomes extreme, the condition is called body dysmorphic disorder (BDD). BDD can begin in adolescence or adulthood, with complaints often focusing on slight "flaws" of the face or head—things that are not obvious to others. Individuals with BDD may spend hours every day thinking about their defect and looking at themselves in mirrors; they may desire and seek repeated cosmetic surgeries. BDD is related to obsessive-compulsive disorder and can lead to depression, social phobia, and suicide if left untreated. Medication and psychotherapy can help people with BDD.

In some cases, body image may bear little resemblance to fact. A person suffering from the eating disorder anorexia nervosa typically has a severely distorted body image believing herself to be fat even when she has become emaciated (see the next section for more on anorexia). Distorted body image is also a hallmark of *muscle dysmorphia,* a disorder experienced by some body builders in which they see themselves as small and out of shape despite being very muscular. People with muscle dysmorphia may let obsessive bodybuilding interfere with their work and relationships. They may also use steroids and other potentially dangerous muscle-building drugs.

To assess your own body image, complete the body image self-test in Lab 8.3.

Acceptance and Change

There are limits to the changes that can be made to body weight and body shape, both of which are influenced by heredity. Knowing when the limits to healthy change have been reached—and learning to accept those limits—is crucial for overall wellness. Women in particular tend to measure self-worth in terms of their appearance; when they don't measure up to an unrealistic cultural ideal, they may see themselves as defective, and their self-esteem falls. The result can be negative body image, disordered eating, or even a full-blown eating disorder (see the box "Gender, Ethnicity, and Body Image").

Weight management needs to take place in a positive and realistic atmosphere. For an obese person, losing as few as 4 kilograms can reduce blood pressure and improve mood. The hazards of excessive dieting and overconcern about body weight need to be countered by a change in attitude. A reasonable weight must take into account a person's weight history, social circumstances, metabolic profile, and psychological well-being.

LO4　8.7 EATING DISORDERS

Problems with body weight and weight control are not limited to excessive body fat. A growing number of people, especially adolescent girls and young women, experience **eating disorders**, characterized by severe disturbances in eating patterns and eating-related behaviour. The major eating disorders are anorexia nervosa, bulimia nervosa, and binge-eating disorder. More than 82 000 Canadians, most of them women, are at risk from suffering from an eating disorder.[12] Many more people have abnormal eating habits and attitudes about food that,

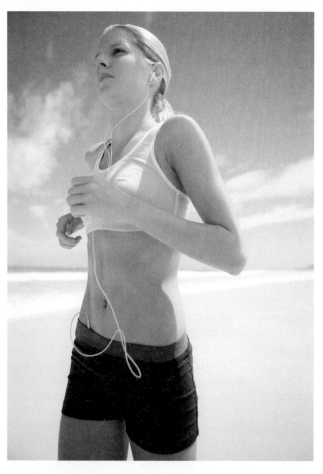

Exercise is a healthy practice, but people with eating disorders sometimes exercise compulsively, building their lives around their workouts. Compulsive exercise can lead to injuries, low body fat, and other health problems.

although not meeting the criteria for a full-blown eating disorder, do disrupt their lives (see the box "Borderline Disordered Eating"). To assess your eating habits, complete Lab 8.3.

Although many different explanations for the development of eating disorders have been proposed, they share one central feature: a dissatisfaction with body image and body weight. Such dissatisfaction is created by distorted thinking, including perfectionistic beliefs, unreasonable demands for self-control, and excessive self-criticism. Dissatisfaction with body weight leads to dysfunctional attitudes about eating, such as fear of fat, preoccupation with food, and problematic eating behaviours. Eating disorders are classified as mental disorders.

Anorexia Nervosa

A person suffering from **anorexia nervosa** does not eat enough food to maintain a reasonable body weight. A BMI of 17.5 or less is sometimes used as a diagnostic criterion for anorexia. Anorexia affects over 38 000 Canadians, 90% of them female. Although it can occur later, anorexia typically develops between the ages of 14 and 25.[13]

People with anorexia have an intense fear of gaining weight or becoming fat. Their body image is distorted so that even when emaciated, they think they are fat. People with anorexia may engage in compulsive behaviours or rituals that help keep them from eating. They also commonly use vigorous and prolonged physical activity to reduce body weight. Although they may express a great interest in food, their own diet becomes more and more extreme. People with anorexia are typically introverted, emotionally reserved, and socially insecure. Their entire sense of self-esteem may be tied up in their evaluation of their body shape and weight.

Anorexia nervosa has been linked to a variety of medical complications, including disorders of the cardiovascular, gastrointestinal, and endocrine systems. Because of extreme weight loss, females with anorexia often stop menstruating. When body fat is virtually gone and muscles are severely wasted, the body turns to its own organs in a desperate search for protein. Death can occur from heart failure caused by electrolyte imbalances. About 1 in 10 women with anorexia dies of starvation, cardiac arrest, or other medical complications—one of the highest death rates for any psychiatric disorder. Depression is also a serious risk, and about half the fatalities relating to anorexia are suicides.[14]

Bulimia Nervosa

A person suffering from **bulimia nervosa** engages in recurrent episodes of binge eating followed by **purging**. Although bulimia usually begins in adolescence or young adulthood, it has recently begun to emerge at increasingly younger (11–12 years) and older (40–60 years) ages.

Research suggests that about 5% of university/college-age women have bulimia.

During a binge, a bulimic person may consume anywhere from 1000 to 60 000 calories. This is followed by an attempt to get rid of the food by purging, usually by vomiting or using laxatives or diuretics. During a binge, people with bulimia feel as though they have lost control and cannot stop or limit how much they eat. Some binge and purge only occasionally; others do so many times every day. Binges may be triggered by a major life change or other stressful event. Binge eating and purging may become a way of dealing with difficult feelings such as anger and disappointment.

The binge-purge cycle of bulimia places a tremendous strain on the body and can have serious health effects, including tooth decay, esophageal damage and chronic hoarseness, menstrual irregularities, depression, liver and kidney damage, and cardiac arrhythmia. Bulimia is often difficult to recognize because sufferers conceal their eating habits and usually maintain a normal weight, although they may experience fluctuations of 4–7 kilograms. About 114 000 Canadian women suffer from bulimia.[15]

Binge-Eating Disorder

Binge-eating disorder is characterized by uncontrollable eating without any compensatory purging behaviours. Common eating patterns are eating more rapidly than normal, eating until uncomfortably full, eating when not hungry, and preferring to eat alone. Uncontrolled eating is usually followed by weight gain and feelings of guilt, shame, and depression. Many people with binge-eating disorder mistakenly see rigid dieting as the only solution to their problem. However, rigid dieting usually causes feelings of deprivation and a return to overeating.

Compulsive overeaters rarely eat because of hunger. Instead, they use food to cope with stress, conflict, and other difficult emotions or to provide solace or entertainment. Binge eaters are almost always obese, so they face all the health risks associated with obesity. In addition, binge eaters may have higher-than-average rates of depression and anxiety. Although Canadian statistics

TERMS

eating disorder A serious disturbance in eating patterns or eating-related behaviour, characterized by a negative body image and concerns about body weight or body fat.

anorexia nervosa An eating disorder characterized by a refusal to maintain body weight at a minimally healthy level and an intense fear of gaining weight or becoming fat; self-starvation.

bulimia nervosa An eating disorder characterized by recurrent episodes of binge eating and then purging to prevent weight gain.

purging The use of vomiting, laxatives, excessive exercise, restrictive dieting, enemas, diuretics, or diet pills to compensate for food that has been eaten and that the person fears will produce weight gain.

Borderline Disordered Eating

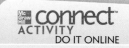
Mc Graw Hill connect™
ACTIVITY
DO IT ONLINE

For every person diagnosed with a full-blown eating disorder, there are many more who don't meet all the criteria but who have eating problems that significantly disrupt their lives. People with borderline disordered eating have some symptoms of eating disorders—for example, excessive dieting, occasional binging or purging—but do not meet the full diagnostic criteria for anorexia, bulimia, or binge-eating disorder.

Meaningful statistics about borderline disordered eating are hard to come by, in part because it is difficult to define exactly when eating habits cross the line between normal and disordered. However, experts feel that many Canadians, particularly women, have at least some unhealthy attitudes and behaviours in relation to food and self-image.

Ideally, our relationship to food should be a happy one. The biological urge to satisfy hunger is one of our most basic drives, and eating is associated with many pleasurable sensations. For some of us, food triggers pleasant memories of good times, family, holidays, and fun. But for too many people, food is a source of anguish rather than pleasure. Eating results in feelings of guilt and self-loathing rather than satisfaction. causing tremendous disruption in the lives of the affected individuals. And experts estimate that as many as one-quarter of people with borderline disordered eating will eventually develop a full eating disorder.

How do you know if you have disordered eating habits? When thoughts about weight and food dominate your life, you have a problem. If you're convinced that your worth as a person hinges on how you look and how much you weigh, it's time to get help. Self-induced vomiting or laxative use after meals, even if only once in a while, is reason for concern. Do you feel compelled to overexercise to compensate for what you've eaten? Do you routinely restrict your food intake and sometimes eat nothing in an effort to feel more in control? These are all danger signs and could mean that you are developing a serious problem. Lab 8.3 can help you determine whether you are at risk for an eating disorder.

What can you do if you suspect you have an eating problem? Eating problems tend to become worse when you cloak them in secrecy. Check with your student health or counselling centre—nearly all universities and colleges have counsellors and medical personnel who can help you or refer you to a specialist if needed. If you are intimidated about asking for help, an easy first step is to learn more about eating problems online by visiting a reliable website; several good resources are listed in the For Further Exploration section at the end of the chapter.

---

have not been collected, binge-eating disorder is the most prevalent eating disorder among Americans with 2–5% of all U.S. adults suffering from the disorder.[16]

Treating Eating Disorders

The treatment of eating disorders must address both problematic eating behaviours and the misuse of food to manage stress and emotions. Treatment for anorexia nervosa first involves averting a medical crisis by restoring adequate body weight; then the psychological aspects of the disorder can be addressed. The treatment of bulimia nervosa or binge-eating disorder involves first stabilizing the eating patterns, then identifying and changing the patterns of thinking that lead to disordered eating. Treatment usually involves a combination of psychotherapy, medication, and medical management. Friends and family members often want to know what they can do to help someone with an eating disorder. For suggestions, see the box "If Someone You Know Has an Eating Disorder . . ."

People with milder patterns of disordered eating may benefit from getting a nutrition checkup with a registered dietician. A professional can help determine appropriate body weight and calorie intake and offer advice on how to budget calories into a balanced, healthy diet.

LO5 8.8 CREATING AN INDIVIDUAL WEIGHT-MANAGEMENT PLAN

Here are some strategies for creating a program of weight management that will last a lifetime.

Assess Your Motivation and Commitment

Before starting your weight-management program, take a fresh look within and assess your motivation and commitment. The point is not only to achieve success but also to guard against frustration, negative changes in self-esteem, and the sense of failure that attends broken resolutions or "yo-yo dieting." Think about the reasons you want to lose weight. Self-focused reasons, such as to feel good about yourself or to have a greater sense of well-being, can often lead to success. Trying to lose weight for others or out of concern for how others view you is a poor foundation for a weight-management program. Make a list of your reasons for wanting to manage your weight and post it in a prominent place.

Set Reasonable Goals

Choose a goal weight or body fat percentage that is both healthy and reasonable. Refer to the calculations you completed in Lab 6.2 to arrive at a goal. Be sure to use Chapter 1 (SMART Goals) as a starting point for setting your goals. Subdivide your long-term goal into a series of short-term goals. Be willing to renegotiate your final goal as your program moves along.

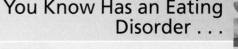
Secrecy and denial are two hallmarks of eating disorders, so it can be hard to know if someone has anorexia or bulimia. Signs that a friend may have anoriexia include sudden weight loss, excessive dieting or exercise, guilt or preoccupation with food and eating, frequent weighing, fear of becoming fat despite being thin, and baggy or layered clothes to conceal weight loss. Signs that someone may have bulimia include excessive eating without weight gain, secretiveness about food (stealing, hiding, or hoarding food), self-induced vomiting (bathroom visits during or after a meal), swollen glands or puffy face, erosion of tooth enamel, and use of laxatives, diuretics, or diet pills to control weight.

If you decide to approach a friend with your concerns, here are some tips to follow:

- Find out about treatment resources in your community. (See For Further Exploration for suggestions.) You may want to consult a professional at your school clinic or counselling centre about the best way to approach the situation.

- Arrange to speak with your friend in a private place, and allow enough time to talk.

- Express your concerns, with specific observations of your friend's behaviour. Expect him or her to deny or minimize the problem and possibly to become angry with you. Stay calm and nonjudgmental, and continue to express your concern.

- Avoid giving simplistic advice about eating habits. Listen if your friend wants to talk, and offer your support and understanding. Give your friend the information you found about where he or she can get help, and offer to go along.

- If the situation is an emergency—if your friend has fainted, for example, or attempted suicide, for example—call 911 for help immediately.

- If you are upset about the situation, consider talking to someone yourself. The professionals at the clinic or counselling centre are there to help you. Remember, you are not to blame for another person's eating disorder.

Assess Your Current Energy Balance

To lose the recommended 0.25–1 kg a week, you'll need to create a negative energy balance of between 1750 and 7000 calories a week, or 250–1000 calories a day. (No diet should reduce calorie intake below 1500 a day for men or 1200 a day for women.) Complete Labs 8.1 and 8.2 to assess your current daily energy needs and to develop strategies for achieving a negative energy balance that will lead to gradual, moderate weight loss. (See the *Common Questions Answered* section of this chapter for guidelines for altering your energy balance to *gain* weight.)

Research clearly shows support for the maintenance of a negative energy balance for success in any weight loss program. In fact, studies examining diet-only versus exercise-only behaviour change programs suggest that either can be an effective method.[17] By the same token, combining diet and exercise to create a negative energy balance has been proven to be even more effective in immediate and long-term weight loss.[18]

Increase Your Level of Physical Activity

To generate a negative energy balance, it's usually best to exercise more rather than eat less. One reason is that dieting reduces RMR, whereas exercise raises it. Furthermore, studies have shown that being physically fit is even more important than weight loss in reducing your mortality risk (see Chapter 6). The key is keeping fit with moderate exercise—Figure 2.1 describes Health Canada's suggestions for adding exercise to your lifestyle.

Table 8.2 lists the calorie costs of selected physical activities; refer to Table 9.1 for examples of different aerobic activities and their intensities.

Make Changes in Your Diet and Eating Habits

If you can't generate a large enough negative calorie balance solely by increasing physical activity, you may want to supplement exercise with some dietary strategies. Don't think of this as "going on a diet"; your goal is to make small changes in your diet that you can maintain for a lifetime. Don't try skipping meals, fasting, or a very-low-calorie diet. These strategies seldom work, and they can have negative effects on your ability to manage your weight and on your overall health. Instead, try monitoring calories or simply cutting portion sizes. Refer back to the box "Lifestyle Strategies for Successful Weight Management" for suggestions.

Put Your Plan into Action

Be systematic in your efforts to change your behaviour, both what you eat and how you exercise. Many of those who are successful at controlling their weight track their progress in writing, enlist the support of others, and think positively.

WRITE DAILY Write down everything you eat, including how many calories it contains. (See Figure 1.6 for one example of a food journal.) Researchers have found that writing down the food choices you make every day increases your commitment and helps you stick to your diet, especially during high-risk times such as holidays, parties, and family gatherings. Writing every day also serves as a reminder to you that losing weight is important.

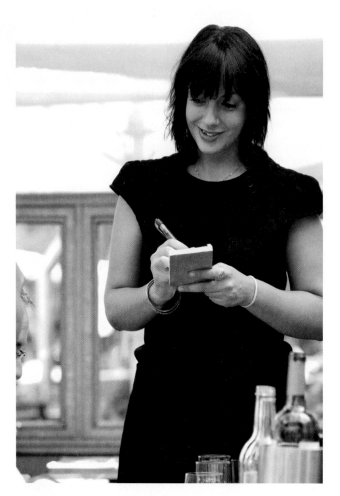

A food journal can be an important part of a weight-management plan.

GET OTHERS TO HELP Enlist friends and family members to help and give them specific suggestions about what you would find helpful. You might, for instance, ask someone to leave you an encouraging voice mail once a day or twice a week, or ask someone to send you reminders by email or phone. Besides asking for regular moral support, find a buddy to work out with you regularly and to be there as an emergency support.

THINK POSITIVELY Give yourself lots of praise and rewards. Think about your accomplishments each day, and congratulate yourself. You can write these positive thoughts in your food journal. If you do slip, stay objective and don't waste time on self-criticism. If you are keeping a journal, you can see the slip for what it is—an easily contained lapse rather than a catastrophic relapse that ends in your losing confidence and control. Remember that as weight loss slows, the weight loss at this slower rate is more permanent than earlier, more dramatic losses.

TIPS FOR TODAY AND THE FUTURE

Many weight management approaches work, but the simplest formula is moderate food intake coupled with regular exercise.

RIGHT NOW YOU CAN

- Assess your weight-management needs. Do you need to gain weight, lose weight, or stay at your current weight?
- List five things you can do to add more lifestyle activity (not exercise) to your daily routine.
- Identify the foods you regularly eat that may be sabotaging your ability to manage your weight.
- Start a journal to identify ways that you plan to incorporate healthy lifestyle choices.

IN THE FUTURE YOU CAN

- Make an honest assessment of your current body image. Is it accurate and fair, or is it unduly negative and unhealthy? If your body image presents a problem, consider getting professional advice on how to view yourself realistically.
- Keep track of your energy needs to determine whether your energy-balance equation is correct. Use this information as part of your long-term weight-management efforts.

Besides keeping track of what you eat, keep track of your formal exercise program and other daily physical activities so you can begin increasing either their intensity or duration. People who succeed in their health program expend lots of energy in physical activity—according to one study, an average of 2700 calories a week. Popular activities are walking, cycling, aerobic dance, and stair climbing.

SUMMARY

- Excess body weight increases the risk of numerous diseases, particularly cardiovascular disease, cancer, and diabetes.
- Although genetic factors help determine a person's weight, the influence of heredity can be overcome.
- Physiological factors involved in the regulation of body weight and body fat include metabolic rate and hormones.

- Energy-balance components that an individual can control are calories taken in and calories expended in physical activity.
- Nutritional guidelines for weight management and wellness include controlling consumption of total calories, unhealthy fats and carbohydrates, and protein; monitoring portion sizes and calorie density; increasing consumption of whole grains, fruits, and vegetables.

How can I safely gain weight?

Just as for losing weight, a program for weight gain should be gradual and should include both exercise and dietary changes. The foundation of a successful and healthy program for weight gain is a combination of strength training and a high-carbohydrate, high-calorie diet. Strength training is critical because it will help you add weight as muscle rather than fat.

Energy balance is also important in a program for gaining weight. You need to consume more calories than your body needs in order to gain weight, but you need to choose those extra calories wisely. Fatty, high-calorie foods may seem like an obvious choice, but consuming additional calories as fat can jeopardize your health and your weight-management program. A diet high in fat carries health risks, including increased risk of cardiovascular disease and certain types of cancer. A better strategy is to consume additional calories as complex carbohydrates from whole grains, fruits, and vegetables. A diet for weight gain should contain about 60–65% of total daily calories from carbohydrates. You probably do not need to be concerned with protein: Although protein requirements increase when you exercise, the protein consumption of most Canadians is already well above the Recommended Nutrient Intake (RNI).

In order to gain primarily muscle weight instead of fat, a gradual program of weight gain is your best bet. Try these strategies for consuming extra calories:

- Don't skip any meals.
- Add two or three snacks to your daily eating routine.
- Try a sports drink or supplement that has at least 60% of calories from carbohydrates, as well as significant amounts of protein, vitamins, and minerals. (But don't use supplements to replace meals, because they don't contain all food components.)

How can I achieve a "perfect" body?

The current cultural ideal of an ultra-thin, ultrafit body is impossible for most people to achieve. A reasonable goal for body weight and body shape must take into account an individual's heredity, weight history, social circumstances, metabolic rate, and psychological well-being. Don't set goals based on movie stars or fashion models. Modern photographic techniques can make people look much different on film or in magazines than they do in person. Many of these people are also genetically endowed with body shapes that are impossible for us to emulate. The best approach is to work with what you've got. Adopting a wellness lifestyle that includes regular exercise and a healthy diet will naturally result in the best possible body shape for you. Obsessively trying to achieve unreasonable goals can lead to problems such as eating disorders, overtraining, and injuries.

- Activity guidelines for weight control emphasize engaging in moderate-intensity physical activity for 150 minutes or more per week; regular, prolonged endurance exercise and weight training can burn a significant number of calories while maintaining muscle mass.
- The sense of well-being that results from a well-balanced diet can reinforce commitment to weight control; improve self-esteem; and lead to realistic, as opposed to negative, self-talk. Successful weight management results in not using food as a way to cope with stress.
- In cases of extreme obesity, weight loss requires medical supervision; in less extreme cases, people can set up individual programs, perhaps getting guidance from reliable books, or they can get help by joining a formal weight-loss program.
- Dissatisfaction with body image and body weight can lead to physical problems and serious eating disorders, including anorexia nervosa, bulimia nervosa, and binge-eating disorder.
- A successful personal plan assesses motivation, sets reasonable and healthy goals, and emphasizes increased activity rather than decreased calories.

FOR FURTHER EXPLORATION

Organizations and Websites

Canadian Obesity Network. Provides news, events, and resources related to obesity in Canada.
http://www.obesitynetwork.ca/

Cyberdiet. Provides a variety of assessment and planning tools as well as practical tips for eating a healthy diet and being physically active.
http://www.cyberdiet.com

Health Canada—Food and Nutrition. Answers questions dealing with food consumption, active lifestyles, and other relevant areas.
http://www.hc-sc.gc.ca/fn-an/index_e.html

MedlinePlus: Obesity and Weight Loss. Provides news and links to reliable information from government agencies and key professional associations.
http://www.nlm.nih.gov/medlineplus/obesity.html
http://www.nlm.nih.gov/medlineplus/weightlossdieting.html

Public Health Agency of Canada. A valuable source of timely, trusted and credible information on healthy living.

http://www.phac-aspc.gc.ca/index-eng.php

WHO: Obesity and Overweight. Provides information on WHO's global strategy on diet and physical activity.

http://www.who.int/dietphysicalactivity

There are also many resources for people concerned about body image and eating disorders:

MedlinePlus: Eating Disorders

http://www.nlm.nih.gov/medlineplus/eatingdisorders.html

National Eating Disorder Information Centre. Resource for information on eating disorders and weight preoccupation.

http://www.nedic.ca/

Women's Body Image and Health

http://www.4woman.gov/bodyimage

See also the listings in Chapters 1, 6, and 7.

LAB 8.1 Calculating Daily Energy Needs

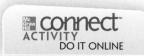

Part I Estimating Current Energy Intake from a Food Record

If your weight is stable, your current daily energy intake is the number of calories you need to consume to maintain your weight at your current activity level. Keep a careful and complete record of everything you eat for one day and then total the calories in all the foods and beverages you consumed. (This calculation can be done by hand or by using a nutrition analysis software program.) Record your total energy intake below:

Current energy intake (from food record): _____ Calories per day

Part II Estimating Daily Energy Requirements Using Food and Nutrition Board Formulas

Many people underestimate the size of their food portions, and so energy goals based on estimates of current calorie intake from food records can be inaccurate. You can also estimate your daily energy needs using the formulas listed below. To use the appropriate formula for your sex, you'll need to plug in the following:

- Age (in years)
- Weight (in pounds)
- Height (in inches)
- Physical activity coefficient (PA) from the table below.

To help estimate your physical activity level, consider the following guidelines: Someone who typically engages in 30 minutes of moderate intensity activity, equivalent to walking 3.2 kilometres in 30 minutes, in addition to the activities in maintaining a sedentary lifestyle is considered "low active;" someone who typically engages in the equivalent of 90 minutes of moderate intensity activity is rated as "active." You might find it helpful to refer back to Lab 2.2 to estimate your physical activity level.

	Physical Activity Coefficient (PA)	
Physical Activity Level	Men	Women
Sedentary	1.00	1.00
Low active	1.12	1.14
Active	1.27	1.27
Very active	1.54	1.45

Estimated Daily Energy Requirement for Weight Maintenance in Men

$$864 - (9.72 \times age) + (PA \times [(6.39 \times weight) + (12.78 \times height)])$$

1. $9.72 \times$ _____ Age (years) = _____

2. $864 -$ _____ Result from step 1 = _____ [result may be a negative number]

3. $6.39 \times$ _____ Weight (pounds) = _____

4. $12.78 \times$ _____ Height (inches) = _____

5. _____ result from step 3 + _____ result from step 4 = _____

6. _____ PA (from table) × _____ result from step 5 = _____

7. _____ result from step 2 + _____ result from

   step 6 = _____ calories per day

Estimated Daily Energy Requirement for Weight Maintenance in Women

$$387 - (7.31 \times \text{age}) + (\text{PA} \times [(4.91 \times \text{weight}) + (16.78 \times \text{height})])$$

1. 7.31 × _____ Age (years) = _____

2. 387 − _____ Result from step 1 = _____ [result may be a negative number]

3. 4.91 × _____ Weight (pounds) = _____

4. 16.78 × _____ Height (inches) = _____

5. _____ result from step 3 + _____ result from step 4 = _____

6. _____ PA (from table) × _____ result from step 5 = _____

7. _____ result from step 2 + _____ result from

   step 6 = _____ calories per day

Daily energy needs for weight maintenance (from formula): _____ calories/day

Part III Determining an Individual Daily Energy Goal for Weight Maintenance

If you calculated values for daily energy needs based on both methods, examine the two values. Some difference is likely—people tend to underestimate their food intake and overestimate their level of physical activity—but if the two values are very far off, check your food record and your physical activity estimate for accuracy and make any necessary adjustments. For an individualized estimate of daily calorie needs, average the two values:

Daily energy needs = (**food record result _____ calories/day + formula result _____ calories/day)**
÷ 2 = _____ calories/day

Using Your Results

How did you score? Are you surprised by the value you calculated for your approximate daily energy needs? If so, is the value higher or lower than you expected?

What should you do next? Enter the results of this lab in the Preprogram Assessment column in Appendix C. If you wish to change your energy balance to lose weight, complete Lab 8.2 to set goals and develop specific strategies for change. (If your goal is weight gain, see the *Common Questions Answered* section of this chapter for basic guidelines.) One of the best ways to tip your energy balance toward weight loss is to increase your daily physical activity. If you include increases in activity as part of your program, then you can use the results of this lab to chart changes in your daily energy expenditure (and needs). Look for ways to increase the amount of time you spend in physical activity, thus increasing your physical activity coefficient. After several weeks of your program, complete this lab again, and enter the results in the Postprogram Assessment column of Appendix C. How do the results compare? Did your program for boosting physical activity show up as an increase in your daily energy expenditure and need?

SOURCE: Estimating Daily Energy Requirements Using Food and Nutrition Board Formulas Part II: Reprinted with permission from *Dietary Reference Intakes for Energy, Carbohydrate, Fiber, Fat, Fatty Acids, Cholesterol, Protein, and Amino Acids (Macronutrients)*. Reprinted with permission from the National Academies Press, Copyright 2005, National Academy of Sciences.

LAB 8.2 Identifying Weight-Loss Goals and Ways to Meet Them

Mc Graw Hill connect
ACTIVITY
DO IT ONLINE

Negative Calorie Balance

Complete the following calculations to determine your weekly and daily negative calorie balance goals and the number of weeks to achieve your target weight.

Current weight _____ kg − target weight (from Lab 6.2) _____ kg = total weight to lose _____ kg

Total weight to lose _____ kg ÷ weight to lose each week _____ kg = time to achieve target weight _____ weeks

Weight to lose each week _____ kg × 7700 cal/kg = weekly negative calorie balance _____ cal/week

Weekly negative calorie balance _____ cal/week ÷ 7 days/week = daily negative calorie balance _____ cal/day

To keep your weight-loss program on schedule, you must achieve the daily negative calorie balance by either decreasing your calorie consumption (eating less) or increasing your calorie expenditure (being more active). A combination of the two strategies will probably be most successful.

Changes in Activity Level

Adding a few minutes of exercise every day is a good way of expending calories. Use the calorie costs for different activities listed in Table 8.2 to plan ways for raising your calorie expenditure level.

Activity	Duration	Calories Used
_____	_____	_____
_____	_____	_____
_____	_____	_____
	Total calories expended:	_____

Changes in Diet

Look closely at your diet from one day, as recorded in Lab 7.2. Identify ways to cut calorie consumption by eliminating certain items or substituting lower-calorie choices. Be realistic in your cuts and substitutions; you need to develop a plan you can live with.

Food Item	Substitute Food item	Calorie Savings
_____	_____	_____
_____	_____	_____
_____	_____	_____
	Total calories expended:	_____

Total calories expended _____ + total calories cut _____ = Total negative calorie balance _____

Have you met your required negative energy balance? If not, revise your dietary and activity changes to meet your goal.

LABORATORY ACTIVITIES

Common Problem Eating Behaviours

For each of the groups of statements that appear below, check those that are true for you. If you check several statements for a given pattern or problem, it will probably be a significant factor in your weight-management program. One possible strategy for dealing with each type of problem is given. For those eating problems you identify as important, add your own ideas to the strategies listed.

1. _____ I often skip meals.

   _____ I often eat a number of snacks in place of a meal.

   _____ I don't have a regular schedule of meal and snack times.

   _____ I make up for missed meals and snacks by eating more at the next meal.

   Problem: Irregular eating habits

   Possible solutions:

   • Write out a plan for each day's meals in advance. Carry it with you and stick to it.

   • _____

   • _____

2. _____ I eat more than one sweet dessert or snack each day.

   _____ I usually snack on foods high in calories and fat (chips, cookies, ice cream).

   _____ I drink regular (not sugar-free) soft drinks.

   _____ I choose types of meat that are high in fat.

   _____ I consume more than one alcoholic beverage a day.

   Problem: Poor food choices

   Possible solutions:

   • Keep a supply of raw fruits or vegetables handy for snacks.

   • _____

   • _____

3. _____ I always eat everything on my plate.

   _____ I often go back for seconds and thirds.

   _____ I take larger helpings than most people.

   _____ I eat up leftovers instead of putting them away.

   Problem: Portion sizes too large

   Possible solutions:

   • Measure all portions with a scale or measuring cup.

   • _____

   • _____

LAB 8.3 Checking for Body Image Problems and Eating Disorders

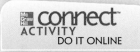

Assessing Your Body Image

	Never	Sometimes	Often	Always
1. I dislike seeing myself in mirrors.	0	1	2	3
2. When I shop for clothing, I am more aware of my weight problem, and consequently I find shopping for clothes somewhat unpleasant.	0	1	2	3
3. I'm ashamed to be seen in public.	0	1	2	3
4. I prefer to avoid engaging in sports or public exercise because of my appearance.	0	1	2	3
5. I feel somewhat embarrassed about my body in the presence of someone of the other sex.	0	1	2	3
6. I think my body is ugly.	0	1	2	3
7. I feel that other people must think my body is unattractive.	0	1	2	3
8. I feel that my family or friends may be embarrassed to be seen with me.	0	1	2	3
9. I find myself comparing myself with other people to see if they are heavier than I am.	0	1	2	3
10. I find it difficult to enjoy activities because I am self-conscious about my physical appearance.	0	1	2	3
11. Feeling guilty about my weight problem preoccupies most of my thinking.	0	1	2	3
12. My thoughts about my body and physical appearance are negative and self-critical.	0	1	2	3

Now add up the number of points you have circled in each column: _____ _____ + _____ + _____ + _____

Score Interpretation

The lowest possible score is 0, and this indicates a positive body image. The highest possible score is 36, and this indicates an unhealthy body image. A score higher than 14 suggests a need to develop a healthier body image.

SOURCE: Nash, J. D. 1997. *The New Maximize Your Body Potential.* Palo Alto, Calif.: Bull Publishing. Reprinted with permission of the publisher.

Eating Disorder Checklist

	Always	Very Often	Often	Sometimes	Rarely	Never
1. I like eating with other people.	0	0	0	1	2	3
2. I like my clothes to fit tightly.	0	0	0	1	2	3
3. I enjoy eating meat.	0	0	0	1	2	3
4. I have regular menstrual periods.	0	0	0	1	2	3
5. I enjoy eating at restaurants.	0	0	0	1	2	3
6. I enjoy trying new rich foods.	0	0	0	1	2	3
7. I prepare foods for others, but do not eat what I cook.	3	2	1	0	0	0
8. I become anxious prior to eating.	3	2	1	0	0	0
9. I am terrified about being overweight.	3	2	1	0	0	0
10. I avoid eating when I am hungry.	3	2	1	0	0	0
11. I find myself preoccupied with food.	3	2	1	0	0	0

12. I have gone on eating binges where I feel that I may not be able to stop.	3	2	1	0	0	0.
13. I cut my food into small pieces.	3	2	1	0	0	0
14. I am aware of the calorie content of foods that I eat.	3	2	1	0	0	0
15. I particularly avoid foods with a high carbohydrate content (bread, potatoes, rice, etc.).	3	2	1	0	0	0
16. I feel bloated after meals.	3	2	1	0	0	0
17. I feel others would prefer me to eat more.	3	2	1	0	0	0
18. I vomit after I have eaten.	3	2	1	0	0	0
19. I feel extremely guilty after eating.	3	2	1	0	0	0
20. I am preoccupied with a desire to be thinner.	3	2	1	0	0	0
21. I exercise strenuously to burn off calories.	3	2	1	0	0	0
22. I weigh myself several times a day.	3	2	1	0	0	0
23. I wake up early in the morning.	3	2	1	0	0	0
24. I eat the same foods day after day.	3	2	1	0	0	0
25. I think about burning up calories when I exercise.	3	2	1	0	0	0
26. Other people think I am too thin.						
27. I am preoccupied with the thought of having fat on my body.	3	2	1	0	0	0
28. I take longer than others to eat my meals.	3	2	1	0	0	0
29. I take laxatives.	3	2	1	0	0	0
30. I avoid foods with sugar in them.	3	2	1	0	0	0
31. I eat diet foods.	3	2	1	0	0	0
32. I feel that food controls my life.	3	2	1	0	0	0
33. I display self-control around food.	3	2	1	0	0	0
34. I feel that others pressure me to eat.	3	2	1	0	0	0
35. I give too much time and thought to food.	3	2	1	0	0	0
36. I suffer from constipation.	3	2	1	0	0	0
37. I feel uncomfortable after eating sweets.	3	2	1	0	0	0
38. I engage in dieting behaviour.	3	2	1	0	0	0
39. I like my stomach to be empty.	3	2	1	0	0	0
40. I have the impulse to vomit after meals.	3	2	1	0	0	0

Now add up the number of points in each column for ____ + ____ + ____ + ____ + ____ + ____
statements 1 through 40: _____

Score Interpretation

The possible range is 0–120. A score higher than 50 suggests an eating disorder. A score between 30 and 50 suggests a borderline eating disorder. A score less than 30 is within the normal range. Among those with normal eating habits, the average score is 15.4.

SOURCE: Garner, D. M., Omstead, M., Polivy, J., Development and Validation of a Multidimensional Eating Disorder Inventory for Anorexia Nervosa and Bulimia. *International Journal of Eating Disorders* 2:15–33, 1983. Copyright © 1983 John Wiley & Sons. Reprinted by permission of John Wiley & Sons, Inc.

Using Your Results

How did you score? Are you surprised by your scores? Do the results of either assessment indicate that you may have a problem with body image or disordered eating?

What should you do next? If your results are borderline, consider trying some of the self-help strategies suggested in the chapter. If body image or disordered eating is a significant problem for you, get professional advice; a physician, therapist, and/or registered dietitian can help. Make an appointment today.

CHAPTER 9

PUTTING TOGETHER A COMPLETE FITNESS PROGRAM

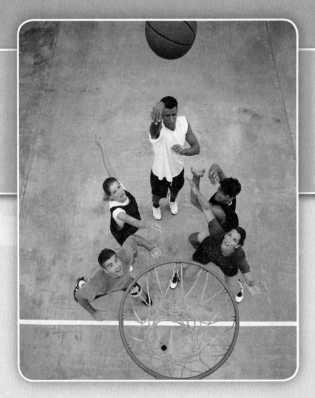

LEARNING OBJECTIVES

After reading this chapter, you should be able to

LO1 List the steps for putting together a successful personal fitness program

LO2 Describe strategies that can help you maintain a fitness program over the long term

LO3 Tailor a fitness program to accommodate special health concerns and different life stages

TEST YOUR KNOWLEDGE

1. **Swimming is a total fitness activity that develops all the components of health-related fitness.**

   True or false?

2. **Older adults should avoid exercise to protect themselves against falls and injuries.**

   True or false?

3. **Participation at a moderate level will burn more calories during which activity?**

   a. soccer
   b. rope skipping
   c. swimming

ANSWERS

1. **FALSE.** Swimming is excellent for developing cardiorespiratory endurance and muscular endurance, but because it is not a weight-bearing activity, it tends to reduce bone density. Swimmers are advised to include weight training in their exercise program to maintain bone mass.

2. **FALSE.** Older adults receive the same health benefits from exercise as younger adults, including improvements in strength, body composition, cardiorespiratory health, flexibility, balance, stability, and cognitive functioning. A far greater danger is posed by inactivity.

3. **B.** Moderate rope skipping burns more calories per minute than soccer or swimming. At a vigorous level of participation, all three are comparable.

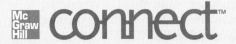

Practise and learn online with Connect.

Understanding the benefits of physical fitness, as explained in Chapters 1–8, is the first step toward creating a well-rounded exercise program. The next challenge is to choose and combine activities into a program that develops all the components of fitness and helps you stay motivated. This chapter presents a step-by-step plan for creating and maintaining a well-rounded program. At the end of this chapter, you'll find sample programs based on popular activities. These programs provide structure that can be helpful if you're beginning an exercise program for the first time.

LO1   9.1 DEVELOPING A PERSONAL FITNESS PLAN

If you're ready to create a complete fitness program based around the activities you enjoy most, begin by preparing the program plan and contract in Lab 9.1. By carefully developing your plan and signing a contract, you'll increase your chances of success. The step-by-step procedure outlined here will guide you through the steps of Lab 9.1 to create an exercise program that's right for you. (See Figure 9.1 for a sample personal fitness program plan and contract.)

1. Set Goals

Ask yourself, "What do I want from my fitness program?" Develop different types of goals—general and specific, long term and short term. General or long-term goals might include things like lowering your risk for chronic disease, improving posture, having more energy, and improving the fit of your clothes.

It's a good idea to also develop some specific, short-term goals based on measurable factors. Specific goals might be

- Raising cardiorespiratory capacity ($\dot{V}O_{2max}$) by 10%
- Reducing the time it takes you to jog 5 kilometres from 22 minutes to 19 minutes
- Increasing the number of push-ups you can do from 15 to 25
- Lowering BMI from 26 to 24.5.

Having specific goals will allow you to track your progress and enjoy the measurable changes brought about by your fitness program. Finally, break your specific goals into several smaller steps (mini-goals), such as those shown in Figure 9.1. (For detailed discussions of goals and goal setting in a behaviour change or fitness program, refer back to Chapters 1 and 2.)

Physical fitness assessment tests—as described in Chapters 3–6—are essential to determining your goals. They help you decide which types of exercise you should emphasize, and they help you understand the relative difficulty of attaining specific goals. If you have health problems, such as high blood pressure, heart disease, obesity,

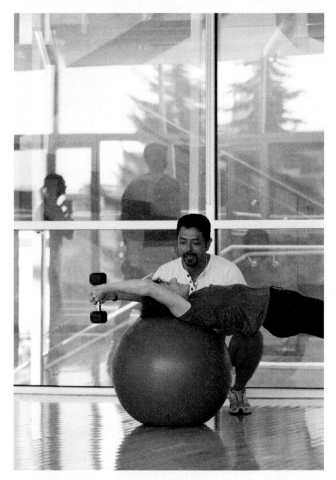

An overall fitness program includes exercises to develop all the components of physical fitness.

or serious joint or muscle disabilities, see your physician before taking assessment tests. Measure your progress by taking these tests about every 3 months.

2. Select Activities

If you have already chosen activities and used the FITT principle to create separate program plans for different fitness components in Chapters 3–5, you can put those plans together into a single program. It's usually best to include exercises to develop each of the health-related components of fitness:

- Cardiorespiratory endurance is developed by activities that involve continuous rhythmic movements of large-muscle groups like those in the legs (see Chapter 3).
- Muscular strength and endurance are developed by training against resistance (see Chapter 4).
- Flexibility is developed by stretching the major muscle groups (see Chapter 5).
- Healthy body composition can be developed by combining a sensible diet and a program of regular exercise, including cardiorespiratory endurance exercise to burn calories and resistance training to build muscle mass (see Chapter 6).

A. I [Tracie Kaufman] am contracting with myself to follow a physical
   (name)
fitness program to work toward the following goals:

Specific or short-term goals

1. Improving cardiorespiratory fitness by raising my $\dot{V}O_{2max}$ from 34 to 37 ml/kg/min
2. Improving upper body muscular strength and endurance rating from fair to good
3. Improving body composition (from 28% to 25% body fat)
4. Improving my tennis game (hitting 20 playable shots in a row against the ball machine)

General or long-term goals

1. Developing a more positive attitude about myself
2. Improving the fit of my clothes
3. Building and maintaining bone mass to reduce my risk of osteoporosis
4. Increasing my life expectancy and reducing my risk for diabetes and heart disease

B. **My program plan is as follows:**

Activities	Components (Check X)					Time	Frequency (Check X)							Intensity*
	CRE	MS	ME	F	BC		M	Tu	W	Th	F	S	S	
Swimming	X	X	X	X	X	35min	X		X		X			140–170 bpm
Tennis	X	X	X	X	X	90min					X			RPE = 13–16
Weight training		X	X	X	X	30min		X		X		X		see Lab 4.3
Stretching				X		25min	X		X		X	X		—

*List your target heart rate range or an RPE value if appropriate.

C. My program will begin on Sept. ⬍ 21 ⬍ My program includes the following schedule
   of mini-goals. For each step in my program, I will give myself the reward listed.

Completing 2 full weeks of program (mini-goal 1)	Oct. ⬍ 5 ⬍	movie with friends (reward)
$\dot{V}O_{2max}$ of 35 ml/kg/min (mini-goal 2)	Nov. ⬍ 2 ⬍	new CD (reward)
Completing 10 full weeks of program (mini-goal 3)	Nov. ⬍ 30 ⬍	new sweater (reward)
Percent body fat of 27% (mini-goal 4)	Dec. ⬍ 22 ⬍	weekend away (reward)
$\dot{V}O_{2max}$ of 36 ml/kg/min (mini-goal)	Jan. ⬍ 18 ⬍	new CD (reward)

D. My program will include the addition of physical activity to my daily routine (such
   as climbing stairs or walking to class):

1. Walking to and from campus job
2. Taking the stairs to dorm room instead of elevator
3. Bicycling to the library instead of driving
4. Doing one active chore a day
5.

E. I will use the following tools to monitor my program and my progress toward
   my goals:

I'll use a chart that lists the number of laps and minutes I swim and the
charts for strength and flexibility from Labs 4.3 & 5.2.

I sign this contract as an indication of my personal commitment to reach my goal.

Tracie Kaufman   Sep. ⬍ 10 ⬍
(your signature)

I have recruited a helper who will witness my contract and

swim with me three days per week

(list any way your helper will participate in your program)

Russell Walker   Sep. ⬍ 10 ⬍
(witness's signature)

FIGURE 9.1 A sample personal fitness program plan and contract.

Although some research indicates that pre-workout stretching can reduce muscle power and interfere with motor control, there are benefits to stretching after running. You can increase flexibility by doing stretching exercises as part of your cool-down.

The Conference Board of Canada reported that Canadians participate in a vast number of sports but tend to concentrate their energy expenditures on a few—ice hockey, golf, baseball, skiing, and soccer are the top 5 sports participated in by Canadians.[1]

Table 9.1 shows the intensity levels of several popular activities that promote health. Check the ratings of the activities you're considering to make sure the program you put together will help you achieve your goals. The Public Health Agency of Canada also provides age-specific recommendations on their website at www.phac-aspc.gc.ca/hp-ps/hl-mvs/pa-ap/index-eng.php.

If you select activities that support your commitment rather than activities that turn exercise into a chore, the right program will be its own incentive for continuing. Consider the following factors in making your choices:

- *Fun and interest.* Your fitness program is much more likely to be successful if you choose activities that you enjoy doing. Start by considering any activities you currently engage in and enjoy. If you want to add a new activity to your program, it is a good idea to try it for a while before committing to it. Table 9.2 shows a number of popular recreational activities you may enjoy. (See the box "Can Stability Balls Be Part of a Safe and Effective Fitness Program?")

- *Your current skill and fitness level.* Although many activities are appropriate for beginners, some sports and activities require a moderate level of skill to obtain fitness benefits. For example, a beginning tennis player will probably not be able to sustain rallies

long enough to develop cardiorespiratory endurance. A better choice might be a walking program while you improve your tennis game. To build skill for a particular activity, consider taking a class or getting some instruction from a coach or fellow participant.

- *Time and convenience.* You are more likely to maintain a long-term exercise program if you can easily fit exercise into your daily routine. As you consider activities, think about whether a special location or facility is required. Can you participate in the activity close to your residence, school, or job? Are the necessary facilities available at convenient times (see Lab 9.2)? Can you participate in the activity year-round, or will you need to find an alternative during the summer or winter? Would a home treadmill make you more likely to exercise regularly?

- *Cost.* Some sports and activities require equipment, fees, or some type of membership investment. If you are on a tight budget, limit your choices to activities that are inexpensive or free. Investigate the facilities on your campus, which you may be able to use at little or no cost. Many activities require no equipment beyond an appropriate pair of shoes.

- *Special health needs.* If you have special exercise needs due to a particular health problem, choose activities that will conform to your needs and enhance your ability to cope. Ask your physician about how best to tailor an exercise program to your particular needs and goals.

Ask Yourself

QUESTIONS FOR CRITICAL THINKING AND REFLECTION

Consider the list of physical activities and sports in Table 9.1. Given your current fitness and skill level, which ones could you reasonably incorporate into your exercise program?

TABLE 9.1 Examples of Different Aerobic Activities and Their Intensities

Moderate-Intensity Activities	Vigorous-Intensity Activities
• Walking briskly (3 miles per hour [5 km/h] or faster, but not race-walking)	• Race-walking, jogging, or running
• Water aerobics	• Swimming laps
• Bicycling slower than 10 miles per hour [16 km/h] per hour	• Singles tennis
• Doubles tennis	• Aerobic dancing
• Ballroom dancing	• Bicycling 10 miles per hour [16 km/h] or faster
• General gardening	• Jumping rope
	• Heavy gardening (continuous digging or hoeing)
	• Hiking uphill or with a heavy backpack

SOURCE: Physical Activity Guidelines Advisory Committee. 2008. *Physical Activity Guidelines Advisory Committee Report, 2008.* Washington, D.C.: U.S. Department of Health and Human Services.

TABLE 9.2 Popular Recreational Activities of Canadians

Activity	Reported by % of Sample
Walking for exercise	71%
Gardening, yard work	49%
Home exercise	33%
Swimming	22%
Bicycling	20%
Social dancing	18%

SOURCE: "Popularity of Physical Recreation Activities of Adults, Age 20+." Statistics Canada, Canadian Community Health Survey, 2005. (www.cflri.ca/media/node/371/tables/pam2005_tables.pdf, p. 117).

3. Set a Target Frequency, Intensity, and Time (Duration) for Each Activity

The next step is to apply the FITT principle and set a starting frequency, intensity, and time (duration) for each type of activity you've chosen (see the summary in Figure 9.2 and the sample in Figure 9.1). Refer to the calculations and plans you completed in Chapters 3–5.

CARDIORESPIRATORY ENDURANCE EXERCISE As noted in earlier chapters, the Public Health Agency of Canada has concluded that most health benefits occur with at least 150 minutes per week of moderate-intensity physical ativity (such as brisk walking) or 75 minutes per week of vigorous-intensity activity (such as jogging). Additional benefits occur with more exercise. An appropriate frequency for cardiorespiratory endurance exercise is 3–5 times per week. For intensity, note your target heart rate zone or RPE value (see Chapter 3). Your target total workout time (duration) should be about 20–60 minutes, depending on the intensity of the activity. You can exercise in a single session or in multiple sessions of 10 or more minutes.

MUSCULAR STRENGTH AND ENDURANCE TRAINING A frequency of at least 2 nonconsecutive days per week for strength training is recommended. As described in Chapter 4, a general fitness strength training program includes 1 or more sets of 8–12 repetitions of 8–10 exercises that work all major muscle groups. For intensity, choose a weight that is heavy enough to fatigue your muscles but not so heavy that you cannot complete the full number of repetitions with proper form. Exercises that use body weight for resistance also build strength and muscle endurance.

FLEXIBILITY TRAINING Stretches should be performed when muscles are warm at least 2–3 days per week (5–7 days per week is ideal). Stretches should be performed for all major muscle groups. For each exercise, stretch to the point of slight tension or mild discomfort and hold the stretch for 15–30 seconds; do 2–4 repetitions of each exercise.

4. Set Up a System of Mini-Goals and Rewards

To keep your program on track, it is important to set up a system of goals and rewards. Break your specific goals into several steps, and set a target date for each step. For example, if one of the goals of an 18-year-old male student's program is to improve upper-body strength and endurance, he could use the push-up test in Lab 4.2 to set intermediate goals. If he can currently perform 15 pushups (for a rating of "very poor"), he might set intermediate goals of 17, 20, 25, and 30 push-ups

FITNESS TIP

Want to lift weights without going to a gym? Try using resistance bands. Research shows that—especially for young women—resistance bands are just as effective as weight machines or free weights for increasing muscular strength.

	Cardiorespiratory endurance training	Strength training	Flexibility training
Frequency	3–5 days per week	2–3 nonconsecutive days per week	2–3 days per week (minimum); 5–7 days per week (ideal)
Intensity	55/65–90% of maximum heart rate	Sufficient resistance to fatigue muscles	Stretch to the point of tension
Time	20–60 minutes in sessions lasting 10 minutes or more	8–12 repetitions of each exercise, 1 or more sets	2–4 repetitions of each exercise, held for 15–30 seconds
Type	Continuous rhythmic activities using large muscle groups	Resistance exercises for all major muscle groups	Stretching exercises for all major joints

FIGURE 9.2 A summary of the FITT principle for the health-related components of fitness.

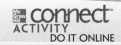

ACTIVITY
DO IT ONLINE

THE EVIDENCE FOR EXERCISE

Can Stability Balls Be Part of a Safe and Effective Fitness Program?

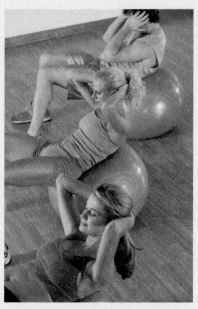

As you create a personalized exercise program, you might consider incorporating a stability ball into your workouts. Stability balls add variety and challenge to a workout and can help you target certain muscle groups more effectively than is possible with some other workout strategies. But what is the real purpose of stability balls, and what is the best way to use them?

When most people think of exercising with stability balls, they think of *core training*—exercises that target the muscles of the trunk. These core muscles, as described in Chapter 5, surround your internal organs and provide support for your spine. The core muscles enable you to stand straight, sit up, twist and bend, and perform countless types of movements, both large and small. If you play any type of competitive sport, from golf to figure skating, your core muscles are essential to your performance. In everyday living, a strong, stable core helps you maintain good posture and balance and provides some protection against injuries.

Core training can be done on a stable surface, such as a floor or bench, or on an unstable surface, such as a stability ball. A stability ball—which is actually an unstable platform—gets its name from the fact that it forces the user's body to stabilize itself to compensate for the ball's instability. Using a stability ball, therefore, is sometimes called *instability training*. Stability ball exercises activate muscle and nerve groups that might not otherwise get involved in the exercise. Depending on the specific exercises being done, instability training improves core strength and enhances the stability of supporting joints throughout the body.

There are many ways to incorporate a stability ball into a typical workout. For example, you can perform crunches or curl-ups while lying on a ball instead of the floor. Lying face-down across a ball provides different leverage points for push-ups. A variety of resistance training exercises can be performed on a stability ball, but experts recommend using dumbbells rather than barbells when lifting weights on a ball.

Although stability balls are an excellent workout tool, they have drawbacks. For example, if you lift weights while resting on a ball instead of a stable bench, much of your muscles' effort is devoted to keeping your body stable, reducing the muscles' ability to exert force. This effort can enhance your overall stability, but it can also slow your gains in strength. Research has shown that some exercises (such as curl-ups) can be more stressful to certain joints and muscles when performed on a ball, at least in some people. Further, there is always a risk of falling off an unstable surface; this can cause serious injury, especially if you are holding weights in your hands.

Finally, while instability training is a valuable aid in building up the core stabilizing muscles, it contributes little to the development of dynamic strength or power in the core. This strength and power is essential to total core fitness (especially in athletes) and must be developed through other types of exercise. For these reasons, many experts recommend instability training as part of an overall exercise program but do not suggest that all exercises be performed on a ball. For example, it's probably more effective to do curl-ups on the floor 2 days per week and on a ball 1 day per week, instead of using the ball every day. If you want to work with stability balls, it's a good idea to join a class where you can learn about this method from a qualified instructor and make sure instability training is appropriate for you.

SOURCES: Behm, D. G., et al. 2010. Canadian Society for Exercise Physiology position stand: The use of instability to train the core in athletic and non-athletic conditioning. *Applied Physiology Nutrition and Metabolism.* 35(1): 109–112; Marshall, P. W., et al. 2010. Electromyographic analysis of upper body, lower body, and abdominal muscles during advanced Swiss ball exercises. *Journal of Strength and Conditioning Research.* 24(6): 1537–1545; and Okada, T., et al. 2011. Relationship between core stability, functional movement, and performance. *Journal of Strength and Conditioning Research.* 25(1): 252–261.

(for a final rating of "fair"). By allowing several weeks between mini-goals and specifying rewards, he'll be able to track his progress and reward himself as he moves toward his final goal. Reaching a series of small goals is more satisfying than working toward a single, more challenging goal that may take months to achieve. For more on choosing appropriate rewards, refer to Chapter 1 and Activity 4 in the Behaviour Change Workbook at the end of the text.

5. Include Lifestyle Physical Activity in Your Program

Daily physical activity is a simple but important way to improve your overall wellness. As part of your fitness program plan, specify ways to be more active during your daily routine. You may find it helpful to first use your health journal to track your activities for several days. Review the records in your journal, identify routine opportunities to be more active, and add these to your program plan in Lab 9.1.

6. Develop Tools for Monitoring Your Progress

A record that tracks your daily progress will help remind you of your ongoing commitment to your program and give you a sense of accomplishment. Figure 9.3 shows you how to create a general program log and record the activity type, frequency, and time (duration). Or if you wish, complete specific activity logs like those in Labs 3.2, 4.3, and 5.2

Name: Tracie Kaufman

Enter time, distance, or another factor (such as heart rate or perceived exertion) to track your progress.

Activity/Date	M	Tu	W	Th	F	Sa	Su	Weekly Total	M	Tu	W	Th	F	Sa	Su	Weekly Total
1 Swimming	730 m		660 m		730 m			2125 m	730 m		730 m		775 m			2240 m
2 Tennis						90 min		90 min						95 min		95 min
3 Weight Training		X		X		X				X		X			X	
4 Stretching	X		X		X	X			X		X	X	X	X		

FIGURE 9.3 A sample program log.

in addition to, or instead of, a general log. Post your log in a place where you'll see it often as a reminder and as an incentive for improvement. If you have specific, measurable goals, you can also graph your weekly or monthly progress toward your goal (Figure 9.4). To monitor the overall progress of your fitness program, you may choose to reassess your fitness every 3 months or so during the improvement phase of your program. Because the results of different fitness tests vary, be sure to compare results for the same assessments over time.

7. Make a Commitment

Your final step in planning your program is to make a commitment by signing a contract. Find a witness for your contract—preferably one who will be actively involved in your program. Keep your contract in a visible spot to remind you of your commitment.

LO2 9.2 PUTTING YOUR PLAN INTO ACTION

Once you've developed a detailed plan and signed your contract, you are ready to begin your fitness program. Refer to the specific training suggestions provided in Chapters 2–5 for advice on beginning and maintaining your program. Many people find it easier to plan a

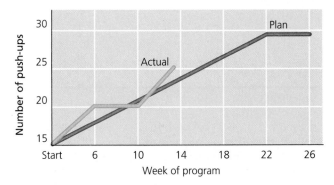

FIGURE 9.4 A sample program progress chart.

program than to put their plan into action and stick with it over time. For that reason, adherence to healthy lifestyle programs has become an important area of study for psychologists and health researchers. The guidelines below and in the next section reflect research into strategies that help people succeed in sticking with an exercise program:

- **Start slowly and increase fitness gradually.** Overzealous exercising can result in discouraging discomforts and injuries. Your program is meant to last a lifetime. The important first step is to break your established pattern of inactivity. Be patient and realistic. Once your body has adjusted to your starting level of exercise, slowly increase the amount of overload. Small increases are the key—achieving a large number of small improvements will eventually result in substantial gains in fitness. It's usually best to increase duration and frequency before increasing intensity.

- **Find an exercise buddy.** The social side of exercise is an important factor for many regular exercisers. Working out with a friend will make exercise more enjoyable and increase your chances of sticking with your program. Find an exercise partner who shares your goals and general fitness level.

- **Ask for support from others.** You have a much greater chance of exercising consistently if you have the support of important people in your life, such as parents, spouse, partner, and friends. Talk with them about your program, and let them know the importance of exercise and wellness in your life. Exercise needs to be a critical component of your day (just like sleeping and eating). Good communication will help others become more supportive of and enthusiastic about the time you spend on your wellness program.

- **Vary your activities.** You can make your program more fun over the long term if you participate in a variety of different activities that you enjoy. You can also add interest by strategies such as varying the routes you take when walking, finding a new tennis or racquetball partner, or switching to a new volleyball or basketball court. Varying your activities,

Getting Your Fitness Program Back on Track

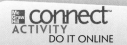
Lapses are a normal part of any behaviour change program. The important point is to move on and avoid becoming discouraged. Try again, and keep trying. Know that continued effort will lead to success.

- Don't judge yourself harshly. Focus on the improvements you've already obtained from your program and how good you feel after exercise—both physically and mentally.

- Visualize what it will be like to reach your goals. Keep these pictures in your mind as an incentive to stick with your program.

- Use your exercise journal to identify thoughts and behaviours that are causing noncompliance. Devise strategies to combat these problematic patterns. If needed, make additional changes in your environment or obtain more social support. Call a friend to walk with you. Put your exercise clothes in your car or backpack.

- Make changes in your plan and reward system to help renew your enthusiasm and commitment to your program. Try changing fitness activities or your exercise schedule. Build in more opportunities to reward yourself.

- Plan ahead for difficult situations. Think about what circumstances might make it tough to keep up your fitness routine. Develop strategies to increase your chances of sticking with your program. For example, devise strategies for your program during vacation, travel, bad weather, and so on.

- If you're in a bad mood or just don't feel like exercising, remind yourself that physical activity is probably the one thing you can do that will make you feel better. Even if you can only do half your scheduled workout, you'll boost your energy, improve your mood, and help keep your program on track.

---

a strategy known as *cross-training*, has other benefits. It can help you develop balanced, total body fitness. For example, by alternating running with swimming, you build both upper- and lower-body strength. Cross-training can reduce the risk of injury and overtraining because the same muscles, bones, and joints are not continuously subjected to the stresses of the same activity. Cross-training can be done either by choosing different activities on different days or by alternating activities within a single workout.

- *Cycle the duration and intensity of your workouts.* Olympic athletes use a training technique called *periodization of training,* meaning that they vary the duration and intensity of their workouts. Sometimes they exercise very intensely; at other times they train lightly or rest. You can use the same technique to improve fitness more quickly and make your training program more varied and enjoyable. For example, if your program consists of walking, weight training, and stretching, pick one day a week for each activity to train a little harder or longer than you normally do. If you usually walk 3 km in 10 minutes per kilometre, increase the pace to 9 minutes per km once a week. If you lift weights twice a week, train more intensely during one of the workouts by using more resistance or performing multiple sets.

- *Adapt to changing environments and schedules.* Most people are creatures of habit and have trouble adjusting to change. Don't use bad weather or a new job as an excuse to give up your exercise program. If you walk in the summer, put on a warm coat and walk in the winter. If you can't go out because of darkness, join a gym and walk on a treadmill.

- *Expect fluctuations and lapses.* On some days, your progress will be excellent, but on others, you'll barely

be able to drag yourself through your scheduled activities. Don't let off-days or lapses discourage you or make you feel guilty. Instead, feel a renewed commitment for your fitness program (see the box "Getting Your Fitness Program Back on Track").

- *Choose other healthy lifestyle behaviours.* Exercise provides huge benefits for your health, but other behaviours are also important. Choose a nutritious diet, and avoid harmful habits like smoking and overconsumption of alcohol. Be sure to stay hydrated with water or other healthy beverages (see the box "Choosing Healthy Beverages"). Don't skimp on sleep, which has a mutually beneficial relationship with exercise. Physical activity improves sleep, and adequate sleep can improve physical performance.

Ask Yourself

QUESTIONS FOR CRITICAL THINKING AND REFLECTION

How do you typically deal with setbacks? For example, if you have trouble getting motivated to study for exams, what strategies do you use to get back on track? Could those strategies work for keeping your fitness program moving forward? If so, how?

WELLNESS TIP

Are you into intervals? Interval training can dramatically boost muscle performance and maximal oxygen consumption, but it doesn't do that much for certain measures of heart health. This is one reason it's important to vary your workouts; blend intervals with higher-volume workouts for optimal results.

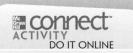
Choosing Healthy Beverages

As discussed in other chapters, it's important to stay hydrated at all times, but especially when you are exercising. Too little water intake can leave you feeling fatigued, reduce your body's performance, and leave you vulnerable to heat-related sicknesses in hot weather. But *what* you drink is as significant as how much you drink, both when you are exercising and when you are going about your normal routine.

The Great Water Controversy

Wherever you see people exercising, you will see bottled water in abundance. For several years, a debate has been raging about the quality and safety of commercially bottled water. Recently, new evidence has emerged showing that most bottled waters are no better for you than regular tap water, and some bottled waters may actually be bad for you.

In a 2008 analysis, the Environmental Working Group found 38 different contaminants in 10 popular brands of bottled water. Contaminants included heavy metals such as arsenic, pharmaceutical residues, and other pollutants commonly found in urban wastewater, and a variety of industrial chemicals.

Many commercially bottled water products are really just tap water drawn from municipal water systems. Such revelations have caused some bottlers to put statements on their products' labels, identifying them as having been drawn from a standard water supply. Although these products are priced many times higher than water from a residential tap, they provide no benefit over standard tap water.

An even bigger issue is that plastic water bottles have become a huge environmental problem, with billions of bottles now filling landfills and floating in the world's oceans. Many kinds of plastic bottles will never decompose at all; at best, some types of plastic take years to biodegrade.

Experts say that when you're exercising, the cheapest and safest way to stay hydrated is to drink filtered tap water. If you need to carry water with you, buy a reusable container (preferably made of stainless steel) that can be cleaned after each use. If you drink from plastic bottles, be sure they are recyclable and dispose of them by recycling.

Other Choices

Instead of water, many people choose to drink carbonated beverages, juice, tea, or flavored water. While these kinds of beverages have their place, it's important not to drink them too often or in large amounts, especially if they are high in sugar or caffeine. Sugary drinks add empty calories to your diet, and caffeine is a psychoactive drug with a variety of side effects.

Regular (nondiet) carbonated beverages are now one of the leading source of calories in the Canadian diet; most people don't count the calories from beverages as part of their daily caloric intake, leading them to underestimate their total intake. For this reason and others, many experts believe that soda consumption is a major factor in the increasing levels of obesity, metabolic syndrome, diabetes, and other chronic diseases among North Americans.

If you're concerned that the liquid portion of your diet is not as healthy as it should be, choose water, 100% fruit juice, low-fat or fat-free milk, or unsweetened herbal tea more often. Avoid regular carbonated beverages, sweetened bottled ice tea, flavoured water, and fruit beverages made with little fruit juice. To make water more appealing, try adding slices of citrus fruit or mixing 100% fruit juice with sparkling water. With some imagination, you can make sure you stay hydrated without consuming excess calories, spending money unnecessarily, or hurting the environment.

SOURCE: Leiba, N., et. al. 2011. The Environmental Working Group's 2011 Bottled Water Scorecard (http://www.ewg.org/bottled-water -2011-home, retrieved April 5, 2011).

LO3 9.3 EXERCISE GUIDELINES FOR LIFE STAGES

A fitness program may also need to be adjusted to accommodate the requirements of different life stages.

Children and Adolescents

Only 7% of Canadian children and youth aged 5–17 are physically active enough to meet Canada's Physical Activity Guidelines of at least 60 minutes of moderate to vigorous physical activity per day.[2] Lack of physical activity has led to alarming increases in overweight and obesity in children and adolescents. If you have children or are in a position to influence children, keep these guidelines in mind:

- Provide opportunities for children and adolescents to exercise every day. Minimize sedentary activities, such as watching television. Children and adolescents should aim for 60 minutes of moderate activity every day.

- During family outings, choose dynamic activities. For example, go for a walk, park away from a mall and then walk to the stores.

- For children younger than 12 years, emphasize skill development and fitness rather than excellence in competitive sports. For adolescents, combine participation and training in lifetime sports with traditional, competitive sports.

- Make sure children are developmentally capable of participating in an activity. For example, catching skills are difficult for young children because their nervous system is not developed enough to fully master the skill. Gradually increase the complexity of the skill once the child has mastered the simpler skill.

- Make sure children get plenty of water when exercising in the heat. Make sure they are dressed properly when doing sports in the cold.

Pregnant Women

Exercise is important during pregnancy, but women should be cautious because some types of exercise can pose increased risk to the mother and the unborn child. Pregnant women should consider these guidelines when exercising:

- See your physician about possible modifications needed for your particular pregnancy.
- Continue mild-to-moderate exercise routines at least three times a week (for most women, this means maintaining an exercise heart rate of 100–160 beats per minute). Avoid exercising vigorously or to exhaustion, especially in the third trimester. Monitor exercise intensity by assessing how you feel rather than by monitoring your heart rate; RPE levels of 11–13 are appropriate.
- Favour non- or low-weight-bearing exercises such as swimming or cycling over weight-bearing exercises, which can carry increased risk of injury.
- Avoid exercise in a supine position—lying on your back—after the first trimester. This position restricts blood flow to the uterus. Also avoid prolonged periods of motionless standing.
- Avoid exercise that could cause loss of balance, especially in the third trimester, and exercise that might injure the abdomen, stress the joints, or carry a risk of falling (such as contact sports, vigorous racquet sports, skiing, and in-line skating).
- Avoid activities involving extremes in barometric pressue, such as scuba diving and mountain climbing.
- Especially during the first trimester, drink plenty of fluids and exercise in well-ventilated areas to avoid heat stress.
- Do 3–5 sets of 10 Kegel exercises daily. These exercises involve tightening the muscles of the pelvic floor for 5–15 seconds. Kegel exercises are thought to help prevent incontinence (involuntary loss of urine) and speed recovery after giving birth.
- After giving birth, resume prepregnancy exercise routines gradually, based on how you feel.

Older Adults

Older people readily adapt to endurance exercise and strength training. Exercise principles are the same as for younger people, but some specific guidelines apply:

- The Public Heath Agency and CSEP recommend that older adults (those over 65 years of age) take part in at least 2.5 hours of moderate-to-vigorous intensity aerobic activity each week.
- For strength training, it is recommended that older adults add bone and muscle strengthening activities involving the major muscle groups at least twice each week.
- Older adults should perform flexibility exercises at least 2 days per week for at least 10 minutes. Exercises that improve balance should also be performed 2 days per week.
- Drink plenty of water and avoid exercising in excessively hot or cold environments. Wear clothes that speed heat loss in warm environments and that prevent heat loss in cold environments.
- Warm up slowly and carefully. Increase intensity and duration of exercise gradually.
- Cool down slowly, continuing very light exercise until the heart rate is below 100 beats per minute.

TIPS FOR TODAY AND THE FUTURE

A complete fitness program includes activities to build and maintain cardiorespiratory endurance, muscular strength and endurance, and flexibility.

RIGHT NOW YOU CAN

- Get a journal to track your daily physical activity and exercise routine.
- Put away your remote control devices—every bit of physical activity can benefit your health.
- Set a firm time for your next workout with your training partner.
- Plan to go to bed 15 minutes earlier than usual.

IN THE FUTURE YOU CAN

- Create a schedule that incorporates your workouts into your daily routine. Each week, update the schedule for the upcoming week.
- Learn more about the importance of sleep to good health. If you consistently have trouble sleeping, consult with your physician about seeing a sleep specialist or undergoing a sleep evaluation.

Should I exercise every day?

Some daily exercise is beneficial, and health experts recommend that you engage in at least 30 minutes of moderate physical activity at least 5 days per week. Back experts suggest that you also do back pain prevention exercises daily. However, if you train intensely every day without giving yourself a rest, you will likely get injured or become overtrained. When strength training, for example, rest at least 48 hours between workouts before exercising the same muscle group. For cardiorespiratory endurance exercise, rest or exercise lightly the day after an intense or long-duration workout. Balancing the proper amount of rest and exercise will help you feel better and improve your fitness faster.

I'm just starting an exercise program. How much activity should I do at first?

Be conservative. Walking is a good way to begin almost any fitness program. At first, walk for approximately 10 minutes, and then increase the distance and pace. After several weeks, you can progress to something more vigorous. Let your body be your guide. If the intensity and duration of a workout seem easy, increase them a little the next time. The key is to be progressive; don't try to achieve physical fitness in one or two workouts. Build your fitness gradually.

What are kickboxing and Tae Bo? Are they effective forms of exercise?

Kickboxing and Tae Bo are group fitness workouts that combine martial arts manoeuvres, boxing moves, and traditional group exercise activities. Participants in martial arts workouts repetitively execute a variety of punches and kicks, building movement combinations that involve the entire body. Workouts are often choreographed to moderately paced popular music and are continuous. Although more research is needed to clarify the actual training effects, the workouts certainly develop cardiovascular endurance, muscular endurance, and flexibility. Because of the potential for injury, classes should be led either by a certified fitness professional who has had ancillary training in teaching martial arts skills or a martial artist with qualifications as a fitness instructor. Other key safety elements include precise skill modelling and verbal instruction, moderate pacing, and an emphasis on health-related fitness development.

SUMMARY

- Steps for putting together a complete fitness program include (1) setting realistic goals; (2) selecting activities to develop all the health-related components of fitness; (3) setting a target frequency, intensity, and time (duration) for each activity; (4) setting up a system of mini-goals and rewards; (5) making lifestyle physical activity a part of the daily routine; (6) developing tools for monitoring progress; and (7) making a commitment.

- In selecting activities, consider fun and interest, your current skill and fitness levels, time and convenience, cost, and any special health concerns.

- Keys to beginning and maintaining a successful program include starting slowly, increasing intensity and duration gradually, finding a buddy, varying the activities and intensity of the program, and expecting fluctuations and lapses.

- Regular exercise is appropriate and highly beneficial for people with special health concerns or in particular stages of life; program modifications may be necessary to maximize safety.

FOR FURTHER EXPLORATION

Organizations and Websites

Canadian Orthopaedic Association. Provides information about injury care and treatment as well as acting as a resource for professionals.
http://www.coa-aco.org/

Healthy Active Kids Canada. Includes resources and information on active children and promotes increased physical activity participation in Canadian children.
http://www.activehealthykids.ca/AboutUs.aspx

Participaction Canada. Source of information for including physical activity in any lifestyle.
http://www.participaction.com/en-us/Get-Moving/Easy-Ways-To-Start.aspx

The Society of Obstetricians and Gynaecologists of Canada. Provides guidelines for promoting healthy pregnancy and postpartum recovery, including exercise during pregnancy.
http://www.sogc.org/index_e.asp

Sample programs based on four different types of cardiorespiratory activities—walking/jogging/running and calisthenics circuit training—are presented below. Be sure to understand if you have a medical risk for exercise (Chapter 2) before choosing a program and if needed, seek professional advice before making your program choice. Each sample program includes regular cardiorespiratory endurance exercise, resistance training, and stretching. Read the descriptions of the programs you're considering, and decide which will work best for you based on your present routine, the potential for enjoyment, and adaptability to your lifestyle. If you choose one of these programs, complete the personal fitness program plan in Lab 9.1, just as if you had created a program from scratch.

No program will produce enormous changes in your fitness level in the first few weeks. Follow the specifics of the program for 3–4 weeks. Then if the exercise program doesn't seem suitable, make adjustments to adapt it to your particular needs. But retain the basic elements of the program that make it effective for developing fitness.

GENERAL GUIDELINES

The following guidelines can help make the activity programs more effective for you.

- **Frequency and time.** To experience training effects, you should exercise for 20–60 minutes at least three times a week.

- **Intensity.** To work effectively for cardiorespiratory endurance training or to improve body composition, you must raise your heart rate into its target zone. Monitor your pulse or use rates of perceived exertion (RPE) to monitor your intensity.

  If you've been sedentary, begin very slowly. Give your muscles a chance to adjust to their increased workload. It's probably best to keep your heart rate below target until your body has had time to adjust to new demands. At first you may not need to work very hard to keep your heart rate in its target zone, but as your cardiorespiratory endurance improves, you will probably need to increase intensity.

- **Interval training.** Some of the sample programs involve continuous activity. Others rely on interval training, which calls for alternating a relief interval with exercise (walking after jogging, for example, or coasting after biking uphill). Interval training is an effective way of progressive overload and improves fitness rapidly (see the box "Interval Training: Pros and Cons" in Chapter 3).

- **Resistance training and stretching guidelines.** For the resistance training and stretching parts of the program, remember the general guidelines for safe and effective exercise. See the summary of guidelines in Figure 9.2.

- **Warm-up and cool-down.** Begin each exercise session with a warm-up suited to your age and level of fitness (3–10 minutes in length). Begin your activity at a slow pace and work up gradually to your target heart rate. Always slow down gradually at the end of your exercise session to bring your system back to its normal state. It's a good idea to do stretching exercises to increase your flexibility after cardiorespiratory exercise or strength training because your muscles will be warm and ready to stretch. More information regarding warm-up and cool-down are included in Chapter 2.

  Follow the guidelines presented in Chapter 3 for exercising in hot or cold weather. Drink enough liquids to stay adequately hydrated, particularly in hot weather.

- **Record keeping.** After each exercise session, record your daily distance or time on a progress chart.

WALKING/JOGGING/RUNNING SAMPLE PROGRAM

Walking is the perfect exercise. It increases longevity, builds fitness, expends calories, prevents weight gain, and protects against heart disease, stroke, and back pain. You don't need to join a gym, and you can walk almost anywhere. People who walk 30 minutes five times per week will lose an average of 5 pounds in 6–12 months—without dieting, watching what they eat, or exercising intensely.

Jogging takes walking to the next level. Jogging only 75 minutes per week will increase fitness, promote weight control, and provide health benefits that will prevent disease and increase longevity. Your ultimate goal for promoting wellness is to walk at a moderate intensity for 150–300 minutes per week or jog at 70% effort or more for 75–150 minutes per week.

It isn't always easy to distinguish among walking, jogging, and running. For clarity and consistency, we'll consider walking to be any on-foot exercise of less than 8 km per hour, jogging any pace between 8 and 12 km per hour, and running any pace faster than that. The faster your pace or the longer you exercise, the more calories you burn (Table 1). The greater the number of calories burned, the higher the potential training effects of these activities. Table 2 contains a sample walking/jogging fitness program.

Equipment and Technique

These activities require no special skills, expensive equipment, or unusual facilities. Comfortable clothing, well-fitted walking or running shoes (see Chapter 3), and a stopwatch or ordinary watch with a second hand are all you need.

When you advance to jogging, use proper technique:

- Run with your back straight and your head up. Look straight ahead, not at your feet. Shift your pelvis forward and tuck your buttocks in.

- Hold your arms slightly away from your body. Your elbows should be bent so that your forearms are parallel to the ground. You may cup your hands, but do not clench your fists. Allow your arms to swing loosely and rhythmically with each stride.

- Let your heel hit the ground first in each stride. Then roll forward onto the ball of your foot and push off for the next stride. If you find this difficult, you can try a more flat-footed style, but don't land on the balls of your feet.

- Keep your steps short by allowing your foot to strike the ground in line with your knee. Keep your knees bent at all times.

- Breathe deeply through your mouth. Try to use your abdominal muscles rather than just your chest muscles to take deep breaths.

- Stay relaxed.

Find a safe, convenient place to walk or jog. Exercise on a trail, path, or sidewalk to stay clear of bicycles and cars. Make sure your clothes are brightly coloured so others can see you easily.

Developing Cardiorespiratory Endurance

The four variations of the basic walking/jogging/running sample program that follow are designed to help you regulate the intensity, duration, and frequency of your program. Use the following guidelines to choose the variation that is right for you.

- *Variation 1: Walking (Starting).* Choose this program if you have medical restrictions, are recovering from illness or surgery, tire easily after short walks, are obese, or have a sedentary lifestyle, and if you want to prepare for the advanced walking program to improve cardiorespiratory endurance, body composition, and muscular endurance.

- *Variation 2: Advanced Walking.* Choose this program if you already can walk comfortably for 30 minutes and if you want to develop and maintain cardiorespiratory fitness, a lean body, and muscular endurance.

- *Variation 3: Preparing for a Jogging Program.* Choose this program if you already can walk comfortably for 30 minutes and if you want to prepare for the jogging/running program to improve cardiorespiratory endurance, body composition, and muscular endurance.

- *Variation 4: Jogging/Running.* Choose this program if you already can jog comfortably without muscular discomfort, if you already can jog for 15 minutes without stopping or 30 minutes with brief walking intervals within your target heart rate range, and if you want to develop and maintain a high level of cardiorespiratory fitness, a lean body, and muscular endurance.

Table 1 Estimated Calories Expended by a 75 kilogram (165-pound) Adult at Different Intensities of Walking and Running for 150 and 300 minutes per week (min/wk)				
	Speed (Kilometres Per Hour)	Speed (Minutes Per Kilometre)	Calories Expended Exercising 150 Min/Wk	Calories Expended Exercising 300 Min/Wk
	Rest	—	190	380
Walking	6.5	9.0	565	1130
	7.8	7.6	620	1240
	10.4	5.8	940	1880
	11.2	5.4	1125	2250
Jogging/Running	13.0	4.6	1500	3000
	15.6	3.8	1875	3750
	18.2	3.3	2155	4310
	20.8	2.6	2530	5060
	26.0	2.3	3000	6000

NOTE: Heavier people will expend slightly more calories, while lighter people will expend slightly fewer.

SOURCE: Adapted from Physical Activity Guidelines Advisory Committee. 2008. *Physical Activity Guidelines Advisory Committee Report, 2008.* Washington, D. C.: U.S. Department of Health and Human Services.

Table 2 Sample Walking/Jogging Fitness Program

Day	Activities
Monday	• **Walking/Jogging:** Walk briskly for 30 minutes or jog for 25 minutes.
	• **Stretching:** Stretch major muscle groups for 10 minutes after exercise. Do each exercise 2 times; hold stretch for 15–30 seconds.
Tuesday	• **Resistance workout:** Using body weight for resistance, perform the following exercises: • Push-ups: 2 sets, 20 reps per set • Pull-ups: 2 sets, 5 reps per set • Unloaded squats: 2 sets, 10 reps per set • Curl-ups: 2 sets, 20 reps per set • Side bridges: 3 sets, 10-second hold (left and right sides) • Spine extensions: 3 sets, 10-second hold (left and right sides)
Wednesday	• Repeat Monday activities.
Thursday	• Repeat Tuesday activities.
Friday	• Repeat Monday activities.
Saturday	• **Rest.**
Sunday	• **Rest.**

Variation 1: Walking (Starting)

FIT—frequency, intensity, and time: Walk at first for 15 minutes at a pace that keeps your heart rate below your target zone. Gradually increase to 30-minute sessions. The distance you travel will probably be 2–4 km. At the beginning, walk every other day. You can gradually increase to daily walking if you want to burn more calories (helpful if you want to change body composition).

Calorie cost: Work up to using 90–135 calories in each session (see Table 1). To increase calorie costs to the target level, walk for a longer time or for a longer distance rather than sharply increasing speed.

Beginning a walking/jogging program: Start slowly if you have not been exercising, are overweight, or are recovering from an illness or surgery. At first, walk for 15 minutes at a slow pace, below your target heart rate zone. Gradually increase to 30-minute sessions. You will probably cover 1.5 to 3 km. At the beginning, walk every other day.

You can gradually increase to walking each day of the week if you want to expend more calories (which is helpful if you want to change body composition). Depending upon your weight, you will expend ("burn") 90–135 calories during each 30-minute walking session. To increase the calories that you expend, walk for a longer time or for a longer distance instead of sharply increasing speed.

Start at the level of effort that is most comfortable for you. Maintain a normal, easy pace and stop to rest as often as you need to. Never prolong a walk past the point of comfort. When walking with a friend (a good motivator), let a comfortable conversation be your guide to pace. If you find that you cannot carry on a conversation without getting out of breath, then you are walking too quickly.

Once your muscles have become adjusted to the exercise program, increase the duration of your sessions by no more than 10% each week. Keep your heart rate just below your target zone. Don't be discouraged by a lack of immediate progress, and don't try to speed things up by overdoing it. Remember that pace and heart rate can vary with the terrain, the weather, and other factors.

Variation 2: Advanced Walking

Advanced walking involves walking more quickly for longer times. You should feel an increased perception of effort, but the exercise intensity should not be too stressful. Vary your pace to allow for intervals of slow, medium, and fast walking. Keep your heart rate toward the lower end of your target zone with brief periods in the upper levels. At first, walk for 30 minutes and increase your walking time gradually until eventually you reach 60 minutes at a brisk pace and can walk 3–6.5 km. Try to walk at least 5 days per week. Vary your program by changing the pace and distance or by walking routes with different terrains and views. You can expect to burn 200–350 calories or more during each advanced walking session.

Variation 3: Preparing for a Jogging Program

Increase the intensity of exercise by gradually introducing jogging into your walking program. During a 3-km walk, for example, periodically jog for 100 m and then resume walking. Increase the number and distance of your jogging segments until you can jog continuously for the entire distance. More physically fit people may be capable of jogging without walking first. However, people unaccustomed to jogging should initially combine walking with short bouts of jogging.

A good strategy is to exercise on a 400-metre track at a local high school or university. Begin by jogging the straight-aways and walking the turns for 800 metres (two laps). Progress to walking 200 metres (half lap) and jogging 200 metres; jogging 400 metres and walking 200 metres; jogging 800 metres, walking 800 metres; and jogging 1200 metres, walking 400 metres. Continue until you can run 3 km without stopping.

Variation 4: Jogging/Running

During the transition to jogging, adjust the ratio of walking to jogging to keep within your target heart rate zone as much as possible. Most people who sustain a continuous jog/run program will find that they can stay within their target heart rate zone with a speed of 9–12 km/h (5–7 minutes per km). Exercise at least every other day. Increasing frequency by doing other activities on alternate days will place less stress on the weight-bearing parts of your lower body than will a daily program of jogging/running.

Developing Muscular Strength and Endurance and Flexibility

Walking, jogging, and running provide muscular endurance workouts for your lower body; they also develop muscular strength of the lower body to a lesser degree. If you'd like to increase your running speed and performance, you might want to focus your program on lower-body exercises. (Don't neglect upper-body strength. It is important for overall wellness.) For flexibility, pay special attention to the hamstrings and quadriceps, which are not worked through their complete range of motion during walking or jogging.

Staying with Your Walking/Jogging Program

Health experts have found that simple motivators such as using a pedometer, walking a dog, parking farther from the office or grocery store, or training for a fun run helped people stay with their programs. Use a pedometer or GPS exercise device to track your progress and help motivate you to increase distance and speed. Accurate pedometers for walking, such as those made by Omron, Yamax, and New Lifestyles, cost $20–$40 and are accurate to about 5%. Sophisticated GPS-based devices made by Polar and Garmin keep track of your exercise speed and distance via satellite, monitor heart rate, and store data that can be downloaded wirelessly to your computer. Several of these units can be plugged into programs such as Google Earth, which can give you a satellite view of your walking or jogging route.

A pedometer can also help you increase the number of steps you walk each day. Most sedentary people take only 2000 to 3000 steps per day. Adding 1000 steps per day and increasing gradually until you reach 10 000 steps can increase fitness and help you manage your weight. Once you reach 10 000 steps, continue to increase the effectiveness of those steps by reducing the time it takes to complete them!

CALISTHENICS CIRCUIT-TRAINING SAMPLE PROGRAM

Calisthenics are rhythmic exercises that typically develop muscular strength, muscular endurance, and flexibility. Because calisthenic exercises require little or no equipment, they can be performed at home or while travelling. As commonly practised, such exercises do not constitute a well-rounded fitness program because they do not develop cardiorespiratory endurance. However, a calisthenics program based on circuit training can be the basis of a complete fitness program.

Circuit training is a system of organizing a series of exercises that are performed consecutively. Exercises for different muscle groups follow one another, providing a well-rounded workout and helping to delay the onset of fatigue. When you have performed all the exercises in this model program, you will have completed one circuit; a workout consists of three trips around the circuit. By performing the exercises continuously and not resting between exercises or circuits, you can develop the cardiorespiratory endurance component of fitness. In addition, some of the individual exercises, such as jumping jacks or running in place, develop cardiorespiratory endurance.

Equipment

To time your exercises (which is required only once, when you create your work description), you need a

clock or watch with a second hand. If you plan to perform calisthenics regularly, it's a good idea to get a pair of cross-training athletic shoes. Choose an exercise area that is well ventilated and comfortable, with enough room for you to do the exercises without interference. You may want to perform the floor exercises (such as curl-ups) on an exercise mat or a non-skid rug.

Technique

To perform a complete calisthenics cross-training circuit, you need to be able to perform the following exercises smoothly:

- *Arm circles.* Stand with your feet shoulder-width apart and your knees slightly bent. Maintain good posture to protect the lower back. Hold your arms out to the side at shoulder height with palms up. Rotate your arms forward in a circular motion. Keep your shoulders down. Halfway through the time limit or work description, reverse the direction of your circles.

- *Push-ups.* Depending on your level of muscular strength and endurance, you can perform either standard push-ups or modified push-ups. For standard push-ups, begin with your body supported by your hands and feet; for modified push-ups, begin with your body supported by your hands and knees. Lower your chest to the floor with your back straight and your fingers pointed forward. Return to the starting position. (See Lab 4.2.)

- *Squats.* Stand with feet shoulder-width apart and toes pointed slightly outward. Keeping your head up and lower back straight, squat down until your thighs are approximately parallel with the floor. Don't let your knees extend out in front of your toes. Hold this position for about 2 seconds. Return to the starting position. (See Lab 4.1 and Lab 4.2.)

- *Curl-ups.* Lie on your back on the floor with your arms folded across your chest, knees bent, and feet on the floor. Curl your trunk up and forward by raising your head and shoulders from the ground. Lower to the starting position. (See Lab 4.2.)

  Alternative instructions (performing curl-ups this way provides better protection for the back during the exercise): Lie on your back on a mat with one knee bent and foot flat on the floor. Place your hands under your lower back and maintain a neutral spine (don't flatten your back to the mat). Curl up as far as possible by contracting the rectus abdominis muscle ("6-pack muscle") rather than your neck and shoulder muscles. As fitness improves, do the exercise with arms folded on your chest. Eventually, place your hands lightly on your forehead, but do not pull on your head and neck.

- *Side leg raises.* Lie on your right side, with your right arm extended flat along the floor in front of your body. Bend your right knee, keeping your knee and thigh in line with your torso. Place your left hand on the floor in front of your chest for balance. Keeping your left leg straight, foot flexed, and toes and knee facing forward (not up), lift your leg 30–60 cm off the floor. Then lower it to the starting position. Do half of your total repetitions on this side, and then do the same number of repetitions on the other side.

- *Heel raises.* Stand with your feet shoulder-width apart and your toes pointed slightly outward. Press down with your toes while lifting your heels. Return to the starting position. Do not bounce. (See Exercise 8 in the free weights portion of the Weight Training Exercises in Chapter 4.)

- *Jumping jacks.* Start with your feet together and your hands at your sides. Jump into a straddle position and clap your hands over your head. Then jump back to the starting position and lower your arms to your sides. Always land with your knees slightly bent. If you prefer a low-impact movement, step to the side into the straddle position and then step back into the starting position; alternate legs.

- *Upper-back flies.* Stand with your feet ½ times shoulder-width apart and your knees slightly bent. Keeping your back straight, lean forward at the hips until your torso is diagonal to the floor. Let your arms hang forward, with elbows slightly bent and hands fisted. Leading with your elbows, open your arms to the side and pull your shoulder blades together. Return to the starting position. Lift your arms smoothly and with resistance; do not bounce or swing them.

- *Lunges.* Begin with your feet shoulder-width apart and your hands at your sides or resting on your shoulders. Step forward onto your right foot until your right thigh is almost parallel to the floor. Your right knee should be directly above your right ankle and should not push out in front of your toes. Bend your left knee and drop it directly below your torso in line with your left ankle; your lower left leg should be about parallel to the floor. (See Exercise 6 in the Flexibility Exercises in Chapter 5.) Return to the starting position, using the gluteal muscles to push off the floor. Contract the abdominals to relieve pressure on your knees and lower back. Alternate legs. (*Note:* Do not perform lunges if you have knee problems.)

- *Back bridges.* Lie on your back with knees bent and arms extended to the side. Tuck your pelvis under and then lift your tailbone, buttocks, and lower back from the floor. Hold for 5–10 seconds, with your weight resting on your feet, arms, and shoulders. Return to the starting position. (See Exercise 10 in the Low Back Exercises in Chapter 5.)

- *Spine extension.* Start on your hands and knees, with your knees below your hips and your hands below your shoulders. Simultaneously raise and straighten your right arm and left leg until they are in line with your spine. Hold this position for 30 seconds. Do not raise either the arm or the leg above spine level (that is, don't arch your back). Return to the starting position and immediately repeat the movement with the left arm and right leg. Do not raise your arms and legs excessively or increase the low back curve by tilting the pelvis. (See Exercise 10 in the free weights portion of the Weight Training Exercises in Chapter 4.)

- *Side bridges.* Lie on your side with your knees bent and your top arm lying alongside your body. Lift your hips so that your weight is supported by your forearm and knees. (See Exercise 11 in the free weights portion of the Weight Training Exercises in Chapter 4). Hold the position for 10 seconds, breathing normally. Repeat on the other side. As you increase fitness, make the exercise more difficult by doing it with straight legs and supporting yourself with your feet and forearm or with your feet and hand (arm extended, elbow straight). (See Lab 5.3.) Hold your spine straight—don't let it sag during the exercise.

- *Running in place.* Run with your knees lifted and land with the ball of your foot first. Follow through by pressing your heel to the floor. If you prefer a low-impact movement, march in place, lifting your knees high. (When you count repetitions of running or marching, count alternate steps.)

Developing Cardiorespiratory Endurance

Calisthenics can help develop cardiorespiratory fitness provided the intensity is moderate to intense. Maximize the cardiorespiratory benefits by moving rapidly between exercises and doing each movement vigorously.

FIT—frequency, intensity, and time: Do the workout 3–5 days per week. Exercise intensely enough to raise your heart rate into the target zone: 65–90% of maximum heart rate or an RPE of 12–18. (If you have been inactive for a long time, start out at a heart rate that is 10–20% below your target zone.) Exercise at an intensity that allows you to comfortably carry on a conversation. Begin by doing the calisthenics circuit one time. As you gain fitness, build up gradually until you can complete 3 circuits (see "As you progress" below).

Calorie cost: To estimate the number of calories you burn, first determine the amount of time it takes to complete a circuit, multiply the calories per minute per kg (.080) by your weight, then multiply that figure by the number of minutes you need to complete one circuit of exercises. For example, assuming you weigh 60 kg and complete a circuit in 15 minutes, you would burn 72 calories per circuit: 60 × .080 (calories per kg for calisthenics training) = 48 × 15 (minutes) = 72 calories burned. To burn more calories, increase your repetitions, work faster, and/or work longer.

At the beginning: Before doing your first full calisthenic workout, you need to set up a work description—the number of repetitions of each exercise you will perform in each circuit. To do this, determine the maximum number of repetitions of each exercise you can perform in the time listed in the following table.

For example, count the maximum number of arm circles you can do in 30 seconds, and record that number in the "Max" column. Rest fully between exercises to obtain true maximums. Once you have filled in the "Max" column, write half of this number in the "Work Description" column labeled "½ Max." Once you have completed this step, you no longer have to worry about timing the individual exercises.

After your work description is set up, perform each circuit as follows:

- Warm up before you begin the circuit by doing some walking, jogging, or easy calisthenics. When you are ready to begin, note your starting time.

- Perform the exercises in order, each for the number of repetitions in the "½ Max" column. Time no longer matters for each exercise; just work steadily.

- Monitor your intensity by checking your heart rate or monitoring your rating of perceived exertion (RPE). Do not rest between exercises unless your heart rate or RPE goes above your target zone.

- Complete three trips around the circuit. In the progress chart on the next page, write the date and total time the three circuits took.

- Cool down.

As you progress: When you can perform three circuits in 20 minutes, increase the number of repetitions (the work description) of each exercise by one-quarter of the present work description. For example, if your current work description for push-ups is 20 repetitions, your new work description will be 25. Record the date and the new work description values in the program plan table.

Developing Muscular Strength and Endurance and Flexibility

If you perform a full range of calisthenic exercises (as described in this program), you can develop muscular strength and endurance in all the major muscle groups of your body. Your gains, however, will not be as significant as those from weight training using free weights or machines (unless you add arm or leg weights to increase resistance). To develop flexibility, stretch during your cool-down, when your muscles are warm.

Work Description

Exercise	Time	Max	½ Max	Date: _____	Date: _____	Date: _____	Date: _____	Date: _____	Date: _____
Arm circles	30 sec								
Jumping jacks	1 min								
Push-ups	1 min								
Squats	1 min								
Curl-ups	1 min								
Side leg raises	1 min								
Heel raises	30 sec								
Upper-back flies	30 sec								
Lunges	1 min								
Back bridges	1 min								
Spine extensions	1 min								
Side bridges	1 min								
Run in place	3 min								

Progress Chart

Date	
Time	

Name _____ Section _____ Date _____

LAB 9.1 A Personal Fitness Program Plan and Contract

connect
ACTIVITY
DO IT ONLINE

A. I, _____, am contracting with myself to follow a physical fitness program to
    (name)

work toward the following goals:

Specific or short-term goals (include current status for each)

1. _____
2. _____
3. _____
4. _____

General or long-term goals

1. _____
2. _____
3. _____
4. _____

B. My program plan is as follows:

Activities	Components (Check ✓)					Frequency (Check ✓)							Intensity*	Time (duration)
	CRE	MS	ME	F	BC	M	Tu	W	Th	F	Sa	Su		

*Conduct activities for achieving CRE goals in your target range for heart rate or RPE.

C. My program will begin on _____. My program includes the following schedule of mini-goals. For each
    (date)

step in my program, I will give myself the reward listed.

_____	_____	_____
(mini-goal 1)	(date)	(reward)

_____	_____	_____
(mini-goal 2)	(date)	(reward)

_____	_____	_____
(mini-goal 3)	(date)	(reward)

_____	_____	_____
(mini-goal 4)	(date)	(reward)

_____	_____	_____
(mini-goal 5)	(date)	(reward)

D. My program will include the addition of physical activity to my daily routine (such as climbing stairs or walking to class):

1. _____
2. _____
3. _____
4. _____
5. _____

E. I will use the following tools to monitor my program and my progress toward my goals:

_____
(list any charts, graphs, or journals you plan to use)

_____

_____

I sign this contract as an indication of my personal commitment to reach my goal.

_____   _____
(your signature)   (date)

I have recruited a helper who will witness my contract and _____

_____

_____

_____   _____
(witness's signature)   (date)

Name _____ Section _____ Date _____

LAB 9.2 Getting to Know Your Fitness Facility

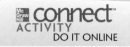

To help create a successful training program, take time out to learn more about the fitness facility you plan to use.

Basic Information

Name and location of facility: _____

Hours of operation: _____

Times available for general use: _____

Times most convenient for your schedule: _____

Can you obtain an initial session or consultation with a trainer to help you create a program? yes _____ no _____

If so, what does the initial planning session involve? _____

_____

Are any of the staff certified? Do any have special training? If yes, list/describe: _____

_____

What types of equipment are available for the development of cardiorespiratory endurance? Briefly list/describe: _____

_____

_____

_____

Are any group activities or classes available? If so, briefly describe: _____

_____

_____

What types of weight training equipment are available for use? _____

_____

Yes   No

_____ _____ Is there a fee for using the facility? If so, how much? $ _____

_____ _____ Is a student ID required for access to the facility?

_____ _____ Do you need to sign up in advance to use the facility or any of the equipment?

_____ _____ Is there typically a line or wait to use the equipment during the times you use the facility?

_____ _____ Is there a separate area with mats for stretching and/or cool-down?

_____ _____ Do you need to bring your own towel?

_____ _____ Are lockers available? If so, do you need to bring your own lock? yes _____ no _____

_____ _____ Are showers available? If so, do you need to bring your own soap and shampoo? yes _____ no _____

_____ _____ Is drinking water available? (If not, be sure to bring your own bottle of water.)

Describe any other amenities, such as vending machines or saunas that are available at the facility.

_____

_____

Information about Equipment

Fill in the specific equipment and exercise(s) that you can use to develop cardiorespiratory endurance and each of the major muscle groups. For cardiorespiratory endurance, list the type(s) of equipment and a sample starting workout: frequency, intensity, time, and other pertinent information (such as a setting for resistance or speed). For muscular strength and endurance, list the equipment, exercises, and indicate the order in which you'll complete them during a workout session.

Cardiorespiratory Endurance Equipment

Equipment	Sample Starting Workout

Muscular Strength and Endurance Equipment

Order	Muscle Groups	Equipment	Exercise(s)
	Neck		
	Chest		
	Shoulders		
	Upper back		
	Front of arms		
	Back of arms		
	Buttocks		
	Abdomen		
	Lower back		
	Front of thighs		
	Back of thighs		
	Calves		
	Other:		
	Other:		

CHAPTER 10

STRESS

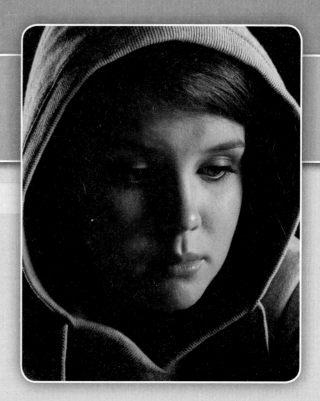

LEARNING OBJECTIVES

After reading this chapter, you should be able to

LO1 Explain what stress is and how people react to it—physically, emotionally, and behaviourally

LO2 Describe the relationship between stress and disease

LO3 List common sources of stress

LO4 Describe techniques for preventing and managing stress

LO5 Put together a plan for successfully managing the stress in your life

TEST YOUR KNOWLEDGE

1. Which of the following events can cause stress?

a. taking out a loan
b. failing a test
c. graduating from university or college
d. watching a hockey game

2. Moderate exercise can stimulate which of the following?

a. analgesia (pain relief)
b. birth of new brain cells
c. relaxation

3. Which of the following can be a result of chronic stress?

a. violence
b. heart attack
c. stroke

ANSWERS

1. **ALL FOUR.** Stress-producing factors can be pleasant or unpleasant and can include physical challenges and goal achievement as well as what are perceived as negative events.

2. **ALL THREE.** Regular exercise is linked to improvement in many dimensions of wellness.

3. **ALL THREE.** Chronic—or ongoing—stress can last for years. People who suffer from long-term stress may ultimately become violent toward themselves or others. They also run a greater than normal risk for certain ailments, especially cardiovascular disease.

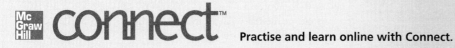

Practise and learn online with Connect.

Like the term *fitness, stress* is a word many people use without really understanding its precise meaning. Stress is popularly viewed as an uncomfortable response to a negative event, which probably describes *nervous tension* more than the cluster of physical and psychological responses that actually constitute stress. In fact, stress is not limited to negative situations; it is also a response to pleasurable physical challenges and the achievement of personal goals. Whether stress is experienced as pleasant or unpleasant depends largely on the situation and the individual. Because learning effective responses to whatever induces stress can enhance psychological health and help prevent a number of serious diseases, stress management is an important part of daily life.

This chapter explains the physiological and psychological reactions that make up the stress response and describes how these reactions can be risks to good health. The chapter also presents ways of managing stress with a personal program or with the help of others.

LO1 10.1 WHAT IS STRESS?

In common usage, *stress* refers to two different things: situations that trigger physical *and* emotional reactions and the reactions themselves. This text, we'll use the more precise term **stressor** for a situation that triggers physical and emotional reactions and the term **stress response** for those reactions. A first date and a final exam are examples of stressors; sweaty palms and a pounding heart are symptoms of the stress response. We'll use the term **stress** to describe the general physical and emotional state that

accompanies the stress response. So, for example, a person taking a final exam experiences stress.

Physical Responses to Stressors

Imagine a near miss: As you step off the curb, a car careens toward you. With just a fraction of a second to spare, you leap safely out of harm's way. In that split second of danger and in the moments following it, you experience a predictable series of physical reactions. Your body goes from a relaxed state to one prepared for physical action to cope with a threat to your life.

Two major control systems in your body are responsible for your physical response to stressors: the nervous system and the endocrine system. Through a variety of rapid chemical reactions affecting almost every part of your body, you are primed to act quickly and appropriately in times of danger.

ACTIONS OF THE NERVOUS SYSTEM The nervous system consists of the brain, spinal cord, and nerves. Part of the nervous system is under voluntary control, as when you tell your arm to reach for a chocolate. The part that is not under conscious supervision—for example, the part that controls the digestion of the chocolate—is known as the **autonomic nervous system.** In addition to digestion, it controls your heart rate, breathing, blood pressure, and hundreds of other functions you normally take for granted.

The autonomic nervous system consists of two divisions.

- The **parasympathetic division** is in control when you are relaxed; it aids in digesting food, storing energy, and promoting growth.
- The **sympathetic division** is activated during times of arousal, including exercise, and when there is an emergency, such as severe pain, anger, or fear.

Sympathetic nerves use the neurotransmitter **norepinephrine** to exert their actions on nearly every organ, sweat gland, blood vessel, and muscle to enable your body to handle an emergency. In general, the sympathetic division commands your body to stop storing energy and instead to mobilize all energy resources to respond to the crisis.

ACTIONS OF THE ENDOCRINE SYSTEM During stress, the sympathetic nervous system triggers the **endocrine system.** This system of glands, tissues, and cells helps control body functions by releasing **hormones** and other chemical messengers into the bloodstream to influence metabolism and other body processes. These chemicals act on a variety of targets throughout the body. Along with the nervous system, the endocrine system helps prepare the body to respond to a stressor.

THE TWO SYSTEMS TOGETHER How do both systems work together in an emergency? Let's go back to your near collision with a car. Both reflexes and higher cognitive areas in your brain quickly make the decision that

TERMS

stressor Any physical or psychological event or condition that produces physical and emotional reactions.

stress response The physical and emotional reactions to a stressor.

stress The collective physiological and emotional responses to any stimulus that disturbs an individual's homeostasis.

autonomic nervous system The branch of the nervous system that controls basic body processes; consists of the sympathetic and parasympathetic divisions.

parasympathetic division A division of the autonomic nervous system that moderates the excitatory effect of the sympathetic division, slowing metabolism and restoring energy supplies.

sympathetic division A division of the autonomic nervous system that reacts to danger or other challenges by almost instantly accelerating body processes.

norepinephrine A neurotransmitter released by the sympathetic nervous system onto specific tissues to increase their function in the face of increased activity; when released by the brain, causes arousal (increased attention, awareness, and alertness); also called *noradrenaline.*

endocrine system The system of glands, tissues, and cells that secretes hormones into the bloodstream to influence metabolism and other body processes.

hormone A chemical messenger produced in the body and transported in the bloodstream to target cells or organs for specific regulation of their activities.

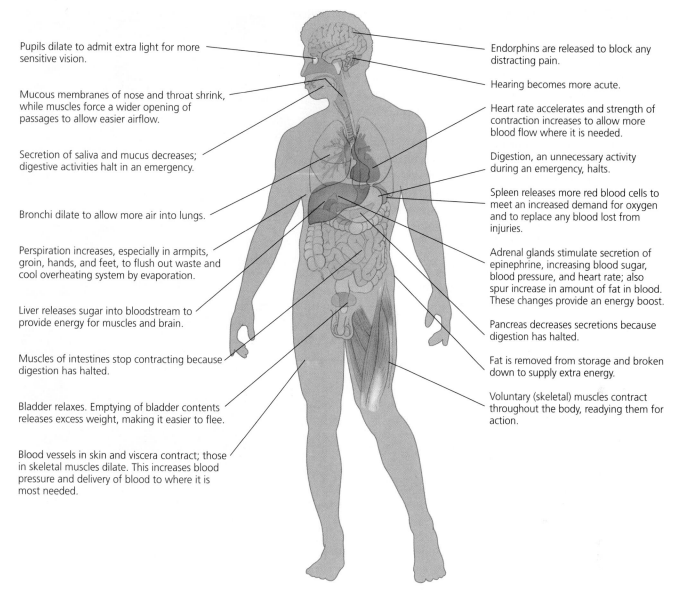

Pupils dilate to admit extra light for more sensitive vision.

Mucous membranes of nose and throat shrink, while muscles force a wider opening of passages to allow easier airflow.

Secretion of saliva and mucus decreases; digestive activities halt in an emergency.

Bronchi dilate to allow more air into lungs.

Perspiration increases, especially in armpits, groin, hands, and feet, to flush out waste and cool overheating system by evaporation.

Liver releases sugar into bloodstream to provide energy for muscles and brain.

Muscles of intestines stop contracting because digestion has halted.

Bladder relaxes. Emptying of bladder contents releases excess weight, making it easier to flee.

Blood vessels in skin and viscera contract; those in skeletal muscles dilate. This increases blood pressure and delivery of blood to where it is most needed.

Endorphins are released to block any distracting pain.

Hearing becomes more acute.

Heart rate accelerates and strength of contraction increases to allow more blood flow where it is needed.

Digestion, an unnecessary activity during an emergency, halts.

Spleen releases more red blood cells to meet an increased demand for oxygen and to replace any blood lost from injuries.

Adrenal glands stimulate secretion of epinephrine, increasing blood sugar, blood pressure, and heart rate; also spur increase in amount of fat in blood. These changes provide an energy boost.

Pancreas decreases secretions because digestion has halted.

Fat is removed from storage and broken down to supply extra energy.

Voluntary (skeletal) muscles contract throughout the body, readying them for action.

FIGURE 10.1   The fight-or-flight reaction.   In response to a stressor, the autonomic nervous system and the endocrine system cause physical changes that prepare the body to deal with an emergency.

you are facing a threat—and your body prepares to meet the danger. Chemical messages and actions of sympathetic nerves cause the release of key hormones, including **cortisol** and **epinephrine.** These hormones trigger a series of profound physiological changes (Figure 10.1), including:

- Heart and respiration rates accelerate to speed oxygen through the body.
- Hearing and vision become more acute.
- The liver releases extra sugar into the bloodstream to boost energy.
- Perspiration increases to cool the skin.
- The brain releases **endorphins**—chemicals that can inhibit or block sensations of pain—in case you are injured.

Taken together, these almost-instantaneous physical changes are called the **fight-or-flight reaction.** They give you the heightened reflexes and strength you need to dodge the car or deal with other stressors. Although these physical changes may vary in intensity, the same

cortisol   A steroid hormone secreted by the cortex (outer layer) of the adrenal gland; also called *hydrocortisone.*

epinephrine   A hormone secreted by the medulla (inner core) of the adrenal gland that affects the functioning of organs involved in responding to a stressor; also called *adrenaline.*

endorphins   Brain secretions that have pain-inhibiting effects.

fight-or-flight reaction   A defence reaction that prepares a person for conflict or escape by triggering hormonal, cardiovascular, metabolic, and other changes.

TERMS

basic set of physical reactions occurs in response to any type of stressor—positive or negative, physical or psychological.

THE RETURN TO HOMEOSTASIS   Once a stressful situation ends, the parasympathetic division of your autonomic nervous system takes command and halts the reaction. It restores **homeostasis**, a state in which blood pressure, heart rate, hormone levels, and other vital functions are maintained within a narrow range of normal. Your parasympathetic nervous system calms your body down, slowing a rapid heartbeat, drying sweaty palms, and returning breathing to normal. Gradually, your body resumes its normal "housekeeping" functions, such as digestion and temperature regulation. Damage that may have been sustained during the fight-or-flight reaction is repaired. The day after you narrowly dodge the car, you wake up feeling fine. In this way, your body can grow, repair itself, and acquire reserves of energy. When the next crisis comes, you'll be ready to respond again, instantly.

THE FIGHT-OR-FLIGHT REACTION IN MODERN LIFE The fight-or-flight reaction is a part of our biological heritage, and it's a survival mechanism that has served humans well. In modern life, however, it is often inappropriate. Many stressors we face in everyday life do not require a physical response—for example, an exam, a mess left by a roommate, or a stop light. The fight-or-flight reaction prepares the body for physical action regardless of whether such action is a necessary or appropriate response to a particular stressor.

Emotional and Behavioural Responses to Stressors

We all experience a similar set of physical responses to stressors, which make up the fight-or-flight reaction. These responses, however, vary from person to person and from one situation to another. People's perceptions of potential stressors—and their reactions to such stressors—also vary greatly. For example, you may feel confident about taking exams but may be nervous about talking to people you don't know, while your roommate may love challenging social situations but may be very nervous about taking tests. Many factors, some external and some internal, help explain these differences.

Your cognitive appraisal of a potential stressor will influence how it is viewed. Two factors that can reduce the magnitude of the stress response are successful prediction and the perception control. For instance, obtaining course syllabi at the beginning of the term allows you to predict the timing of major deadlines and exams. Having this predictive knowledge also allows you to exert some control over your study and recreation plans and can thus help reduce the stress caused by exams.

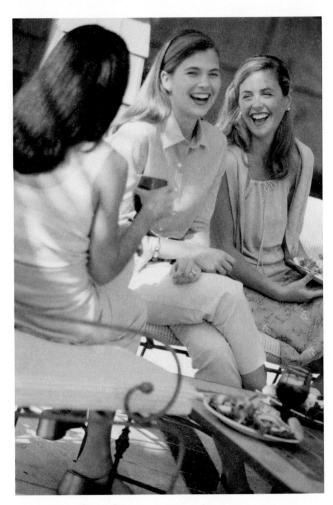

A person's emotional and behavioural responses to stressors depend on many different factors, including personality, gender, and cultural background. Research suggests that women are more likely than men to respond to stressors by seeking social support, a pattern referred to as tend-and-befriend.

Cognitive appraisal is highly individual and strongly related to emotions. The facts of a situation—Who? What? Where? When?—typically are evaluated fairly consistently from person to person. Evaluation with respect to personal outcome, however, varies: What does this mean for me? Can I do anything about it? Will it improve or worsen? If an individual perceives a situation as exceeding her or his ability to cope, the result can be

WELLNESS TIP

Chronic stress not only harms your health, it can make you age faster. A study of women who were long-term caregivers to very sick children revealed that, over time, the women's bodies lost their ability to create new red blood cells. On average, these women were physically 10 years older than their actual chronological age. This is one reason it pays to learn to manage stress, especially when you're young!

negative emotions and an inappropriate stress response. If, on the other hand, a person perceives a situation as a challenge that is within her or his ability to manage, more positive and appropriate responses are likely. A moderate level of stress, if coped with appropriately, can help promote optimal performance (Figure 10.2).

EFFECTIVE AND INEFFECTIVE RESPONSES Common emotional responses to stressors include anxiety, depression, and fear. Although emotional responses are determined in part by inborn personality or temperament, we often can moderate or learn to control them. Coping techniques are discussed later in the chapter.

Behavioural responses to stressors—controlled by the **somatic nervous system,** which manages our conscious actions—are entirely under our control. Effective behavioural responses such as talking, laughing, exercising, meditating, learning time-management skills, and finding a more compatible roommate can promote wellness and enable us to function at our best. Ineffective behavioural responses to stressors include overeating, expressing hostility, and using tobacco, alcohol, or other drugs.

PERSONALITY AND STRESS Some people seem to be nervous, irritable, and easily upset by minor annoyances; others are calm and composed even in difficult situations. Scientists remain unsure just why this is or how the brain's complex emotional mechanisms work. But **personality,** the sum of behavioural and emotional tendencies, clearly affects how people perceive and react to stressors. To investigate the links among personality, stress, and overall wellness, researchers have looked at different constellations of characteristics, or "personality types."

- *Type A.* People with Type A personality are often described as ultracompetitive, controlling, impatient, aggressive, and even hostile. Type A people have a higher perceived stress level and more problems coping with stress. They react explosively to stressors and are upset by events that others would consider only annoyances. Studies indicate that certain characteristics of the Type A pattern—anger, cynicism, and hostility—increase the risk of heart disease.

- *Type B.* The Type B personality is relaxed and contemplative. Type B people are less frustrated by daily events and more tolerant of the behaviour of others.

- *Type C.* The Type C personality is characterized by difficulty expressing emotions, anger suppression, feelings of hopelessness and despair, and an exaggerated stress response to minor cognitive stressors. This heightened response may be related to impaired immune functions.

Studies of Type A and C personalities suggest that expressing your emotions is beneficial but that habitually expressing exaggerated stress responses or hostility is unhealthy.

Researchers have also looked for personality traits that enable people to deal more successfully with stress. One such trait is hardiness, a particular form of optimism. People with a hardy personality view potential stressors as challenges and opportunities for growth and learning, rather than as burdens. Hardy people perceive fewer situations as stressful, and their reaction to stressors tends to be less intense. They are committed to their activities, have a sense of inner purpose and an inner locus of control, and feel at least partly in control of their lives.

You probably can't change your basic personality, but you can change your typical behaviours and patterns of thinking and develop positive coping strategies. You can also use stress management techniques like those described later in the chapter.

GENDER AND STRESS Our gender role—the activities, abilities, and behaviours our culture expects of us based on our sex—can affect our experience of stress. Some behavioural responses to stressors, such

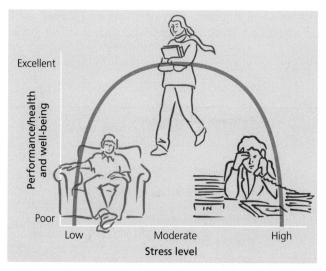

FIGURE 10.2 Stress level, performance, and well-being. A moderate level of stress challenges individuals in a way that promotes optimal performance and well-being. Too little stress, and people are not challenged enough to improve; too much stress, and the challenges become stressors that can impair physical and emotional health.

homeostasis A state of stability and consistency in a person's physiological functioning.

somatic nervous system The branch of the peripheral nervous system that governs motor functions and sensory information, largely under conscious control.

personality The sum of behavioural, cognitive, and emotional tendencies.

TERMS

QUESTIONS FOR CRITICAL THINKING AND REFLECTION

Think of the last time you faced a significant stressor. How did you respond? List the physical, emotional, and behavioural reactions you felt. Did these responses help you deal with the stress, or did they interfere with your efforts to handle it?

as crying or openly expressing anger, may be deemed more appropriate for one gender than the other. Strict adherence to gender roles can thus place limits on how a person responds to stress and can itself become a source of stress. Adherence to traditional gender roles can also affect the perception of a potential stressor. For example, if a man derives most of his sense of self-worth from his work, retirement may be a more stressful life change for him than for a woman whose self-image is based on several different roles.

Although both men and women experience the fight-or-flight physiological response to stress, women are more likely to respond behaviourally with a pattern of "tend-and-befriend"—nurturing friends and family and seeking social support and social contacts. Rather than becoming aggressive or withdrawing from difficult situations, women are more likely to create and enhance their social networks in ways that reduce stress.

PAST EXPERIENCES Past experiences can profoundly influence the evaluation of a potential stressor. Consider an individual who has had a bad experience giving a speech in the past. He or she is much more likely to perceive an upcoming speech as stressful than someone who has had positive public speaking experiences. Effective behavioural responses, such as careful preparation and visualizing success, can help overcome the effects of negative past experiences.

The Stress Experience as a Whole

Physical, emotional, and behavioural responses to stressors are intimately interrelated. The more intense the emotional response, the stronger the physical response. Effective behavioural responses can lessen stress; ineffective ones only worsen it. Sometimes people have such intense responses to stressors or such ineffective coping techniques that they need professional help. (Table 10.1 lists some of the symptoms of excess stress.) More often, however, people can learn to handle stressors on their own.

LO2 10.2 STRESS AND WELLNESS

The role of stress in health and disease is complex, and much remains to be learned about the exact mechanisms by which stress influences health. However, mounting evidence suggests that stress can increase vulnerability to numerous ailments. Several theories have been proposed to explain the relationship between stress and disease.

The General Adaptation Syndrome

Biologist Hans Selye was one of the first scientists to develop a comprehensive theory of stress and disease. Based on his work in the 1930s and 1940s, Selye coined the term **general adaptation syndrome (GAS)** to describe what he believed is a universal and predictable response pattern to all stressors. Some stressors are pleasant, such as attending a party, or unpleasant, such as a bad grade.

TABLE 10.1 Symptoms of Excess Stress

Physical Symptoms	Emotional Symptoms	Behavioural Symptoms
Dry mouth	Anxiety or edginess	Crying
Excessive perspiration	Depression	Disrupted eating habits
Frequent illnesses	Edginess	Disrupted sleeping habits
Gastrointestinal problems	Fatigue	Harsh treatment of others
Grinding of teeth	Hypervigilance	Problems communicating
Headaches	Impulsiveness	Sexual problems
High blood pressure	Inability to concentrate	Social isolation
Pounding heart	Irritability	Increased use of tobacco, alcohol, or other drugs
Stiff neck or aching lower back	Trouble remembering things	

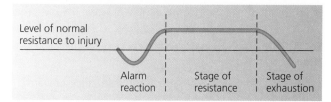

FIGURE 10.3 **The general adaptation syndrome.** During the alarm phase, a lower resistance to injury is evident. With continued stress, resistance to injury is actually enhanced. With prolonged exposure to repeated stressors, exhaustion sets in, with a return of low resistance levels seen during acute stress.

SOURCE: Insel, P. M., and W. T. Roth, 2004. *Core Concepts in Health,* 9th ed. 2004 update. Copyright © 2004 The McGraw-Hill Companies, Inc. Reprinted with permission of The McGraw-Hill Companies, Inc.

In the GAS theory, stress triggered by a pleasant stressor **eustress**; stress triggered by an unpleasant stressor **distress.** The sequence of physical responses associated with GAS (Figure 10.3). is the same for both eustress and distress and occurs in three stages:

- *Alarm.* The alarm stage includes the complex sequence of events brought on by the fight-or-flight reaction. During this stage, the body is more susceptible to disease or injury because it is geared up to deal with a crisis. Someone in this phase may experience headaches, indigestion, anxiety, and disrupted sleeping and eating patterns.

- *Resistance.* With continued stress, the body develops a new level of homeostasis in which it is more resistant to disease and injury than normal. During this stage, a person can cope with normal life and added stress.

- *Exhaustion.* The first two stages of GAS require a great deal of energy. If a stressor persists, or if several stressors occur in succession, general exhaustion results. This is not the sort of exhaustion people complain of after a long, busy day. Rather it's a life-threatening type of physiological exhaustion.

Allostatic Load

Although GAS is still viewed as a key contribution to the understanding of stress, some aspects of it are now outdated. For example, increased susceptibility to disease after repeated or prolonged stress is now thought to be due to the effects of the stress response itself rather than to a depletion of resources (exhaustion stage). In particular, long-term overexposure to such stress hormones as cortisol has been linked with health problems. Further, although physical stress reactions promote homeostasis (resistance stage), they also have negative effects on the body.

The long-term wear and tear of the stress response is called the **allostatic load.** An individual's allostatic load depends on many factors, including genetics, life

experiences, and emotional and behavioural responses to stressors. A high allostatic load may be due to frequent stressors, poor adaptation to common stressors, an inability to shut down the stress response, or imbalances in the stress response of different body systems. High allostatic load has been linked with heart disease, high blood pressure, obesity, and reduced brain and immune system functioning. In other words, when your allostatic load exceeds your ability to cope, you are more likely to get sick.

Psychoneuroimmunology

One of the most fruitful areas of current research into the relationship between stress and disease is **psychoneuroimmunology (PNI).** PNI is the study of the interactions among the nervous system, the endocrine system, and the immune system. The underlying premise of PNI is that stress, through the actions of the nervous and endocrine systems, impairs the immune system and thereby affects health.

There is a complex network of nerve and chemical connections between the nervous and endocrine systems and the immune system. We have already seen the profound physical effects of hormones and other chemical messengers released during the stress response. These compounds also influence the immune system by affecting the number and efficiency of immune system cells, or lymphocytes.

The nervous, endocrine, and immune systems share other connections. Scientists have identified hormone-like substances called *neuropeptides* that appear to translate emotions into physiological events. Neuropeptides are produced and received by both brain and immune cells, so that the brain and the immune system share a

general adaptation syndrome (GAS) A pattern of stress responses consisting of three stages: alarm, resistance, and exhaustion.

eustress Stress resulting from a pleasant stressor.

distress Stress resulting from an unpleasant stressor.

allostatic load The long-term negative impact of the stress response on the body.

psychoneuroimmunology (PNI) The study of the interactions among the nervous, endocrine, and immune systems.

TERMS

TAKE CHARGE

Overcoming Insomnia

Most people can overcome insomnia by discovering the cause of poor sleep and taking steps to remedy it. Insomnia that lasts for more than 6 months and interferes with daytime functioning requires consultation with a physician. Sleeping pills are not recommended for chronic insomnia because they can be habit-forming; they also lose their effectiveness over time.

If you're bothered by insomnia, try the following:

- Determine how much sleep you need to feel refreshed the next day, and don't sleep longer than that.

- Go to bed at the same time every night and, more important, get up at the same time every morning, 7 days a week, regardless of how much sleep you got. Don't nap more than 30 minutes per day.

- Exercise regularly, but not too close to bedtime. Your metabolism needs at least 6 hours to slow down after exercise.

- Avoid tobacco and caffeine late in the day, and alcohol before bedtime (it causes disturbed, fragmented sleep).

- If you take any medications (prescription or not), ask your doctor or pharmacist if they interfere with sleep.

- Have a light snack before bedtime; you'll sleep better if you're not hungry.

- Use your bed only for sleep. Don't eat, read, study, or watch television in bed.

- Establish a relaxing bedtime routine that helps you unwind and lets your brain know it's time to go to sleep. Read, listen to music, or practise a relaxation technique. Don't lie down in bed until you're sleepy.

- If you don't fall asleep in 15–20 minutes, or if you wake up and can't fall asleep again, get out of bed, leave the room if possible, and do something monotonous until you feel sleepy. Try distracting yourself with imagery instead of counting sheep; imagine yourself on a pleasant vacation or enjoying some beautiful scenery.

- If sleep problems persist, ask your doctor for a referral to a sleep specialist in your area. You may be a candidate for a sleep study—an overnight evaluation of your sleep pattern that can uncover many sleep-related disorders.

Ask Yourself

QUESTIONS FOR CRITICAL THINKING AND REFLECTION

Have you ever felt so much stress that you felt ill in some way? If so, what were your symptoms? How did you handle them? Did the experience affect the way you reacted to other stressful events?

biochemical "language," which also happens to be the language of emotions. The biochemical changes accompanying particular emotions can strongly influence the functioning of the immune system.

Links Between Stress and Specific Conditions

Although much remains to be learned, it is clear that people who have unresolved chronic stress in their lives or who handle stressors poorly are at risk for a wide range of health problems. In the short term, the problem might just be a cold, a stiff neck, or a stomachache. Over the long term, the problems can be more severe, such as cardiovascular disease or impairment of the immune system.

CARDIOVASCULAR DISEASE The stress response profoundly affects the cardiovascular system. During the stress response, heart rate increases and blood vessels constrict, causing blood pressure to rise. Chronic

high blood pressure is a major cause of atherosclerosis, a disease in which the lining of the blood vessels becomes damaged and caked with fatty deposits. These deposits can block arteries, causing heart attacks and strokes (see Chapter 11).

Recent research suggests that certain types of emotional responses increase a person's risk of cardiovascular disease. People who exhibit extreme increases in heart rate and blood pressure in response to emotional stressors, may face an increased risk of cardiovascular problems.[1]

ALTERED FUNCTIONING OF THE IMMUNE SYSTEM PNI research helps explain how stress affects the immune system. Some of the health problems linked to stress-related changes in immune function include vulnerability to colds and other infections, asthma and allergy attacks, susceptibility to cancer, and flare-ups of chronic diseases such as genital herpes and HIV infection.

OTHER HEALTH PROBLEMS Many other health problems may be caused or worsened by uncontrolled stress, including the following:

- Digestive problems such as stomachaches, diarrhea, constipation, irritable bowel syndrome, and ulcers
- Tension headaches and migraines
- Insomnia and fatigue (see the "Overcoming Insomnia" box)
- Injuries, including on-the-job injuries caused by repetitive strain

- Menstrual irregularities, impotence, and pregnancy complications
- Psychological problems, including depression, anxiety, panic attacks, eating disorders, and post-traumatic stress disorder (PTSD), which afflicts people who have suffered or witnessed severe trauma

LO3 10.3 COMMON SOURCES OF STRESS

Being able to recognize potential sources of stress is an important step in successfully managing the stress in our lives.

Major Life Changes

Any major change in your life that requires adjustment and accommodation can be a source of stress. Early adulthood and the university/college years are typically associated with many significant changes, such as moving out of the family home, establishing new relationships, setting educational and career goals, and developing a sense of identity and purpose. Even changes typically thought of as positive—graduation, job promotion, marriage—can be stressful.

Clusters of life changes, particularly those that are perceived negatively, may be linked to health problems in some people. Personality and coping skills are important moderating influences, however. People with a strong support network and a stress-resistant personality are less likely to become ill in response to major life changes than people with fewer resources.

Daily Hassles

Although major life changes are undoubtedly stressful, they seldom occur regularly. Researchers have proposed that minor problems—life's daily hassles, such as losing your keys or wallet—can be an even greater source of stress because they occur much more often.

People who perceive hassles negatively are likely to experience a moderate stress response every time they are faced with one. Over time, this can take a significant toll on health. Studies indicate that for some people, daily hassles contribute to a general decrease in overall wellness.

University/College Stressors

University or college is a time of major life changes and abundant minor hassles. For many students, university/college means being away from home for the first time, or you may be adding extra responsibilities to a life already filled with job and family. In 2003 the American College Health Association interviewed over 19 000 students with results showing that stress was self-reported to be the greatest impediment to academic performance.[2] A 2001 University of Alberta study found that university/college students saw finding a meaningful career, and academic and financial concerns as the greatest stressors on student life.[3]

Nearly all students share stresses like the following:

- *Academic stressors.* Exams, grades, and an endless workload await every university/college student but can be especially troublesome for young students just out of high school.
- *Interpersonal stressors.* Most students are more than just students; they are also friends, children, employees, spouses, parents, and so on. Managing relationships while juggling the rigors of university/college life can be daunting, especially if some friends or family are less than supportive.
- *Time pressures.* Class schedules, assignments, and deadlines are an inescapable part of university/college life. But these time pressures can be drastically compounded for students who also have a job and/or family responsibilities.
- *Financial concerns.* The majority of university/college students need financial aid not just to cover the cost of tuition but to survive from day to day while in school. For many, university/college life isn't possible without a job, and the pressure to stay afloat financially competes with academic and other stressors.
- *Worries about the future.* As university/college life comes to an end, students face the reality of life after university/college. This means thinking about a career, choosing a place to live, and leaving the friends and routines of school behind.

Job-Related Stressors

In recent surveys, 30% of Canadians rate their jobs as the key source of stress in their lives. Tight schedules and overtime leave less time to exercise, socialize, and engage in other stress-proofing activities. Only a third of the Canadian workforce report working the standard 40-hour work week while about a quarter spend 50 hours or more per week at their job. This is a 10% increase from 10 years ago.[4] Worries about job performance, salary, and job security and interactions with bosses, coworkers, and customers can contribute to stress. High levels of job stress are also common for people who are left out of important decisions relating to their jobs. When workers are given the opportunity to shape how their jobs are performed, job satisfaction goes up and stress levels go down.

If job-related (or education-related) stress is severe or chronic, the result can be *burnout*, a state of physical, mental, and emotional exhaustion. Burnout occurs most often in highly motivated and driven individuals who come to feel that their work is not recognized or that they are not accomplishing their goals. People in the helping professions—teachers, social workers, caregivers, police officers, and so on—are also prone to burnout. For some people who suffer from burnout, a vacation or leave of absence may be appropriate. For others, a reduced work schedule, better communication with superiors, or a change in job goals may be necessary. Improving time-management skills can also help.

Interpersonal and Social Stressors

Although social support is a key buffer against stress, your interactions with others can themselves be a source of stress. Your relationships with family members and old friends may change as you develop new interests and as the course of your life changes.

The community and society in which you live can also be major sources of stress. Social stressors include prejudice and discrimination. You may feel stress as you try to relate to people of other ethnic or socioeconomic groups. As a member of a particular ethnic group, you may feel pressure to assimilate into mainstream society. If English or French is not your first language, you face the added burden of conducting many daily activities in a language with which you may not be completely comfortable.

Other Stressors

Environmental stressors—external conditions or events that cause stress—include loud noises, unpleasant smells, industrial accidents, violence, and natural disasters. Internal stressors are found not in our interactions with our environment but within ourselves. We put pressure on ourselves to reach personal goals and then evaluate our progress and performance. Physical and emotional states such as illness and exhaustion are other examples of internal stressors.

LO4 10.4 MANAGING STRESS

What can you do about these effects of stress? A great deal. By pursuing a wellness lifestyle—being physically active, eating well, getting enough sleep, and so on—and by learning simple ways to identify and moderate individual stressors, you can control the stress in your life. (There are also some stress-management practices you should avoid; see the following section on "Counterproductive Strategies for Coping with Stress").

Counterproductive Strategies for Coping with Stress

University/college students develop a variety of habits in response to stress—some of them ineffective and even unhealthy. Here are a few unhealthy coping techniques to avoid:

- *Alcohol:* A few drinks might make you feel at ease, and getting drunk may help you forget the stress in your life—but any relief alcohol provides is temporary. Binge drinking and excessive alcohol consumption are not effective ways to handle stress, and using alcohol to deal with stress puts you at risk for all the short-term and long-term problems associated with alcohol abuse.

- *Tobacco:* The nicotine in cigarettes and other tobacco products can make you feel relaxed and may even increase your ability to concentrate. Tobacco, however, is highly addictive and smoking causes cancer, heart disease, sexual problems, and many other health problems. Tobacco is one of the leading preventable causes of death in Canada.

- *Other drugs:* Altering your body chemistry in order to cope with stress is a strategy that has many pitfalls. Caffeine raises cortisol levels and blood pressure and disrupts sleep. Marijuana can elicit panic attacks with repeated use, and some research suggests that it heightens the body's stress response.

- *Binge eating:* Eating can induce relaxation, which reduces stress. Eating as a means of coping with stress, however, may lead to weight gain and to binge eating, a risky behaviour associated with eating disorders.

There is one other problem with these methods of fighting stress; that is, none of them addresses the actual cause of the stress in your life. To combat stress in a healthy way, learn some of the stress-management techniques described in this chapter.

Exercise

Researchers have found that people who exercise regularly react with milder physical stress responses before, during, and after exposure to stressors and that their overall sense of well-being increases as well

Ask Yourself

QUESTIONS FOR CRITICAL THINKING AND REFLECTION

What are the top two or three stressors in your life right now? Are they new to your life—as part of your university/college experience—or are they stressors you've experienced in the past? Do they include both positive and negative experiences (eustress and distress)?

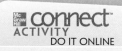

Does Exercise Improve Mental Health?

The overall conclusion from the many papers that have investigated the association between physical activity and mental health is that exercise—even modest activity such as taking a daily walk—can help combat a variety of mental health problems. For example, studies found that regular physical activity protects against depression and the onset of major depressive disorders; it can also reduce symptoms of depression in otherwise healthy people. Other studies found that physical activity protects against anxiety and the onset of anxiety disorders (such as specific phobia, social phobia, generalized anxiety, and panic disorder); it also helps reduce symptoms in people affected with anxiety disorders.

Physical activity can enhance feelings of well-being in some people, which may provide some protection against psychological distress. Overall, physically active people are about 25–30% less likely to feel distressed than inactive people. Regardless of the number, age, or health status of the people being studied, those who were active managed stress better than their inactive counterparts.

Researchers have also looked at specific aspects of the activity-stress association. For example, one study found that taking a long walk can be effective at reducing anxiety and blood pressure. Another showed that a brisk walk of as little as 10 minutes' duration can leave people feeling more relaxed and energetic for up to 2 hours. People who took three brisk 45-minute walks each week for 3 months reported that they perceived fewer daily hassles and had a greater sense of general wellness.

The findings are not surprising. The stress response mobilizes energy resources and readies the body for physical emergencies. If you experience stress and do not exert yourself physically, you are not completing the energy cycle. You may not be able to exercise while your daily stressors are occurring, but you can be active later in the day. Such activity allows you to expend the nervous energy you have built up and trains your body to return more readily to homeostasis after stressful situations.

Scientists have not determined how much physical activity is needed to effectively manage stress, but it's safe to say that the amount required varies with the individual. If you are an easygoing person who doesn't let life's minor hassles get to you, you may require significantly less activity for stress management than a hard-charging Type A personality who reacts hotly to any stressor. Regardless, experts believe that the more active you are, the more stress-relieving benefits you will enjoy. But studies show that you don't have to increase your fitness to decrease stress levels. Simply being active can make most people feel less stressed, whether or not they are trying to improve their fitness.

Physical activity also helps you sleep better, and consistently sound sleep is critical to managing stress. According to the National Sleep Foundation, about two-thirds of us have trouble sleeping at least a few nights a week, and 41% say they have difficulty sleeping virtually every night. There are about 70 known sleep disorders, and disordered sleep is associated with a variety of physical and neurological problems, including health problems relating to stress. Although only a few small-scale studies have been done on the relationship between physical activity and sleep, most experts have concluded that regular activity promotes better sleep and provides some protection against sleep interruptions such as insomnia and sleep apnea. Consistent, restful sleep is now regarded as a protective factor in disorders such as depression, anxiety, obesity, and heart disease.

SOURCES: Physical Activity Guidelines Advisory Committee. 2008. *Physical Activity Guidelines Advisory Committee Report, 2008.* Washington, D.C.: U.S. Department of Health and Human Services; and National Sleep Foundation. 2011. *2011 Sleep in America Poll: Summary of Findings.* Washington, D.C.: National Sleep Foundation.

THE EVIDENCE FOR EXERCISE

(see the box "Does Exercise Improve Mental Health?"). Although even light exercise can have a beneficial effect, an integrated fitness program can have a significant impact on stress.

For some people, however, exercise can become just one more stressor in a highly stressed life. People who exercise compulsively risk overtraining, a condition characterized by fatigue, irritability, depression, and diminished athletic performance. An overly strenuous exercise program can even make a person sick by compromising immune function. For the details of a safe and effective exercise program, refer to Chapter 9.

Nutrition

A healthy, balanced diet will supply the energy needed to cope with stress. In addition, eating wisely will enhance your feelings of self-control and self-esteem. Avoiding or limiting caffeine is also important in stress management. Although one or two cups of coffee a day probably won't hurt you, caffeine is a mildly addictive stimulant that leaves some people jittery, irritable, and unable to sleep; consuming caffeine during stressful situations can raise blood pressure and increase levels of cortisol. (For more on sound nutrition and for advice on evaluating dietary supplements, many of which are marketed for stress, see Chapter 7.)

Sleep

Adults need 7–9 hours of sleep every night to stay healthy and perform their best. Getting enough sleep isn't just good for you physically; adequate sleep also improves mood, fosters feelings of competence and self-worth, enhances mental functioning, and supports emotional functioning.

SLEEP AND STRESS Stress hormone levels in the bloodstream vary throughout the day and are related to sleep patterns. Peak concentrations of these hormones

Building Social Support

Meaningful connections with others can play a key role in stress management and overall wellness. A sense of isolation can lead to chronic stress, which in turn can increase one's susceptibility to temporary illnesses like colds and to chronic illnesses like heart disease. Although the mechanism isn't clear, social isolation can be as significant to mortality rates as factors like smoking, high blood pressure, and obesity.

There is no single best pattern of social support that works for everyone. However, research suggests that having a variety of types of relationships may be important for wellness. Here are some tips for strengthening your social ties:

- **Foster friendships.** Keep in regular contact with your friends. Offer respect, trust, and acceptance, and provide help and support in times of need. Express appreciation for your friends.

- **Keep your family ties strong.** Stay in touch with the family members you feel close to. Participate in family activities and celebrations. If your family doesn't function well as a support system for its members, create a second "family" of people with whom you have built meaningful ties.

- **Get involved with a group.** Do volunteer work, take a class, attend a lecture series, join a religious group. These types of activities can give you a sense of security, a place to talk about your feelings or concerns, and a way to build new friendships. Choose activities that are meaningful to you and that include direct involvement with other people.

- **Build your communication skills.** The more you share your feelings with others, the closer the bonds between you will become. When others are speaking, be a considerate and attentive listener.

Individual relationships change over the course of your life, but it's never too late to build friendships or become more involved in your community. Your investment of time and energy in your social network will pay off—in a brighter outlook now, and in better health and well-being for the future.

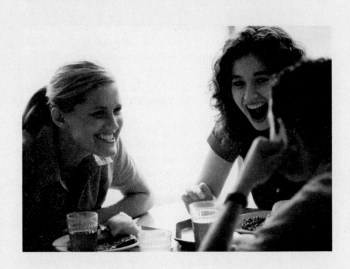

SOURCE: "Friends can be good medicine." 1998. As found in the *Mind/Body Newsletter* 7(1): 3–6.

occur in the early morning, followed by a slow decline during the day and evening. Concentrations return to peak levels during the final stages of sleep and in the early morning hours.

Even though stress hormones are released during sleep, it is the lack of sleep that has the greatest impact on stress. The Better Sleep Council of Canada reported that one third of Canadians are unable to sleep at night at least once per week as a result of stress. In someone who is suffering from sleep deprivation (not getting enough sleep over time), mental and physical processes deteriorate steadily. A sleep-deprived person experiences headaches, feels irritable, is unable to concentrate, and is more prone to forgetfulness. Poor-quality sleep has long been associated with stress and depression. A small 2008 study of female university/college students further associated sleep deprivation with an increased risk of suicide.

Acute sleep deprivation slows the daytime decline in stress hormones, so evening levels are higher than normal. A decrease in total sleep time also causes an increase in the level of stress hormones. Together, these changes may cause an increase in stress hormone levels throughout the day and may contribute to physical and mental exhaustion. Extreme sleep deprivation can lead to hallucinations and other psychotic symptoms, as well as to a significant increase in heart attack risk.

Social Support

Sharing fears, frustrations, and joys make life richer and seems to contribute to the well-being of body and mind. One study of university/college students found that students are more likely to exercise if they have social support for that activity, and that the social support that women prefer differs from that of men. In fact, women showed a greater preference for social support from family members while social support from friends was more encouraging for men.[5] Other studies have shown that married people have greater satisfaction with life and a healthier cardiovascular system than single people.[6] The crucial common denominator in all these findings is the meaningful connection with others. For more on developing and maintaining your social network, see the box "Building Social Support."

Spiritual wellness means different things to different people. For many, it involves developing a set of guiding beliefs, principles, or values that give purpose and meaning to life. It helps people achieve a sense of wholeness within themselves and in their relationships with others. Spiritual wellness influences people on an individual level, as well as on a community level, where it can bond people together through compassion, love, forgiveness, and self-sacrifice.

There are many paths to spiritual wellness. One of the most common in our society is organized religion. The major religions provide paths for transforming the self in ways that can lead to greater happiness and serenity and reduce feelings of anxiety and hopelessness. For example, in Christianity salvation follows turning away from the selfish ego to God's sovereignty and grace, where a joy is found that frees the believer from anxious self-concern and despair. Islam is the word for a kind of self-surrender leading to peace with God. Buddhism teaches how to detach oneself from selfish desire, leading to compassion for the suffering of others and freedom from fear-engendering illusions. Judaism emphasizes the social and ethical redemption the Jewish community can experience if it follows the laws of God.

Religions teach specific techniques for achieving these transformations of the self: prayer, both in groups and in private; meditation; the performance of rituals and ceremonies symbolizing religious truths; and good works and service to others. Religious organizations also usually offer social and material support to members who might otherwise be isolated.

Spiritual wellness does not require participation in organized religion. Many people find meaning and purpose in other ways. By spending time in nature or working on environmental issues, people can experience continuity with the natural world. Spiritual wellness can come through helping others in one's community or by promoting human rights, peace and harmony among people, and opportunities for human development on a global level. Other people develop spiritual wellness through art or through their personal relationships.

How would you define spiritual wellness and its role in your life? What beliefs and practices do you associate with your sense of spiritual wellness? To achieve overall well-being, it is important to take time out to consider what you can do to help your spiritual side grow and flourish.

Communication

How do you communicate your wishes and needs to others? Communicating in an assertive way that respects the rights of others as well as your own rights can prevent potentially stressful situations from getting out of control.

Some people have trouble either telling others what they need or saying no to the needs of others. They may suppress their feelings of anger, frustration, and resentment, and they may end up feeling taken advantage of or suffering in unhealthy relationships. At the other extreme are people who express anger openly and directly by being verbally or physically aggressive or indirectly by making critical, hurtful comments to others. Their abusive behaviour pushes other people away, so they also have problems with relationships.

Good communication skills can help everyone form and maintain healthy relationships. If you typically suppress your feelings, you might want to take an assertiveness training course that can help you identify and change your patterns of communication. If you have trouble controlling your anger, you can benefit from learning anger management strategies; see the box "Dealing with Anger."

Striving for Spiritual Wellness

Spiritual wellness is associated with greater coping skills and higher levels of overall wellness. It is a very personal wellness component, and there are many ways to develop it (see the box "Paths to Spiritual Wellness"). Researchers have linked spiritual wellness to longer life expectancy, reduced risk of disease and faster recovery, and improved emotional health. Although spirituality is difficult to study, and researchers

WELLNESS TIP

In a stressful situation, do you ever stop and count to 10? If not, you should. It works! In the few seconds it takes to count to 10, you can calm your mind, get your breathing under control, slow your heart rate, and lower your blood pressure. In effect, that quick 10-count can offset the stress reaction and help you avoid making things worse.

aren't sure how or why spirituality seems to improve health, several explanations have been offered. Lab 10.3 includes exercises designed to help you build spiritual wellness.

Confiding in Yourself Through Writing

Keeping a diary is like confiding in someone else, except that you are confiding in yourself. This form of coping with severe stress may be especially helpful for those who are shy or introverted and find it difficult to open up to others. Although writing about traumatic and stressful events may have a short-term negative effect on mood, over the long term, stress is reduced and positive changes in health occur. A key to promoting health and well-being through journaling is to write about your emotional responses to stressful events. Set aside a special time each day or week to write down your feelings about stressful events in your life.

Time Management

Learning to manage your time successfully can be crucial to coping with everyday stressors. Overcommitment, procrastination, and even boredom are significant

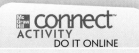

TAKE CHARGE

Dealing with Anger

Anger is a natural response to something we perceive as a betrayal, injustice, threat, or other wrong—whether real or imagined. We may respond physically with faster heart and breathing rates, increased muscle tension, a knot in the stomach, trembling, or a red face. When anger alerts us that something is wrong, it is a useful emotion that can lead to constructive change. When anger leads to loss of control and to aggression, it causes problems.

According to current popular wisdom, it's healthy to express your feelings, including anger. However, research has shown that people who are overtly hostile are at higher risk for heart disease and heart attacks than calmer people. In addition, expressing anger in thoughtless or out-of-control ways can damage personal and professional relationships.

People who experience rage or explosive anger are particularly at risk for negative repercussions. Some of these people may have *intermittent explosive disorder,* characterized by aggressiveness that is impulsive and out of proportion to the stimulus. Explosive anger renders people temporarily unable to think straight or act in their own best interests. Counselling can help very angry people learn how to manage their anger.

In dealing with anger, it is important to distinguish between a reasonable degree of self-assertiveness and a gratuitous expression of aggression. When you are *assertive,* you stand up for your own rights at the same time that you respect the rights of others. When you are *aggressive,* you violate the rights of others.

Managing Your Own Anger

What are the best ways to handle anger? If you find yourself in a situation where you are getting angry, answer these questions:

- Is the situation important enough to get angry about?

- Are you truly justified in getting angry?

- Is expressing your anger going to make a positive difference?

If the answer to all these questions is yes, then calm, assertive communication may be appropriate. Use "I" statements to express your feelings ("I would like . . . ," "I feel . . ."), and listen respectfully to the other person's point of view. Don't attack verbally or make demands; try to negotiate a constructive, mutually satisfying solution.

If you answer no to any of the questions, try to calm yourself. First, reframe the situation by thinking about it differently. Try these strategies:

- Don't take it personally—maybe the driver who cut you off simply didn't see you.

- Look for mitigating factors—maybe the classmate who didn't say hello was preoccupied with money concerns.

- Practise empathy—try to see the situation from the other person's point of view.

- Ask questions—clarify the situation by asking what the other person meant. Avoid defensiveness.

- Focus on the present—don't let this situation trigger thoughts of past incidents that you perceive as similar.

Second, calm your body down.

- Use the old trick of counting to 10 before you respond.

- Concentrate on your breathing, and take long, slow breaths.

- Imagine yourself in a beautiful, peaceful place.

- If needed, take a longer cooling-off period by leaving the situation until your anger has subsided.

Dealing with Other People's Anger

If someone you are with becomes very angry, try these strategies:

- Respond asymmetrically—remain calm. Don't get angry in response.

- Apologize if you think you are to blame. (Don't apologize if you don't think you are to blame.)

- Validate the other person by acknowledging that he or she has some reason to be angry. However, don't accept verbal abuse.

- Focus on the problem and ask what can be done to alleviate the situation.

- If the person cannot be calmed, disengage from the situation, at least temporarily. After a time-out, attempts at rational problem solving may be more successful.

Warning Signs of Violence

Violence is never acceptable. The following behaviours over a period of time suggest the potential for violence:

- A history of making threats and engaging in aggressive behaviour

- Drug or alcohol abuse

- Gang membership

- Access to or fascination with weapons

- Feelings of rejection or aloneness; the feeling of constantly being disrespected; victimization by bullies

- Withdrawal from usual activities and friends; poor school performance

- Failure to acknowledge the rights of others

The following are immediate warning signs of violence:

- Daily loss of temper or frequent physical fighting

- Significant vandalism or property damage

- Increased risk-taking behaviour; increased drug or alcohol abuse

- Threats or detailed plans to commit acts of violence

- Pleasure in hurting animals

- The presence of weapons

Don't spend time with someone who shows these warning signs of violence. Ask someone in authority or an experienced professional for help.

stressors for many people. Along with gaining control of nutrition and exercise to maintain a healthy energy balance, time management is an important element in a wellness program. Try these strategies for improving your time-management skills:

- **Set priorities**. Divide your tasks into three groups: essential, important, and trivial. Focus on the first two. Ignore the third.
- **Schedule tasks for peak efficiency**. You've undoubtedly noticed you're most productive at certain times of the day (or night). Schedule as many of your tasks for those hours as you can and stick to your schedule.
- **Set realistic goals and write them down**. Attainable goals spur you on. Impossible goals, by definition, cause frustration and failure. Fully commit yourself to achieving your goals by putting them in writing.
- **Budget enough time**. For each project you undertake, calculate how long it will take to complete. Then tack on another 10–15%, or even 25%, as a buffer.
- **Break up long-term goals into short-term ones**. Instead of waiting for or relying on large blocks of time, use short amounts of time to start a project or keep it moving.
- **Visualize achieving your goals**. By mentally rehearsing your performance of a task, you will be able to reach your goal more smoothly.
- **Keep track of the tasks you put off**. Analyze the reasons why you procrastinate. If the task is difficult or unpleasant, look for ways to make it easier or more fun. For example, if you find the readings for one of your classes particularly difficult, choose an especially nice setting for your reading and then reward yourself each time you complete a section or chapter.
- **Consider doing your least-favourite tasks first**. Once you have the most unpleasant ones out of the way, you can work on the projects you enjoy more.
- **Consolidate tasks when possible**. For example, try walking to the store so that you run your errands and exercise in the same block of time.
- **Identify quick transitional tasks**. Keep a list of 5- to 10-minute tasks you can do while waiting or between other tasks, such as watering your plants, doing the dishes, or checking a homework assignment.
- **Delegate responsibility**. Asking for help when you have too much to do is no cop-out; it's good time management. Just don't delegate to others the jobs you know you should do yourself.
- **Say no when necessary**. If the demands made on you don't seem reasonable, say no—tactfully, but without guilt or apology.

- **Give yourself a break**. Allow time for play—free, unstructured time when you ignore the clock. Don't consider this a waste of time. Play renews you and enables you to work more efficiently.
- **Avoid your personal "time sinks."** You can probably identify your own time sinks, activities like watching television, surfing the Internet, or talking on the phone that consistently use up more time than you anticipate and put you behind schedule. Some days, it may be best to avoid problematic activities altogether; for example, if you have a big paper due, don't sit down for a 5-minute TV break if it is likely to turn into a 2-hour break. Try a 5-minute walk if you need to clear your head.
- **Stop thinking or talking about what you're going to do, and just do it!** Sometimes the best solution for procrastination is to stop waiting for the right moment and just get started. You will probably find that things are not as bad as you feared, and your momentum will keep you going.

For more help with time management, complete Activity 10 in the Behaviour Change Workbook at the end of the text.

Cognitive Techniques

Certain thought patterns and ways of thinking, including ideas, beliefs, and perceptions, can contribute to stress and have a negative impact on health. The Transactional Model of Stress and Coping (Lazarus and Folkman, 1984) is just one model that examines our cognitive abilities where stress is concerned. This model suggests that we will cognitively appraise whether the stress that we enocunter threatens our well-being. We are then able to determine whether or not we have the resources to meet the demands of that stressor. Lazarus and Folkman suggest that if we appraise the stress as a challenge, that allows us to view the stress in a positive way and to realize that we can overcome and prosper.

Other habits of mind, if practised with patience and consistency, can help break unhealthy thought patterns. Here are some suggestions that might help us appraise situations more positively.

- Monitor your self-talk and attempt to minimize hostile, critical, suspicious, and self-deprecating thoughts (see the box "Realistic Self-Talk").
- Modify expectations; they often restrict experience and lead to disappointment. Try to accept life as it comes.
- Live in the present; clear your mind of old debris and fears for the future so you can enjoy life as it is now.
- "Go with the flow." Accept what you can't change; forgive faults; be flexible.

Cultivating your sense of humour is another key cognitive stress management technique. Even a fleeting smile

Got a problem that's causing you stress? Solve it! Problem solving is a skill—one that requires practice and patience, but one that can pay off in a more balanced, less stressful life. Think of a problem that's bugging you right now, and take the following steps to solve it:

1. Define the problem in a sentence or two. Write it down.

2. List the problem's cause. There may be more than one.

3. List some potential solutions. Don't stop with one or the most obvious one. Write down several options.

4. For each solution, list the potential positive and negative consequences. Be thorough.

5. Choose the solution you think will work best, or will have the fewest negative consequences.

6. List the steps you'll need to take to carry out your solution.

7. Get started with the list of steps you just made. Don't delay unless you have to.

8. As you work on solving the problem, pause occasionally and reevaluate. Revise your approach, if necessary.

If you can't seem to solve a problem on your own, get help. Talk to someone who knows you well, or get help from a counsellor, and work through these steps again. Any problem can be solved, but some may just be too big to handle on your own.

---

produces changes in your autonomic nervous system that can lift your spirits. Hearty laughter triggers the release of endorphins, and after a good laugh, your muscles go slack and your pulse and blood pressure dip below normal—you are relaxed.

Relaxation Techniques

The **relaxation response** is a physiological state characterized by a feeling of warmth and quiet mental alertness. This response is the opposite of the fight-or-flight reaction. When the relaxation response is triggered by a relaxation technique, heart rate, breathing, and metabolism slow down; blood flow to the brain and skin increases; and brain waves shift from an alert beta rhythm to a relaxed alpha rhythm.

The techniques described in this section and in the box "Relaxation Through Meditation" are among the most popular techniques and the easiest to learn. All these techniques take practice, so it may be several weeks before the benefits become noticeable in everyday life.

PROGRESSIVE RELAXATION In this simple relaxation technique, you tense, then relax the muscles of the body one by one. Also known as deep muscle relaxation, this technique addresses the muscle tension that occurs when the body is experiencing stress. Consciously relaxing tensed muscles sends a message to other body systems to reduce the stress response.

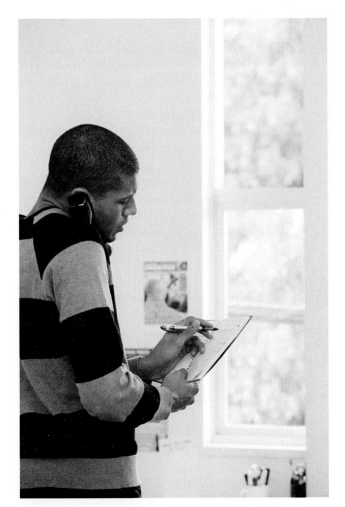

Managing the many commitments of adult life—including work, school, and relationships—can sometimes feel overwhelming and produce a great deal of stress. Time-management skills, including careful scheduling with a datebook or handheld computer, can help people cope with busy days.

TERMS

relaxation response A physiological state characterized by a feeling of warmth and quiet mental alertness.

Realistic Self-Talk

Do your patterns of thinking make events seem worse than they truly are? Do negative beliefs about yourself become self-fulfilling prophecies? Substituting realistic self-talk for negative self-talk can help you build and maintain self-esteem and cope better with the challenges in your life. Here are some examples of common types of distorted, negative self-talk, along with suggestions for more accurate and rational responses.

Cognitive Distortion	Negative Self-Talk	Realistic Self-Talk
Focusing on negatives	School is so discouraging—nothing but one hassle after another.	School is pretty challenging and has its difficulties, but there certainly are rewards. It's really a mixture of good and bad.
Expecting the worst	Why would my boss want to meet with me this afternoon if not to fire me?	I wonder why my boss wants to meet with me. I guess I'll just have to wait and see.
Overgeneralizing	(After getting a poor grade on a paper) Just as I thought—I'm incompetent at everything.	I'll start working on the next paper earlier. That way, if I run into problems, I'll have time to consult with the TA.
Minimizing	I won the speech contest, but none of the other speakers was very good. I wouldn't have done as well against stiffer competition.	It may not have been the best speech I'll ever give, but it was good enough to win the contest. I'm really improving as a speaker.
Blaming others	I wouldn't have eaten so much last night if my friends hadn't insisted on going to that restaurant.	I overdid it last night. Next time I'll make different choices.
Expecting perfection	I should have scored 100% on this test. I can't believe I missed that one problem through a careless mistake.	Too bad I missed one problem through carelessness, but overall I did very well on this test. Next time I'll be more careful.

SOURCE: Based on W. Schafer. 1999. *Stress Management for Wellness,* 4th ed. Copyright © 2000 Wadsworth, a part of Cengage Learning, Inc. Reproduced by permission (http://www.cengage.com/permissions).

To practise progressive relaxation, begin by inhaling as you contract your right fist. Then exhale as you release your fist. Repeat. Contract and relax your right bicep. Repeat. Do the same using your left arm. Then, working from forehead to feet, contract and relax other muscles. Repeat each contraction at least once, inhaling as you tense and exhaling as you relax. To speed up the process, tense and relax more muscles at one time—for example, both arms simultaneously. With practice you'll be able to relax quickly by simply clenching and releasing only your fists.

VISUALIZATION Visualization, also known as using imagery, is so effective in enhancing sports performance that it has become part of the curriculum at training camps for Canadian Olympic athletes. This same technique can be used to induce relaxation, to help change habits, or to improve performance on an exam, on stage, or on a playing field.

To practise visualization, imagine yourself floating on a cloud, sitting on a mountaintop, or lying in a meadow. Try to identify all the perceptible qualities of the environment—sight, sound, temperature, smell, and so on. Your body will respond as if your imagery were real.

An alternative is to close your eyes and imagine a deep purple light filling your body. Then change the colour into a soothing gold. As the colour lightens, so should your distress. Imagery can also enhance performance: Visualize yourself succeeding at a task that worries you.

DEEP BREATHING Your breathing pattern is closely tied to your stress level. Deep, slow breathing is associated with relaxation. Rapid, shallow, often irregular breathing occurs during the stress response. With practice, you can learn to slow and quiet your breathing pattern, thereby also quieting your mind and relaxing your body. Try one of the breathing techniques described in the box "Breathing for Relaxation" for on-the-spot tension relief, as well as for long-term stress reduction.

LISTENING TO MUSIC Music can relax us. It has been shown to influence pulse, blood pressure, and the electrical activity of muscles. Listening to soothing, lyrical music can lessen depression, anxiety, and stress levels. To experience the stress-management benefits of music

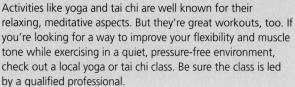

FITNESS TIP

Activities like yoga and tai chi are well known for their relaxing, meditative aspects. But they're great workouts, too. If you're looking for a way to improve your flexibility and muscle tone while exercising in a quiet, pressure-free environment, check out a local yoga or tai chi class. Be sure the class is led by a qualified professional.

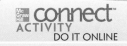
DIMENSIONS OF DIVERSITY

Techniques for managing stress by inducing the relaxation response have been developed in many cultures over the centuries. One such technique is yoga, described in Chapter 5. Another technique that has become popular in North America is meditation.

At its most basic level, meditation, or self-reflective thought, involves quieting or emptying the mind to achieve deep relaxation. Some practitioners of meditation view it on a deeper level as a means of focusing concentration, increasing self-awareness, and bringing enlightenment to their lives. Meditation has been integrated into the practices of several religions—Buddhism, Hinduism, Confucianism, Taoism—but it is not a religion itself, nor does its practice require any special knowledge, belief, or background.

There are many styles of meditation, based on different ways of quieting the mind. Here is a simple, practical technique for eliciting the relaxation response using one style:

1. Pick a word, a phrase, or an object to focus on. You can choose a word or phrase that has a deep meaning for you, but any word or phrase will work. Some meditators prefer to focus on their breathing.

2. Sit comfortably in a quiet place. Close your eyes if you're not focusing on an object.

3. Relax your muscles.

4. Breathe slowly and naturally. If you're using a focus word or phrase, silently repeat it each time you exhale. If you're using an object, focus on it as you breathe.

5. Keep your attitude passive. Disregard thoughts that drift in.

6. Continue for 10–20 minutes once or twice a day.

7. After you've finished, sit quietly for a few minutes with your eyes closed, then open. Then stand up.

Allow relaxation to occur at its own pace; don't force it. Don't be surprised if you can't tune your mind out for more than a few seconds at a time. It's nothing to get angry about. The more you ignore the intrusions, the easier it will become. If you want to time your session, peek at a watch or clock occasionally, but don't set a jarring alarm.

Although you'll feel refreshed even after the first session, it may take a month or more to get noticeable results. Be patient. Eventually, the relaxation response become so natural that it occurs spontaneously or on demand when you sit quietly for a few moments.

yourself, set aside a time to listen. Choose music you enjoy and selections that make you feel relaxed.

Other Techniques

Other stress-management techniques, such as biofeedback, hypnosis and self-hypnosis, and massage, require a partner or professional training or assistance. As with the relaxation techniques presented, all take practice, and it may be several weeks before the benefits are noticeable.

Biofeedback helps people reduce their response to stress by enabling them to become more aware of their level of physiological arousal. In biofeedback, some measure of stress—perspiration, heart rate, skin temperature, or muscle tension—is mechanically monitored, and feedback is given using sound (a tone or music), light, or a meter or dial. With practice, people begin to exercise conscious control over their physiological stress responses. The point of biofeedback training is to develop the ability to transfer the skill to daily life without the use of electronic equipment. Biofeedback initially requires the help of a therapist, stress counsellor, or technician.

LO5 10.5 GETTING HELP

You can use the principles of behavioural self-management described in Chapter 1 to create a stress-management program tailored specifically to your needs. The starting point of a successful program is to listen to your body. When you learn to recognize the stress response and the emotions and thoughts that accompany it, you'll be in a position to take charge of how you handle stress. Labs 10.1 and 10.2 can guide you in identifying and finding ways to cope with stress-inducing situations.

If you feel you need guidance beyond the information in this text, excellent self-help guides can be found in bookstores or the library; helpful websites are listed in For Further Exploration at the end of the chapter; and most university/college campuses have counselling services that assist students in dealing with stresses that may be specific to them.

Some people also find it helpful to express their feelings in a journal. Grappling with a painful experience in this way provides an emotional release and can help you develop more constructive ways of dealing with similar situations in the future.

Peer Counselling and Support Groups

If you still feel overwhelmed despite efforts to manage your stress, you may want to seek outside help. Peer counselling, often available through the student health centre or counselling centre, is usually staffed by people with special training that emphasizes maintaining confidentiality. Peer counsellors can steer those seeking help to appropriate campus and community resources or just offer sympathetic listening.

Diaphragmatic Breathing

1. Lie on your back with your body relaxed.

2. Place one hand on your chest and one on your abdomen. (You will use your hands to monitor the depth and location of your breathing.)

3. Inhale slowly and deeply through your nose into your abdomen. Your abdomen should push up as far as is comfortable. Your chest should expand only a little and only in conjunction with the movement of your abdomen.

4. Exhale gently through your mouth.

Tension-Release Breathing

1. Lie down or sit in a chair and get comfortable.

2. Take a slow, deep breath into your abdomen. Inhale through your nose. Try to visualize the air moving to every part of your body. As you breathe in, say to yourself, "Breathe in relaxation."

3. Exhale through your mouth. Visualize tension leaving your body. Say to yourself, "Breathe out tension."

There are many variations on these techniques. For example, sit in a chair and raise your arms, shoulders, and chin as you inhale; lower them as you exhale. Or slowly count to 4 as you inhale, then again as you exhale.

Many yoga experts suggest breathing rhythmically, in time with your own heartbeat. Relax and listen closely for the sensation of your heart beating, or monitor your pulse while you breathe. As you inhale, count to 4 or 8 in time with your heartbeat, then repeat the count as you exhale. Breathing in time with soothing music can work well, too.

Experts suggest inhaling through the nose and exhaling through the mouth. Breathe slowly, deeply, and gently. To focus on breathing gently, imagine a candle burning a few inches in front of you. Try to exhale softly enough to make the candle's flame flicker, not hard enough to blow it out.

Practice is important, too. Perform your chosen breathing exercise two or more times daily, for 5–10 minutes per session.

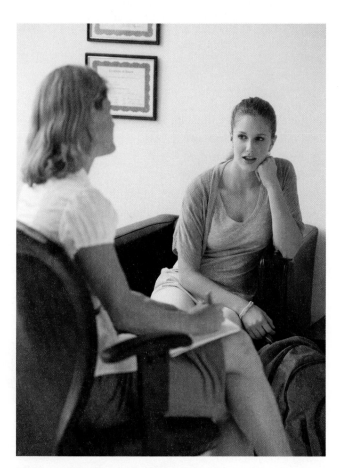

Many people seek help from professional therapists when dealing with stress-related problems.

Support groups are typically organized around a particular issue or problem: all group members might be entering a new school, re-entering school after an interruption, struggling with single parenting, experiencing eating disorders, or coping with particular kinds of trauma. Simply voicing concerns that others share can relieve stress.

Professional Help

Psychotherapy, especially a short-term course of sessions, can also be tremendously helpful in dealing with stress-related problems. Not all therapists are right for all people, so it's a good idea to shop around for a compatible psychotherapist with reasonable fees. (See the box "Choosing and Evaluating Mental Health Professionals.")

Is It Stress or Something More Serious?

Most of us have had periods of feeling down when we become pessimistic, anxious, less energetic, and less able to enjoy life. Such feelings and thoughts can be normal responses to the ordinary challenges of life. Symptoms that may indicate a more serious problem that requires professional help include the following:

- Depression, anxiety, or other emotional problems begin to interfere seriously with school or work performance or in getting along with others.

- Suicide is attempted or is seriously considered.

Choosing and Evaluating Mental Health Professionals

University and college students are usually in a good position to find convenient, affordable mental health care. Larger schools typically have both health services that employ psychiatrists and psychologists, and counselling centres staffed by professionals and peer counsellors. Resources in the community may include a school of medicine, a hospital, and a variety of professionals who work independently. It's a good idea to get recommendations from physicians, clergy, friends who have been in therapy, or community agencies rather than to pick a name at random.

Financial considerations are also important. Find out how much different services will cost and which ones are covered by medicare. If you're not adequately covered by your provincial health plan, don't let that stop you from getting help; investigate low-cost alternatives on campus and in your community. The cost of treatment is linked to how many therapy sessions will be needed, which in turn depends on the type of therapy and the nature of the problem. Psychological therapies focusing on specific problems may require 8 or 10 sessions at weekly intervals. Therapies aiming for psychological awareness and personality change can last months or years.

Deciding whether a therapist is right for you will require meeting the therapist in person. Before or during your first meeting, find out about the therapist's background and training:

- Does she or he have a degree from an appropriate professional school?
- Has she or he had experience treating people with problems similar to yours?
- How much will therapy cost? Or is it free?

You have a right to know the answers to these questions and should not hesitate to ask them. After your initial meeting, evaluate your impressions:

- Does the therapist seem like a warm, intelligent person who would be able to help you and is interested in doing so?
- Are you comfortable with the personality, values, and beliefs of the therapist?
- Is he or she willing to talk about the techniques to be used? Do these techniques make sense to you?

If you answer yes to these questions, this therapist may be satisfactory for you. If you feel uncomfortable—and you're not in need of emergency care—it's worthwhile to set up one-time consultations with one or two others before you make up your mind. Take the time to find someone who feels right for you.

Later in your treatment, evaluate your progress:

- Are you being helped by the treatment?
- If you are displeased, is it because you aren't making progress or because therapy is raising difficult, painful issues you don't want to deal with?
- Can you express dissatisfaction to your therapist? Such feedback can improve your treatment.

If you're convinced your therapy isn't working or is harmful, thank your therapist for her or his efforts and find another.

- Symptoms such as hallucinations, delusions, incoherent speech, or loss of memory occur.
- Alcohol or drugs are used to the extent that they impair normal functioning; finding or taking drugs occupies much of the week; or reducing the dosage leads to psychological or physical withdrawal symptoms.

Depression is of particular concern because severe depression is linked to suicide, the second leading cause of death among Canadians between the ages of 15 to 25.[7] In some cases, depression, like severe stress, is a clear-cut reaction to a specific event, such as the loss of a loved one or failing in school or work. In other cases, no trigger event is obvious. Symptoms of depression include the following:

- Negative self-concept
- Pervasive feelings of sadness and hopelessness
- Loss of pleasure in usual activities
- Poor appetite and weight loss
- Insomnia or disturbed sleep
- Restlessness or fatigue
- Thoughts of worthlessness and guilt
- Trouble concentrating or making decisions
- Thoughts of death or suicide

Not all of these symptoms are present in everyone who is depressed, but most do experience a loss of interest or pleasure in their usual activities. Warning signs of suicide include expressing the wish to be dead; revealing

Ask yourself

QUESTIONS FOR CRITICAL THINKING AND REFLECTION

What percentage of your daily stress is time-related? How effective are your time management skills? Identify one thing you can start doing right now to manage your time better, and describe how you can apply it to one aspect of your daily routine.

Are there any relaxation techniques I can use in response to an immediate stressor?

Yes. Try the deep breathing techniques described in the chapter, and try some of the following to see which work best for you:

- Do a full-body stretch while standing or sitting. Stretch your arms out to the sides and then reach them as far as possible over your head. Rotate your body from the waist. Bend over as far as is comfortable for you.
- Do a partial session of progressive muscle relaxation. Tense and then relax some of the muscles in your body. Focus on the muscles that are stiff or tense. Shake out your arms and legs.
- Take a short, brisk walk (3–5 minutes). Breathe deeply.
- Engage in realistic self-talk about the stressor. Mentally rehearse dealing successfully with the stressor. As an alternative, focus your mind on some other activity.

- Briefly reflect on something personally meaningful. In one study of college students, researchers found that self-reflection on important personal values prior to a stressful task reduces the hormonal response to the stressor.

Can stress cause headaches?

Stress is one possible cause of the most common type of headache, the tension headache. About 90% of headaches are tension headaches, characterized by a dull, steady pain, usually on both sides of the head. It may feel as though a band of pressure is tightening around the head, and the pain may extend to the neck and shoulders. Acute tension headaches may last from hours to days, while chronic tension headaches may occur almost every day for months or even years. Stress, poor posture, and immobility are leading causes of tension headaches. There is no cure, but the pain can be relieved with over-the-counter painkillers; many people also try such therapies as massage, relaxation, hot or cold showers, and rest. Stress is also one possible trigger of migraine headaches, which are typically characterized by throbbing pain (often on one side of the head), heightened sensitivity to light and noise, visual disturbances such as flashing lights, nausea, and fatigue.

If your headaches are frequent, keep a journal with details about the events surrounding each one. Are your tension headaches associated with late nights, academic deadlines, or long periods spent sitting at a computer? Are migraines associated with certain foods, stress, fatigue, specific sounds or odours, or (in women) menstruation? If you can identify the stressors or other factors that are consistently associated with your headaches, you can begin to gain more control over the situation. If you suffer persistent tension or migraine headaches, consult your physician.

contemplated suicide methods; increasing social withdrawal and isolation; and a sudden, inexplicable lightening of mood (which can indicate the person has finally decided to commit suicide).

If you are severely depressed or know someone who is, expert help from a mental health professional is essential. Most communities have emergency help available, often in the form of a hotline telephone counselling service, and many universities and colleges have health services and counselling centres that can provide help. Treatments for depression and many other psychological disorders are highly effective.

TIPS FOR TODAY AND THE FUTURE

For the stress you can't avoid, develop a range of stress-management techniques and strategies.

RIGHT NOW YOU CAN

- Practise deep breathing for 5 to 10 minutes.
- Visualize a relaxing, peaceful place and imagine yourself experiencing it as vividly as possible. Stay there as long as you can.
- Do some stretching exercises, such as those described in Chapter 5.
- Get out your datebook and schedule what you'll be doing the rest of today and tomorrow. Pencil in a short walk and a conversation with a friend.

IN THE FUTURE YOU CAN

- Take a class or workshop that can help you overcome a source of stress, such as one in assertiveness training or time management.
- Find a way to build relaxing time into every day. Just 15 minutes of meditation, stretching, or massage can induce the relaxation response.

- Stress is the collective physiological and emotional response to any stressor. Physiological responses to stressors are the same for everyone.

- The autonomic nervous system and the endocrine system are responsible for the body's physical response to stressors. The sympathetic nervous system mobilizes the body and activates key hormones of the endocrine system, causing the fight-or-flight reaction. The parasympathetic system returns the body to homeostasis.

- Behavioural responses to stress are controlled by the somatic nervous system and fall under a person's conscious control.

- The general adaptation syndrome model and research in psychoneuroimmunology contribute to our understanding of the links between stress and disease. People who have many stressors in their lives or handle stress poorly are at risk for cardiovascular disease, impairment of the immune system, and many other problems.

- Potential sources of stress include major life changes, daily hassles, school- and job-related stressors, and interpersonal and social stressors.

- Positive ways of managing stress include regular exercise, good nutrition, support from other people, clear communication, spiritual wellness, effective time management, cognitive techniques, and other relaxation techniques.

- If a personal program for stress management doesn't work, peer counselling, support groups, and psychotherapy are available.

FOR FURTHER EXPLORATION

Organizations and Websites

American College Health Association. Includes a reference to the National College Health Assessment (NCHA) assessment tool.
http://www.acha.org

American Psychological Association. Provides information on stress management and psychological disorders.
202-336-5500; 800-964-2000 (referrals)
http://www.apa.org
http://helping.apa.org

Association for Applied Psychophysiology and Biofeedback. Provides information and links about biofeedback.
http://www.aapb.org

Canadian Association for Suicide Prevention. Working to reduce suicide and its impact on Canadians.
http://www.suicideprevention.ca/

Canadian Centre for Occupational Health and Safety. Source of information for the promotion of a safe working environment.
http://www.ccohs.ca

Canadian Institute of Stress. Founded by Drs. Hans Selye and Richard Erle, the institute offers a number of tools and educational programs for the workplace, home, and others.
http://www.stresscanada.org/

Canadian Mental Health Association. Promotes good mental health for all including those experiencing mental illness.
http://www.cmha.ca

Harvard Mind-Body Medical Institute. Provides information about stress management and relaxation techniques.
http://www.mbmi.org

The Humor Project. A clearinghouse for information and practical ideas related to humour.
518-587-8770
http://www.humorproject.com

Interactive Budgeting Worksheet. An interactive calculator designed to help students balance income and expenses.
http://www.ed.gov/offices/OSFAP/DirectLoan/BudgetCalc/
budget.html

National Sleep Foundation. Works to help the public understand sleep and sleep disorders through the support of sleep-related research, education, and advocacy.
http://www.sleepfoundation.org

Student Counselling Virtual Pamphlet Collection. Links to online pamphlets from student counselling centres at colleges and universities; topics include stress, sleep, and time management.
http://counseling.uchicago.edu/vpc/

LAB 10.1 Identifying Your Stress Level and Key Stressors

McGraw Hill connect
ACTIVITY
DO IT ONLINE

How Much Stress Do You Suffer From?

To help determine how much stress you experience on a daily basis, answer the following questions.

How many of the symptoms of excess stress in the list below do you experience frequently?_____

Symptoms of Excess Stress

Physical Symptoms
Dry mouth
Excessive perspiration
Frequent illnesses
Gastrointestinal problems
Grinding of teeth
Headaches
High blood pressure
Pounding heart
Stiff neck or aching lower back

Emotional Symptoms
Anxiety or edginess
Depression
Fatigue
Hypervigilance
Impulsiveness
Inability to concentrate
Irritability
Trouble remembering things

Behavioural Symptoms
Crying
Disrupted eating habits
Disrupted sleeping habits
Harsh treatment of others
Problems communicating
Sexual problems
Social isolation
Increased use of tobacco,
  alcohol, or other drugs

Yes **No**

_____ _____ 1. Are you easily startled or irritated?
_____ _____ 2. Are you increasingly forgetful?
_____ _____ 3. Do you have trouble falling or staying asleep?
_____ _____ 4. Do you continually worry about events in your future?
_____ _____ 5. Do you feel as if you are constantly under pressure to produce?
_____ _____ 6. Do you frequently use tobacco, alcohol, or other drugs to help you relax?
_____ _____ 7. Do you often feel as if you have less energy than you need to finish the day?
_____ _____ 8. Do you have recurrent stomachaches or headaches?
_____ _____ 9. Is it difficult for you to find satisfaction in simple life pleasures?
_____ _____ 10. Are you often disappointed in yourself and others?
_____ _____ 11. Are you overly concerned with being liked or accepted by others?
_____ _____ 12. Have you lost interest in intimacy or sex?
_____ _____ 13. Are you concerned that you do not have enough money?

Experiencing some of the stress-related symptoms or answering yes to a few questions is normal. However, if you experience a large number of stress symptoms or you answered yes to a majority of the questions, you are likely experiencing a high level of stress. Take time out to develop effective stress-management techniques. Many coping strategies that can aid you in dealing with your university/college stressors are described in this chapter. Additionally, your school's counselling centre can provide valuable support.

Weekly Stress Log

Now that you are familiar with the signals of stress, complete the weekly stress log to map patterns in your stress levels and identify sources of stress. Enter a score for each hour of each day according to the ratings listed below.

	A.M.							P.M.												
	6	7	8	9	10	11	12	1	2	3	4	5	6	7	8	9	10	11	12	*Average*
Monday																				
Tuesday																				
Wednesday																				
Thursday																				
Friday																				
Saturday																				
Sunday																				
Average																				

Ratings: 1 = No anxiety; general feeling of well-being
2 = Mild anxiety; no interference with activity
3 = Moderate anxiety; specific signal(s) of stress present
4 = High anxiety; interference with activity
5 = Very high anxiety and panic reactions; general inability to engage in activity

To identify daily or weekly patterns in your stress level, average your stress rating for each hour and each day. For example, if your scores for 6:00 A.M. are 3, 3, 4, 3, and 4, with blanks for Saturday and Sunday, your 6:00 A.M. rating would be 17 ÷ 5, or 3.4 (moderate to high anxiety). Finally, calculate an average weekly stress score by averaging your daily average stress scores. Your weekly average will give you a sense of your overall level of stress.

Using Your Results

How did you score? How high are your daily and weekly stress scores? Are you at all surprised by your score for average stress level?

Are you satisfied with your stress rating? If not, set a specific goal:

What should you do next? Enter the results of this lab in the Preprogram Assessment column in Appendix C. If you've set a goal for improvement, begin by using your log to look for patterns and significant time periods in order to identify key stressors in your life. Below, list any stressors that caused you a significant amount of discomfort this week; these can be people, places, events, or recurring thoughts or worries. For each, enter one strategy that would help you deal more successfully with the stressor; examples of strategies might include practising an oral presentation in front of a friend or engaging in positive self-talk.

Next, begin to put your strategies into action. In addition, complete Lab 10.2 to help you incorporate lifestyle stress-management techniques into your daily routine.

LAB 10.2 Stress Management Techniques

Connect ACTIVITY DO IT ONLINE

Part I Lifestyle Stress Management

For each of the areas listed in the table below, describe your current lifestyle as it relates to stress management. For example, do you have enough social support? How are your exercise and nutrition habits? Is time management a problem for you? For each area, list two ways that you could change your current habits to help you manage your stress. Sample strategies might include calling a friend before a challenging class, taking a short walk before lunch, and buying and using a datebook to track your time.

	Current lifestyle	Lifestyle change #1	Lifestyle change #2
Social support system			
Exercise habits			
Nutrition habits			
Time management techniques			
Self-talk patterns			
Sleep habits			

Part II Relaxation Techniques

Choose two relaxation techniques described in this chapter (progressive relaxation, visualization, deep breathing, meditation, yoga, tai chi, massage, listening to music). If a taped recording is available for progressive relaxation or visualization, these techniques can be performed by your entire class as a group.

List the techniques you tried.

1. _____

2. _____

How did you feel before you tried these techniques?

_____

_____

_____

What did you think or how did you feel during each of the techniques you tried?

1. _____

_____

_____

2. _____

_____

_____

How did you feel after you tried these techniques?

_____

_____

_____

LAB 10.3 Developing Spiritual Wellness

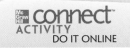

To develop spiritual wellness, it is important to take time out to think about what gives meaning and purpose to your life and what actions you can take to support the spiritual dimension of your life.

Look Inward

This week, spend some quiet time alone with your thoughts and feelings. Slow the pace of your day, remove your watch, turn your phone off, and focus on your immediate experience. Try one of the following activities or develop another that is meaningful to you and that contributes to your sense of spiritual well-being.

- *Spend time in nature.* Experience continuity with the natural world by spending solitary time in a natural setting. Watch the sky (day or night), a sunrise, or a sunset; listen to waves on a shore or wind in the trees; feel the breeze on your face or raindrops on your skin; smell the grass, brush, trees, or flowers. Open all your senses to the beauty of nature.

- *Experience art, architecture, or music.* Spend time with a work of art or architecture or a piece of music. Choose one that will awaken your senses, engage your emotions, and challenge your understanding. Take a break and then repeat the experience to see how your responses change the second time.

- *Express your creativity.* Set aside time for a favourite activity, one that allows you to express your creative side. Sing, draw, paint, play a musical instrument, sculpt, build, dance, cook, garden—choose an activity in which you will be so engaged that you will lose track of time. Strive for feelings of joy and exhilaration.

- *Engage in a personal spiritual practice.* Pray, meditate, do yoga, chant. Choose a spiritual practice that is familiar to you or try one that is new. Tune out the outside world and turn your attention inward, focusing on the experience.

In the space below, describe the personal spiritual activity you tried and how it made you feel—both during the activity and after.

Reach Out

Spiritual wellness can be a bond among people and can promote values such as altruism, forgiveness, and compassion. Try one of the following spiritual activities that involve reaching out to others.

- *Share writings that inspire you.* Find two writings that inspire, guide, and comfort you—passages from sacred works, poems, quotations from literature, songs. Share them with someone else by reading them aloud and explaining what they mean to you.

- *Practise kindness.* Spend a day practising small acts of personal kindness for people you know as well as for strangers. Compliment a friend, send a card, let someone go ahead of you in line, pick up litter, do someone else's chores, help someone with packages, say please and thank you, smile.

- *Perform community service.* Foster a sense of community by becoming a volunteer. Find a local nonprofit group and offer your time and talent. Mentor a youth, work at a food bank, support a literacy project, help build low-cost housing, visit seniors in a nursing home. You can also work on national or international issues by writing letters to your elected representatives and other officials.

In the space below, describe the spiritual activity you performed and how it made you feel—during the activity and after. Include details about the writings you chose or the acts of kindness or community service you performed.

Keep a Journal

One strategy for continuing on the path toward spiritual wellness is to keep a journal. Use a journal to record your thoughts, feelings, and experiences; to jot down quotes that engage you; to sketch pictures and write poetry about what is meaningful to you. Begin your spiritual journal today.

LAB 10.4 Time Management Skills

One method of reducing stress may be to examine the ways that you spend your time. Effectively spending time means that you are able to prioritize your daily activities and accomplish those things that are most important to you. Meeting deadlines, due dates, and preparing for classes and exams are all things that many students consider important.

Log Your Time

- Log your daily activities for a span of three days.
- For each day, use a table similar to Table A below to record your activities, the total time you spend on each activity (in half-hour units) and to indicate the priority level of each.
- Your priority levels are:
  - A—activities that MUST GET DONE that day
  - B—activities you would like to get done, but if you cannot complete them that day, they can wait until the next day.
  - C—activities that NEVER should have been done on that day

Table A

Activity:	Time Spent (in ½ hour blocks)	Priority level:

Total the time you spent on each of A, B, and C activities for all three days and record below. Note that the total of all three days should add up to 72 hours.

"A" Activities = _____ hours

"B" Activities = _____ hours

"C" Activities = _____ hours

Next, begin to put your priorities and strategies into action. Complete Lab 10.2 to help you incorporate lifestyle stress-management techniques into your daily routine.

CHAPTER 11

CARDIOVASCULAR HEALTH

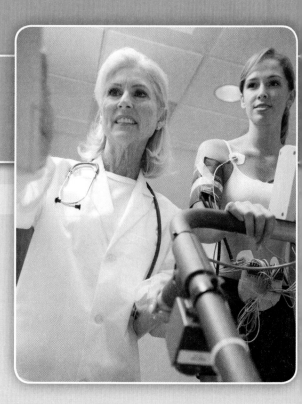

LEARNING OBJECTIVES

After reading this chapter, you should be able to

LO1 Discuss the major forms of cardiovascular disease and how they develop

LO2 Describe the controllable and uncontrollable risk factors associated with cardiovascular disease

LO3 List the steps you can take now to lower your personal risk of developing cardiovascular disease

TEST YOUR KNOWLEDGE

1. **Women are about as likely to die of cardiovascular disease as they are to die of breast cancer.**

   True or false?

2. **How much earlier, on average, do sedentary people develop heart disease compared with people who exercise?**

   a. 6 months
   b. 2 years
   c. 6 years

3. **Which of the following foods would be a good choice for promoting heart health?**

   a. whole grains
   b. salmon
   c. bananas

ANSWERS

1. **FALSE.** Cardiovascular disease kills far more. Among Canadian women, more than 1 in 3 deaths are due to CVD and about 1 in 25 is due to breast cancer. In addition, more women than men die each year from cardiovascular disease.

2. **C.** Both endurance exercise and strength training improve cardiovascular health.

3. **ALL THREE.** Whole grains (whole wheat, oatmeal, rye, barley, and brown rice), foods with omega-3 fatty acids (salmon), and foods high in potassium and low in sodium (bananas) all improve cardiovascular health.

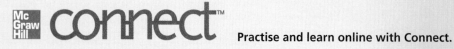

Practise and learn online with Connect.

Cardiovascular disease (CVD) is the leading cause of death in Canada (see Table 1.2, ranks 2–4); one-third of all Canadians alive today will die from CVD. Much of the incidence of CVD is attributable to the Canadian way of life. Too many Canadians are overweight and sedentary, smoke cigarettes, manage stress ineffectively, have uncontrolled high blood pressure or high cholesterol levels, and don't know the signs of CVD. Not all risk factors for CVD are controllable—some people have an inherited tendency toward high cholesterol levels, for example—but many are within the control of the individual.

This chapter explains the major forms of CVD, including hypertension, atherosclerosis, and stroke. It also considers the factors that put people at risk for CVD. Most important, it explains the steps individuals can take to protect their hearts and promote cardiovascular health throughout their lives.

LO1 11.1 MAJOR FORMS OF CARDIOVASCULAR DISEASE

As the leading cause of death in Canada, cardiovascular diseases kill over 73 000 people a year in this country alone. The financial burden of CVD, including the costs of medical treatments and lost productivity, exceeds $20 billion annually. Although the main forms of CVD are interrelated and have elements in common, we treat them separately here for the sake of clarity. Hypertension, which is both a major risk factor and a form of CVD, is discussed later in the chapter.

Atherosclerosis

Atherosclerosis is a form of arteriosclerosis, or thickening and hardening of the arteries. In atherosclerosis, arteries become narrowed by deposits of fat, cholesterol, and other substances. The process begins when the cells lining the arteries (endothelial cells) become damaged,

often through a combination of factors such as smoking, high blood pressure, and deposits of oxidized LDL particles. The body's response to this damage results in inflammation and changes in the artery lining. Deposits, called **plaques**, accumulate on artery walls; the arteries lose their elasticity and their ability to expand and contract, restricting blood flow. Once narrowed by a plaque, an artery is vulnerable to blockage by blood clots (Figure 11.1). The risk of life-threatening clots and heart attacks increases if the fibrous cap covering a plaque ruptures.

If the heart, brain, and/or other organs are deprived of blood, and oxygen it carries, the effects of atherosclerosis can be deadly. Coronary arteries, which supply the heart with blood, are particularly susceptible to plaque buildup, a condition called **coronary heart disease (CHD)**, or *coronary artery disease.* The blockage of a coronary artery causes a heart attack. If a cerebral artery (leading to the brain) is blocked, the result is a stroke. The main risk factors for atherosclerosis are cigarette smoking, physical inactivity, high levels of blood cholesterol, high blood pressure, and diabetes. Although the actual causes of atherosclerosis are complicated and not completely understood, physicians will work with patients to adjust lifestyle and prescribe medications, surgery, or other procedures as needed.

cardiovascular disease (CVD) A collective term for various diseases of the heart and blood vessels.

atherosclerosis A form of CVD in which the inner layers of artery walls are made thick and irregular by plaque deposits; arteries become narrowed, and blood supply is reduced.

plaque A deposit of fatty (and other) substances on the inner wall of the arteries.

coronary heart disease (CHD) Heart disease caused by atherosclerosis in the arteries that supply blood to the heart muscle; also called *coronary artery disease.*

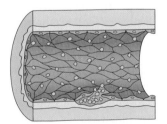

Plaque buildup begins when endothelial cells lining the arteries are damaged by smoking, high blood pressure, oxidized LDL, and other causes; excess cholesterol particles collect beneath these cells.

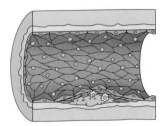

In response to the damage, platelets and other types of cells collect at the site; a fibrous cap forms, isolating the plaque within the artery wall. An early-stage plaque is called a fatty streak.

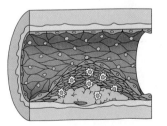

Chemicals released by cells in and around the plaque cause further inflammation and buildup; an advanced plaque contains LDL, white blood cells, connective tissue, smooth muscle cells, platelets, and other compounds.

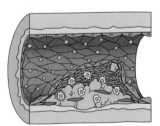

The narrowed artery is vulnerable to blockage by clots. The risk of blockage and heart attack rises if the fibrous cap cracks (probably due to destructive enzymes released by white blood cells within the plaque).

FIGURE 11.1 Stages of plaque development.

Heart Disease and Heart Attacks

Although a **heart attack,** or myocardial infarction (MI), may come without warning, it is usually the end result of a long-term disease process. The heart requires a steady supply of oxygen-rich blood to function properly (Figure 11.2). If one of the coronary arteries that supplies blood to the heart becomes blocked by a blood clot, a heart attack results. A heart attack caused by a clot is called a *coronary thrombosis*. During a heart attack, part of the heart muscle (myocardium) may die from lack of oxygen.

Chest pain called **angina pectoris** is a signal that the heart isn't getting enough oxygen to supply its needs. Although not actually a heart attack, angina—felt as an extreme tightness in the chest and heavy pressure behind the breastbone or in the shoulder, neck, arm, hand, or back—is a warning that the heart is overloaded.

If the electrical impulses that control heartbeat are disrupted, the heart may beat too quickly, too slowly, or in an irregular fashion, a condition known as **arrhythmia.** The symptoms of arrhythmia range from imperceptible to severe and even fatal. **Sudden cardiac death,** also called *cardiac arrest,* is most often caused by an arrythmia called *ventricular fibrillation,* a kind of "quivering" of the ventricle that makes it ineffective in pumping blood. If ventricular fibrillation continues for more than a few minutes, it is fatal. Cardiac defribillation, in which an electrical shock is delivered to the heart, can jolt the heart into a more efficient rhythm.

Not all heart attacks involve sharp chest pain. Women, in particular, are more likely to have different symptoms—shortness of breath, weakness, unusual fatigue, cold sweat, dizziness, and nausea. If symptoms of heart trouble do occur, it is critical to contact the emergency

medical service or go immediately to the nearest hospital or clinic with a 24-hour emergency cardiac facility (see the box "What to Do in Case of Heart Attack, Stroke, or Cardiac Arrest"). Many experts also suggest that the heart attack victim chew and swallow one adult aspirin tablet (325 mg); aspirin has an immediate anticlotting effect. If someone having a heart attack gets to the emergency room quickly enough, a clot-dissolving agent can be injected to dissolve a clot in the coronary artery, reducing the amount of damage to the heart muscle.

Physicians have a variety of diagnostic tools and treatments for heart disease. A patient may undergo a stress or exercise test, in which he or she runs on a treadmill or pedals a stationary cycle while being monitored with an electrocardiogram (ECG or EKG). Certain characteristic changes in the heart's electrical activity while it is under stress can reveal particular heart problems, such as restricted blood flow to the heart muscle. Tools that allow the physician to visualize a patient's heart and arteries include magnetic resonance imaging (MRI), electron-beam computed tomography (EBC), echocardiograms, and angiograms.

If tests indicate a problem or if a person has already had a heart attack, several treatments are possible. Along with a low-fat diet, regular exercise, and smoking cessation, many patients are also advised to take aspirin daily to reduce clotting and inflammation. However, there is a mounting body of evidence to show that daily aspirin therapy may be ineffective in preventing first-time heart attacks or strokes, even in patients at high risk for such events. Aspirin therapy has been shown to prevent subsequent heart attacks and strokes in people who have already had one. Prescription drugs can also help reduce the strain on the heart. *Balloon angioplasty,* a common surgical treatment, involves threading a catheter with an inflatable balloon tip through a coronary artery until it reaches the area of blockage; the balloon is then inflated, flattening the plaque and widening the arterial opening. Many surgeons permanently implant coronary stents—flexible stainless steel tubes—to prop the artery open and prevent reclogging after angioplasty. In *coronary bypass surgery,* healthy blood vessels from the person are grafted to coronary arteries to detour or bypass the blocked portion of the coronaty artery.

Stroke

A **stroke,** also called a *cerebrovascular accident (CVA),* occurs when the blood supply to the brain is cut off. If brain cells are deprived of blood for more than a few

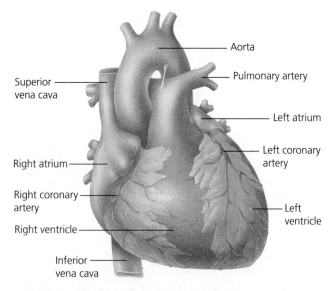

FIGURE 11.2 Blood supply to the heart. Blood is supplied to the heart from the right and left coronary arteries, which branch off the aorta. If a coronary artery becomes blocked by plaque buildup or a blood clot, a heart attack occurs; part of the heart muscle may die due to lack of oxygen.

Aorta

Pulmonary artery

Superior vena cava

Left atrium

Left coronary artery

Right atrium

Right coronary artery

Left ventricle

Right ventricle

Inferior vena cava

minutes, they die. Once brain cells begin dying, about 2 million cells are lost every minute that blood flow is not restored. Prompt treatment of stroke can greatly decrease the risk of permanent disability.

A stroke may be caused by a blood clot that blocks an artery (ischemic stroke) or by a ruptured blood vessel (hemorrhagic stroke). Ischemic strokes are often caused by atherosclerosis or certain types of arrhythmia. Hemorrhagic strokes may occur if there is a weak spot in an artery wall or following a head injury. The interruption of the blood supply to any area of the brain prevents the nerve cells there from functioning, in some cases, causing death. Nerve cells control sensation and most body movements; depending on the area of the brain that is affected, a stroke may cause paralysis, walking disability, speech impairment, or memory loss. Of the over 50 000 Canadians who have strokes each year, 15% will die and close to 75% will suffer some lasting disability.[1]

Effective treatment requires the prompt recognition of symptoms and correct diagnosis of the type of stroke that has occurred. Treatment may involve the use of clot-dissolving and antihypertensive drugs. Even if brain tissue has been damaged or destroyed, nerve cells in the brain can make new pathways, and some functions can be taken over by other parts of the brain.

Many people have strokes, however, without knowing it, so they do not realize they may need treatment or to be evaluated for the risk of a full-blown stroke in the future. These people suffer *silent cerebral infarcts*, more commonly known as "silent strokes." Silent strokes do not cause any noticeable symptoms while they are occurring. Although they may be mild, silent strokes leave their victims at a higher risk for subsequent and more serious strokes later in life. They also contribute to loss of mental and cognitive skills. In 2008, a study of MRI scans of 2000 elderly people revealed that 11% of the subjects had brain damage from one or more strokes but did not realize they had ever had a stroke. A 2009 study suggested that silent strokes may be five times more prevalent than full-blown strokes in people under age 65.

Congestive Heart Failure

The heart's pumping mechanism can be damaged by a number of conditions, including high blood pressure, heart attack, atherosclerosis, **rheumatic fever,** or birth defects. When the heart cannot maintain its regular pumping rate and force, fluids begin to back up. When extra fluid seeps through capillary walls, edema (swelling) results, usually in the legs and ankles, but sometimes in other parts of the body as well. Fluid can collect in the lungs and interfere with breathing, particularly when a person is lying down. This condition is called *pulmonary edema,* and the entire process is known as **congestive heart failure.** Treatment includes reducing the workload on the heart, modifying salt intake, and using drugs that help the body eliminate excess fluid.

Ask Yourself

QUESTIONS FOR CRITICAL THINKING AND REFLECTION

Has anyone you know ever had a heart attack? If so, was the onset gradual or sudden? Were appropriate steps taken to help the person (for example, call 911, give CPR, or use an AED? Do you feel comfortable dealing with a cardiac emergency? If not, what can you do to improve your readiness?

LO2 11.2 RISK FACTORS FOR CARDIOVASCULAR DISEASE

Researchers have identified a variety of factors associated with an increased risk of developing CVD. They are grouped into two categories: major risk factors and contributing risk factors. Some major risk factors, such as diet, exercise habits, and use of tobacco, are linked to controllable aspects of lifestyle and can therefore be changed. Others, such as age, sex, and heredity, are beyond an individual's control. (You can evaluate your personal CVD risk factors in Part I of Lab 11.1.)

CVD Risk Factors That Can Be Altered

The Canadian Heart Health Initiative and the Heart and Stroke Foundation of Canada have identified 6 major risk factors for CVD that can be changed. These are tobacco use, high blood pressure, unhealthy blood cholesterol levels, physical inactivity, obesity, diabetes. Also identified as alterable are triglyceride levels, psychological and social factors and drug use. Most Canadians, including young adults, have major risk factors for CVD. For example, among adult Canadians, close to 35% have

heart attack   Damage to, or death of, heart muscle, resulting from a failure of the coronary arteries to deliver enough blood to the heart; also known as *myocardial infarction* (MI).

angina pectoris   A condition in which the heart muscle does not receive enough blood, causing severe pain in the chest and often in the arm and shoulder.

arrhythmia   A change in the normal pattern of the heartbeat.

sudden cardiac death   A nontraumatic, unexpected death from sudden cardiac arrest, most often due to arrhythmia; in most instances, victims have underlying heart disease.

stroke   An impeded blood supply to some part of the brain resulting in the destruction of brain cells; also called *cerebrovascular accident (CVA).*

rheumatic fever   A disease, mainly of children, characterized by fever, inflammation, and pain in the joints; often damages the heart muscle, a condition called rheumatic heart disease.

congestive heart failure   A condition resulting from the heart's inability to pump out all the blood that returns to it. Blood backs up in the veins leading to the heart, causing an accumulation of fluid in various parts of the body.

TERMS

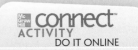

TAKE CHARGE

What to Do in Case of Heart Attack, Stroke, or Cardiac Arrest

Heart Attack Some heart attacks are sudden and intense, but most heart attacks start slowly, with mild pain or discomfort. Often people affected aren't sure what's wrong and wait too long before getting help. Here are signs that can mean a heart attack is happening:

- **Chest discomfort.** Most heart attacks involve discomfort in the centre of the chest that lasts more than a few minutes, or that goes away and comes back. It can feel like uncomfortable pressure, squeezing, fullness, or pain.

- **Discomfort in other areas of the upper body.** Symptoms can include pain or discomfort in one or both arms, the back, neck, jaw, or stomach.

- **Shortness of breath.** This may occur with or without chest discomfort.

- **Other signs.** These may include breaking out in a cold sweat, nausea, vomiting, or lightheadedness.

As with men, women's most common heart attack symptom is chest pain or discomfort. However, women are somewhat more likely than men to experience some of the other common symptoms, particularly shortness of breath, nausea or vomiting, and back or jaw pain.

If you or someone you're with has chest discomfort, especially with one or more of the other signs, don't wait more than 5 minutes before seeking help.

Calling 911 is almost always the fastest way to get lifesaving treatment. Emergency medical services (EMS) staff can begin treatment when they arrive—up to an hour sooner than if someone gets to the hospital by car. The staff are also trained to revive someone whose heart has stopped. Patients with chest pain who arrive by ambulance usually receive faster treatment at the hospital, too.

If you are the one having symptoms and you can't access EMS, have someone drive you to the hospital right away. Don't drive yourself unless you have absolutely no other option.

Stroke The Heart and Stroke Foundation says these are the warning signs of stroke:

- **Weakness**—sudden loss of strength or sudden numbness in the face, arm, or leg even if temporary.

- **Trouble speaking**—sudden difficulty speaking or understanding or sudden confusion, even if temporary.

- **Vision problems**—sudden trouble with vision, even if temporary.

- **Headache**—sudden severe and unusual headache.

- **Dizziness**—sudden loss of balance, especially with any of the above signs.

If you experience any of these symptoms, CALL 9-1-1 or your local emergency number immediately. Health Canada has approved the clot-busting drug called tPA to be used within 3 hours from the time symptoms begin. However, emerging science is now showing that tPA could be effective up to 4½ hours afterward. As a result, the Canadian Stroke Strategy has issued new Canadian Best Practices Recommendations for Stroke Care, which have included this new treatment time. Still, it will be up to the attending emergency doctors to determine when tPA may be administered or if it is appropriate to the situation.

Cardiac Arrest Cardiac arrest strikes immediately and without warning. Here are the signs:

- Sudden loss of responsiveness. No response to gentle shaking. No movement or coughing.

- No normal breathing. The victim does not take a normal breath for several seconds.

- No signs of circulation. No pulse or blood pressure.

If cardiac arrest occurs, call 911 or your local emergency number immediately and begin CPR immediately (visit your local Heart and Stroke Foundation, or http://www.heartandstroke.ca, to find out how to sign up to become certified in CPR). If an automated external defibrillator (AED) is available and someone trained to use it is nearby, involve her or him.

SOURCE: American Heart Association, 2010. *Heart Attack, Stroke, and Cardiac Arrest Warning Signs.* Reprinted with permission (http://www.americanheart.org). Copyright © 2010 American Heart Association.

---

high cholesterol levels,[2] 25% have hypertension,[3] 19% smoke,[4] and more than 32% are overweight.[5]

TOBACCO USE Your risk of developing CVD increases with the length and intensity of your exposure to cigarette smoke. Smokers are 2 to 4 times more likely to develop CVD than non-smokers. In addition, Canadians who smoke have a 70% greater chance of dying from CVD than non-smokers. Women who smoke double their risk for cervical cancer, triple their risk of dying from CVD and are 5 times more likely to die from a stroke than women who do not smoke.[6]

Smoking harms the cardiovascular system in several ways:

- It damages the linings of arteries.
- It reduces the level of *high-density lipoproteins (HDL)*, or "good" cholesterol.
- It raises the levels of triglycerides and *low-density lipoproteins (LDL)*, or "bad" cholesterol.
- Nicotine increases blood pressure and heart rate.
- The carbon monoxide in cigarette smoke displaces oxygen in the blood, reducing the amount of oxygen available to the body.

- Smoking causes **platelets** to stick together in the blood stream, leading to clotting.
- Smoking speeds the development of fatty deposits in the arteries.

You don't have to smoke to be affected. Environmental tobacco smoke (ETS), or second-hand smoke in high concentrations has been linked to the development of cardiovascular disease. ETS and high cholesterol levels act together to damage the cells that line artery walls. While exposure to ETS is a growing concern, measuring our exposure to ETS is not a simple task. Currently there is no easy method of assessing risk but recent research has concluded that some combination of body fluid evaluation (urine, blood, saliva) combined with parental recall information may be the optimal method of assessing ETS exposure in children.

HIGH BLOOD PRESSURE High blood pressure, or **hypertension,** is a risk factor for many forms of cardiovascular disease, including heart attacks and strokes, and is itself considered a form of CVD. Blood pressure, the force exerted by the blood on blood vessel walls, is created by the pumping action of the heart. High blood pressure occurs when too much force is exerted against the walls of the arteries. Short periods of high blood pressure—such as in response to excitement or exertion—are normal, but chronic high blood pressure is a health risk.

Blood pressure is measured with a stethoscope and a *sphygmomanometer* (see Chapter 3). At home, you can track your own blood pressure by using an inexpensive blood pressure monitor (see the box "Digital Tools for Heart Health"). Blood pressure is expressed as two numbers—for example, 120 over 80—and measured in millimetres of mercury. The first and larger number is the systolic blood pressure; the second is the diastolic blood pressure. A normal blood pressure reading for a healthy young adult is in the ranges of 115–120 systolic over 75–80 diastolic; CVD risk increases when blood pressure rises above this level. Canadian Hypertension Guidelines define high blood pressure in adults as equal to or greater than 140 over 90.

High blood pressure results from either an increased output of blood by the heart or, most often, increased resistance to blood flow in the arteries. The latter condition can be caused by the constriction of smooth muscle surrounding the arteries or by atherosclerosis, a disease process that causes arteries to become clogged and narrowed. High blood pressure also scars and hardens arteries, making them less elastic and further increasing blood pressure. When a person has high blood pressure, the heart

must work harder than normal to force blood through the narrowed and stiffened arteries, straining both the heart and the arteries. Eventually the strained heart weakens and tends to enlarge, which weakens it even more.

High blood pressure is often called a "silent killer" because it usually has no symptoms. A person may have hypertension for years without realizing it. But during that time, it damages vital organs and increases the risk of heart attack, congestive heart failure, stroke, kidney failure, and blindness. In fact, the Heart and Stroke Foundation of Canada reports that high blood pressure is the most important controllable risk factor for stroke.

Hypertension is common, occurring in about 1 in 4 adults. Its incidence rises dramatically with age; however, it can occur among children and young adults. A condition referred to as *prehypertension,* systolic and diastolic pressures just below hypertension levels (120 to 139/80 to 89 mm Hg), has been identified as an additional risk factor for CVD.[7] There are currently no statistics identifying the number of Canadians suffering from prehypertension. In most cases, prehypertension and hypertension cannot be cured, but they can be controlled. The key to avoiding the complications of prehypertension and hypertension is to have your blood pressure checked regularly and to follow your physician's advice about lifestyle changes and medication.

Lifestyle changes are recommended for everyone with prehypertension and hypertension. These lifestyle changes include:

- weight reduction
- regular physical activity
- a healthy diet—the DASH diet is recommended; it emphasizes fruits, vegetables, and whole grains—foods that are rich in potassium and fibre, both of which may reduce blood pressure. Sodium restriction is also helpful.
- moderate consumption of alcohol.

Many people are "self-sensitive," meaning that their blood pressure will decrease significantly when salt intake is restricted. Most experts feel that restricting sodium intake is a good strategy for all people—whether they have hypertension or not. Health Canada guidelines state that adequate intake of sodium is 1500 mg per day, or about two-thirds of a teaspoon of salt; the upper intake limit is set at 2300 mg per day, or about 1 teaspoon of salt. Recently released Statistics Canada data suggest that Canadians consume, on average, nearly 3100 mg of salt a day, though that figure is actually low because it does not include the salt people add to their food.[8] Recent research has shown that lowering your blood pressure

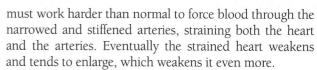

WELLNESS TIP

Always relax a few minutes before checking your blood pressure; doing so will help your blood pressure settle to its normal level. You may get a false reading if you take your blood pressure when you're agitated or moving around.

platelets Cell fragments in the blood that are necessary for the formation of blood clots.

hypertension Sustained abnormally high blood pressure.

Digital Tools for Heart Health

Do you ever check your own heart rate or blood pressure? For people who have heart disease or certain risk factors, tracking these vital signs can become routine. Fortunately, there are plenty of electronic devices available that make it easy to check your heart rate and blood pressure.

Heart Rate Monitors

As described in Chapter 3, there are many kinds of commercially available heart rate monitors. Although these devices are typically meant for use while exercising, they can also give you an accurate count of your resting heart rate. Knowing your resting heart rate can be important for several reasons. For example, a consistently high resting heart rate can be a sign of trouble or indicate that you need to improve your level of cardiorespiratory fitness.

Heart rate monitors usually feature a strap that goes around the user's chest and a watch-like device worn on the arm. The strap contains one or more sensors that gauge the wearer's heartbeat and transmit the information to the wrist device. Smaller, one-piece monitors are also available; some of these devices are worn on the wrist and measure the pulse in the wrist, and even smaller monitors can be worn on a finger (your index finger, for example, has its own measurable pulse).

Simple heart rate monitors display only your current heart rate, but more full-featured models can display other types of information and recall previous readings for comparison.

Blood Pressure Monitors

A home blood pressure monitor is an electronic version of the sphygmomanometer you've seen in doctors' offices. A home monitor features an inflatable arm strap, an inflating bulb, and a monitoring device. These parts are interconnected by flexible air hoses. You place the strap around your upper arm, squeeze the bulb a few times to inflate the strap, and then wait. As the strap slowly releases air, the device checks your pulse and your blood pressure. The monitor displays your diastolic/systolic blood pressure reading on a screen, in the familiar "120/80" format, along with your pulse rate in beats per minute.

Though relatively inexpensive, home blood pressure monitors are typically accurate and widely recommended by doctors for patients with hypertension or prehypertension. If you purchase a blood pressure monitor, take it to your doctor to make sure it provides the same readings as his or her professionally calibrated equipment.

In fact, it's a good idea to talk to your doctor before monitoring your heart rate or blood pressure. Your doctor can tell if it's necessary (and it may not be if you're in overall good health); if your doctor thinks it's a good idea, he or she can give you baseline readings and advice on the proper way to monitor yourself. Your doctor will also tell you when you should be concerned about a reading, and what to do when you are concerned.

---

through healthy lifestyle changes improves cardiovascular health even if your current blood pressure is already below 140 over 90. For people whose blood pressure isn't adequately controlled with lifestyle changes, medication is prescribed.

UNHEALTHY CHOLESTEROL LEVELS Cholesterol is a fatty, waxlike substance that circulates through the bloodstream and is an important component of cell membranes, sex hormones, vitamin D, the fluid that coats the lungs, and the protective sheaths around nerves. Adequate cholesterol is essential for the proper functioning of the body. Excess cholesterol, however, can clog arteries and increase the risk of CVD (Figure 11.3). Your liver manufactures cholesterol; you also get cholesterol from foods.

Good Versus Bad Cholesterol Cholesterol is carried in protein-lipid packages called **lipoproteins.** Lipoproteins can be thought of as shuttles that transport cholesterol to and from the liver through the circulatory system. **Low-density lipoproteins (LDLs)** shuttle cholesterol from the liver to the organs and tissues that require it. LDL is known as "bad" cholesterol because if there is more than the body can use, the excess is deposited in the blood vessels. LDL that accumulates and becomes trapped in artery walls may be oxidized by free radicals, speeding inflammation and damage to artery walls and increasing the likelihood that an artery will become blocked, causing a heart attack or stroke. **High-density lipoproteins (HDLs),** or "good" cholesterol, shuttle unused cholesterol back to the liver for recycling. By removing cholesterol from blood vessels, HDL helps protect against atherosclerosis.

Recommended Blood Cholesterol Levels The risk for CVD increases with increasing blood cholesterol levels, especially LDL. The Heart and Stroke Foundation of Canada does not advocate cholesterol testing for all Canadians. Rather, those with a strong family history of elevated cholesterol or premature heart disease and those who have other coronary heart disease risk factors should consider having their cholesterol levels tested on a

TERMS

lipoproteins Protein-and-lipid substances in the blood that carry fats and cholesterol; classified according to size, density, and chemical composition.

low-density lipoprotein (LDL) A lipoprotein containing a moderate amount of protein and a large amount of cholesterol; "bad" cholesterol.

high-density lipoprotein (HDL) A lipoprotein containing relatively little cholesterol that helps transport cholesterol out of the arteries; "good" cholesterol.

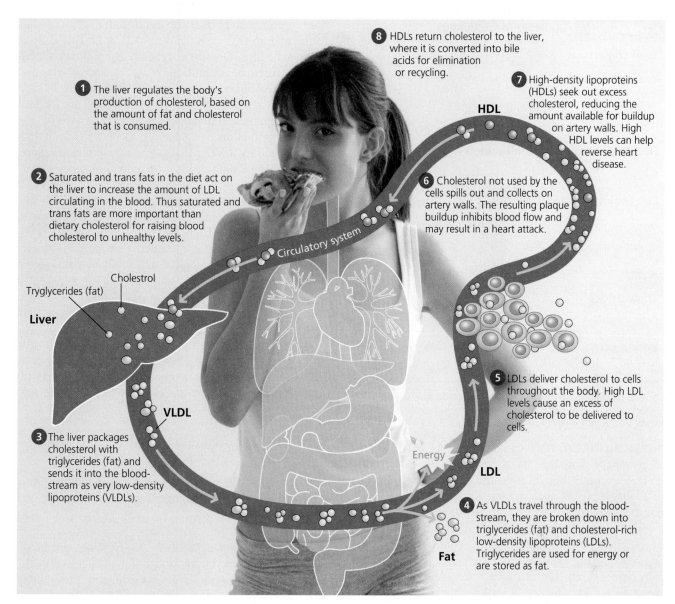

① The liver regulates the body's production of cholesterol, based on the amount of fat and cholesterol that is consumed.

② Saturated and trans fats in the diet act on the liver to increase the amount of LDL circulating in the blood. Thus saturated and trans fats are more important than dietary cholesterol for raising blood cholesterol to unhealthy levels.

Cholestrol

Tryglycerides (fat)

Liver

③ The liver packages cholesterol with triglycerides (fat) and sends it into the blood-stream as very low-density lipoproteins (VLDLs).

VLDL

Circulatory system

⑧ HDLs return cholesterol to the liver, where it is converted into bile acids for elimination or recycling.

⑦ High-density lipoproteins (HDLs) seek out excess cholesterol, reducing the amount available for buildup on artery walls. High HDL levels can help reverse heart disease.

HDL

⑥ Cholesterol not used by the cells spills out and collects on artery walls. The resulting plaque buildup inhibits blood flow and may result in a heart attack.

⑤ LDLs deliver cholesterol to cells throughout the body. High LDL levels cause an excess of cholesterol to be delivered to cells.

Energy

LDL

④ As VLDLs travel through the blood-stream, they are broken down into triglycerides (fat) and cholesterol-rich low-density lipoproteins (LDLs). Triglycerides are used for energy or are stored as fat.

Fat

FIGURE 11.3 Travels with cholesterol.

regular basis. You should visit your doctor to assess your need for a cholesterol test. The recommended test is a lipoprotein profile that measures total cholesterol, LDL cholesterol, HDL cholesterol, and triglycerides (another blood fat). General cholesterol and triglyceride guidelines are given in Table 11.1. In general, high LDL, total cholesterol, and triglyceride levels, and low HDL levels are associated with a high risk for CVD; lowering LDL, total cholesterol and triglycerides can lower risk. Raising HDL is important because a high HDL level seems to offer protection from CVD even in cases where total cholesterol is high, especially for women.

As shown in Table 11.1, LDL levels below 3.5 mmol/L and total cholesterol levels below 5.2 mmol/L are desirable. It is estimated that close to 45% of Canadians have total cholesterol levels of 5.2 mmol/L or higher.[9] The CVD risk associated with elevated cholesterol levels also depends on other factors. For example, an above optimal

level of LDL would be of more concern for an individual who also smoked and had high blood pressure than for an individual without these additional CVD risk factors.

Improving Cholesterol Levels Your primary goal should be to reduce LDL to healthy levels. Important dietary changes for reducing LDL levels include substituting unsaturated for saturated and trans fats and increasing fibre intake. Decreasing saturated and trans fats is particularly important because they promote the production and excretion of cholesterol by the liver. Exercising regularly and eating more fruits, vegetables, and whole grains also help. Many experts believe that cholesterol-lowering foods may be most effective when eaten in combination rather than separately. You can raise your HDL levels by exercising regularly, losing weight if you are overweight, quitting smoking, and altering the amount and type of fat you consume.

TABLE 11.1 Cholesterol Guidelines

Total Cholesterol

Ideal:	less than 5.2 mmol/L
Borderline High:	5.2 to 6.2 mmol/L
High:	6.2 mmol/L or more

HDL Cholesterol (Good Cholesterol)

Desired:	more than 1.5 mmol/L

LDL Cholesterol (Bad Cholesterol)

Ideal:	less than 3.3 mmol/L
Borderline High:	3.4 to 4.1 mmol/L
High:	4.1 to 4.9 mmol/L

Triglycerides

Ideal:	less than 1.7 mmol/L
Borderline High:	1.7 to 2.2 mmol/L
High:	2.3 to 5.6 mmol/L

SOURCE: Cholesterol Guidelines, Mayo Clinic http://www.mayoclinic.com/ health/cholesterol-levels/CL00001 HYPERLINK "http://www.mayoclinic.com/" www.mayoclinic.com, Used with permission.

PHYSICAL INACTIVITY   Close to 60% of Canadians are so sedentary that they are at high risk for developing CVD. Exercise is thought to be the closest thing we have to a "magic bullet" against heart disease. It lowers CVD risk by helping decrease blood pressure, increase HDL levels, maintain desirable weight, improve the condition of the blood vessels, and prevent or control diabetes. In fact, introducing exercise to your daily routine dramatically reduces your risk for stroke.[10] One study found that women who accumulated at least 3 hours of brisk walking each week cut their risk of heart attack and stroke by more than half. (See Chapter 3 for more information on the physical and psychological effects of exercise.)

OBESITY   The risk of death from CVD is two to three times higher in obese people (BMI > 30) than it is in lean people (BMI 18.5–24.9), and for every 5-unit increment of BMI, a person's risk of death from coronary heart disease increases by 30%. Excess weight increases the strain on the heart by contributing to high blood pressure and high cholesterol. It can also lead to diabetes, another CVD risk factor (see next section). As discussed in Chapter 6,

FITNESS TIP

Weight training should be part of any fitness program, but it can raise your blood pressure, at least temporarily. Be sure to balance weight training with aerobic exercise, which can lower blood pressure over the long term.

distribution of body fat is also significant: Fat that collects in the abdomen is more dangerous than fat that collects around the hips. Obesity in general, and abdominal obesity in particular, is significantly associated with narrowing of the coronary arteries, even in young adults in their twenties. A sensible diet and regular exercise are the best ways to achieve and maintain a healthy body weight. For someone who is overweight, even modest weight reduction can reduce CVD risk by lowering blood pressure, improving cholesterol levels, and reducing diabetes risk.

DIABETES   As described in Chapter 6, diabetes is a disorder in which the metabolism of glucose is disrupted, causing a buildup of glucose in the bloodstream. People with diabetes are at increased risk for CVD, partly because elevated blood glucose levels can damage the lining of arteries, making them more vulnerable to atherosclerosis; diabetics also often have other risk factors, including hypertension, obesity, unhealthy cholesterol and triglyceride levels, and platelet and blood coagulation abnormalities. Even people whose diabetes is under control face an increased risk of CVD. Therefore, careful control of other risk factors is critical for people with diabetes. People with pre-diabetes also face a significantly increased risk of CVD.

Contributing Risk Factors That Can Be Changed

Various other CVD risk factors can be changed, including triglyceride levels, psychological and social factors, and drug use.

HIGH TRIGLYCERIDE LEVELS   Triglycerides are blood fats that are obtained from food and manufactured by the body. High triglyceride levels are a reliable predictor of heart disease, especially if associated with other risk factors, such as low HDL levels, obesity, and diabetes. Factors contributing to elevated triglyceride levels include excess body fat, physical inactivity, cigarette smoking, type 2 diabetes, excess alcohol intake, very high carbohydrate diets, and certain diseases and medications.

A full lipid profile should include testing and evaluation of triglyceride levels (see Table 11.1). For people with borderline high triglyceride levels, increased physical activity and weight reduction can help bring levels down into the healthy range; for people with high triglycerides, drug therapy may be needed. Limiting alcohol use and quitting smoking are also helpful.

PSYCHOLOGICAL AND SOCIAL FACTORS   Many of the psychological and social factors that influence other areas of wellness are also important risk factors for CVD.

- *Stress.* Excessive stress can strain the heart and blood vessels over time and contribute to CVD. A full-blown stress response causes blood vessels to constrict and blood pressure to rise. Blood platelets

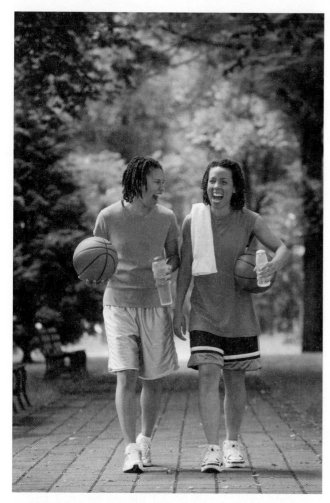

Stress and social isolation can increase risk of cardiovascular disease. A strong social support network improves both heart health and overall wellness.

CVD.[12] If you have high levels of hostility (complete the self-assessment in Lab 11.1), refer to Chapter 10 for ways to manage stress and handle anger.

- *Suppressing psychological distress.* Consistently suppressing anger and other negative emotions may also be hazardous to a healthy heart. People who hide psychological distress tend to have a higher rate of heart disease than people who experience similar distress but share it with others. People with so-called Type D personalities tend to be pessimistic, negative, and unhappy and to suppress these feelings.

- *Depression and anxiety.* Both mild and severe depression are linked to an increased risk of CVD. Researchers have also found a strong association between anxiety disorders and an increased risk of death from heart disease, particularly sudden death from heart attack.

- *Social isolation.* People with little social support are at higher risk of dying from CVD than people with close ties to others. Studies suggest that religious commitment has a positive effect on heart health, perhaps because of the strong community provided by membership. A strong social support network is a major antidote to stress. Friends and family members can also promote and support a healthy lifestyle.

- *Low socioeconomic status.* Low socioeconomic status and low educational attainment also increase risk for CVD, probably because of a variety of factors, including lifestyle, response to stress, and access to health care.

Major Risk Factors That Can't Be Changed

A number of major risk factors for CVD cannot be changed: heredity, aging, being male, ethnicity, and C-reactive protein.

HEREDITY   Multiple genes contribute to the development of CVD and its risk factors. Having an unfavourable set of genes increases your risk, but risk is modifiable by lifestyle factors such as whether you smoke, exercise, or eat a healthy diet. People who inherit a tendency for CVD are not destined to develop it, but they may have to work harder than other people to prevent it.

AGING   The risk of heart attack increases dramatically after age 65. Over 90% of Canadians over the age of 65 have at least one major risk factor for CVD and the highest percentage of Canadians with two or more risk factors falls in this age demographic.[13] For people over 55, the incidence of stroke increases by close to 30% in each successive decade. However, many people in their thirties and forties, especially men, have heart attacks.

become more likely to cluster, possibly enhancing the formation of artery-clogging clots. Stress can trigger abnormal heart rhythms, with potentially fatal consequences. People sometimes also adopt unhealthy habits such as smoking or overeating as a means of dealing with severe stress. In fact, one study has identified stressful areas of life such as finances, home life, and major life events as prominent events that increase our risk for CVD.[11]

- *Chronic hostility and anger.* Certain traits in the hard-driving "Type A" personality—hostility, cynicism, and anger—are associated with increased risk of heart disease. People with a quick temper, a persistently hostile outlook, and a cynical, mistrusting attitude toward life experience the stress response more intensely and frequently than do more relaxed, trusting individuals. When they encounter the irritations of daily life, their blood pressure rises, their blood vessels constrict, and their level of stress hormones increases much more than is the case for their relaxed counterparts. Over time, these effects may damage arteries and promote

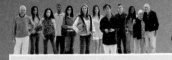

Gender and CVD

CVD is the leading cause of death for all North Americans, but significant differences exist between men and women in the incidence, diagnosis, and treatment of this deadly disease.

CVD has been thought of as a "man's disease," but it actually kills about the same number of women as it does men. The difference lies in the types of CVD that women versus men die from; with most women dying from stroke and congestive heart failure (failure of the heart to pump blood), while more men die from heart attacks and coronary artery diseases such as atherosclerosis. For women, CVD typically does not develop until after age 50. The hormone estrogen, produced naturally by a woman's ovaries until menopause, improves blood lipid concentrations and other CVD risk factors. For the last several decades, many physicians encouraged menopausal women to take hormone replacement therapy (HRT) to relieve menopause symptoms and presumably to reduce their risk of CVD. However, recent studies have found that HRT may actually *increase* a woman's risk for heart disease and other health problems. For this reason, the use of HRT for the prevention of chronic diseases such as CVD may not be recommended for some women.

When women do have heart attacks, they are more likely than men to die within a year. One reason is that since they develop heart disease at older ages, they are more likely to have other health problems that complicate treatment. Women also have smaller hearts and arteries than men, possibly making diagnosis and surgery more difficult. In addition, medical personnel appear to evaluate and treat women less aggressively than men. Women presenting with CVD are just as likely as men to report chest pain, but they are also likely to report non-chest-pain symptoms, which may obscure their diagnosis. These symptoms include fatigue, weakness, shortness of breath, nausea, vomiting, and pain in the abdomen, neck, jaw, and back. A woman who experiences these symptoms should be persistent in seeking accurate diagnosis and appropriate treatment.

Careful diagnosis of cardiac symptoms is also key in avoiding unnecessary invasive procedures in cases of stress cardiomyopathy ("broken heart syndrome"), which occurs much more commonly in women than in men. In this condition, hormones and neurotransmitters associated with a severe stress response stun the heart, producing heart-attack-like symptoms and decreased pumping function of the heart, but no damage to the heart muscle. Typically, the condition reverses quickly.

Women should be aware of their CVD risk factors and consult with a physician to assess their risk and determine the best way to prevent CVD.

SOURCE: Heart and Stroke Foundation. 2005. Heart Attack and Stroke Warning Signs (http://ww2.heartandstroke.ca). Copyright© 2005 Heart and Stroke Foundation. Reprinted with permission.

BEING MALE Although CVD is the leading killer of both men and women in Canada. Canadian men show a greater prevalence (than women) of risk factors for CVD such as hypertension and obesity.[14] Estrogen production, highest during the childbearing years, may offer pre-menopausal women some protection against CVD (see the box "Gender and CVD").

ETHNICITY Death rates from heart disease vary among ethnic groups in Canada. The 1999 First Nations and Inuit Regional Health Survey found the self-reported rate of CVD in this group to be approximately three times higher than that in the Canadian population as a whole.[15] Another recent study examined Canadians of European, South Asian, and Chinese origin and found that Canadians of both European and South Asian origin had relatively high rates of CVD. Overall trends among the groups suggested that mortality rates from CVD were converging in the three groups—suggesting that lifestyle and environmental factors may be playing a role.[16] In fact, the Heart and Stroke Foundation of Canada reports that as immigrant groups begin to adopt more and more unhealthy lifestyle habits, their risk for CVD increases.[17] The rate at which immigrants are adopting those unhealthy habits is nearing and in some cases, has surpassed, that of those born in Canada (Figure 11.4).

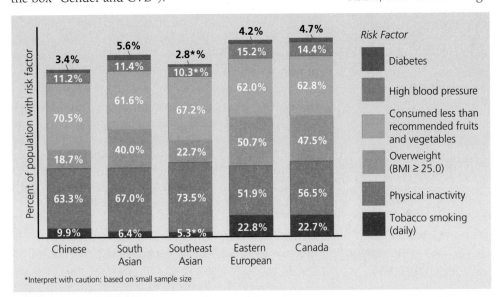

*Interpret with caution: based on small sample size

FIGURE 11.4 **Risk factors for heart disease and stroke among adults aged 20+ years of various ethnic backgrounds, Canada, 2000.**

SOURCE: "Risk Factors for Heart Disease and Stroke Among Adults Aged 20+ Years of Various Ethnic Backgrounds, Canada, 2000," Statistics Canada, *Canadian Community Health Survey.*

C-REACTIVE PROTEIN High levels of a substance called C-reactive protein (CRP), which is released into the bloodstream during the inflammatory response, may be a marker for a substantially elevated risk for heart attack and stroke. CRP may be released when an artery is injured by smoking, cholesterol, infectious agents, or other factors. Lifestyle changes and certain drugs can reduce CRP levels. Statin drugs, widely prescribed to lower cholesterol, also decrease inflammation; this may be one reason that statin drugs seem to lower CVD risk even in people with normal blood lipid levels.

Possible Risk Factors Currently Being Studied

In recent years, a number of other possible risk factors for cardiovascular disease have been identified.

Elevated blood levels of homocysteine, an amino acid that may damage the lining of blood vessels, are associated with an increased risk of CVD. Men generally have higher homocysteine levels than women, as do individuals with diets low in folic acid, vitamin B-12, and vitamin B-6. Most people can lower homocysteine levels easily by adopting a healthy diet rich in fruits, vegetables, and grains and by taking supplements if needed.

High levels of a specific type of LDL called lipoprotein(a), or Lp(a), have been identified as a possible risk factor for coronary heart disease (CHD), especially when associated with high LDL or low HDL levels. Lp(a) levels have a strong genetic component and are difficult to treat. LDL particles differ in size and density, and people with a high proportion of small, dense LDL particles—a condition called LDL pattern B—also appear to be at greater risk for CVD. Exercise, a low-fat diet, and certain lipid-lowering drugs may help lower CVD risk in people with LDL pattern B.

Several infectious agents, including *Chlamydia pneumoniae, cytomegalovirus,* and *Helicobacter pylori,* have also been identified as possible risk factors. Infections may damage arteries and lead to chronic inflammation. Another marker for higher risk is fibrinogen, a protein involved in blood clotting.

Certain CVD risk factors are often found in a cluster referred to as *metabolic syndrome* or *insulin resistance syndrome.* As described in Chapter 6, symptoms of metabolic syndrome include abdominal obesity, high blood pressure, high triglycerides, low HDL cholesterol, high blood pressure, and high blood glucose levels. More than 25% of Canadian adults have metabolic syndrome, with the highest rate (41%) found among First Nations' people.[18] Weight control, physical activity, and a diet rich in unsaturated fats and fibre is recommended for people with metabolic syndrome. Exercise is especially important because it increases insulin sensitivity even if it doesn't produce weight loss.

Ask yourself

QUESTIONS FOR CRITICAL THINKING AND REFLECTION

What risk factors do you have for cardiovascular disease? Which ones are factors you have control over, and which are factors you can't change? If you have risk factors you cannot change (such as a family history of CVD), were you aware that you can make lifestyle adjustments to reduce your risk? Do you think you will make them? Why or why not?

LO3 11.3 PROTECTING YOURSELF AGAINST CARDIOVASCULAR DISEASE

You can take several important steps right now to lower your risk of developing CVD in the future (Figure 11.5). Reducing CVD risk factors when you are young can pay off with many extra years of life and health.

Eat Heart-Healthy

For most Canadians, changing to a heart-healthy diet involves cutting total fat intake, substituting unsaturated fats for saturated and trans fats, and increasing intake of whole grains and fibre.

DECREASED FAT AND CHOLESTEROL INTAKE Health Canada recommends that all Canadians adopt a diet in which total fat consumption is no more than 30% of total daily calories, with no more than one-third of those fat calories (10% of total daily calories) coming from saturated fat. For people with heart disease or high LDL levels, a total fat intake of 25–35% of total daily calories and a saturated fat intake of less than 7% of total calories is recommended. This higher total fat allowance is helpful for people who also have high triglyceride and low HDL levels. Diets rich in high-glycemic-index carbohydrates may lower HDL levels and raise levels of triglycerides and glucose in some people, including those with metabolic syndrome. For this group, then, a diet slightly higher in unsaturated fats is allowed, while saturated fats are further restricted.

Saturated fat is found in animal products, palm and coconut oil, and hydrogenated vegetable oils, which are also high in trans fats. Saturated and trans fats influence the production and excretion of cholesterol by the liver,

Do More	Do Less
• Eat a diet rich in fruits, vegetables, whole grains, and low-fat or fat-free dairy products. Eat five to nine servings of fruits and vegetables each day.	• Don't use tobacco in any form: cigarettes, spit tobacco, cigars and pipes, bidis and clove cigarettes.
• Eat several servings of high-fibre foods each day.	• Limit consumption of fats, especially trans fats and saturated fats.
• Eat two or more servings of fish per week; try a few servings of nuts and soy foods each week.	• Limit consumption of salt to no more than 2300 mg of sodium per day (1500 mg if you have or are at high risk for hypertension).
• Choose unsaturated fats rather than saturated and trans fats.	• Avoid exposure to environmental tobacco smoke.
• Be physically active; do both aerobic exercise and strength training on a regular basis.	• Avoid excessive alcohol consumption— no more than one drink per day for women and two drinks per day for men.
• Achieve and maintain a healthy weight.	
• Develop effective strategies for handling stress and anger. Nurture old friendships and family ties, and make new friends; pay attention to your spiritual side.	• Limit consumption of cholesterol, added sugars, and refined carbohydrates.
• Obtain recommended screening tests and follow your physician's recommendations.	• Avoid excess stress, anger, and hostility.

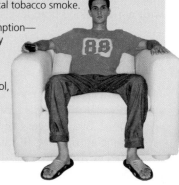

FIGURE 11.5 Strategies for reducing your risk of cardiovascular disease.

so decreasing intake of these fats is the most important dietary change you can make to improve cholesterol levels. Animal products contain cholesterol as well as saturated fat, and it is recommended that most Canadians limit dietary cholesterol intake to no more than 300 mg per day; for people with heart disease or high LDL levels, the suggested daily limit is 200 mg.

INCREASED FIBRE INTAKE Fibre traps the bile acids the liver needs to manufacture cholesterol and carries them to the large intestine, where they are excreted. It also slows the production of proteins that promote blood clotting. Fibre may interfere with the absorption of dietary fat and may also help you cut total food intake because foods rich in insoluble fibre tend to be filling. To obtain the recommended 25–38 grams of dietary fibre a day, choose a diet rich in whole grains, fruits, and vegetables. Good sources of fibre include oatmeal, some breakfast cereals, barley, legumes, and most fruits and vegetables.

SODIUM AND POTASSIUM INTAKE The recommended limit for sodium intake is 2300 milligrams per day; for population groups at special risk, including those with hypertension, middle-aged and older adults, and some ethnic groups, the recommended limit is 1500 milligrams

per day. To limit sodium intake, read food labels carefully, and avoid foods particularly high in sodium; foods that are fresh, less processed, and less sodium-dense are good choices. Adequate potassium intake is also important in the control of blood pressure. Good food sources include leafy green vegetables like spinach and beet greens, root vegetables like white and sweet potatoes, vine fruits like cantaloupe and honeydew melon, winter squash, bananas, many dried fruits, and tomato sauce.

ALCOHOL Moderate alcohol consumption may lower the risk of CHD among middle-aged and older adults. (Moderate means no more than one drink per day for women and two drinks per day for men.) For most people under age 45, however, the risks of alcohol use probably outweigh any health benefit. If you do drink, do so moderately, with food and at times when drinking will not put you or others at risk.

DASH A dietary plan that reflects many of the suggestions described here was released as part of a study called Dietary Approaches to Stop Hypertension, or DASH. This is the DASH diet plan:

- 7–8 servings a day of grains and grain products
- 4–5 servings a day of vegetables
- 4–5 servings a day of fruits
- 2–3 servings a day of low-fat or nonfat dairy products
- 2 or fewer servings a day of meats, poultry, and fish
- 4–5 servings a *week* of nuts, seeds, and legumes
- 2–3 servings a day of added fats, oils, and salad dressings
- 5 servings a *week* of snacks and sweets

WELLNESS TIP

Oatmeal can actually lower your level of LDL cholesterol. Oatmeal contains soluble fibre, which prevents LDL particles from entering the bloodstream.

How Does Exercise Affect CVD Risk?

CONNECT ACTIVITY DO IT ONLINE

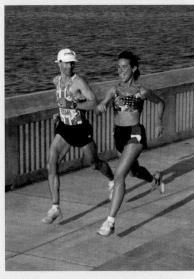

Regular exercise directly and indirectly benefits your cardiovascular health and can actually help you avoid having a heart attack or stroke. The evidence comes from dozens of large-scale, population-based studies conducted over the past several decades. There is so much evidence about the cardiovascular health benefits of exercise, in fact, that physicians regard physical activity as a magic bullet against heart disease.

As with all-cause mortality, physical activity has an inverse relationship with cardiovascular health, meaning that the more exercise you get, the less likely you are to develop or die from CVD. Compared to sedentary individuals, people who engage in regular, moderate physical activity lower their risk of CVD by 20% or more. People who get regular, vigorous exercise reduce their risk of CVD by 30% or more. This positive benefit applies regardless of gender, age, race, or ethnicity.

Most studies focus on various aerobic endurance exercises, such as walking, running on a treadmill, or biking. As noted in Chapter 1, the type of exercise performed is less important than the amount of energy expended during the activity. The greater the energy expenditure, the greater the health benefits. In three different studies conducted between 1999 and 2002, for example, researchers focused on women of various ages who walked for exercise. All three studies showed that the women's relative risk of CVD dropped as they expended more and more energy by walking.

Exercise affects heart health via many mechanisms, all of which are being studied. For example, exercise helps people lose weight and improve body composition. Weight loss can improve heart health by reducing the amount of stress on the heart. Changing body composition to a more positive ratio of fat to fat-free mass boosts resting metabolic rate. Exercise directly strengthens the heart muscle itself, and it improves the balance of fats in the blood by boosting HDL and reducing LDL and triglyceride levels.

Exercise can also prevent metabolic syndrome and reverse many of its negative effects on the body. For example, exercise improves the health and function of the endothelial cells—the inner lining of the arteries. These cells secrete nitric oxide, which regulates blood flow, improves nerve function, strengthens the immune system, enhances reproductive health, and suppresses inflammation. Exercise training also improves the function of cell sodium-potassium pumps, which regulate fluid and electrolyte balance and cellular communication throughout the body.

One of the clearest positive effects of exercise is on hypertension. Many studies, involving thousands of people, have shown that physical activity reduces both systolic and diastolic blood pressure. These studies showed that people who engaged in regular aerobic exercise lowered their resting blood pressure by 2–4%, on average. Lowered blood pressure itself reduces the risk of other kinds of cardiovascular disease.

Fewer studies have been conducted on exercise and risk of stroke. Even with limited evidence, however, there appears to be a similar inverse relationship between physical activity and stroke. According to a handful of studies, the most physically active people reduced their risk of both ischemic and hemorrhagic strokes by up to 30%. Although this benefit appears to apply equally to men and women, there is not sufficient evidence that it applies equally across races or ethnicities.

Of course, exercise isn't possible for everyone and may actually be dangerous for some people. Anyone who has CVD or serious risk factors for heart disease should work with their physician to determine whether or how to exercise.

THE EVIDENCE FOR EXERCISE

SOURCES: Cornelissen, V. A., and R. H. Fagard. 2005. Effect of resistance training on resting blood pressure: A meta-analysis of randomized controlled trials. *Journal of Hypertension* 23(2): 251–259; Physical Activity Guidelines Advisory Committee. 2008. *Physical Activity Guidelines Advisory Committee Report, 2008.* Washington, D.C.: U.S. Department of Health and Human Services; Schnohr, P., et al. 2006. Long-term physical activity in leisure time and mortality from coronary heart disease, stroke, respiratory diseases, and cancer. The Copenhagen City Heart Study. *European Journal of Cardiovascular Prevention and Rehabilitation* 13(2): 173–179; and Williams, M. A., et al. 2007. Resistance exercise in individuals with and without cardiovascular disease: 2007 update: A scientific statement from the American Heart Association Council on Clinical Cardiology and Council on Nutrition, Physical Activity, and Metabolism. *Circulation* 116(5): 572–584.

The DASH diet also follows the dietary recommendations for lowering one's risk of cancer, osteoporosis, and heart disease.

Exercise Regularly

You can significantly reduce your risk of CVD with a moderate amount of physical activity (see the box "How Does Exercise Affect CVD Risk?"). A formal exercise program can provide even greater benefits. The information in Chapters 2–5 and 9 can help you create and implement a complete exercise program that meets your needs for fitness and prevention of chronic disease.

Avoid Tobacco

The number-one risk factor for CVD that you can control is smoking. If you smoke, quit. If you don't, don't start. The majority of people who start don't believe they will become hooked, but most do. If you live or work with people who smoke, encourage them to quit—for their sake and yours. If you find yourself breathing in smoke, take steps to prevent or stop this exposure. Quitting smoking will significantly reduce your CVD risk, but studies show that smoking and exposure to ETS may permanently increase the rate of plaque formation in arteries.

I know what foods to avoid to prevent CVD, but are there any foods I should eat to protect myself from CVD?

The most important dietary change for CVD prevention is a negative one: cutting back on foods high in saturated and trans fat. However, certain foods can be helpful. The positive effects of unsaturated fats, soluble fibre, and alcohol on heart health were discussed earlier in the chapter. Other potentially beneficial foods include those rich in the following:

- *Omega-3 fatty acids*. Found in fish, shellfish, and some nuts and seeds, omega-3 fatty acids reduce clotting and inflammation and may lower the risk of fatal arrhythmia.

- *Folic acid, vitamin B-6, and vitamin B-12*. These vitamins may affect CVD risk by lowering homocysteine levels; see Table 7.2 for a list of food sources.

- *Plant stanols and sterols*. Plant stanols and sterols, found in some types of trans-free margarines and other products, reduce the absorption of cholesterol in the body and help lower LDL levels.

- *Soy protein*. Replacing some animal protein with soy protein can lower LDL cholesterol. Soy-based foods include tofu, tempeh, and soy-based beverages.

- *Calcium*. Diets rich in calcium may help in preventing hypertension and possibly stroke by reducing insulin resistance and platelet aggregation. Low-fat or nonfat dairy products are rich in calcium; refer to Chapter 7 for other sources.

The advice I hear from the media about protecting myself from CVD seems to be changing all the time. What am I supposed to believe?

Health-related research is now described in popular newspapers and magazines rather than just medical journals, meaning that more and more people have access to the information. Researchers do not deliberately set out to mislead or confuse people. However, news reports may oversimplify the results of research studies, leaving out some of the qualifications and questions the researchers present with their findings. In addition, news reports may not differentiate between a preliminary finding and a result that has been verified by a large number of long-term studies. And researchers themselves must strike a balance between reporting promising preliminary findings to the public, thereby allowing people to act on them, and waiting 10–20 years until long-term studies confirm (or disprove) a particular theory.

Although you cannot become an expert on all subjects, there are some general strategies you can use to assess the health advice that appears in the media; see the box "Evaluating Health News."

What's a heart murmur, and is it dangerous?

A heart murmur is an extra or altered heart sound heard during a routine

Know and Manage Your Blood Pressure

Currently, nearly 43% of the 5 million Canadians with hypertension are not even aware that they may have blood pressure problems.[19] If you have no CVD risk factors, have your blood pressure measured at least once every 2 years; yearly tests are recommended if you have other risk factors. If your blood pressure is high, follow your physician's advice on lowering it.

Know and Manage Your Cholesterol Levels

Everyone age 20 and over should have a lipoprotein profile—which measures total cholesterol, HDL, LDL, and triglyceride levels—at least once every five years. Your goal for LDL depends in part on how many of the following major risk factors you have: cigarette smoking, high blood pressure, low HDL cholesterol (less than 0.9 mmol/L), a family history of heart disease, and age above 45 years for men and 55 years for women. For some people, adopting therapeutic lifestyle changes (TLC)—weight management, increased physical activity, and dietary changes—is enough to lower cholesterol levels. For others, medications may also be needed.

Develop Ways to Handle Stress and Anger

To reduce the psychological and social risk factors for CVD, develop effective strategies for handling the stress in your life. Shore up your social support network, and, if anger and hostility are problems for you, try some of the techniques described in Chapter 10 for managing stress and anger.

medical exam. The source is often a problem with one of the heart valves that separate the chambers of the heart. Congenital defects and certain infections can cause abnormalities in the valves. The most common heart valve disorder is mitral valve prolapse (MVP), which occurs in about 4% of the population. MVP is characterized by a "billowing" of the mitral valve, which separates the left ventricle and left atrium, during ventricular contraction; in some cases, blood leaks from the ventricle into the atrium. Most people with MVP have no symptoms; they are able to exercise and live as long as people without MVP.

MVP can be confirmed with echocardiography. Treatment is usually unnecessary, although surgery may be needed in the rare cases where leakage through the faulty valve is severe. Experts disagree over whether patients with MVP should take antibiotics prior to dental procedures, a precautionary step used to prevent bacteria, which may be dislodged into the bloodstream during some types of dental and surgical procedures, from infecting the defective valve. Most often, only those patients with significant blood leakage are advised to take antibiotics.

Although MVP usually requires no treatment, more severe heart valve disorders can impair blood flow through the heart. Treatment depends on the location and severity of the problem. More serious defects may be treated with surgery to repair or replace a valve.

How does stress contribute to cardiovascular disease?

With stress, the brain tells the adrenal glands to secrete cortisol and other hormones and neurotransmitters, which in turn activate the sympathetic nervous system—causing the fight-or-flight response. This response increases heart rate and blood pressure so that more blood is distributed to the heart and other muscles in anticipation of physical activity. Blood glucose concentrations and cholesterol also increase to provide a source of energy, and the platelets become activated so that they will be more likely to clot in case of injury. Such a response can be adaptive if you're being chased by a hungry lion but may be more detrimental than useful if you're sitting at a desk taking an exam or feeling frustrated by a task given to you by your boss.

If you are healthy, you can tolerate the cardiovascular responses that take place during stress, but if you already have CVD, stress can lead to adverse outcomes such as abnormal heart rhythms, heart attacks, and sudden cardiac death. It has long been known that an increase in heart rhythm problems and deaths is associated with acute mental stress. For example, the rate of potentially life-threatening arrhythmias in patients who already had underlying heart disease doubled during the month after the September 11 terrorist attacks; this increase was not limited to people in close proximity to Manhattan.

Because avoiding all stress is impossible, having healthy mechanisms to cope with it is your best defence. Instead of adopting unhealthy habits such as smoking, drinking, or overeating to deal with stress, try healthier coping techniques such as exercising, getting enough sleep, and talking to family and friends.

Ask Yourself

QUESTIONS FOR CRITICAL THINKING AND REFLECTION

Do you know what your blood pressure and cholesterol levels are, on average? If not, is there a reason you don't know? Is there something preventing you from getting this information about yourself? How can you motivate yourself to have these easy but important health checks?

TIPS FOR TODAY AND THE FUTURE

Because cardiovascular disease is a long-term process that can begin when you're young, it's important to develop heart-healthy habits early in life.

RIGHT NOW YOU CAN

- Make an appointment to have your blood pressure and cholesterol levels checked.
- List the key stressors in your life, and decide what to do about the ones that bother you most.
- Plan to replace one high-fat item in your diet with one that is high in fibre. For example, replace a doughnut with a bowl of whole-grain cereal or a cup of yogurt with fruit.

IN THE FUTURE YOU CAN

- Track your eating habits for one week, then compare them to the DASH eating plan. Make adjustments to bring your diet closer to the DASH recommendations.
- Sign up for a class in CPR. A CPR certification equips you with valuable life-saving skills you can use to help someone who is choking, having a heart attack, or experiencing cardiac arrest. Many CPR classes also include training in the use of an AED.

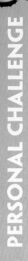

Getting to Know Your Pulse Rate

Do you know what your resting pulse rate is? It's easy to find out, and it can be useful information for you and your doctor. Chapter 3 provides instructions for checking your own pulse. Practise a few times, and then check your resting pulse rate each day for 7 consecutive days. Write the results here:

Day	Time	Pulse
1.	_____	_____
2.	_____	_____
3.	_____	_____
4.	_____	_____
5.	_____	_____
6.	_____	_____
7.	_____	_____

Be sure to rest for at least 10 minutes before checking your resting pulse rate, and don't check your pulse right after eating (some foods can increase your heart rate temporarily). For most people, a resting pulse rate between 60 and 100 beats per minute is considered normal. Very fit people may have a slower resting pulse rate.

SUMMARY

- The major controllable risk factors for CVD are smoking, hypertension, unhealthy cholesterol levels, a sedentary lifestyle, obesity, and diabetes.

- Contributing factors for CVD that can be changed include high triglyceride levels, inadequate stress management, a hostile personality, depression, anxiety, lack of social support, and poverty.

- Major risk factors that can't be changed are heredity, aging, being male, and ethnicity.

- Hypertension weakens the heart and scars and hardens arteries, causing resistance to blood flow. It is defined as blood pressure equal to or higher than 140 over 90.

- Atherosclerosis is a progressive hardening and narrowing of arteries that can lead to restricted blood flow and even complete blockage.

- Heart attacks, strokes, and congestive heart failure are the results of a long-term disease process; hypertension and atherosclerosis are usually involved.

- Reducing heart disease risk involves eating a heart-healthy diet, exercising regularly, avoiding tobacco, managing blood pressure and cholesterol levels, handling stress and anger, and knowing your risk factors.

FOR FURTHER EXPLORATION

Organizations and Websites

Canadian Cardiovascular Society. Includes research-based information on cardiovascular issues.
http://www.ccs.ca

Dieticians of Canada. Website devoted to the provision of nutrition information for professionals and consumers.
http://www.dieticians.ca

Franklin Institute Science Museum/The Heart: An On-Line Exploration. An online museum exhibit containing information on the structure and function of the heart, how to monitor your heart's health, and how to maintain a healthy heart.
http://www.fi.edu/biosci/heart.html

Heart and Stroke Foundation of Canada. Provides information on the prevention and control of heart disease and stroke. Includes risk assessments and articles for reducing the risks associated with heart disease and stroke.
http://www.heartandstroke.ca

HeartInfo—Heart Information Network. Provides information for heart patients and others interested in identifying and reducing their risk factors for heart disease; includes links to many related sites.
http://www.heartinfo.org

MedlinePlus: Heart and Circulation Topics. Provides links to reliable sources of information on cardiovascular health.
http://www.nlm.nih.gov/medlineplus/heartandcirculation.html

See also the listings for Chapters 8 and 10.

Evaluating Health News

Canadians face an avalanche of health information from newspapers, magazines, books, and television programs. It's not always easy to decide what to believe. The following questions can help you evaluate health news:

1. *Is the report based on research or on an anecdote?* Information or recommendations based on one or more carefully designed research studies has more validity than one person's experiences.

2. *What is the source of the information?* A study in a respected publication has been reviewed by editors and other researchers in the field—people who are in a position to evaluate the merits of a study and its results. Information put forth by government agencies and national research organizations is also usually considered reliable.

3. *How big was the study?* A study that involves many subjects is more likely to yield reliable results than a study involving only a few people. Another indication that a finding is meaningful is if several different studies yield the same results.

4. *Who were the people involved in the study?* Research findings are more likely to apply to you if you share important characteristics with the subjects of the study. For example, the results of a study on men over age 50 who smoke may not be particularly meaningful for a 30-year-old non-smoking woman. Even less applicable are studies done in test tubes or on animals.

5. *What kind of study was it?* Epidemiological studies involve observation or interviews in order to trace the relationships among lifestyle, physical characteristics, and diseases. Although epidemiological studies can suggest links, they cannot establish cause-and-effect relationships. Clinical or interventional studies involve testing the effects of different treatments on groups of people who have similar lifestyles and characteristics. They are more likely to provide conclusive evidence of a cause-and-effect relationship. The best interventional studies share the following characteristics:

   • *Controlled.* A group of people who receive the treatment is compared with a matched group who do not receive the treatment.

   • *Randomized.* The treatment and control groups are selected randomly.

   • *Double-blind.* Researchers and participants are unaware of who is receiving the treatment.

   • *Multicentre.* The experiment is performed at more than one institution.

6. *What do the statistics really say?* First, are the results described as "statistically significant"? If a study is large and well designed, its results can be deemed statistically significant, meaning there is less than a 5% chance that the findings resulted from chance. Second, are the results stated in terms of relative or absolute risk? Many findings are reported in terms of relative risk—how a particular treatment or condition affects a person's disease risk. Consider the following examples of relative risk:

   • According to some estimates, taking estrogen without progesterone can increase a postmenopausal woman's risk of dying from endometrial cancer by 233%.

   • Giving antiviral medication to HIV-infected pregnant women reduces prenatal transmission of HIV by 90%.

   The first of these two findings seems far more dramatic than the second—until one also considers *absolute risk,* the actual risk of the illness in the population being considered. The absolute risk of endometrial cancer is 0.3%; a 233% increase based on the effects of estrogen raises it to 1%, a change of 0.7%. Without treatment, about 25% of infants born to HIV-infected women will be infected with HIV; with treatment, the absolute risk drops to about 2%, a change of 23%. Because the absolute risk of an HIV-infected mother passing the virus to her infant is so much greater than a woman's risk of developing endometrial cancer (25% compared with 0.3%), a smaller change in relative risk translates into a much greater change in absolute risk.

7. *Is new health advice being offered?* If the media report new guidelines for health behaviour or medical treatment, examine the source. Government agencies and national research foundations usually consider a great deal of evidence before offering health advice. Above all, use common sense, and check with your physician before making a major change in your health habits based on news reports.

LAB 11.1 Cardiovascular Health

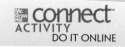

Part I CVD Risk Assessment

Your chances of suffering a heart attack or stroke before age 55 depend on a variety of factors, many of which are under your control. To help identify your risk factors, circle the response for each risk category that best describes you.

1. Sex and Age

   0 Female age 55 or younger; male age 45 or younger

   2 Female over age 55; male over age 45

2. Heredity/Family History

   0 Neither parent suffered a heart attack or stroke before age 60.

   3 One parent suffered a heart attack or stroke before age 60.

   7 Both parents suffered a heart attack or stroke before age 60.

3. Smoking

   0 Never smoked

   3 Quit more than 2 years ago and lifetime smoking is less than 5 pack-years*

   6 Quit less than 2 years ago and/or lifetime smoking is greater than 5 pack-years*

   8 Smoke less than ½ pack per day

   13 Smoke more than ½ pack per day

   15 Smoke more than 1 pack per day

4. Environmental Tobacco Smoke

   0 Do not live or work with smokers

   2 Exposed to ETS at work

   3 Live with smoker

   4 Both live and work with smokers

5. Blood Pressure
   (If available, use the average of the last three readings.)

   0 120/80 or below

   1 121/81–130/85

   3 Don't know blood pressure

   5 131/86–150/90

   9 151/91–170/100

   13 Above 170/100

6. Total Cholesterol

0	Lower than 5.2	4	5.8–5.9
1	5.3–5.4	5	6.0–6.1
2	Don't know	6	Over 6.2
3	5.5–5.7		

7. HDL Cholesterol

   0 Over 0.9 mmol/L

   1 0.7–0.8

   2 Don't know HDL

   12 Lower than 0.9

8. Exercise

   0 Exercise three times a week

   1 Exercise once or twice a week

   2 Occasional exercise less than once a week

   7 Rarely exercise

9. Diabetes

   0 No personal or family history

   2 One parent with diabetes

   6 Two parents with diabetes

   9 Type 2 diabetes

   13 Type 1 diabetes

10. Body Mass Index (kg/m2)

    0 <23.0

    1 23.0–24.9

    2 25.0–28.9

    3 29.0–34.9

    5 35.0–39.9

    7 ≥40.0

11. Stress

    0 Relaxed most of the time

    1 Occasionally stressed and angry

    2 Frequently stressed and angry

    3 Usually stressed and angry

Scoring

Total your risk factor points. Refer to the list below to get an approximate rating of your risk of suffering an early heart attack or stroke.

Score	Estimated Risk
Less than 20	Low risk
20–29	Moderate risk
30–45	High risk
Over 45	Extremely high risk

*Pack-years can be calculated by multiplying the number of packs you smoked per day by the number of years you smoked. For example, if you smoked a pack and a half a day for 5 years, you would have smoked the equivalent of 1.5 × 5 = 7.5 pack-years.

Part II Hostility Assessment

Are you too hostile? To help answer that question, Duke University researcher Redford Williams, M.D., has devised a short self-test. It is not a scientific evaluation, but it does offer a rough measure of hostility. Are the following statements true or false for you?

1. I often get annoyed at checkout cashiers or the people in front of me when I'm waiting in line.
2. I usually keep an eye on the people I work or live with to make sure they do what they should.
3. I often wonder how homeless people can have so little respect for themselves.
4. I believe that most people will take advantage of you if you let them.
5. The habits of friends or family members often annoy me.
6. When I'm stuck in traffic, I often start breathing faster and my heart pounds.
7. When I'm annoyed with people, I really want to let them know it.
8. If someone does me wrong, I want to get even.
9. I'd like to have the last word in any argument.
10. At least once a week, I have the urge to yell at or even hit someone.

According to Williams, five or more "true" statements suggest that you're excessively hostile and should consider taking steps to mellow out.

Using Your Results

How did you score?

(1) What is your CVD risk assessment score? Are you at all surprised by your score?

Are you satisfied with your CVD risk rating? If not, set a specific goal: _____

(2) What is your hostility assessment score? Are you at all surprised by the result?

Are you satisfied with your hostility rating? If not, set a specific goal: _____

What should you do next? Enter the results of this lab in the Preprogram Assessment column in Appendix C. (1) If you've set a goal for the overall CVD risk assessment score, identify a risk area that you can change, such as smoking, exercise, and stress. Then list three steps or strategies for changing the risk area you've chosen.
Risk area: _____
Strategies for change:

(2) If you've set a goal for the hostility assessment score, review the anger management strategies in Chapter 10 and select several that you will try to use to manage your own angry responses. Strategies for anger management:

Next, begin to put your strategies into action. After several weeks of a program to reduce CVD risk or hostility, do this lab again and enter the results in the Postprogram Assessment column of Appendix C. How do the results compare?

SOURCES: CVD risk assessment adapted from Insel, P. M., and W. T. Roth. 2008. *Core Concepts in Health,* 10th ed, Update. Copyright © 2008 The McGraw-Hill Companies, Inc. Reprinted with permission of The McGraw-Hill Companies, Inc.; and Hostility quiz from *Life Skills,* by Virginia Williams and Redford B. Williams. New York: Times Books. Reprinted by permission of the authors.

CHAPTER 12

CANCER

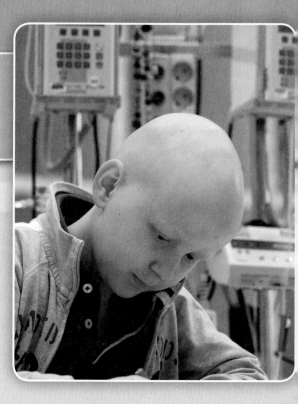

LEARNING OBJECTIVES

After reading this chapter, you should be able to

LO1 Explain what cancer is and how it spreads

LO2 List and describe common cancers—their risk factors, signs and symptoms, treatments, and approaches to prevention

LO3 Discuss some of the causes of cancer and how they can be avoided or minimized

LO4 List specific actions you can take to lower your risk of cancer

TEST YOUR KNOWLEDGE

1. **Eating which of these foods may help prevent cancer?**

   a. chili peppers
   b. broccoli
   c. oranges

2. **Using a sunscreen with an SPF rating of 15 means that you**

   a. can stay in the sun for 15 minutes without getting burned.
   b. can stay in the sun 15 times longer without getting burned than if you didn't use it.
   c. are protected against the full range of ultraviolet (UV) radiation.

3. **The use of condoms during sexual intercourse can prevent cancer in women.**

   True or false?

ANSWERS

1. **ALL THREE.** These and many other fruits and vegetables are rich in phytochemicals, naturally occurring substances that may have anticancer effects.

2. **B.** Choose a sunscreen that has an SPF rating of 15 or higher and that protects against both UVA and UVB rays. Apply it generously; most people use less than half the recommended amount.

3. **TRUE.** The primary cause of cervical cancer is infection with the human papillomavirus (HPV), a sexually transmitted pathogen. The use of condoms can prevent HPV infection.

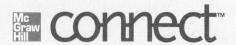

Practise and learn online with Connect.

Cancer causes more than 70 000 deaths in Canada each year, and it is the most common cause of death. Evidence indicates that more than 60% of all cancers in Canada could be prevented by simple changes in lifestyle.[1] Tobacco use is responsible for about one-third of all cancer deaths. Diet and exercise, including their relationship with obesity, account for another similar proportion of cancer deaths[2] (see Figure 12.1).

LO1 12.1 WHAT IS CANCER?

Cancer is the abnormal, uncontrolled growth of cells, which, if left untreated, can ultimately cause death.

Tumours

Most cancers take the form of tumours, although not all tumours are cancerous. A **tumour** (or neoplasm) is simply a mass of tissue that serves no physiological purpose. It can be benign, like a wart, or malignant, like most lung cancers.

Benign tumours (noncancerous tumours) are made up of cells similar to the surrounding normal cells and are enclosed in a membrane that prevents them from penetrating neighbouring tissues. They are dangerous only if their physical presence interferes with body functions.

The term **malignant tumour** is synonymous with cancer. A malignant tumour, or cancer, is capable of invading surrounding structures, including blood vessels, the **lymphatic system,** and nerves. It can also spread to distant sites via the blood and lymphatic circulation. A few cancers, like leukemia (cancer of the blood) do not produce a mass but still have the fundamental property of rapid, uncontrolled growth of cells.

Every case of cancer begins as a change in a cell that allows it to grow and divide when it should not. A malignant cell divides without regard for normal control mechanisms and gradually produces a mass of abnormal cells, or a tumour. It takes about a billion cells to make a mass the size of a pea, so a single tumour cell must go through many divisions, often taking years, before the tumour grows to a noticeable size. Eventually a tumour produces a sign or symptom that is detected. In an accessible location, a tumour may be felt as a lump. In less accessible locations, a tumour may be noticed only after considerable growth has taken place and may then be detected only by an indirect symptom—for instance, a persistent cough or unexplained bleeding or pain.

Metastasis

Metastasis, the spreading of cancer cells, occurs because cancer cells do not stick to each other as strongly as normal cells do and therefore may not remain at the site of the *primary tumour,* the original location. They break away and can pass through the lining of lymph or blood vessels to invade nearby tissue. They can also drift to distant parts of the body, where they establish new colonies of cancer cells. This travelling and seeding process is called *metastasizing,* and the new tumours are called *secondary tumours,* or *metastases.*

This ability of cancer cells to metastasize makes early cancer detection critical. To control the cancer, every cancerous cell must be removed. Once cancer cells enter either the lymphatic system or the bloodstream, it is extremely difficult to stop their spread.

LO2 12.2 COMMON CANCERS

The Canadian Cancer Society estimates that more than 177 800 Canadians were diagnosed with cancer in 2011 and of those, 75 000 will die from the disease. Health Canada reports that the majority of new cases are diagnosed in those between aged 20–59 and those over 70.[3]

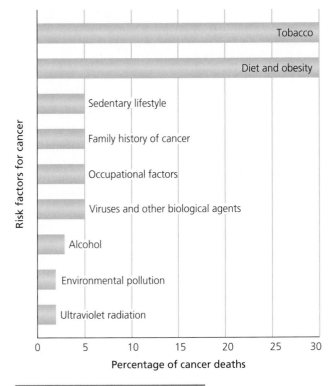

VITAL STATISTICS

FIGURE 12.1 Percentage of all cancer deaths linked to risk factors.

SOURCE: Harvard Center for Cancer Prevention. 1996. Harvard Reports on Cancer Prevention. Vol. 1: Human Causes of Cancer. *Cancer Causes and Control* 7(Suppl. 1).

TERMS

cancer Abnormal, uncontrolled multiplication of cells.

tumour A mass of tissue that serves no physiological purpose; also called a *neoplasm.*

benign tumour A tumour that is not cancerous.

malignant tumour A tumour that is cancerous and capable of spreading.

lymphatic system A system of vessels that returns proteins, lipids, and other substances from fluid in the tissues to the circulatory system.

metastasis The spread of cancer cells from one part of the body to another.

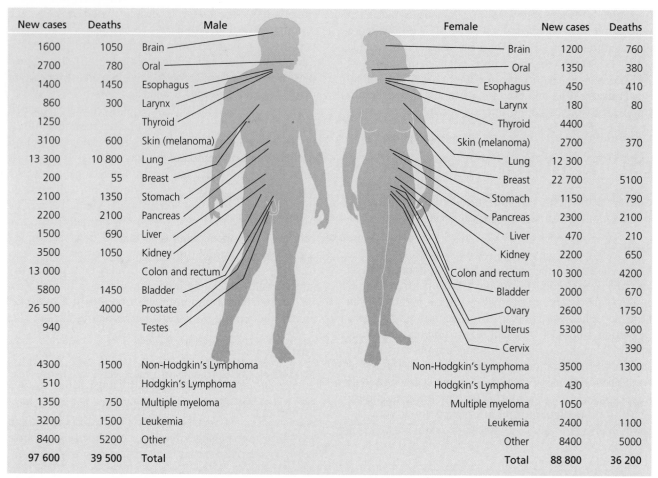

New cases	Deaths	Male		Female	New cases	Deaths
1600	1050	Brain		Brain	1200	760
2700	780	Oral		Oral	1350	380
1400	1450	Esophagus		Esophagus	450	410
860	300	Larynx		Larynx	180	80
1250		Thyroid		Thyroid	4400	
3100	600	Skin (melanoma)		Skin (melanoma)	2700	370
13 300	10 800	Lung		Lung	12 300	
200	55	Breast		Breast	22 700	5100
2100	1350	Stomach		Stomach	1150	790
2200	2100	Pancreas		Pancreas	2300	2100
1500	690	Liver		Liver	470	210
3500	1050	Kidney		Kidney	2200	650
13 000		Colon and rectum		Colon and rectum	10 300	4200
5800	1450	Bladder		Bladder	2000	670
26 500	4000	Prostate		Ovary	2600	1750
940		Testes		Uterus	5300	900
				Cervix		390
4300	1500	Non-Hodgkin's Lymphoma		Non-Hodgkin's Lymphoma	3500	1300
510		Hodgkin's Lymphoma		Hodgkin's Lymphoma	430	
1350	750	Multiple myeloma		Multiple myeloma	1050	
3200	1500	Leukemia		Leukemia	2400	1100
8400	5200	Other		Other	8400	5000
97 600	39 500	Total		Total	88 800	36 200

FIGURE 12.2 Estimated New Cases and Deaths for Cancers by Sex, Canada, 2012.

SOURCE: Analysis by: Chronic Disease Surveillance and Monitoring Division, CCDPC, Public Health Agency of Canada. Data sources: Canadian Cancer Registry and Canadian Vital Statistics Death databases at Statistics Canada. Canadian Cancer Society: *Canadian Cancer Statistics* 2012

WELLNESS TIP

If you smoke, find a way to stop. There are many options for quitting smoking. See online Chapter 14: Substance Use and Abuse for advice on giving up tobacco.

Cancer is an intriguing disease in that it has many origins, affects numerous parts of the body, and treatment for the different kinds of cancer can vary. Figure 12.2 above clearly describes those areas of the body that cancer can strike and the rate of death from those cancer sites.

Lung Cancer

Lung cancer is the most common cause of cancer death in Canada; it was responsible for about 18 216 deaths in 2006 alone.

TERMS

carcinogen Any substance that causes cancer.
chemotherapy The treatment of cancer with chemicals that selectively destroy cancerous cells.

The chief risk factor for lung cancer is tobacco smoke, which accounts for 30% of all cancers.[4] When smoking is combined with exposure to other environmental **carcinogens,** such as asbestos particles, the risk of cancer can be multiplied by a factor of 10 or more. But the smoker is not the only one at risk. Long-term exposure to environmental tobacco smoke (ETS), or secondhand smoke, also increases risk for lung cancer. The risk for lung cancer is 20% greater for non-smokers exposed to secondhand smoke than for people who are unexposed. The 2000–2001 Canadian Community Health Survey reported that 28% of Canadians are exposed to ETS.

Symptoms of lung cancer do not usually appear until the disease has advanced to the invasive stage. Signals such as a persistent cough, chest pain, or recurring bronchitis may be the first indication of a tumour's presence. Lung cancer is most often treated by some combination of surgery, radiation, and **chemotherapy;** if all the tumour cells can be removed or killed, a cure is possible. Unfortunately, lung cancer is usually detected only after it has begun to spread, and only about 15% of lung cancer patients are alive 5 years after diagnosis.[5]

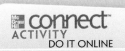
How to Examine Your Breasts

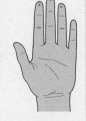

The best time to examine your breasts is when the breasts are not tender or swollen. Women who are pregnant or breastfeeding or have breast implants can also choose to examine their breasts regularly. Women who examine their breasts should have their technique reviewed by their health care professional during their clinical breast exams (CBEs). It is acceptable for women to choose not to do BSE or to do BSE occasionally. Women who choose not to do BSE should still be aware of their breasts and report any changes to their health care professional without delay.

How To Examine Your Breasts

- Lie down and place your right arm behind your head. The exam is done while lying down because when lying down, the breast tissue spreads evenly over the chest wall and it is as thin as possible, making it much easier to feel all the breast tissue.

- Use the finger pads of the three middle fingers on your left hand to feel for lumps in the right breast. Use overlapping dime-sized circular motions of the finger pads to feel the breast tissue.

- Use three different levels of pressure to feel all the breast tissue. Light pressure is needed to feel the tissue closest to the skin; medium pressure to feel a little deeper; and firm pressure to feel the tissue closest to the chest and ribs. A firm ridge in the lower curve of each breast is normal. If you're not sure how hard to press, talk with your doctor or nurse. Use each pressure level to feel the breast tissue before moving on to the next spot.

- Move around the breast in a up-and-down pattern starting at an imaginary line drawn straight down your side from the underarm and moving across the breast to the middle of the chest bone (sternum and breastbone). Be sure to check

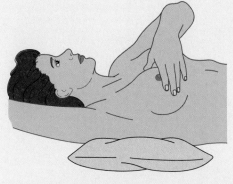

the entire breast area going down until you feel only ribs and up to the neck or collar bone (clavicle).

- Repeat the exam on your left breast using the finger pads of the right hand.

- While standing in front of a mirror with your hands pressing firmly down on your hips, look at your breasts for any changes of size, shape, contour, or dimpling. (The pressing down on the hips position contracts the chest wall muscles and enhances any breast changes.) Continue to look for changes with your arms down at your sides and then with your arms raised up over your head with your palms pressed together.

- Examine each underarm while sitting up or standing and with your arm only slightly raised so you can easily feel in this area. Raising your arm straight up tightens the tissue in this area and makes it very difficult to examine.

The Monthly Breast Self-Exam information is currently being reviewed and updated by the Canadian Breast Cancer Foundation (CBCF). Please go to http://www.cbcf.org for the new guide.

SOURCE: American Cancer Society's website (http://www.cancer.org, 2011). Copyright © 2011 American Cancer Society, Inc. Reprinted with permission.

Colon and Rectal Cancer

Another common cancer in Canada is colorectal cancer. It is the second leading cause of cancer death, after lung cancer, in both men and women. Age is a key risk factor, with more than 90% of cases diagnosed in people age 50 and older.[6] This is likely the result of recommended colorectal examinations (i.e., colonoscopy) yearly in those with a higher than average risk of colorectal cancer, or those over 50 years of age. Many cancers arise from preexisting polyps, small growths on the wall of the colon that may gradually develop into malignancies. The tendency to form colon polyps appears to be determined by specific genes, and about 15–30% of colon cancers may be due to inherited gene mutations.

Lifestyle also affects colon cancer risk. Regular physical activity reduces risk; obesity increases risk.

Although the mechanisms are unclear, high intake of red meat, smoked meat and fish, and simple sugars appears to increase risk, as does excessive alcohol consumption and smoking. Protective lifestyle factors may include a diet rich in fruits, vegetables, and whole grains; adequate intake of folic acid, calcium, magnesium, and vitamin D; regular use of nonsteroidal anti-inflammatory drugs such as aspirin and ibuprofen; and, in women, use of oral contraceptives.

Young polyps and early-stage cancers can be removed before they spread. Because polyps may bleed as they progress, the standard warning signs of colon cancer are bleeding from the rectum or a change in bowel habits. A stool blood test, performed during a routine physical exam, can detect small amounts of blood in the stool long before obvious bleeding would be noticed. The Canadian Cancer Society (CCS) recommends that this

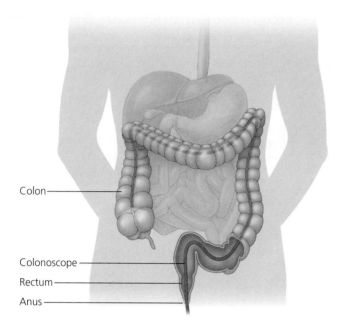

Colon

Colonoscope

Rectum

Anus

FIGURE 12.3 Colonoscopy.

examination be performed annually after age 50 (earlier for people with a family history of the disease). Another test is the colonoscopy, in which a flexible fibre-optic device is inserted through the rectum, allowing the colon to be examined and polyps to be removed (Figure 12.3). Studies show that screening could reduce the occurrence of colorectal cancer by 80%, but only about half of adults undergo these tests.

Surgery is the primary method of treatment. The 5-year survival rate is 90% for colon and rectal cancers detected early and 64% overall.

Breast Cancer

Breast cancer is the most common cancer in women and is second to lung cancer in the number of cancer deaths among women. In men, breast cancer occurs only rarely. In Canada, about 1 woman in 9 will develop breast cancer in her lifetime.

RISK FACTORS There is a strong genetic factor in breast cancer. A woman who has two close relatives with breast cancer is 4 to 6 times more likely to develop the disease than a woman who has no close relatives with breast cancer. However, only about 15% of cancers occur in women with a family history of it.

> **TERMS**
>
> **mammogram** A low-dose X-ray of the breasts used for the early detection of breast cancer.
>
> **biopsy** The removal and examination of a small piece of body tissue for the purpose of diagnosis.
>
> **ultrasonography** An imaging method in which inaudible high-pitched sound (ultrasound) is bounced off body structures to create an image on a monitor.

Other risk factors include:

- experiencing early onset menstruation or late-onset menopause
- late onset of menopause
- having no children or having a first child after age 30
- current use of hormone replacement therapy
- being obese
- using alcohol

The female hormone estrogen may be a common element in some of these risk factors. Estrogen promotes cell growth in responsive tissues, such as the breast and uterus, so any factor that increases estrogen exposure may raise the risk of breast cancer. Fat cells also produce estrogen, and estrogen levels are higher in obese women. Alcohol can increase estrogen in the blood as well.

PREVENTION Although some risk factors cannot be changed, important lifestyle risk factors can be controlled. Eating a low-fat, vegetable-rich diet, exercising regularly, limiting alcohol intake, and maintaining a healthy body weight can minimize the chance of developing breast cancer, even for women at risk from family history or other factors. Some research has also found that long-term use of aspirin and other nonsteroidal anti-inflammatory drugs reduces risk, possibly by affecting estrogen synthesis.

DETECTION The early detection of breast cancer is promoted through a three-part approach:

1. *Mammography:* A **mammogram** is a low-dose breast X ray that can spot breast abnormalities before physical symptoms arise. A newer type of mammography, called *digital mammography,* may provide more accurate results in some women, as may magnetic resonance imaging (MRI). The Canadian Cancer Society recommends that women over 50 get a mammogram every 2 years.

2. *Clinical breast exams:* Women between the ages of 20 and 39 should have a clinical breast exam about every 3 years. Women over 40 should have one every year.

3. *Breast self-exams:* By doing breast self-exams (BSEs), a woman can become familiar with her breasts and alert her physician to any changes (see the nearby box "How to Examine Your Breasts"). Although the ACS encourages all women to perform regular breast self-exams, many women elect not to do them, fearing they may not perform them correctly. When women learn proper self-exam technique from a health care professional, however, they are much more likely to regularly examine their breasts. Women who choose to do self-exams should begin at age 20.

If any of these methods detects a lump in the breast, it can be **biopsied** or scanned by **ultrasonography** to determine whether it is cancerous. In 90% of cases, the lump is found to be harmless.

TREATMENT If the lump is cancerous, one of several surgical treatments may be used, ranging from a lumpectomy (removal of the lump and surrounding tissue) to a mastectomy (removal of the breast). Chemotherapy or radiation may also be used to eradicate as many cancerous cells as possible.

Several new drugs have been developed for preventing and treating breast cancer. These include selective estrogen-receptor modulators (SERMs), which act like estrogen in some tissues but block estrogen's effects in others. The two best-known SERMs are tamoxifen and raloxifene. Another category of drug, called trastuzumab (Herceptin), is a special type of antibody that binds to a specific cancer-related target in the body. Regardless of the treatments used, social support can also affect a patient's psychological and physical wellness.

If the tumour is discovered early, before it has spread to the adjacent lymph nodes, the patient with breast cancer has about a 98% chance of surviving more than 5 years.

Prostate Cancer

The prostate gland is situated at the base of the bladder in men. It produces seminal fluid; if enlarged, it can block the flow of urine. Prostate cancer is the most common cancer in men and the second leading cause of cancer death in men. An estimated 25 500 new cases of prostate cancer were diagnosed in 2011.[7]

Age is the strongest predictor of the risk of prostate cancer, with about 75% of cases diagnosed in men over the age of 65. Inherited genetic predisposition may be responsible for 5–10% of cases; men with a family history of the disease should be vigilant about screening. Diets high in calories, dairy products, refined grains, and animal fats and low in plant foods (especially vegetable fibre) have been implicated as possible culprits, as have obesity, inactivity, and a history of sexually transmitted infections. Type 2 diabetes and insulin resistance are also associated with prostate cancer. Diet may be an important means of preventing prostate cancer. Soy foods, tomatoes, and cruciferous vegetables are being investigated for their possible protective effects.

Some cases are first detected by rectal examination during a routine physical exam. During this exam, a physician feels the prostate through the rectum to determine if the gland is enlarged or if lumps are present. Ultrasound and biopsy may also be used to detect and diagnose prostate cancer. A specialized test, called the **prostate-specific antigen (PSA) blood test**, is commonly used to detect prostate cancer and can be useful,

but the test is controversial because it can yield false-positive results. The Canadian Cancer Society recommends that men over 50 discuss the benefits of rectal exams and PSA testing with their physician. Men at high risk for the disease (such as African Canadian men and men with a close relative who have been diagnosed with prostate cancer) should begin annual testing at 40.

If the tumour is malignant, the prostate is usually removed surgically. However, a small, slow-growing tumour in an older man may be treated with watchful waiting because he is more likely to die from another cause before his cancer becomes life-threatening. A less invasive treatment involves radiation of the tumour by surgically implanting radioactive seeds in the prostate gland. The use of drugs to block the male hormone androgen is showing a great deal of promise when used in tandem with radiation therapy, resulting in lower death rates among test subjects. Androgen may encourage the growth of prostate cancer, so anti-androgen therapy is already commonly used against prostate cancer. The 5-year survival rate for all stages of prostate cancer is now nearly 100%.

Cancers of the Female Reproductive Tract

Because the uterus, cervix, and ovaries are subject to similar hormonal influences, the cancers of these organs can be discussed as a group.

CERVICAL CANCER Cervical cancer is at least in part a sexually transmitted disease. Most cases of cervical cancer stem from infection by the human papillomavirus (HPV), which causes genital warts and is transmitted during unprotected sex. Smoking and prior infection with the STIs herpes and chlamydia are other possible risk factors in cervical cancer.

Cervical cancer can be prevented by avoiding infection with HPV; sexual abstinence, mutually monogamous sex with an uninfected partner, or regular use of condoms can reduce the risk of HPV infection (see online Chapter 15 for more on HPV and other STIs).

Recently, some provinces began offering a vaccine (Gardasil) that protects against four types of HPV viruses. The vaccine can help prevent cervical cancer as

prostate-specific antigen (PSA) blood test A diagnostic test for prostate cancer that measures blood levels of prostate-specific antigen (PSA)

TERMS

well as cancers of the vagina and vulva. The vaccine is recommended for all girls ages 11–12; the recommendation also allows vaccinations of girls as young as 9 and women up to age 26.

Screening for the changes in cervical cells that precede cancer is done chiefly by means of the **Pap test.** During a pelvic exam, loose cells are scraped from the cervix, spread on a slide, stained for easier viewing, and examined under a microscope to see whether they are normal in size and shape. If cells are abnormal, a condition commonly referred to as *cervical dysplasia,* the Pap test is repeated at intervals. In about one-third of cases, the cellular changes progress toward malignancy. If this happens, the abnormal cells must be removed, either surgically or by destroying them with an ultracold (cryoscopic) probe or localized laser treatment. In more advanced cases, treatment may involve chemotherapy, radiation, or hysterectomy (surgical removal of the uterus).

The Canadian Cancer Society recommends that women who are sexually active start having regular Pap tests by the age of 21 and have the tests every 1 to 3 years, depending on your previous test results.

UTERINE OR ENDOMETRIAL CANCER   Cancer of the lining of the uterus, or endometrium, most often occurs after age 55. The risk factors are similar to those for breast cancer. The use of oral contraceptives, which combine estrogen and progestin, appears to provide protection. Endometrial cancer is usually detectable by pelvic examination. It is treated surgically, commonly by hysterectomy (removal of the uterus). Radiation and chemotherapy may be used as well.

OVARIAN CANCER   There are no approved screening tests to conclusively detect ovarian cancer so it is often diagnosed late in its development. Recent research investigating the detection of substances (called biomarkers) found in greater concentrations in tumours has discovered that cancer-antigen 125 (CA125) may be present in greater concentration in ovarian cells than other cells. Like other testing options such as routine exams (i.e., pelvic exams or ultrasound), CA125 testing has not been proven conclusive in screening for ovarian cancer. The risk factors for ovarian cancer are similar to those for breast and endometrial cancer. Anything that lowers a woman's lifetime number of ovulation cycles—pregnancy, breast-feeding, or use of oral contraceptives—reduces the risk of ovarian cancer.

In 2007, the Gynecologic Cancer Foundation announced that scientists had reached a consensus on symptoms of ovarian cancer: bloating, pelvic or abdominal pain, difficulty eating or feeling full quickly, and urinary problems (urgency or frequency). Women who

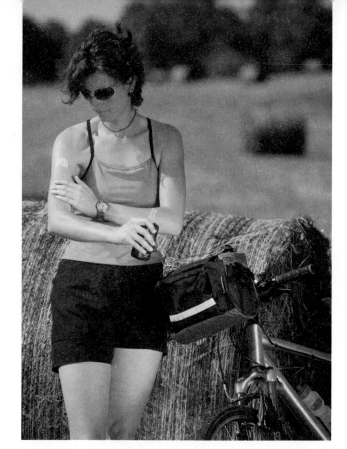

Sunscreen protects against skin cancer as well as sunburns.

experience these symptoms almost daily for a few weeks should see their physician. Some ovarian cancers are also detected through regular pelvic exams, sometimes with ultrasound imaging of the ovaries. Ovarian cancer is treated by surgical removal of one or both ovaries, the fallopian tubes, and the uterus.

Skin Cancer

Skin cancer is the most common cancer of all when cases of the highly curable forms are included in the count. Almost all cases of skin cancer can be traced to excessive exposure to **ultraviolet (UV) radiation** from the sun, including longer-wavelength ultraviolet A (UVA) and shorter-wavelength ultraviolet B (UVB) radiation. UVB radiation causes sunburns and can damage the eyes and immune system. UVA is less likely to cause a sunburn, but it damages connective tissue and leads to premature aging of the skin. Tanning lamps and tanning salon beds emit mostly UVA radiation. Both solar and artificial sources of UVA and UVB radiation are human carcinogens that cause skin cancer.

Both severe, acute sun reactions (sunburns) and chronic low-level sun reactions (suntans) can lead to skin cancer. The American Academy of Dermatology suggests that the risk of skin cancer doubles in people who have had five or more sunburns in their lifetime. People with fair skin have less natural protection against skin damage from the sun and a higher risk of developing skin cancer than people with naturally dark skin. Severe sunburns in

TERMS

Pap test   A scraping of cells from the cervix for examination under a microscope to detect cancer.

ultraviolet (UV) radiation   Light rays of a specific wavelength, emitted by the sun; most UV rays are blocked by the ozone layer in the upper atmosphere.

childhood have been linked to a greatly increased risk of skin cancer in later life, so children in particular should be protected. Other risk factors include having many moles, particularly large ones, spending time at high altitudes, and a family history of the disease.

There are three main types of skin cancer, named for the types of skin cell from which they develop. **Basal cell** and **squamous cell carcinomas** together account for about 95% of the skin cancers diagnosed each year. They are usually found in chronically sun-exposed areas, such as the face, neck, hands, and arms. They usually appear as pale, waxlike, pearly nodules, or red, scaly, sharply outlined patches. These cancers are often painless, although they may bleed, crust, and form an open sore.

Melanoma is by far the most dangerous skin cancer because it spreads so rapidly. It can occur anywhere on the body, but the most common sites are the back, chest, abdomen, and lower legs. A melanoma usually appears at the site of a preexisting mole. The mole may begin to enlarge, become mottled or varied in colour (colours can include blue, pink, and white), or develop an irregular surface or irregular borders. Tissue invaded by melanoma may also itch, burn, or bleed easily.

To protect yourself against skin cancer avoid overexposure to UV radiation. People of every age, including babies and children, need to be protected from the sun (see the box "Sunscreen and Sun-Protective Clothing"). You can help with early detection by making it a habit to examine your skin regularly. Most of the spots, freckles, moles, and blemishes on your body are normal. But if you notice an unusual growth, discolouration, or sore that does not heal, see your physician or a dermatologist immediately. The characteristics that may signal that a skin lesion is a melanoma are illustrated in Figure 12.4.

If you do have an unusual skin lesion, your physician will examine it and possibly perform a biopsy. If the lesion is cancerous, it is usually removed surgically, a procedure that can almost always be performed in the physician's office using a local anesthetic. Treatment is usually simple and successful when the cancer is caught early.

Oral Cancer

Oral cancer—cancers of the lip, tongue, mouth, and throat—can be traced principally to cigarette, cigar, or pipe smoking; the use of smokeless (spit) tobacco; and excessive consumption of alcohol. These risk factors work together to multiply a person's risk of oral cancer. The incidence of oral cancer is more than twice as great in men as in women and most frequent in men over 40. Oral cancers are fairly easy to detect but often hard to cure. The primary methods of treatment are surgery and radiation.

Testicular Cancer

Testicular cancer is relatively rare, accounting for less than 1% of cancers in men. Testicular cancer is much more common among Caucasians than Latin, Asian, or

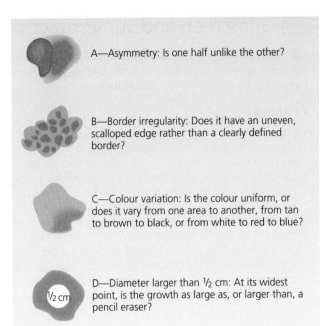

A—Asymmetry: Is one half unlike the other?

B—Border irregularity: Does it have an uneven, scalloped edge rather than a clearly defined border?

C—Colour variation: Is the colour uniform, or does it vary from one area to another, from tan to brown to black, or from white to red to blue?

½ cm

D—Diameter larger than ½ cm: At its widest point, is the growth as large as, or larger than, a pencil eraser?

FIGURE 12.4   The ABCD test for melanoma.   To see a variety of photos of melanoma and benign moles, visit the National Cancer Institute's Visual Online site (http://visualsonline.cancer.gov).

WELLNESS TIP

The Skin Cancer Foundation recommends that everyone see their physician at least once a year for a head-to-toe skin evaluation. Depending on individual risk factors, some people may need to have their skin checked more frequently.

African Canadians. Men with undescended testicles are at increased risk for testicular cancer, and for this reason the condition should be corrected in early childhood. Self-examination may help in the early detection of testicular cancer (see the box "Testicle Self-Examination"). Tumours are treated by surgical removal of the testicle and, if the tumour has spread, by chemotherapy.

Other Cancers

Several other cancers affect thousands of people each year. Some have identifiable risk factors, but the causes of others are still under investigation.

- *Pancreatic cancer* is usually well advanced before symptoms become noticeable, and no effective cure is available. About 3 out of 10 cases are linked to smoking. Other risk factors include being male, African Canadian, or over age 60; having a family history of pancreatic cancer; having diabetes; being inactive and obese; and eating a diet high in fat and meat and low in vegetables.

---

basal cell carcinoma   Cancer of the deepest layers of the skin.
squamous cell carcinoma   Cancer of the surface layers of the skin.
melanoma   A malignant tumour of the skin that arises from pigmented cells, usually a mole.

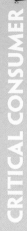

Sunscreen and Sun-Protective Clothing

With consistent use of the proper clothing, sunscreens, and common sense, you can lead an active outdoor life *and* protect your skin against most sun-induced damage.

Clothing

- Wear long-sleeved shirts and long pants. Dark-coloured, tightly woven fabrics provide reasonable protection from the sun. Another good choice is clothing made from special sun-protective fabrics; these garments have an Ultraviolet Protection Factor (UPF) rating, similar to the SPF for sunscreens. For example, a fabric with a UPF rating of 20 allows only one-twentieth of the sun's UV radiation to pass through. There are three categories of UPF protection: A UPF of 15–24 provides "good" UV protection, a UPF of 25–39 provides "very good" protection, and a UPF of 40–50 provides "excellent" protection. By comparison, typical shirts provide a UPF of only 5–9, a value that drops when clothing is wet.

- Consider washing some extra sun protection into your current wardrobe. A new laundry additive adds UV protection to ordinary fabrics; it is recommended by the Skin Cancer Foundation.

- Wear a hat. Your face, ears, neck, and scalp are especially vulnerable to the sun's harmful effects, making hats an essential weapon in the battle against sun damage. A good choice is a broad-brimmed hat or a legionnaire-style cap that covers the ears and neck. You still need to wear sunscreen on your face even if you are wearing a hat.

- Sunglasses are a good protective piece of clothing for the eyes. Health Canada suggests that if you spend a lot of time outdoors, you should wear sunglasses that block both UVA and UVB rays. Long-term exposure can damage the retina and can increase the risk for blindness in those over the age of 60.

Sunscreen

- Use a sunscreen and lip balm with a sun protection factor (SPF) of 15 or higher. (An SPF rating refers to the amount of time you can stay out in the sun before you burn, compared with not using sunscreen; for example, a product with an SPF of 15 would allow you to remain in the sun without burning 15 times longer, on average, than if you didn't apply sunscreen.) If you're fair-skinned, have a family history of skin cancer, are at high altitude, or will be outdoors for many hours, use a sunscreen with a high SPF (30+).

- Choose a broad-spectrum sunscreen that protects against both UVA and UVB radiation. The SPF rating of a sunscreen currently applies only to UVB, but a number of ingredients, especially titanium dioxide and zinc oxide, are effective at blocking most UVA radiation. Use a water-resistant sunscreen if you swim or sweat quite a bit. If you have sensitive skin, you may need to try several brands before finding one that doesn't irritate your skin. If you have acne, look for a sunscreen that is labelled "noncomedogenic," which means that it will not cause pimples.

- Shake sunscreen before applying. Apply it 30 minutes before exposure to allow it time to bond to the skin. Reapply sunscreen frequently and generously to all sun-exposed areas (many people overlook their temples, ears, and sides and backs of their necks). Most people use less than half as much as they need to attain the full SPF rating. One ounce of sunscreen is enough to cover an average-size adult in a swimsuit. Reapply sunscreen 15–30 minutes after sun exposure begins and then every 2 hours after that and/or following activities, such as swimming, that could remove sunscreen.

- If you're taking medications, ask your physician or pharmacist about possible reactions to sunlight or interactions with sunscreens. Medications for acne, allergies, and diabetes are just a few of the products that can trigger reactions. If you're using sunscreen and an insect repellent containing DEET, use extra sunscreen (DEET may decrease sunscreen effectiveness).

- Don't let sunscreens give you a false sense of security. Most of the sunscreens currently on the market allow considerable UVA radiation to penetrate the skin, with the potential for causing skin cancers (especially melanoma), as well as wrinkles and other forms of skin damage.

Time of Day and Location

- Avoid sun exposure between 10 a.m. and 4 p.m., when the sun's rays are most intense. Clouds allow as much as 80% of UV rays to reach your skin. Stay in the shade when you can.

- Consult the day's UV Index, which predicts UV levels on a 0–10 + scale, to get a sense of the amount of sun protection you'll need; take special care on days with a rating of 5 or above. UV Index ratings are available in local newspapers, from the television, or from certain websites.

- Be aware that UV rays can penetrate at least 1 metre in water. Thus, swimmers should wear water-resistant sunscreens. Snow, sand, water, concrete, and white-painted surfaces are also highly reflective.

Tanning Salons and Sunless Tanning Products

- Stay away from tanning salons! Despite advertising claims to the contrary, the lights used in tanning parlours are damaging to your skin. Tanning beds and lamps emit mostly UVA radiation, increasing your risk of premature skin aging (such as wrinkles) and skin cancer.

- If you really want a tan, consider using sunless self-tanning lotions. Lotions, creams, and sprays containing the colour additive dihydroxyacetone (DHA) are approved for tanning. (Some tanning accelerators and tanning pills have not been approved because these products have not been proven to be safe or effective.) DHA is for external use only and should not be inhaled, swallowed, or used around the eyes. Tanning salons that offer spraying or misting with DHA need to ensure that customers are protected from exposure to the eyes, lips, and mucous membranes as well as internal exposure. Most sunless tanning products do not contain sunscreen, so if you use them in the sun, be sure to wear sunscreen.

SOURCE: Health Canada, *Healthy Living.* Available online at http://www.hc-sc.gc.ca/hl-vs/sun-sol/protect-protegez/index-eng.php.

The best time to perform a testicular self-exam is after a warm shower or bath, when the scrotum is relaxed. First, stand in front of a mirror and look for any swelling of the scrotum. Then, examine each testicle with both hands. Place the index and middle fingers under the testicle and the thumbs on top; roll the testicle gently between the fingers and thumbs. Don't worry if one testicle seems slightly larger than the other—that's common. Also, expect to feel the epididymis, the soft, sperm-carrying tube at the rear of the testicle.

Perform the self-exam each month. If you find a lump, swelling, or nodule, consult a physician right away. The abnormality may not be cancer, but only a physician can make a diagnosis. Other possible signs of testicular cancer include a change in the way a testicle feels, a sudden collection of fluid in the scrotum, a dull ache in the lower abdomen or groin, a feeling of heaviness in the scrotum, or pain in a testicle or the scrotum.

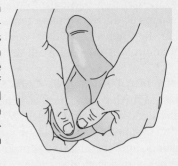

SOURCES: Testicular Cancer Resource Center. 2009. *How to Do a Testicular Self Examination* (http://www.acor.org/tcrc/tcexam.html, retrieved May 17, 2011); and National Cancer Institute. 2009. *Testicular Cancer* (http://www.cancer.gov/cancertopics/types/testicular, retrieved May 17, 2011).

- *Bladder cancer* is 2.5 times more common in men as in women, and smoking is the key risk factor. The first symptoms are likely to be blood in the urine and/or increased frequency of urination. These symptoms can also signal a urinary tract infection but should trigger a visit to a physician, who can evaluate the possibility of cancer.
- *Kidney cancer* usually occurs in people over 50; smoking and obesity are mild risk factors, as is a family history of the disease. Symptoms may include fatigue, pain in the side, and blood in the urine.
- *Brain cancer* commonly develops for no apparent reason and can arise from most of the cell types that are found in the brain. One of the few established risk factors for brain cancer is ionizing radiation, such as X rays of the head. Symptoms are often nonspecific and include headaches, fatigue, behavioural changes, and sometimes seizures. Some brain tumours are curable by surgery or by radiation and chemotherapy, but most are not.
- *Leukemia,* cancer of the white blood cells, starts in the bone marrow but can then spread to the lymph nodes, spleen, liver, other organs, and central nervous system. Most people with leukemia have no known risk factors. About 20% of cases of adult leukemia are related to smoking; other possible risk factors include radiation and certain chemicals and infections. Most symptoms occur because leukemia cells crowd out the production of normal blood cells; the result can be fatigue, anemia, weight loss, and increased risk of infection.
- *Lymphoma* is a form of cancer that begins in the lymph nodes and then may spread to almost any part of the body. There are two types—Hodgkin's disease and non-Hodgkin's lymphoma (NHL). NHL is the more common and more deadly form of the disease; risk factors for NHL are not well understood but may include genetic factors, radiation, and certain chemicals and infections.

LO3 12.3 RISK FACTORS FOR CANCER

Although scientists do not know everything about what causes cancer, they have identified genetic, environmental, and lifestyle factors that may influence your risk for cancer. There are usually several steps in the transformation of a normal cell into a cancer cell, and different factors may work together in the development of cancer.

The Role of DNA

Heredity and genetics are important factors in a person's risk of cancer. Certain genes may predispose some people to cancer, and specific gene mutations have been associated with cancer.

DNA BASICS The nucleus of each cell in your body contains 23 pairs of **chromosomes,** which are made up of tightly packed coils of **DNA** (deoxyribonucleic acid).

chromosomes The threadlike bodies in a cell nucleus that contain molecules of DNA; most human cells contain 23 pairs of chromosomes.

DNA Deoxyribonucleic acid, a chemical substance that carries genetic information.

TERMS

Each chromosome contains thousands of **genes**; you have about 25 000 genes in all. Each of your genes controls the production of a particular protein. By making different proteins at different times, genes can act as switches to alter the ways a cell works. Some genes are responsible for controlling the rate of cell division.

DNA MUTATIONS AND CANCER A *mutation* is any change in the makeup of a gene. Some mutations are inherited; others are caused by environmental agents known as *mutagens*. Mutagens include radiation, certain viruses, and chemical substances in the air we breathe. (When a mutagen also causes cancer, it is called a *carcinogen*.) Some mutations are the result of copying errors that occur when DNA replicates itself as part of cell division.

A mutated gene no longer contains the proper code for producing its protein. It usually takes several mutational changes before a normal cell takes on the properties of a cancer cell. Genes in which mutations are associated with the conversion of a normal cell into a cancer cell are known as **oncogenes.** In their undamaged form, many oncogenes play a role in controlling or restricting cell growth; they are called *tumour suppressor genes.* Mutational damage to suppressor genes releases the brake on growth and leads to rapid and uncontrolled cell division—a precondition for the development of cancer.

An example of an inherited mutated oncogene is BRCA1 (breast cancer gene 1): Women who inherit a damaged copy of this suppressor gene face a significantly increased risk of breast and ovarian cancer.

In most cases, however, mutational damage occurs after birth. For example, only about 5–10% of breast cancer cases can be traced to inherited copies of a damaged BRCA1 gene. In addition, lifestyle factors are important even for those who have inherited a damaged suppressor gene. Testing and identification of hereditary cancer risks can be helpful for some people, especially if it leads to increased attention to controllable risk factors and better medical screening.

CANCER PROMOTERS Substances known as cancer promoters make up another important piece of the cancer puzzle. They don't directly produce DNA mutations, but they accelerate the growth of cells, which means less time for a cell to repair DNA damage caused by other factors. Estrogen, which stimulates cellular growth in the female reproductive organs, is an example of a cancer promoter. Although much still needs to be learned about the role of genetics in cancer, it's clear that minimizing mutation damage to our DNA will lower our risk of many cancers. Unfortunately, a great many substances produce cancer-causing mutations, and we can't escape them all. By identifying the important carcinogens and understanding how they produce their effects, we can help keep our DNA intact and avoid activating "sleeping" oncogenes.

Dietary Factors

Diet is one of the most important factors in cancer prevention, but it is also one of the most complex and controversial. Your food choices affect your cancer risk by both exposing you to potentially dangerous compounds and depriving you of potentially protective ones. The following sections examine some of the dietary factors that may affect cancer risk.

DIETARY FAT AND MEAT Diets high in fat and meat appear to contribute to certain cancers, including colon, stomach, and prostate. As is true with heart disease, certain types of fats may be riskier than others. Diets favouring omega-6 poly-unsaturated fats are associated with a higher risk of certain cancers than are diets favouring the omega-3 forms commonly found in fish and canola oil. (See Chapter 7 for more information on types of fatty acids.)

ALCOHOL Alcohol is associated with an increased incidence of several cancers. For example, an average alcohol intake of three drinks a day is associated with a doubling in the risk of breast cancer. Alcohol and tobacco interact as risk factors for oral cancer. Heavy users of both alcohol and tobacco have a risk for oral cancer up to 15 times greater than that of people who don't drink or use tobacco.

FRIED FOODS Scientists have found high levels of the chemical acrylamide (a probable human carcinogen) in starch-based foods that have been fried or baked at high temperatures, including french fries and certain types of snack chips and crackers. Studies are ongoing, but, in 2005, the World Health Organization urged food companies to work to lower the acrylamide content of foods to reduce any risk to public health. Acrylamide levels vary widely in foods, and there are currently no warnings against eating specific foods. The wisest course may be to consume a variety of foods and avoid overindulging in any single class of foods, particularly items like french fries and potato chips, which may contain other unhealthy substances such as saturated and trans fats. You can also limit your exposure to acrylamide by not smoking; you get much more of the chemical from smoking than from food.

FIBRE Various potential cancer-fighting actions have been proposed for fibre, but none has been firmly established. Although further study is needed to clarify the relationship between fibre intake and cancer risk, experts still recommend a high-fibre diet for its overall positive effect on health.

TERMS

gene A section of a chromosome that contains the instructions for making a particular protein; the basic unit of heredity.

oncogene A gene involved in the transformation of a normal cell into a cancer cell.

TABLE 12.1 Foods with Phytochemicals

Food	Phytochemical	Potential Anticancer Effects
Chili peppers (*Note:* Hotter peppers contain more capsaicin.)	Capsaicin	Neutralizes effect of nitrosamines; may block carcinogens in cigarette smoke from acting on cells
Oranges, lemons, limes, onions, apples, berries, eggplant	Flavonoids	Act as antioxidants; block access of carcinogens to cells; suppress malignant changes in cells; prevent cancer cells from multiplying
Citrus fruits, cherries	Monoterpenes	Help detoxify carcinogens; inhibit spread of cancer cells
Cruciferous vegetables (broccoli, cabbage, bok choy, cauliflower, kale, brussels sprouts, collards)	Isothiocyanates	Boost production of cancer-fighting enzymes; suppress tumour growth; block effects of estrogen on cell growth
Garlic, onions, leeks, shallots, chives	Allyl sulfides	Increase levels of enzymes that break down potential carcinogens; boost activity of cancer-fighting immune cells
Grapes, red wine, peanuts	Resveratrol	Acts as an antioxidant; suppresses tumour growth
Green, oolong, and black teas (*Note:* Drinking burning hot tea may *increase* cancer risk.)	Polyphenols	Increase antioxidant activity; prevent cancer cells from multiplying; help speed excretion of carcinogens from body
Orange, deep yellow, red, pink, and dark green vegetables; some fruits	Carotenoids	Act as antioxidants; reduce levels of cancer-promoting enzymes; inhibit spread of cancer cells
Soy foods, whole grains, flax seeds, nuts	Phytoestrogens	Block effects of estrogen on cell growth; lower blood levels of estrogen
Whole grains, legumes	Phytic acid	Binds iron, which may prevent it from creating cell-damaging free radicals

FRUITS AND VEGETABLES Canada's Food Guide encourage individuals to eat a plant-based diet containing numerous servings of vegetables and fruits every day, and to choose whole grains over processed grains. A massive number of epidemiological studies provide evidence that high consumption of fruits and vegetables reduces the risk of many cancers. Exactly which constituents of fruits and vegetables are responsible for reducing cancer risk is not clear, but researchers have identified many mechanisms by which food components may act against cancer. Some may prevent carcinogens from forming in the first place or block them from reaching or acting on target cells. Others boost enzymes that detoxify carcinogens and render them harmless. Still other anti-cancer agents act on cells that have already been exposed to carcinogens, slowing the development of cancer or starving cancer cells of oxygen and nutrients by cutting off their blood supply.

Some essential nutrients have been found to act against cancer. For example, vitamin C, vitamin E, selenium, and the **carotenoids** (vitamin A precursors) may help block the initiation of cancer by acting as **antioxidants.** Antioxidants prevent **free radicals** from damaging DNA. See the National Cancer Institute website for research on the many ways that we are examining the impact of antioxidants (http://www.cancer.gov/cancertopics/factsheet/antioxidantsprevention). Vitamin C may also block the conversion of nitrates (food preservatives) into cancer-causing agents. Folic acid may inhibit the transformation

of normal cells into malignant cells and strengthen immune function. Calcium inhibits the growth of cells in the colon and may slow the spread of potentially cancerous cells.

Many other anticancer agents in the diet fall under the broader heading of **phytochemicals,** substances in plants that help protect against chronic diseases (see Table 12.1 above). One of the first to be identified was sulforaphane, a compound found in broccoli.

To increase your intake of potential cancer fighters, eat a wide variety of fruits, vegetables, legumes, and grains (see Lab 12.1). Don't rely on supplements; studies suggest that vitamins and antioxidants taken in

carotenoid Any of a group of yellow-to-red plant pigments; some can be converted to vitamin A by the liver, and many act as antioxidants or have other anticancer effects. The carotenoids include beta-carotene, lutein, lycopene, and zeaxanthin.

antioxidant A substance that can lessen the breakdown of food or body constituents; actions include binding oxygen and donating electrons to free radicals.

free radicals Electron-seeking compounds that can react with fats, proteins, and DNA, damaging cell membranes and mutating genes in their search for electrons; produced through chemical reactions in the body and through exposure to environmental factors such as sunlight and tobacco smoke.

phytochemical A naturally occurring substance found in plant foods that may help prevent chronic diseases such as cancer and heart disease; *phyto* means plant.

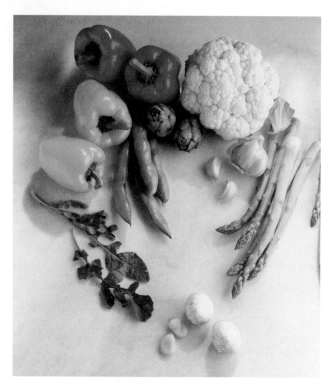

Your food choices significantly affect your risk of cancer. Red bell peppers, chili peppers, and garlic are just a few of the foods containing cancer-fighting phytochemicals.

supplement form (even the widely touted vitamins B, C, D, and E, folic acid, and calcium) do not prevent cancer. Isolated phytochemicals may be harmful if taken in high doses, and it is likely that the anticancer effects of many foods are the result of many chemical substances working in combination.

Obesity and Inactivity

It is important to maintain a healthy weight throughout life by balancing caloric intake with physical activity and achieving and maintaining a healthy weight if currently overweight or obese. Several common types of cancer (colon, breast,[8] endometrium, kidney, prostate) are associated with being overweight or obese,[9] and research has shown a relationship between increased physical activity and a reduction in cancer risk in these forms of cancer (see the box "How Does Exercise Affect Cancer Risk?").

Metabolic Syndrome

Scientists have long believed that metabolic syndrome (described in Chapter 6) might be associated with various types of cancer. New evidence supports this belief. For example, a 2008 study concluded that people with metabolic syndrome have a 75% higher risk of developing colorectal cancer than people without metabolic syndrome. Anyone with metabolic syndrome is advised

to eat a heart-healthy diet, exercise regularly, and make sure their blood pressure and cholesterol levels are under control.

Carcinogens in the Environment

Some carcinogens occur naturally in the environment, like the sun's UV rays. Others are synthetic substances that show up occasionally in the general environment but more often in the work environments of specific industries.

INGESTED CHEMICALS The food industry uses preservatives and other additives to prevent food from becoming spoiled or stale. Some of these compounds are antioxidants and may actually decrease any cancer-causing properties the food might have. Other compounds, like the nitrates and nitrites found in beer and ale, ham, bacon, hot dogs, and lunch meats, are potentially more dangerous. Although nitrates and nitrites are not themselves carcinogenic, they can combine with dietary substances in the stomach and be converted to nitrosamines, which are highly potent carcinogens. Foods cured with nitrites, as well as those cured by salt or smoke, have been linked to esophageal and stomach cancer, and they should be eaten only in modest amounts. Similarly, people who regularly eat charred or very well done meat may increase their risk of pancreatic cancer by 60–70%, compared to people who rarely eat over-cooked meat. A long-term study by the University of Minnesota confirmed the results of previous studies, which showed that charred meat contains a number of carcinogens, most notably compounds called heterocyclic amines (HAs). HAs are created when certain amino acids in meat are burned at high temperatures. The compound is created whether meat is over-cooked through grilling, barbecuing, broiling, or pan-frying.

ENVIRONMENTAL AND INDUSTRIAL POLLUTION The best available data indicate that less than 2% of cancer deaths are caused by general environmental pollution, such as substances in our air and water. Exposure to carcinogenic materials in the workplace is a more serious problem. Occupational exposure to specific carcinogens may account for up to 5% of cancer deaths. With increasing industry and government regulations, industrial sources of cancer risk should continue to diminish.

RADIATION All sources of radiation are potentially carcinogenic, including medical X rays, radioactive substances (radioisotopes), and UV radiation from the sun, sunlamps, and tanning beds. Most physicians and dentists are quite aware of the risk of radiation, and successful efforts have been made to reduce the amount of radiation needed for mammography, dental X rays, and other necessary medical X rays.

Based on the information in this chapter, how many cancer risks can you identify in your life? For example, do you smoke? Are you sedentary? Do you eat a lot of processed foods? Remember that risk factors can be hereditary or environmental, and environmental risk factors can include behaviours like smoking or working in a toxic environment. Consider the risk factors identified in the text, and list three risk factors that you are exposed to regularly or daily.

1. _____
2. _____
3. _____

Next, list steps you can take to reduce each of these risk factors. Target your steps to each specific risk factor.

1. _____
2. _____
3. _____

Finally, expand your thinking. Can you identify any cancer risk factors that exist in your community? If so, identify one such risk factor and think of ways people in your community can work together to reduce or eliminate that risk.

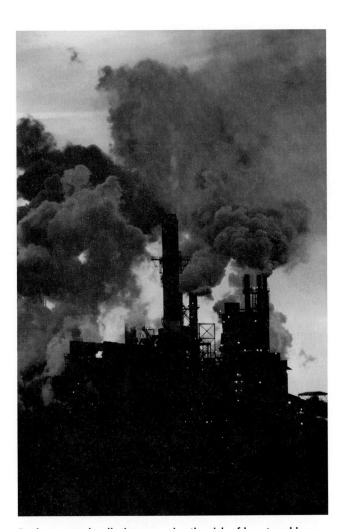

Environmental pollution can raise the risk of heart and lung diseases, but it appears to account for only 2% of cancer deaths.

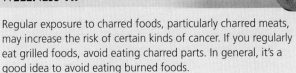

WELLNESS TIP

Regular exposure to charred foods, particularly charred meats, may increase the risk of certain kinds of cancer. If you regularly eat grilled foods, avoid eating charred parts. In general, it's a good idea to avoid eating burned foods.

MICROBES   About 15% of the world's cancers are caused by microbes, including viruses, bacteria, and parasites, although the percentage is much lower in developed countries like Canada. As discussed earlier, certain types of HPV cause many cases of cervical cancer. Other microbes linked to cancer include the *Helicobacter pylori* bacterium, which can cause both stomach ulcers and stomach cancer. The Epstein-Barr virus, best known for causing mononucleosis, is also suspected of contributing to Hodgkin's disease, cancer of the pharynx, and some stomach cancers. Human herpes virus 8 has been linked to Kaposi's sarcoma and certain types of lymphoma. Hepatitis virus B and C together cause as many as 80% of the world's liver cancers.

LO4   12.4 PREVENTING CANCER

Your lifestyle choices can radically lower your cancer risks, so you *can* take a practical approach to cancer prevention. Here are some guidelines:

- *Avoid tobacco.* Smoking is responsible for 80–90% of lung cancers and for about 30% of all cancer deaths. The carcinogenic chemicals in smoke are transported throughout the body in the bloodstream, making smoking a carcinogen for many forms of cancer other than lung cancer. The use of spit tobacco increases the

How Does Exercise Affect Cancer Risk?

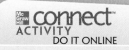
ACTIVITY DO IT ONLINE

THE EVIDENCE FOR EXERCISE

According to statistics from the International Agency for Research on Cancer (IARC), as many as 25% of cancers are due to overweight, obesity, and physical inactivity. Increasing levels of physical activity can potentially ward off several types of cancer.

The links between exercise and cancer prevention are not entirely clear. However, experts have associated increased physical activity and a reduced risk of several specific types of cancer. Studies show, for example, that people who do moderate aerobic exercise for 3–4 hours per week reduce their risk of colon cancer by 30%. Women who do the same amount of exercise can reduce their risk of breast cancer by as much as 40%. (Some studies suggest that women who meet certain criteria can reduce their breast cancer risk up to 80%.) Evidence also shows that, when compared with sedentary people, active people can reduce their risk of lung cancer (20%), endometrial cancer (30%), and ovarian cancer (20%). Researchers are continually trying to establish similar connections between exercise and other types of cancer.

As with all-cause mortality and cardiovascular disease, physical activity appears to have an inverse relationship with the types of cancer just listed. That is, the more you exercise, the lower your risk of developing these kinds of cancer. Energy balance also seems to be a factor, at least in relation to a few types of cancer, meaning that people who burn at least as many calories as they take in may further reduce their risk of some cancers. This positive effect may be due to the fact that reducing body fat (through exercise and a healthy diet) lowers the chemical and hormonal activities of adipose (fat) tissue—activities that may encourage some cancers to develop.

In addition to reducing the biological influences of adipose tissue, physical activity is known to reduce the inflammatory response and to boost immune function. Chronic inflammation,

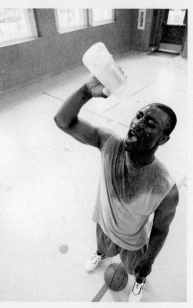

which can have many causes, leaves body tissues more vulnerable to infection. The immune system is the body's first line of defense against cancer, so supporting immune function through exercise may help prevent some cancers.

Emerging data also indicate that physical activity can help improve health outcomes in people who have cancer or are cancer survivors. For example, physical activity appears to restore cardiorespiratory fitness at least to some degree in patients whose heart muscles have been weakened by cancer treatments. This positive outcome was found in 13 separate studies, many of which found significant improvements in heart function among cancer survivors who performed moderate-intensity exercise for 20–40 minutes three times per week. The benefits were similar across several forms of aerobic exercise, including walking, yoga, and tai chi. Additionally, a handful of studies have found that exercise improves muscular strength and endurance and flexibility in patients whose muscles and joints have been weakened by cancer treatments.

SOURCES: Doyle, C., et al. 2006. Nutrition and physical activity during and after cancer treatment: An American Cancer Society guide for informed choices. *CA: A Cancer Journal for Clinicians* 56(6): 323–353; Irwin, M. L., and S. T. Mayne. 2008. Impact of nutrition and exercise on cancer survival. *Cancer Journal* 14(6): 435–441; Morris, G. S., et al. 2009. Pulmonary rehabilitation improves functional status in oncology patients. *Archives of Physical Medicine and Rehabilitation* 90(5): 837–841; and Physical Activity Guidelines Advisory Committee. 2008. *Physical Activity Guidelines Advisory Committee Report, 2008.* Washington, D.C.: U.S. Department of Health and Human Services.

---

risk of cancers of the mouth, larynx, throat, and esophagus. It's also important to avoid exposure to ETS.

- **Control diet and weight.** About one-third of all cancers are in some way linked to what we eat. Choose a low-fat, plant-based diet containing a wide variety of fruits, vegetables, and whole grains rich in phytochemicals. Drink alcohol only in moderation, if at all. Maintain a healthy weight.

- **Exercise.** Regular exercise is linked to lower rates of colon and other cancers. It also helps control weight.

- **Protect skin from the sun.** Almost all cases of skin cancer are sun-related. Wear protective clothing when you're out in the sun and use a sunscreen with an SPF rating of 15 or higher. Don't go to tanning salons.

- **Avoid environmental and occupational carcinogens.** Try to avoid occupational exposure to carcinogens and don't smoke; the cancer risks of many of these agents increase greatly when combined with smoking.

Your first line of defence against cancer involves the lifestyle changes described in this chapter. Your second line of defence against cancer is early detection. It is recommended that you stay alert for any of the seven major warning signs illustrated in Figure 12.5; you can remember these with the acronym CAUTION. The appearance of any of these warning signs, although not a sure indication of cancer, should send you to your physician. The Canadian Cancer Society recommends routine tests to screen for common cancers (see Table 12.2).

Coping with Cancer

If you suffer from cancer or know someone who does, see For Further Exploration at the end of the chapter for tips on how to receive or provide support.

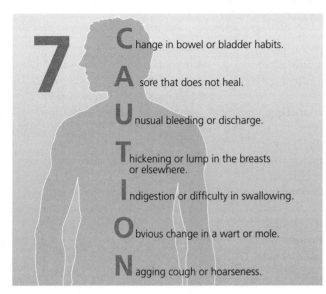

7

Change in bowel or bladder habits.

A sore that does not heal.

Unusual bleeding or discharge.

Thickening or lump in the breasts or elsewhere.

Indigestion or difficulty in swallowing.

Obvious change in a wart or mole.

Nagging cough or hoarseness.

FIGURE 12.5 The seven major warning signs of cancer.

A growing body of research also suggests that we can take an active role in preventing many cancers by adopting a wellness lifestyle.

RIGHT NOW YOU CAN

- If you are a woman, do a breast self-exam; if you are a man, do a testicular self-exam.
- Buy multiple bottles of sunscreens and put them in places where you will most likely see them, such as your backpack, gym bag, or car.
- Check the cancer screening guidelines below, and make sure you are up to date on your screenings.

IN THE FUTURE YOU CAN

- Learn where to find information about daily UV radiation levels in your area, and learn how to interpret the information. Many local newspapers and television stations (and their websites) report current UV levels every day.
- Gradually add foods with abundant phytochemicals to your diet, choosing from the list shown in Table 12.1.

TABLE 12.2 Screening Guidelines for the Early Detection of Cancer in Asymptomatic People

Site	Recommendation
Breast	Clinical breast exams are recommended for all women over the age of 40 every year. Beyond the age of 50, women should also have a mammogram every 2 years and those over 70 should discuss an individualized screening program with their physician. Women at increased risk (e.g., family history, genetic tendency, past breast cancer) should talk with their physicians about the benefits and limitations of starting mammography screening earlier, having additional tests (i.e., breast ultrasound or MRI), or having more frequent exams.
Colorectal	Beginning at age 50, men and women should have a fecal occult blood test (FOBT) every 2 years. Follow-up for a positive test could include a colonoscopy, double contrast barium enema (an X ray of the large intestine) and sigmoidoscopy.
Prostate	Beginning at age 50, men should consult with their physicians about the potential benefits and risks of using the Prostate Specific Antigen (PSA) and digital rectal examinations (DRE) for the early detection of prostate cancer.
Testicular	All men, from age 15 onward, should perform a testicular self-examination each month.
Cervical	Sexually active women over the age of 21 should have a Pap test and pelvic examination every 1 to 3 years, depending upon the screening guidelines in your province. Women who are not sexually active should still continue to have a Pap test. Women who have had a hysterectomy should discuss the need for a Pap test with their physician.
Skin	Check your skin regularly and ensure that you or someone else checks those "hard to see" places such as your back, back of your neck, ears, and back of your legs. **What should you watch for?** • Changes in a birthmark or mole such as shape, colour, size, or surface. • New growths on your skin—pale, pearly nodules that may grow larger and crust, or red, scaly, sharply defined patches. • Sores that do not heal. • Patches of skin that bleed, ooze, swell, itch, or become red and bumpy.

SOURCE: Canadian Cancer Society. 2011 (http://www.cancer.ca).

What is a biopsy?

A biopsy is the removal and examination of a small piece of body tissue. Biopsies enable cancer specialists to carefully examine cells that are suspected of having turned cancerous. Some biopsies are fairly simple to perform, such as those on tissue from moles or skin sores. Other biopsies may require the use of a needle or probe to remove tissue from inside the body, such as in the breast or stomach.

How is cancer treated?

The ideal cancer therapy would kill or remove all cancer cells while leaving normal tissue untouched. Sometimes this is almost possible, as when a surgeon removes a small superficial tumour of the skin. Usually a tumour is less accessible, and some combination of treatments is necessary. Current treatments for cancer are based primarily on the following:

- *Surgery.* Sometimes the organ containing the tumour is not essential for life and can be partially or completely removed. Surgery is less effective when cancer involves widely distributed cells (such as in the case of leukemia) or when the cancer has already metastasized.
- *Chemotherapy.* Cancer cells can be killed by administering drugs that interfere chemically with their growth. Although chemotherapy is targeted at rapidly dividing cancer cells, it can also affect cells in normal tissue, leading to unpleasant side effects.
- *Radiation.* In radiation therapy, a beam of X rays or gamma rays is directed at the tumour, killing the cancer cells. Radiation destroys both normal and cancerous cells but can usually be precisely directed at the tumour.

Some experimental techniques that also show promise for some particular types of cancer include the following:

- *Bone marrow transplants.* Healthy bone marrow cells from a compatible donor are transplanted following the elimination of the patient's bone marrow by radiation or chemotherapy. Transplants of stem cells may provide a solution to the problem of donor incompatibility. These unique, unspecialized cells can divide and produce many specialized cell types, including bone marrow cells. Stem cells can be grown outside the body and then transplanted back into the cancer patient, allowing for safe repopulation of bone marrow.
- *Vaccines and genetically modified immune cells.* These enhance the reaction of a patient's own immune system.
- *Anti-angiogenesis agents.* These starve tumours by blocking their blood supply.
- *Proteasome inhibitors.* Proteasomes help control the cell cycle—the process through which cells divide. If proteasomes malfunction, as is often the case in cancer cells, then cells may begin multiplying out of control. Proteasome inhibitors block the action of proteasomes, halting cell division and killing the cells. One proteasome inhibitor is now being used against certain cancers, and other such drugs are in development.
- *Enzyme activators/blockers.* Normal cells die after dividing a given number of times. Scientists believe that the enzyme caspase triggers the death of normally functioning cells. In cancer cells, caspase activity may be blocked. Conversely, if the enzyme telomerase becomes active in cancer cells, the life/death cycle stops and the cells duplicate indefinitely. In effect, inactive caspase or active telomerase may make cancer cells "immortal." Researchers are studying compounds that can either activate caspase or deactivate telomerase; either type of drug might lead cancer cells to self-destruct. No such drugs are now in clinical use.

In the future, gene sequencing techniques may allow treatments to be targeted at specific cancer subtypes, much as specific antibiotics are now used to treat specific bacterial diseases.

SUMMARY

- Cancer is an abnormal and uncontrollable growth of cells or tissue; cancer cells can metastasize.
- Lung cancer kills more people than any other type of cancer; tobacco smoke is the primary cause.
- Colon and rectal cancer is linked to age, heredity, and a diet low in fruits and vegetables.
- Breast cancer has a genetic component, but lifestyle and hormones are also factors. Prostate cancer is chiefly a disease of aging; diet, heredity, and ethnicity are other risk factors.
- Cancers of the female reproductive tract include cervical, uterine, and ovarian cancer. Cervical cancer is linked to HPV infection; the Pap test is an effective screening test.
- Melanoma is the most serious form of skin cancer; excessive exposure to UV radiation in sunlight is the primary cause.
- Oral cancer is caused primarily by smoking, excess alcohol consumption, and use of spit tobacco.
- Testicular cancer can be detected early through self-examination.

- The genetic basis of some cancers appears to be mutational damage to suppressor genes, which normally limit cell division.

- Cancer-promoting dietary factors include meat, certain types of fat, and alcohol. Dietary elements that may protect against cancer include antioxidants and phytochemicals. An inactive lifestyle is associated with some cancers.

- Some carcinogens occur naturally in the environment; others are manufactured substances. Occupational exposure is a risk for some workers.

- All sources of radiation are potentially carcinogenic, including X rays, UV rays of the sun, and radon gas.

- Strategies for preventing cancer include avoiding tobacco; eating a varied, moderate diet and controlling weight; exercising regularly; protecting skin from the sun; avoiding exposure to environmental and occupational carcinogens; staying alert for cancer warning signs; and getting recommended cancer-screening tests.

FOR FURTHER EXPLORATION

Organizations and Websites

Canadian Breast Cancer Foundation. Provides information and resources on and in support of breast cancer research.
   http://www.cbcf.org

Canadian Cancer Society. Provides a wide range of free materials on the prevention and treatment of cancer.
   http://www.cancer.ca

Canadian Cancer Society Research Institute. Provides information on treatment options, screening, clinical trials, and newly approved drugs.
   http://ncic.cancer.ca

EPA/Sunwise. Provides information about the UV Index and the effects of sun exposure, with links to sites with daily UV Index ratings for U.S. and international cities.
   http://www.epa.gov/sunwise/uvindex.html

Harvard Centre for Cancer Prevention: Your Cancer Risk. Includes interactive risk assessments as well as tips for preventing common cancers.
   http://www.diseaseriskindex.harvard.edu/update/

MedlinePlus: Cancers. Provides links to reliable cancer information.
   http://www.nlm.nih.gov/medlineplus/cancers.html

Skin Cancer Foundation. Provides information relating to skin cancer.
   http://www.skincancer.org

Terry Fox Foundation. Advocates for research support and development.
   http://www.terryfoxrun.org

LAB 12.1 Cancer Prevention

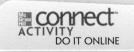

This lab looks at two areas of cancer prevention over which you have a great deal of individual control—diet and sun exposure. For a detailed personal risk profile for many specific types of cancer, complete the assessments at the Washington University School of Medicine's "Your Disease Risk" site (http://www.yourdiseaserisk.wustl.edu).

Part I Eating Cancer Fighting Foods

Track your diet for 3 days, recording the number of servings from each of the following groups that you consume.

Day 1	Day 2	Day 3	*Potential Cancer Fighters*
_____	_____	_____	Orange, deep yellow, pink, and red vegetables and some fruits (for example, apricots, cantaloupe, carrots, corn, grapefruit, mangoes, nectarines, papayas, red and yellow bell peppers, sweet potatoes, pumpkin, tomatoes and tomato sauce, watermelon, winter squash such as acorn or butternut)
_____	_____	_____	Dark-green leafy vegetables (for example, broccoli rabe, chard, kale, romaine and other dark lettuces, spinach; beet, collard, dandelion, mustard, and turnip greens)
_____	_____	_____	Cruciferous vegetables (for example, bok choy, broccoli, brussels sprouts, cabbage, cauliflower, kohlrabi, turnips)
_____	_____	_____	Citrus fruits (for example, grapefruit, lemons, limes, oranges, tangerines)
_____	_____	_____	Whole grains (for example, whole-grain bread, cereal, and pasta; brown rice; oatmeal; whole-grain corn; barley; popcorn; bulgur)
_____	_____	_____	Legumes (for example, peas, lentils, and beans, including fava, navy, kidney, pinto, black, and lima beans)
_____	_____	_____	Berries (for example, strawberries, raspberries, blackberries, blueberries)
_____	_____	_____	Garlic and other allium vegetables (for example, onions, leeks, chives, scallions, shallots)
_____	_____	_____	Soy products (for example, tofu, tempeh, soy milk, miso, soybeans)
_____	_____	_____	Other cancer-fighting fruits (for example, apples, cherries, cranberries or juice, grapes, kiwifruit, pears, plums, prunes, raisins)
_____	_____	_____	Other cancer-fighting vegetables (for example, asparagus, beets, chili peppers, eggplant, green peppers, radishes)
_____	_____	_____	**Daily Totals (Average for three days: _____)**

The goal is to eat at least 7 (for women) or 8 (for men) servings of cancer-fighting fruits and vegetables each day; the more servings, the better.

Note: Research is ongoing, and this list of cancer fighters is not comprehensive. Remember, nearly all fruits, vegetables, and grains are healthy, disease-fighting dietary choices.

Part II Skin Cancer Risk Assessment

Your risk of skin cancer from the ultraviolet radiation in sunlight depends on several factors. Take the quiz that follows to see how sensitive you are. The higher your UV-risk score, the greater your risk of skin cancer—and the greater your need to take precautions against too much sun. Score 1 point for each true statement:

_____ 1. I have blond or red hair.

_____ 2. I have light-coloured eyes (blue, gray, green).

_____ 3. I freckle easily.

_____ 4. I have many moles.

_____ 5. I had two or more blistering sunburns as a child.

_____ 6. I spent lots of time in a tropical climate as a child.

_____ 7. I have a family history of skin cancer.

_____ 8. I work outdoors.

_____ 9. I spend a lot of time in outdoor activities.

_____ 10. I like to spend as much time in the sun as I can.

_____ 11. I sometimes go to a tanning parlour or use a sunlamp.

_____ **Total Score**

Score	Risk of skin cancer from UV radiation
0	Low
1–3	Moderate
4–7	High
8–11	Very high

Using Your Results

How did you score?

(1) How close did you come to the goal of eating 7–9 or more servings of cancer fighters each day? Are you at all surprised by your results?

Are you satisfied with your diet in terms of cancer prevention? If not, set a specific goal for a target number of servings of cancer-fighting fruits and vegetables: _____

(2) What is your skin cancer risk assessment score? Are you at all surprised by the result? Does it indicate that you are at high or very high risk? Do you feel you need to take action because of your risk level?

What should you do next? Enter the results of this lab in the Preprogram Assessment column in Appendix C.

(1) If you've set a goal for the diet and cancer portion of the lab, select a target number of additional cancer fighters from the list to try over the next few days; list the foods below, along with your plan for incorporating them into your diet (as a side dish, as a snack, on a salad, as a substitute for another food, etc.).

Cancer fighter to try:

_____

_____

_____

_____

Plan for trying:

_____

_____

_____

_____

(2) You cannot control all of your risk factors for skin cancer, but you can control your behaviour with regard to sun exposure. Keep a journal to track your behaviour on days when you are outdoors in the sun for a significant period of time. Compare your behaviour with the recommendations for skin cancer prevention described in the chapter. Record such information as time of day, total duration of exposure, UV index for the day, clothing worn, type and amount of sunscreen used, frequency of sunscreen applications, and so on. From this record, identify ways to improve your behaviour to lower your risk of skin cancer. Put together a behaviour change plan.

Next, begin to put your strategies into action. After several weeks of a program to improve your diet or reduce your UV exposure, do this lab again and enter the results in the Postprogram Assessment column of Appendix C. How do the results compare?

SOURCE: Part II: Skin Cancer Risk Assessment adapted from Shear, N. 1996. "What's Your UV-risk Score?" Copyright © 1996 by the Consumers Union of the United States, Inc., Yonkers, NY 10703-1057, a nonprofit organization. Reprinted with permission from the author.

CHAPTER 13

WELLNESS FOR LIFE

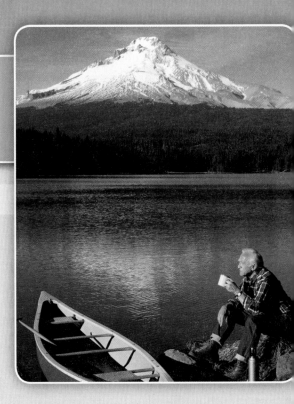

LEARNING OBJECTIVES

After reading this chapter, you should be able to

LO1 List the characteristics, skills, and behaviours that support successful relationships and families

LO2 Explain what individuals can do to promote healthy aging

LO3 Discuss strategies for effective self-care and effective use of the health care system

LO4 Describe the role that the environment plays in personal wellness and the steps individuals can take to preserve and restore the environment

TEST YOUR KNOWLEDGE

1. **Married people tend to be healthier and to live longer than unmarried people.**

   True or false?

2. **Most of the energy used by a standard incandescent light bulb is converted into light.**

   True or false?

3. **The world's population is increasing at an annual rate of**

   a. 0.76 million
   b. 7.6 million
   c. 76 million

ANSWERS

1. **TRUE.** One explanation is that marriage encourages healthy behaviours. Surveys have found that married people are more likely to wear safety belts, be physically active, and not smoke.

2. **FALSE.** About 90% of the energy used by a standard bulb is wasted because it is given off as heat, not light. If each Canadian replaced one incandescent bulb with a compact fluorescent, the yearly energy savings would equal the total production of four nuclear power plants. Fluorescent lights are, however, said to contain higher levels of mercury which can pose problems for landfills when these bulbs are thrown away.

3. **C.** The world's population currently stands at about 6.6 billion and is growing at a rate of about 76 million people per year—about 150 people per minute. The United Nations projects that the planet's population will reach 10 billion by the year 2200.

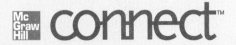

Practise and learn online with Connect.

The goal of this book has been to introduce the concept of wellness and to provide the knowledge and skills you need to live a fit and well lifestyle. Knowing the facts about the effects of your actions on your health enables you to make informed choices. Using behavioural self-management enables you to make important lifestyle changes. This chapter briefly addresses some other skills that are important for a lifetime of wellness: developing and maintaining meaningful interpersonal relationships, meeting the challenges of aging, using the health care system intelligently, and understanding environmental health.

LO1 13.1 DEVELOPING SUCCESSFUL INTERPERSONAL RELATIONSHIPS

Human beings need social relationships; we cannot thrive as solitary creatures (see the box "Intimate Relationships Are Good for Your Health"). Nor could the human species survive if adults didn't cherish and support each other, if we didn't form strong mutual attachments with our infants, and if we didn't create families in which to raise children. Simply put, people need people.

Although people are held together in relationships by a variety of factors, the foundation of many relationships is that ability to give and love. Love in its many forms—romantic, passionate, platonic, parental—is the wellspring from which much of life's meaning and delight flows. In our culture, it binds us together as partners, parents, children, and friends. Just as important, we also need to develop a healthy relationship to ourselves, which includes the ability to self-sooth, to regulate our emotions, and to be alone with ourselves at times.

Forming Relationships

Intimate relationships satisfy many human needs, including the need for approval and affirmation, for companionship, for a sense of belonging, and for sexual expression. Many of society's needs are also fulfilled by relationships, particularly the need to nurture and socialize children within that society.

SELF-CONCEPT AND SELF-ESTEEM To have successful relationships, we must first accept and feel good about ourselves. A positive self-concept and a healthy level of self-esteem are rooted in childhood, in the relationships we had with our parents and other family members. As adults, we probably have a sense that we're basically lovable, worthwhile people if, as children, we felt loved, valued, and respected. Our ways of relating to each other—that is, our adult styles of loving—may also be rooted in childhood. People who are secure in

their intimate relationships probably had a secure, trusting attachment to their mother, father, or other parenting figure.

Even if people's earliest experiences and relationships were less than ideal, they can still establish satisfying relationships in adulthood. That's because humans are resilient and flexible; they have the capacity to change their ideas, beliefs, and behaviour patterns. They can learn how to improve their self-esteem, communicate better, and resolve interpersonal conflicts. Although it helps to have a good start in life, it may be even more important to begin again, right from where you are.

FRIENDSHIP The first relationships we form outside the family are friendships. With members of either the same or the other sex, friendships give people the opportunity to share themselves and discover others. Friendships usually include these characteristics:

- *Companionship.* Friends are relaxed and happy in each other's company. They have common values and interests and spend time together.
- *Respect.* Good friends respect each other's feelings and opinions and work to resolve their differences without demeaning or insulting each other. They also show their respect by being honest with one another.
- *Acceptance.* Friends feel free to be themselves and express their feelings spontaneously without fear of ridicule or criticism.
- *Help.* Sharing time, energy, and even material goods is important to friendship. Friends know they can rely on each other in times of need.
- *Trust.* Friends are secure in the knowledge that they will not intentionally hurt each other.
- *Loyalty.* Friends can count on each other. They stand up for each other in both word and deed.
- *Mutuality.* Friends retain their individual identities, but they share the ups and downs in each other's lives—"what affects you affects me."
- *Reciprocity.* There is give and take between friends, along with the feeling that both share joys and burdens more or less equally over time.

Friendships are often more stable and longer lasting than intimate partnerships. Friends are often more accepting and less critical than lovers, probably because their expectations are different. Like love relationships, friendships bind society together, providing people with emotional support and buffering them from stress.

LOVE AND INTIMACY Intimate love relationships are among the most profound human experiences. They may not give people perfect happiness, but they do tend to give life much of its meaning. For most adults, love, sex, and commitment are closely linked ideals in intimate relationships. Love reflects the positive

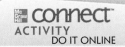
TAKE CHARGE

Intimate Relationships Are Good for Your Health

Research studies consistently underscore the importance of strengthening your family and social ties to help maintain emotional and physical wellness. Living alone, or simply feeling alone, can have a negative effect on both your state of mind and your physical health. Married people, on average, live longer than unmarried people—whether single, divorced, or widowed—and they score higher on measures of mental health. Findings suggest that there are intrinsic benefits to marriage.

People with strong social ties are less likely to become ill and tend to recover more quickly if they do. The benefits of intimate relationships have been demonstrated for a range of conditions: People with strong social support are less likely to catch colds. They recover better from heart attacks and live longer with heart disease. Of men with prostate cancer, those who are married live significantly longer than those who are single, divorced, or widowed.

What is it about social relationships that supports wellness? Friends and partners may encourage and reinforce healthy habits, such as exercising, eating right, and seeing a physician when needed. In times of illness, a loving partner can provide both practical help and emotional support. Feeling loved, esteemed, and valued brings comfort at a time of vulnerability, reduces anxiety, and mitigates the damaging effects of stress.

Although good relationships may help the sick get better, bad relationships may have the opposite effect. The impact of

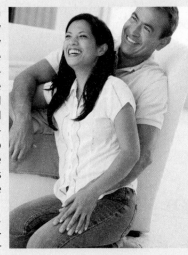

relationship quality on the course of illness may be partly explained by effects on the immune system: A study of married couples whose fighting went beyond normal conflict and into criticism and name-calling found them to have weaker immune responses than couples whose arguments were more civil.

Marriage, of course, isn't the only support system available. Whether married or single, if you have supportive people in your life, you are likely to enjoy better physical and emotional health than if you feel isolated and alone. So when you start planning lifestyle changes to improve your health and well-being, don't forget to nurture your relationships with family and friends. Relationships are powerful medicine.

---

factors that draw people together and sustain them in a relationship—trust, caring, respect, loyalty, interest in the other, and concern for the other's well-being. Sex brings excitement and passion to the relationship, adding fascination and pleasure. Commitment, the determination to continue, reflects the stable factors that help maintain the relationship—responsibility, reliability, and faithfulness. Although love, sex, and commitment are related, they are not necessarily connected. One can exist without the others. Despite the various permutations of the three, most people long for a special relationship that contains them all.

When two people fall in love, their relationship at first is likely to be characterized by high levels of passion and rapidly increasing intimacy. In time, passion decreases as the partners become familiar with each other. The diminishing of passionate love is often experienced as a crisis in a relationship. If a quieter, more lasting love fails to emerge, the relationship will likely break up, and each person will search for another who will once again ignite his or her passion.

But love does not necessarily have to be passionate. When intensity diminishes, partners often discover a more enduring love. They can now move from absorption in each other to a relationship that includes external goals and projects, friends, and family. In this kind of more secure love, satisfaction comes not just from the relationship but also from achieving other creative

objectives, such as work or child rearing. The key to successful relationships isn't in intensity but in transforming passion into an intimate love, based on closeness, caring, and the promise of a shared future.

CHOOSING A PARTNER   Although the pool of potential partners for a relationship may appear huge, most people pair with someone who lives in the same geographic area and who is similar in ethnic and socioeconomic background, educational level, lifestyle, physical appearance, and other traits. In simple terms, people often select partners like themselves.

Although differences add interest to a relationship, similarities increase the chances of a relationship's success. Perhaps the most important question two people can ask is, "How much do we have in common?" If there are major differences, partners should ask, first, "How accepting of differences are we?" and, second, "How well do we communicate?" Acceptance and communication skills go a long way toward making a relationship work, no matter how different the partners.

Because the Internet is a good tool for locating others who share hobbies and interests, people are increasingly looking to cyberspace to find friends and even intimate partners. Most North Americans, hoever, find romantic partners through some form of dating. They narrow the field through a process of getting to know each other. Dating often revolves around a mutually enjoyable activity, such as seeing a movie or having dinner. Casual dating might evolve into steady or exclusive dating, then engagement, and possibly marriage.

For many young people today, traditional dating has given way to a more casual form of getting together in groups. Greater equality between the sexes is at the root of this change. People go out in groups rather than strictly as couples, and each person pays their way. Two people may begin to spend more time together, but often in the group context. If sexual involvement develops, it is more likely to be based on friendship, respect, and common interests than on expectations related to gender roles. In this model, mate selection may progress from getting together to living together to marrying.

Communication

The key to developing and maintaining any type of intimate relationship is good communication. Most of the time, we don't actually think about communicating; we simply talk and behave naturally. But when problems arise—when we feel other people don't understand us or when someone accuses us of not listening—we become aware of our limitations or, more commonly, what we think are other people's limitations. Miscommunication creates frustration and distances us from our friends and partners.

As much as 65% of face-to-face communication is nonverbal. Even when we're silent, we're communicating. We send messages when we look at someone or look away, lean forward or sit back, smile or frown. Especially important forms of nonverbal communication are touch, eye contact, and proximity. If someone we're talking to touches our hand or arm, looks into our eyes, and leans toward us when we talk, we get the message that the person is interested in us and cares about what we're saying. If a person keeps looking around the room while we're talking or takes a step backward, we get the impression the person is uninterested or wants to end the conversation. It's important, when sending messages, to make sure our body language agrees with our words. When our verbal and nonverbal messages don't correspond, we send a mixed message.

COMMUNICATION SKILLS Three keys to good communication in relationships are self-disclosure, listening, and feedback.

- *Self-disclosure* involves revealing personal information that we ordinarily wouldn't reveal because of the risk involved. It usually increases feelings of closeness and moves the relationship to a deeper level of intimacy.
- *Listening* is a rare skill. Good listening skills require that we spend more time and energy trying to fully understand another person's "story" and less time judging, evaluating, blaming, advising, analyzing,

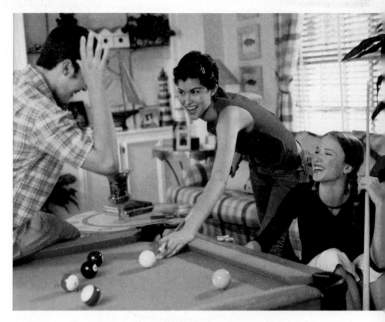

For many college/university students today, group activities have replaced dating as a way to meet and get to know potential partners.

or trying to control. Empathy, warmth, respect, and genuineness are qualities of skillful listeners. Attentive listening encourages friends or partners to share more and, in turn, to be attentive listeners. To connect with other people and develop real emotional intimacy, listening is essential.

- *Feedback*, a constructive response to another's self-disclosure, is the third key to good communication. Giving positive feedback means acknowledging that the friend's or partner's feelings are valid—no matter how upsetting or troubling—and offering self-disclosure in response. Self-disclosure and feedback can open the door to change, whereas other responses block communication and change.

For tips on improving your skills, see the box "Guidelines for Effective Communication."

CONFLICT AND CONFLICT RESOLUTION Conflict is natural in intimate relationships. No matter how close two people become, they still remain separate individuals with their own needs, desires, past experiences, and ways of seeing the world. Conflict itself isn't dangerous to a relationship; it may simply indicate that the relationship is growing. But if it isn't handled in a constructive way, it will damage—and ultimately destroy—the relationship.

Conflict is often accompanied by anger—a natural emotion, but one that can be difficult to handle. If we express anger, we run the risk of creating distrust, fear, and distance. If we act it out without thinking things through, we can cause the conflict to escalate. If we suppress it, it turns into resentment and hostility. The best

Guidelines for Effective Communication

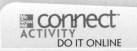

Getting Started

- When you want to have a serious discussion with your partner, choose an appropriate time and place. Find a time when you will not be interrupted and a private place.

- Face your partner and maintain eye contact. Use nonverbal feedback to show that you are interested and involved in the communication process.

Being an Effective Speaker

- State your concern or issue as clearly as you can.

- Use "I" statements—statements about how *you* feel—rather than statements beginning with "You," which tell another person how you think he or she feels. When you use "I" statements, you are taking responsibility for your feelings. "You" statements are often blaming or accusatory and will probably get a defensive or resentful response. The statement "I feel unloved," for example, sends a clearer, less blaming message than the statement "You don't love me."

- Focus on a specific behaviour rather than on the whole person. Be specific about the behaviour you like or don't like. Avoid generalizations beginning with "You always" or "You never." Such statements make people feel defensive.

- Make constructive requests. Opening your request with "I would like" keeps the focus on your needs rather than your partner's supposed deficiencies.

- Avoid blaming, accusing, and belittling. Even if you are right, you have little to gain by putting your partner down. Studies have shown that when people feel criticized or attacked, they are less able to think rationally or solve problems constructively.

- Ask for action ahead of time. Tell your partner what you would like to have happen in the future; don't wait for him or her to blow it and then express anger or disappointment.

Being an Effective Listener

- Provide appropriate nonverbal feedback (nodding, smiling, and so on).

- Don't interrupt.

- Develop the skill of reflective listening. Don't judge, evaluate, analyze, or offer solutions (unless asked to do so). Your partner may just need to have you there in order to sort out feelings. By jumping in right away to "fix" the problem, you may actually be cutting off communication.

- Don't give unsolicited advice. Giving advice implies that you know more about what a person needs to do than he or she does; therefore, it often evokes anger or resentment.

- Clarify your understanding of what your partner is saying by restating it in your own words and asking if your understanding is correct.

- Be sure you are really listening, not off somewhere in your mind rehearsing your reply. Try to tune in to your partner's feelings as well as the words.

- Let your partner know that you value what she or he is saying and want to understand. Respect for the other person is the cornerstone of effective communication.

---

way to handle anger in a relationship is to recognize it as a symptom of something that requires attention and needs to be changed. When angry, partners should back off until they calm down and then come back to the issue later and try to resolve it rationally. Negotiation will help dissipate the anger so the conflict can be resolved. (See Chapter 10 for additional strategies for managing anger.) Some basic strategies are useful in successfully negotiating with a partner:

1. *Clarify the issue.* Take responsibility for thinking through your feelings and discovering what's really bothering you. Agree that one partner will speak first and have the chance to speak fully while the other listens. Then reverse the roles. Try to understand the other partner's position fully by repeating what you've heard and asking questions to clarify or elicit more information.

2. *Find out what each person wants.* Ask your partner to express her or his desires. Don't assume you know what your partner wants and speak for her or him. Clarify and summarize.

3. *Identify alternatives for getting each person what he or she wants.* Practise brainstorming to generate a variety of options.

4. *Decide how to negotiate.* Work out some agreements or plans for change: For example, agree that each partner will do one task; or that one partner will do a task in exchange for something she or he wants.

5. *Solidify the agreements.* Go over the plan verbally and write it down, if necessary, to ensure that you both understand and agree to it.

6. *Review and renegotiate.* Decide on a time frame for trying out the new plan and set a time to discuss how it's working. Make adjustments as needed.

Marriage

The primary functions and benefits of marriage are those of any intimate adult relationship, including affection, personal affirmation, companionship, sexual fulfillment, and emotional growth. Marriage may also provide a structural framework in which to raise children, and it affords some provision for the future. By committing themselves to their relationship by getting married, people also establish themselves with lifelong companions as well as some insurance for their later years.

Although we might like to believe otherwise, love is not enough to make a successful marriage. Couples have to be strong and successful in their relationship before marriage. The following relationship characteristics appear to be the best predictors of a happy marriage:

- The partners have realistic expectations about their relationship.
- Each feels good about the personality of the other.
- They communicate well.
- They have effective ways of resolving conflicts.
- They agree on religious/ethical values.
- They have an egalitarian role relationship.
- They have a good balance of individual versus joint interests and leisure activities.

Coping with the challenges of marriage requires that couples be committed to remaining married through the inevitable ups and downs of the relationship. They need to be tolerant of each other's imperfections, keep their sense of perspective and their sense of humour, and be willing and able to put energy into providing and sustaining mutually sufficient levels of intimacy, sexual satisfaction, and commitment.

Successful Families

Family relationships are another important part of a healthy life. Researchers have proposed that six major qualities or themes appear in strong families.

1. *Commitment.* The family is very important to its members; sexual fidelity between partners is included in commitment.

2. *Appreciation.* People care about one another and express that caring. The home is a positive place to be.

3. *Communication.* People spend time listening to one another and enjoying one another's company. They talk about disagreements and attempt to solve problems.

4. *Time together.* People do things together, often simple activities that don't cost money.

5. *Spiritual wellness.* The family promotes sharing, love, and compassion for other human beings.

6. *Coping with stress and crisis.* When faced with illness, death, marital conflict, or other crises, family members pull together, seek help, and use other coping strategies to meet the challenge.

Partners in committed relationships and members of strong families often go to counselling centres. They know that the smartest thing to do in some situations is to get help. Many counselling resources are available, including marriage and family counsellors, clergy, psychologists, and other trained professionals.

WELLNESS TIP

Remember that modest changes in lifestyle maintained over the long term are more beneficial than dramatic changes that last only a few weeks. Long-term maintenance of behaviour change is challenging.

LO2 13.2 MEETING THE CHALLENGES OF AGING

Aging is a normal process of development that occurs over the entire life span. Although youth is not entirely a state of mind, your attitude toward life and your attention to your health significantly influence the satisfaction you derive from life, especially when new physical and mental challenges occur in later years. If you take charge of your health during young adulthood, you can exert greater control over the physical and mental aspects of aging, and you can respond better to events that might be out of your control. With foresight and energy, you can shape a creative, graceful, and even triumphant old age.

What Happens as You Age?

Aging results from biochemical processes that aren't yet fully understood. Physiological changes are caused by a combination of gradual aging and injury from disease. Because most organ systems have an excess capacity for performing their functions, the body's ability to function is not affected until damage is fairly extensive. Studies of healthy people indicate that general functioning remains essentially constant until after age 70. Even so, a fair number of older Canadians describe themselves as being in poor health (Table 13.1)

Some of the physical changes that accompany aging are these:

- Skin becomes looser, drier, and less elastic.
- The ability to hear high-pitched and certain other sounds declines in most people.

TABLE 13.1	Canadian Self-Rated Health, 2005			
	Excellent	**Very good**	**Good**	**Fair or poor**
12–24 years	24	44	27	5
25–54 years	25	40	27	8
55+ years	15	30	32	22

SOURCE: Calculations by HRSDC based on Statistics Canada. Self-rated health, by age group and sex, household population aged 12 and over, Canada, provinces, territories, health regions (June 2005 boundaries) and peer groups, every 2 years (CANSIM Table 105-0422). Ottawa, Statistics Canada, 2006.

- *Presbyopia*, the inability of the eyes to focus sharply on nearby objects, occurs gradually in most people beginning in their forties. The eyes require more time to adapt to dark conditions, and depth perception may become distorted.
- The sensations of taste and smell diminish somewhat.
- Cells at the base of hair follicles produce progressively less pigment and eventually die. (Hair is thickest at age 20; individual hair shafts shrink after that.)
- Bone mass is lost and muscles become weaker, although both of these changes can be minimized significantly through regular exercise, a proper diet, and other measures.
- The heart pumps less blood with each beat, and maximum heart rate drops. Most of the other changes in the cardiovascular system that are associated with aging can be largely controlled through lifestyle.
- Sexual response slows, but an active and satisfying sex life can continue for both men and women throughout life.

The cumulative effects of these physical changes result in an increase in susceptibility to chronic health conditions such as those described in Chapters 11 and 12. In addition, the more we age, the more likely we are to suffer from more than just one chronic health condition.[1] (See Figure 13.1.)

Life-Enhancing Measures

Many of the characteristics associated with aging aren't due to aging at all. They are the result of neglect and abuse of our bodies and minds. These assaults lay the foundation for later mental problems and chronic conditions. You can prevent, delay, lessen, or even reverse some of the changes associated with aging through good health habits. A few simple things you can do every day will make a vast difference to your health, your appearance, and your energy and vitality.

- *Challenge your mind.* Creativity and intelligence remain stable in healthy individuals. Staying involved in learning as a lifelong process can help you stay sharp and retain all your mental abilities.
- *Plan for social changes.* Social roles change over time and require a period of adjustment. Retirement and an "empty nest" confer the advantage of increased leisure time, but many people do not know how to enjoy it. Throughout life, cultivate interests and hobbies you enjoy, both alone and with others, so that you can continue to live an active and rewarding life in your later years. Volunteering in your community can enhance self-esteem and allow you to be a contributing member of society (see the box "Help Yourself by Helping Others").
- *Develop physical fitness.* Exercise enhances both psychological and physical health. A 2006 study showed that elderly people who burned extra calories through daily activity had a much lower

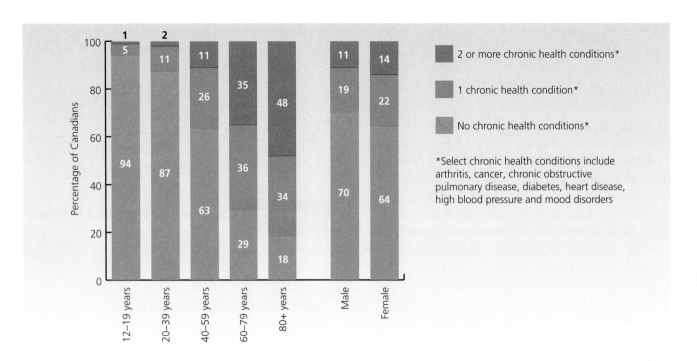

FIGURE 13.1   Chronic health conditions among youth and adults in Canada, 2005.

SOURCE: Broemeling, A. M., Weston, D. E., and Prebtani, F. (2008). Population patterns of chronic health conditions, co-morbidity and healthcare use in Canada. *Healthcare Quarterly,* 11(3): 70–76.

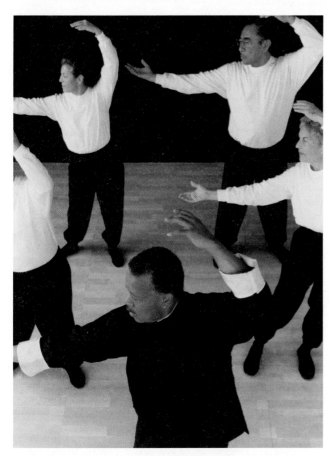

Managing stress is one of the challenges of aging. These people practise stress management and relaxation through taijiquan, an activity that also helps them maintain physical fitness.

mortality rate than their peers who did not exercise. Even in people over 80, endurance and strength training can improve balance, flexibility, and physical functioning and reduce the potential for dangerous falls (see the box "Can Exercise Delay the Effects of Aging?").

- *Eat wisely.* A varied diet with special attention to calorie intake and nutrient density improves health at every age. (See Chapter 7 for detailed information on nutrition.)
- *Maintain a healthy body composition.* Sensible eating habits and an active lifestyle can help you maintain a healthy body composition throughout your life.

Ask Yourself

QUESTIONS FOR CRITICAL THINKING AND REFLECTION

How do you envision your old age? Do you want it to resemble the old age of older adults you know now, or do you want it to be different? What specific attributes and abilities will make your old age happy and productive? What are you doing now to ensure that you will be able to reach your goals?

- *Control drinking and overdependence on medications.* Alcohol abuse ranks with depression as a common hidden mental health problem, affecting 10% of older adults. The problem is often not identified because the effects of alcohol or drug addiction can mimic disease, such as Alzheimer's disease. Don't use alcohol to relieve anxiety or emotional pain; don't take medications when safer forms of treatment are available.
- *Don't smoke.* The average pack-a-day smoker can expect to live about 12 years less than a nonsmoker and to be susceptible to disabilities that affect the quality of life. Premature balding, skin wrinkling, and osteoporosis are also associated with smoking.
- *Recognize and reduce stress.* Don't wear yourself out through lack of sleep, abuse of drugs, or overwork. Practise relaxation and stress management using the techniques described in Chapter 10.

Other strategies for successful aging include getting regular physical examinations to detect treatable diseases, protecting your skin and eyes from the sun, and avoiding extremely loud noises to protect your hearing.

LO3 13.3 USING THE HEALTH CARE SYSTEM INTELLIGENTLY

Just as people can prevent many illnesses through healthy lifestyle choices, they can also avoid many visits to the medical clinic by managing their own health care—by gathering information, soliciting advice, making their own decisions, and taking responsibility for following through. People who manage their own health care are informed partners in medical care; they also practise safe, effective self-care.

How can you develop this self-care attitude and take a more active role in your own health care? First, you have to learn to identify and manage medical problems. Second, you have to learn how to make the health care system work for you. This section will help you become more competent in both of these areas.

Managing Medical Problems

The first step in managing medical problems is observing your body and assessing your symptoms. Symptoms—pain, fever, coughing, diarrhea, and so on—are signals that something isn't working right. Many self-tests are available to help you evaluate medical problems at home: blood pressure monitoring equipment, blood sugar tests for those with diabetes, pregnancy tests, self-tests for urinary tract infections, and more than a dozen other do-it-yourself kits and devices. Careful self-observation and the selective use of self-tests can help provide you with the type of information you need to make informed self-care decisions and participate more actively in your care.

Can Exercise Delay the Effects of Aging?

As people age, they often experience declines in functional health—the ability to perform the tasks of everyday life—and related declines in the quality of life. According to the Human Resources and Skills Development Canada, about 22% of Canadians over age 55 report their health as only "fair" or "poor." Similarly, according to a U.S. Medicare survey, 31% of men and 42% of women age 65–74 reported some sort of mobility limitation in 2003 (meaning they had difficulty walking one-quarter mile or .4 kilometre).

Can physical activity and exercise combat the degenerative effects of aging in middle-aged and older adults? The evidence indicates that they can. In reviewing the research, the U.S. government's Physical Activity Guidelines Advisory Committee concluded that physical activity can prevent or delay the onset of limitations and declines in functional health in older adults, can maintain or improve functional health in those who already have limitations, and can reduce the incidence of falls and fall-related injuries.

One mechanism by which physical activity prevents declines in functional health is through maintenance or improvement of the physiological capacities of the body, such as aerobic power, muscular strength, and balance—in other words, through improvements in physical fitness. Declines in these physiological capacities occur with biological aging and are often compounded by disease-related disability. But evidence shows that older adults who participate in regular aerobic exercise are 30% less likely than inactive individuals to develop functional limitations (such as a limited ability to walk or climb stairs) or role limitations (such as a limited ability to be the family grocery shopper). Although studies found that both physical activity and aerobic fitness were associated with reduced risk of functional limitations, aerobic fitness was associated with a greater reduction of risk. Evidence also suggests that regular physical activity is safe and beneficial for older adults who already have functional limitations.

An example is a 2006 study called the Lifestyle Interventions and Independence for Elders Pilot trial, involving 424 men and women age 70–89 years. Participants were divided into a multimodal exercise group and a health education (control) group. Those in the exercise group participated in aerobic activity (primarily walking), strength training (focusing on the lower limbs), and flexibility exercises over the course of a year. The study found that, compared with the control group, the individuals in the exercise group significantly improved their physical performance and their walking speed. Also observed in the exercise group was an apparent trend toward reduced risk of major mobility disability. Another study, the 2005 Women's Health and Aging Study, found that older women who walked at least 8 blocks per week had better health and functioning after 1 year than did nonwalkers.

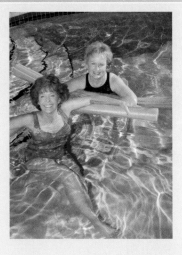

In addition, numerous studies have shown that regular exercise—particularly strength training, balance training, and flexibility exercises—can improve muscular strength, muscular endurance, and stability and provide some protection against falls. Falls are a leading cause of injury among people over age 65, affecting nearly 1.4 million older Canadians per year. In many cases, serious falls lead to long-term hospitalization or nursing home stays. Whether through direct injury or related complications, falls are a significant cause of death for older Canadians. Aerobic activity, especially walking, also helps reduce risk of falls, and some evidence indicates that tai chi exercise programs are beneficial as well. Regular exercise not only reduces the incidence of falls but also greatly enhances mobility, allowing older people to live more independently and with greater confidence.

Of course, physical activity throughout life helps prevent such chronic conditions as cardiovascular disease, stroke, diabetes, and arthritis, all of which cause disability in older adults. Research also shows that regular physical activity can reduce anxiety and depression in older adults. Exercise stimulates blood flow to the brain and can even increase brain mass, helping the brain to function more efficiently and improving memory. Some evidence indicates that exercise may stave off mental decline and the occurrence of age-related dementia.

Current physical activity recommendations for older adults from the Public Health Agency of Canada include moderate- to vigorous-intensity aerobic activity, strength training, and flexibility exercises, as well as balance exercises for older adults at risk for falls. Unfortunately, a large percent of Canadians age 65 and older (63% of women and 51% of men) do not get the recommended amounts of physical activity, and many get no exercise at all beyond the activities of daily living. Older adults are the least active group of Canadians. Although it is important to exercise throughout life, the evidence indicates that older adults who become more active even late in life can experience improvements in physical fitness and functional health. It is never too late to start enjoying the benefits of regular physical activity.

SOURCES: Human Resources and Skills Development Canada. 2012 (http://www4.hrsdc.gc.ca/.3ndic.1t.4r@-eng.jsp?iid=10, retrieved January 30, 2012); Pahor, M., et al. 2006. Effects of a physical activity intervention on measures of physical performance: Results of the Lifestyle Interventions and Independence for Elders Pilot (LIFE-P) study. *Journal of Gerontology Biological Sciences and Medical Sciences* 61(11): 1157–1165; Paterson, D. H., et al. 2007. Aging and physical activity: Evidence to develop exercise recommendations for older adults. *Canadian Journal of Public Health* 98 (Suppl. 2): S69–S108; Physical Activity Guidelines Advisory Committee. 2008. *Physical Activity Guidelines Advisory Committee Report,* 2008. Washington, D.C.: Physical Activity Monitors, 2008. Available at http://www.cflri.ca/node/82, retrieved January 30, 2012, U.S. Department of Health and Human Services; Simonsick, E. M., et al. 2005. Just get out the door! Importance of walking outside the home for maintaining mobility: Findings from the Women's Health and Aging Study. *Journal of the American Geriatrics Society* 53(2): 198–203; and U.S. Department of Health and Human Services, Centers for Medicare & Medicaid Services. 2006. *Medicare Current Beneficiary Survey* (http://www.cms.hhs.gov/MCBS, retrieved January 30, 2012).

Volunteering can enhance emotional, social, spiritual, and physical wellness. Surveys and studies indicate that the sense of purpose, service, and the feelings of generosity and kindness that go with helping others may be as important a consideration for wellness as good nutrition and regular exercise. A 2006 study followed sedentary older people who joined a volunteer group called Experience Corps. The subjects' volunteer activities resulted in many of the same benefits as regular exercise, such as increased energy and vitality. Older adults who volunteer have higher levels of emotional and social wellness and lower rates of death.[2] In a national survey of volunteers from all fields, helpers reported the following benefits:

- "Helper's high"—physical and emotional sensations such as sudden warmth, a surge of energy, and a feeling of euphoria that occur immediately after helping.

- Feelings of increased self-worth, calm, and relaxation.

- A perception of greater physical health.

- Fewer colds and headaches, improved eating and sleeping habits, and some relief from the pain of chronic diseases such as asthma and arthritis.

In helping others, we focus on things other than our own problems, and we get a special kind of attention from the people we help. Helping others can also expand our perspective and enhance our appreciation for our own lives. Helping improves mood, banishes the blues, and may benefit physical health by providing a temporary boost to the immune system and by combatting stress and hostile feelings linked to the development of chronic disease.

No matter what your age, to get the most out of helping, keep the following guidelines in mind:

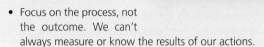

- Remember that helping others doesn't require a huge time commitment or a change of career.

- Choose an activity that involves personal contact. Work with a group to form bonds with other helpers who support your interests and efforts.

- Focus on the process, not the outcome. We can't always measure or know the results of our actions.

- Practise random acts of kindness. Smile, let people go ahead of you in line, pick up litter, and so on.

- Adopt a pet. Several studies suggest that pet owners enjoy better health, perhaps by feeling needed or by having a source of unconditional love.

- Avoid burnout. Recognize your own limits, pace yourself, and try not to feel guilty or discouraged.

In addition to benefiting you, volunteering has the added bonus of increasing the well-being of others. It fosters a sense of community and can provide some practical help for many of the problems facing our society today.

SOURCES: Musick, M. A., A. R. Herzog, and J. S. House. 1999. Volunteering and mortality among older adults. *Journal of Gerontology: Social Sciences* 54B(3): 5173; and Sobel, D. S., and R. Ornstein. 1996. *The Healthy Mind, Healthy Body Handbook*. Los Altos, Calif.: DRx Publishers.

KNOWING WHEN TO SEE A PHYSICIAN In most cases, and with sufficient time and rest, the body heals itself. The decision to seek professional assistance for a symptom is generally guided by the nature of the symptom and by your own history of medical problems. If you're unsure about a symptom, call your physician.

Seek professional assistance for any symptom that is severe, unusual, persistent, or recurrent. Medical emergencies requiring a trip to the nearest hospital emergency room include broken bones, severe burns, deep wounds, uncontrollable bleeding, chest pain, loss of consciousness, poisoning or drug overdose, and difficulty breathing.

SELF-TREATMENT In most cases, your body can itself relieve your symptoms and heal a disorder. The prescriptions filled by your body's internal pharmacy are frequently the safest and most effective treatment. Patience and careful self-observation (watchful waiting) are often the best choices in self-treatment.

Nondrug options are often highly effective. For example, massage, ice packs, and neck exercises may be at times more helpful than drugs in relieving headaches and other pains. Adequate rest is just one of the many nondrug options for preventing or relieving many common health problems. For a variety of disorders either caused or aggravated by stress, the treatment of choice may be relaxation, visualization, humour, changing negative thoughts, and other stress-management strategies (see Chapter 10). Before reaching for medications, consider all of your nondrug options.

Nonprescription, or **over-the-counter (OTC) medications** play an important part in our health care system.

over-the-counter (OTC) medication A medication or medical product that a consumer can purchase without a prescription.

TERMS

Many OTC drugs are highly effective in relieving symptoms and sometimes curing illnesses. Common OTC drugs include antihistamines, expectorants, cough suppressants, pain relievers, and other products.

Any drug can have side effects. These simple guidelines will help you use medicines safely and effectively:

- Always read drug labels and follow directions.
- Do not exceed the recommended dosage or length of treatment unless your physician approves.
- Because OTC drugs, prescription drugs, and herbal remedies can interact, let your physician or pharmacist know before taking more than one type of drug or health remedy at the same time.
- Select medications with one active ingredient rather than combination products. Using single-ingredient products allows you to adjust the dosage of each medication separately for optimal symptom relief; you'll also avoid potential side effects from drugs you don't really need.
- Never take or give a drug from an unlabelled container or in the dark when you can't read the label.
- If you are pregnant, are nursing, or have a chronic medical condition, consult your physician before self-medicating.
- Store medications in a safe place out of the reach of children; avoid locations where dampness or heat might ruin them. Dispose of all expired medications.
- Use special caution with aspirin. Because of an association with a rare but serious problem known as Reye's syndrome, aspirin should not be used for children or adolescents who may have the flu, chicken pox, or any other viral illness.

Getting the Most Out of Medical Care

Although many health problems can be self-treated, many others require treatment by trained professionals. The key to using the health care system effectively is good communication with your physician and other members of the health care team.

THE CANADIAN HEALTH CARE SYSTEM Canada has a government-funded, national health care system based on principles from the Canada Health Act that reinforce a health care system that is:

- universally available to permanent residents
- comprehensive in the services it covers
- accessible without income barriers
- portable within and outside the country
- publicly administered

Each province and territory is responsible for administering its own health care plan and for providing medically necessary services such as prescription drugs, dental care, optometric services, to name a few. In an effort to provide efficient services, some provinces/territories have chosen to introduce their own supplemental plans (i.e., drug plan) while others have chosen to partner with private insurers such as Blue Cross.

The cost of health care in Canada is supplemented by federal and provincial/territorial taxes that all residents are required to pay. In addition, some provinces/territories, like Ontario, collect a health care premium from each of its residents. Recently, some provinces/territories have introduced P3s, or "private-public-partnerships," which represent a way for private companies to use public funds in serving patients who may be willing to pay for services. P3s have proven to be controversial in nature and it remains to be seen whether a "tiered" system of health care will be created by these initiatives.

COMMUNICATING WITH YOUR PHYSICIAN When interacting with health care providers, you should be assertive in a firm but not aggressive manner. Feel free to ask questions, express your concerns, and be persistent. Strategies for good communication include the following:

- *Before the visit.* Make a written list of your questions and concerns; include notes about your symptoms. Bring a list of all medications (prescription and non-prescription) you are taking, or bring them with you to the office.
- *During the visit.* Present your major concerns at the beginning of the visit. Be specific and concise. Try to be as open and honest as you can in sharing your thoughts, feelings, and fears. It is particularly important to be truthful about your concerns so as to receive the best possible advice from your physician. If you're not sure about something your physician has said, ask to go over it again. If appropriate, ask your physician to write down her or his instructions or to recommend reading material.
- *At the end of the visit.* In your own words, briefly state what you understood the physician to say about your problem and what you're supposed to do. Make sure you understand what the next steps are.

OBTAINING APPROPRIATE SCREENING TESTS Another important part of preventive health care is regular screening for various conditions and diseases. Be sure to follow the cholesterol and blood pressure testing recommendations provided in Chapter 11, the cancer screening guidelines given in Chapter 12, and the sexually transmitted infection (STI) screening and testing recommendations given in online Chapter 15. If you have symptoms, or if you are at risk for a particular disease, see your physician to discuss your needs.

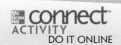

Avoiding Health Care Fraud and Quackery

Consumers waste billions of dollars on unproven, fraudulently marketed, and sometimes useless or even harmful health care products and treatments. In addition, those with serious medical problems may waste valuable time before seeking proper treatment. Health care fraud is a business that sells false hope. It preys on people who are victims of diseases that have no medical cure and on people who want shortcuts to weight loss or improvements to personal appearance.

The first rule of thumb for evaluating any health claim is that if it sounds too good to be true, it probably is. Also, be on the lookout for the typical phrases and marketing techniques fraudulent promoters use to deceive consumers:

- The product is advertised as a quick and effective cure-all for a wide range of ailments.

- The promoters use words like *scientific breakthrough, miraculous cure, secret ingredient,* or *ancient remedy.* Also remember that just because a product is described as "natural" or unprocessed does not necessarily mean it's safe.

- The promoter claims the government or the medical profession has conspired to suppress the product.

- The advertisement includes undocumented case histories claiming amazing results.

- The product is advertised as available from only one source, and payment is required in advance.

- The promoter promises a no-risk "money-back guarantee." Be aware that many fly-by-night operators are not around to respond to your request for a refund.

To check out a particular product, talk to a physician or another health care professional and to family members and friends. Be wary of treatments offered by people who tell you to avoid talking to others. Check with the Better Business Bureau to see whether other consumers have lodged complaints about the product or the product's marketer. You can also check with the appropriate health professional group. For example, check with the Canadian Diabetes Association or the National Arthritis Foundation if the products are promoted for diabetes or arthritis. Take special care with products and devices sold online; the broad reach of the Internet, combined with the ease of setting up and removing websites, makes online sellers particularly difficult to regulate.

SOURCES: Federal Trade Commission. 2001. "Miracle" Health Claims: Add a Dose of Skepticism (http://www.ftc.gov/bcp/conline/pubs/health/frdheal.htm, retrieved December 14, 2002); and Kurtzweil, P. 1999. How to spot health fraud. *FDA Consumer*, November/December.

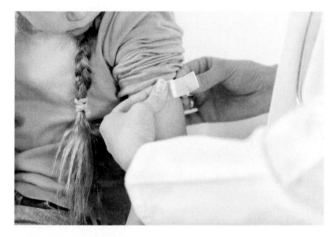

Your health care provider is the best source of reliable information about any prescription or OTC medication you may need to take.

USING COMPLEMENTARY AND ALTERNATIVE MEDICINE

Complementary and alternative medicine (CAM) is defined as those therapies or practices that do not form part of conventional, or mainstream, health care and medical practice as taught in most medical schools and offered in most hospitals. The inclusion of the term *complementary* indicates that most people use such approaches in addition to conventional medical treatments rather than in their place. Consumer surveys

show that more and more people are using various forms of CAM. In Canada, the Fraser Institute reports that 73% of Canadians claim to have used at least one CAM in their lives. The most common forms reportedly used by Canadians were chiropractic (36%), relaxation techniques and massage (23% each), and prayer (21%). Despite their growing popularity, many CAM practices remain controversial, and you need to be critically aware of safety issues (see the box "Avoiding Health Care Fraud and Quackery" above).

Because there is less information available about CAM therapies, as well as less regulation of associated products and providers, it is important for consumers to take an active role. The National Centre for Complementary and Alternative Medicine (NCCAM), which is a part of the National Institutes of Health, advises consumers not to seek CAM therapies without first visiting a conventional health care provider for an evaluation and diagnosis of their symptoms. It's usually best to try conventional treatments that have been shown to be beneficial for your condition. If you are thinking of trying any alternative therapies, it is critically important

complementary and alternative medicine (CAM) Therapies or practices that are not part of conventional or mainstream health care and medical practice as taught in most North American medical schools and available at most North American health care facilities.

TERMS

to talk with your physician or pharmacist to avoid any dangerous interactions. For example, some dietary supplements block or enhance the actions of prescription and over-the-counter drugs. Areas to discuss with your physician include the following:

- **Safety**: Is there anything unsafe about the treatment in general or for you specifically? Are there safety issues you should be aware of?
- **Effectiveness**: Is there any research about the use of the therapy for your condition?
- **Timing**: Is the immediate use of a conventional treatment indicated?
- **Cost**: Is the therapy likely to be very expensive, especially in light of the potential benefit?

You can also get information from individual CAM practitioners and from schools, professional organizations, and provincial licensing boards. Ask about education, training, licensing, and certification. When talking with a CAM practitioner, ask for a full description of the therapy and any potential side effects, how long the therapy should continue before it can be determined if it is beneficial, and how much it will cost. Tell the practitioner about any conventional treatments you are receiving. If anything a CAM practitioner recommends directly conflicts with advice from your physician, discuss it with your physician before making any major changes in any current treatment regimen or in your lifestyle.

Ask Yourself

QUESTIONS FOR CRITICAL THINKING AND REFLECTION

Drug manufacturers use television and magazine advertising to sell their products directly to consumers, telling them, "Ask your doctor about . . ." Has such an ad ever led you to believe you had a condition you didn't know you had? Or informed you about a treatment you didn't know existed? What do you think are the advantages and disadvantages of direct-to-consumer advertising?

You can investigate CAM therapies on your own by going to the library or doing research online, although caution is in order when using websites for the various forms of CAM. A good place to start are the websites of government agencies like Health Canada and of universities and hospitals that conduct government-sponsored research on CAM approaches.

LO4 13.4 ENVIRONMENTAL HEALTH

Because of the close relationship between human beings and the environment, even the healthiest lifestyle can't protect a person from the effects of polluted air, contaminated water, or a nuclear power plant mishap. Environmental health encompasses all the interactions between humans and the environment and the health consequences of these interactions.

Environmental health still focuses on such longstanding concerns as clean air and water, food inspection, and waste disposal, but in recent years its focus has expanded and become more complex. Many of the health challenges of the twenty-first century will involve protecting the environment from the by-products of human activity. Technological advances and rapid population growth have increased the ability of humans to affect and damage the environment. Water supplies are being depleted; landfills are filling up; toxic wastes threaten to contaminate both soil and water; and air pollution is altering the Earth's atmosphere and climate. Today there is a growing recognition that we hold the world in trust for future generations and for other forms of life. Our responsibility is to pass on an environment no worse—and preferably better—than the one we enjoy today.

Population Growth

The rapid expansion of the human population, particularly during the past 50 years, is generally believed to be responsible for most of the stress humans put on the environment. At the beginning of the first century A.D., there were about 300 million people alive. By the seventeenth century, the world's population had gradually increased to 500 million. But then it started to rise exponentially, zooming to 1 billion by about 1800, to 2 billion by 1930, and then doubling again in just 40 years. The world's population, currently about 6.6 billion, is increasing at a rate of about 76 million per year—150 per minute. The United Nations now projects that world population will continue to increase dramatically until it levels off above 10 billion people in 2200. Most of this growth will take place in the developing world, where population growth rates remain high. With so many people consuming and competing for the Earth's resources, it is difficult for societies to provide such basics as clean air and water and to work toward a better environment.

Environmental health may seem like a global challenge, but each person has a unique impact on our planet's health. In fact, there are ways to measure the environmental impact of your individual lifestyle.

For an estimate of how much land and water your lifestyle requires, take the Ecological Footprint quiz at http://www.myfootprint.org. You can also determine your "carbon footprint" at the Global Footprint Network web site (http://www.footprintnetwork.org/en/index.php/GFN/page/calculators) or at the Nature Conservancy website (http://www.nature.org/initiatives/climatechange/calculator/?src=l12).

Go online and take one or all of these quizzes, and compare your results with the results of your classmates. Then identify ways you can reduce the size of your ecological and carbon footprints, both as an individual and as a class.

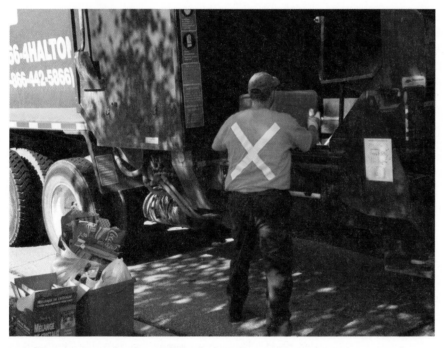

Recycling paper, cans, bottles, and plastics conserves resources, saves energy, and keeps large amounts of solid wastes out of landfills. Many communities have curbside recycling; others have drop-off sites.

Ask Yourself

QUESTIONS FOR CRITICAL THINKING AND REFLECTION

How often do you think about the environment's impact on your personal health? In what ways do your immediate surroundings (your home, neighbourhood, school, workplace) affect your well-being? In what ways do you influence the health of your personal environment?

Although population trends are difficult to influence, many countries recognize the importance of population management. A key goal of population management is to improve the conditions of people's lives so they feel less pressure to have large families. Research indicates that improved health, better education, and increased opportunities for women in the economic, political, and social realms work together with family planning and improved access to effective contraception to cut fertility rates and uncontrolled population growth.

Pollution

Many modern environmental problems are problems of pollution—contaminants in the environment that may pose a health risk. Air pollution is not a human invention—it can be caused by a forest fire, a dust storm, a pollen bloom, or the eruption of a volcano—but it is magnified by human activities, particularly the burning of fossil fuels like coal and gasoline. Air pollution can cause illness and death if pollutants become concentrated for a period of several days or weeks. Increased amounts of carbon monoxide and other pollutants and decreased amounts of oxygen in the air put extra strain on people suffering from heart or respiratory illnesses.

Two atmospheric problems have surfaced in recent years that may have long-range effects on human health.

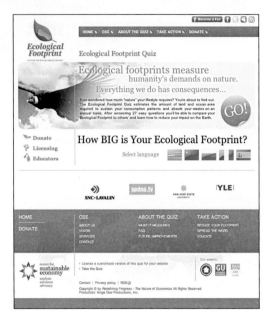

Recycling is a simple but effective way to help protect the environment.

THE GREENHOUSE EFFECT AND GLOBAL WARMING

The gradual raising of the temperature of the lower atmosphere of the Earth is called the greenhouse effect. Warming occurs as a result of the burning of fossil fuels, which releases "greenhouse gases." Experts differ on their estimate of how much temperatures will rise in the near future but agree that continuing temperature change could melt polar ice caps, raise the level of the sea, and change weather patterns. The full health implications of such an increase are not fully known.

As consumers, we can all participate in the reduction of global warming and the greenhouse effect by:

- reducing waste, recycling, and using reusable products instead of disposables.
- Drive less (i.e., walk or bicycle) or drive smart, (i.e., hybrid vehicles, properly inflated tires),
- Use the 'off' switch on lights and electronics when they aren't in use,
- Use less (i.e., less heat, less air conditioning, less hot water) or buy energy-efficient products.

THINNING OF THE OZONE LAYER

The ozone layer in the Earth's atmosphere is being destroyed primarily by chlorofluorocarbons (CFCs), industrial chemicals used in coolants, propellants, solvents, and foaming agents. The ozone layer absorbs ultraviolet (UV) radiation from the sun. As this layer becomes too thin or disappears in spots, increased exposure to UV light may cause more cases of skin cancer, increase the incidence of cataracts and blindness, and impair immune system functioning. It may also interfere with photosynthesis and cause lower crop yields.

Other forms of pollution pose problems as well. Chemical substances, including lead, asbestos, pesticides, and

Ask Yourself

QUESTIONS FOR CRITICAL THINKING AND REFLECTION

What are your views on the issue of climate change? Do you believe it is a real problem, or that it has been overly hyped by the media and some politicians and activist groups? How do you support your views?

hundreds of other products, can cause illness and death. Radiation, whether from the sun, X rays, nuclear power plants, or other sources, can cause cancer, chromosome damage, sterility, and other health problems. Even noise pollution—loud or persistent noise in the environment—can cause hearing loss and stress.

What Can You Do?

Faced with an array of complex and confusing environmental issues, you may feel overwhelmed and conclude that there isn't anything you can do. This isn't true. People can take many actions to limit their negative impact on the environment and to promote environmentally sound practices in the social and political arenas. If everyone made individual changes in his or her life, the impact would be tremendous. Refer to the box "What You Can Do for the Environment" for actions you can take.

Assuming responsibility for your actions in relation to the environment isn't very different from assuming responsibility for your own health behaviours. It involves knowledge, awareness, insight, motivation, and commitment. The same strategies that work to change personal health behaviours can be used to change environment-related behaviours.

13.5 FIT AND WELL FOR LIFE

Adopting a wellness lifestyle is the most important thing you can do to ensure a high quality of life for yourself, now and in the future. The first chapter of this book described a behaviour change program that can be used to change problem behaviours and move toward wellness. Subsequent chapters have provided information on important areas of wellness—physical fitness, weight management, nutrition, stress management, cardiovascular health, and cancer. As you learned about these aspects of wellness and assessed your own status in relation to

FITNESS TIP

Exercising in polluted outdoor air can actually reduce lung function, at least temporarily. When the air quality outside is bad, exercise indoors.

What You Can Do for the Environment

TAKE CHARGE

- Ride your bike, walk, use public transportation, or carpool in a fuel-efficient vehicle instead of driving.

- Keep your car tuned up and well maintained.

- Make sure your residence is well insulated.

- Use compact fluorescent lightbulbs instead of incandescent bulbs to save energy.

- Buy energy-efficient appliances and use them only when necessary.

- Run the washing machine or dishwasher only when they have full loads.

- Buy products with the least amount of packaging you can, or buy products in bulk. Avoid disposable products. Buy recycled or recyclable products.

- Recycle newspapers, glass, cans, paper, and other recyclable items.

- Store food in glass jars and reusable plastic containers rather than plastic wrap.

- Take your own bag along when you go shopping.

- Dispose of household hazardous wastes according to instructions.

- Take showers rather than baths to save water.

- Install sink faucet aerators, water-efficient showerheads, and water-displacement devices in toilets.

- Don't let the water run when you're brushing your teeth, shaving, or hand-washing clothes or dishes.

- Buy products and services from environmentally responsible corporations. Don't buy products made from endangered species.

- Join or support organizations working on environmental causes.

- Vote for political candidates who support environmentally sound practices. Communicate with your elected representatives about environmental issues.

---

each of them, you probably identified personal behaviours that fell short of the ideal. Take the opportunity now (if you haven't already) to consider which of these behaviours you can begin to change. As you do so, let's review the basics of behaviour change.

- Choose one behaviour to change at a time. Begin with something simple.
- Make sure your motivation and commitment are sufficient to carry you through to success. If they're not, review the health consequences of not changing this behaviour.
- Follow the five-step program outlined in Chapter 1: (1) monitor your behaviour and gather data; (2) analyze the data and identify patterns; (3) set realistic, specific goals; (4) devise a strategy or plan of action; (5) make a personal contract.
- Build rewards into the plan.
- Make sure the new behaviour is enjoyable and fits into your routine.
- Get support from family and friends.
- Forgive yourself when you slip. Don't blame yourself or others or undermine yourself by feeling guilty.
- Expect to succeed. Use positive self-talk to create a new self-image—one that includes your new behaviour.

You live in a world in which your own choices and actions have a tremendous impact on your health. Don't let the broad scope of wellness be an excuse for apathy;

instead, let it be a call to action. The time to start making changes in your lifestyle—to start becoming fit and well—is right now!

TIPS FOR TODAY AND THE FUTURE

On every level, from personal to planetary, we can all take an active role in shaping our environment and our level of wellness—now and in the future.

RIGHT NOW YOU CAN

- Call someone you care about and let her or him know how important the relationship is to you. (Don't wait for a special occasion or a crisis!)
- Contact a nonprofit group in your community and offer your time and talent; choose a cause that fits your values and would benefit most from your specific talents.
- Research any alternative or complementary practice or product you are using to find out if it is considered safe.
- Turn the lights off in any unoccupied rooms. Turn the heat down a few degrees and put on a sweater, or turn the air conditioner off and change into shorts.

IN THE FUTURE YOU CAN

- Stay mentally challenged by taking up a new hobby (such as chess) or learning a new language.
- As your existing lightbulbs burn out, replace them with compact fluorescent bulbs, which last longer and use much less electricity than standard incandescent bulbs.
- Have your car checked to make sure it runs efficiently and produces the least amount of emissions possible.

SUMMARY

- Individual and social needs are fulfilled by interpersonal relationships. Self-esteem, trust, and communication skills are the essential elements for building and maintaining good relationships.

- Friendships are characterized by companionship, respect, acceptance, help, trust, loyalty, mutuality, and reciprocity.

- Intimate love relationships encompass love, sex, and long-term commitment. Passion normally decreases with time and is replaced by closeness, caring, shared goals, and family activities.

- Communication skills and conflict resolution are especially important to successful relationships.

- Strong families are characterized by commitment, appreciation, communication, time spent together, spiritual wellness, and the ability to cope with stress and crisis.

- Many of the changes associated with aging are the result of an unhealthy lifestyle. There are many things that people can do to prevent, delay, lessen, or reverse these changes.

- Managing one's own health care involves identifying and managing medical problems and making the best use of the existing health care system.

- Self-care means knowing which symptoms need professional attention and understanding how to self-treat responsibly, with or without over-the-counter and prescription drugs.

- The best use of the health care system requires good communication with physicians and regular medical screenings. Consumers need to use critical thinking skills when considering complementary and alternative therapies.

- Today's environmental health challenges include protecting the environment from the by-products of human activity. Overpopulation contributes to environmental problems, including pollution. Individual actions to minimize negative environmental effects can have a tremendous impact.

FOR FURTHER EXPLORATION

Organizations, Hotlines, and Websites

Active Living Coalition for Older Adults. Promotes a healthy lifestyle for older adults in Canada. Funded by Health Canada and the Public Health Agency of Canada.
http://www.alcoa.ca/e/index.htm

Alberta Centre for Active Living. Presents research and promotes a physically active lifestyle for all segments of the community.
http://www.centre4activeliving.ca/

Canadian Centre for Activity and Aging. From research to practice, this centre is run through the University of Western Ontario and is interested in enhancing the lives of Canadian adults.
http://www.uwo.ca/actage/

Canadian Complementary Medical Association. Is a network of Canadian physicians, residents, and medical students with an interest in complementary and alternative medical therapies.
http://www.ccmadoctors.ca/

Canadian Interdisciplinary Network for CAM Research. Facilitates completion and promotion of research in the area.
http://www.incamresearch.ca/

Canadian Medical Association (CMA). Provides information about physicians, including their training, licensure, and board certification; the website provides recent medical news, advice for consumers, and links to related sites.
http://www.cma.ca

Many national and international organizations work on environmental health problems. A few of the largest and best known are listed below.

Greenpeace:
800-326-0959; http://www.greenpeace.org

National Wildlife Federation:
800-822-9919; http://www.nwf.org

The Nature Conservancy:
703-841-5300; http://www.tnc.org

Sierra Club:
415-977-5500; http://www.sierraclub.org

LAB 13.1 Looking to the Future: Your Values, Goals, and Lifestyle

Your Values

1. List the personality traits or characteristics that you most value—for example, friendly, patient, successful, outgoing, cooperative, loyal to family and friends, respectful of diversity. These can be characteristics of your own or of others.

2. List the activities and accomplishments that you most value—for example, making lots of money, getting good grades, spending time with friends, making your own decisions. These can be accomplishments of your own or of others, or goals you have for the future.

Your Goals and Aspirations

1. Describe the person you want to become. What is the purpose of your life? What is its meaning? What are you trying to accomplish?

2. What significant goals have you yet to realize? These can be creating something or having a particular experience.

3. What can you do to help reach these goals and become the person you want to become? What would you most like to change about yourself?

4. What do you want your life to be like in 5 years? In 10 years? In 20 years?

Your Lifestyle

1. Keeping your values and goals in mind—along with what you've learned from this text about the effects of lifestyle on wellness—examine your current lifestyle. Are you doing everything you can now to enhance the quality of your life in the future? Does your current lifestyle reflect your values and goals? List 10 positive behaviours you engage in now that will help you maintain wellness throughout your life and achieve your goals; examples might include exercising regularly, taking a yoga class to manage stress, maintaining close relationships with family and friends, drinking alcohol moderately or not at all, not smoking, and always wearing a safety belt. Next to each behaviour, list how it helps you achieve wellness and your long-term goals.

2. Next, list your current habits and behaviours that detract from wellness and may keep you from acting in accordance with your values and achieving your goals. For example, if you smoke, you may not be able to participate in your favourite recreational activities as you get older. You may also find that smoking goes against your values because the habit has a significant amount of control over your daily routine (loss of control and freedom), and you negatively affect the health of those you care about by exposing them to environmental tobacco smoke.

Lifestyle Management: Now and in the Future

1. Briefly describe the behaviour change plan(s) you worked on during this course. What behaviour(s) did you target? How successful was your program for behaviour change? Do you think you'll be able to maintain your healthier behaviour(s) in the future?

2. How would you rate your wellness status now? Has it improved in recent weeks or months? Are you more aware of your behaviour and its effect on your level of wellness? Look back at the lab activities you completed for Chapter 1. Has your lifestyle improved? Have you moved up the wellness continuum? If you haven't already retaken some of the assessment lab activities, do so now to check your progress (see Appendix C).

3. List several behaviours that could be targets for behaviour change in the future (see the list you prepared under item 2 in the previous section). Think about which of these behaviours you might want to try to change now. Begin working through the steps in Chapter 1 (and the Behaviour Change Workbook). Every positive change is a step toward wellness.

NUTRITIONAL CONTENT OF COMMON FOODS

For this food composition table, foods are listed within the following groups, corresponding to Canada's Food Guide to Healthy Eating: (1) grain products (2) fruits and vegetables (3) milk products (4) meat and alternatives; and (5) other foods.

Data are provided for a variety of nutrients. For planning and easy reference, complete the following chart with your approximate daily goals or limits; refer to the Nutrition Resources section at the end of Chapter 7. Fill in the daily totals that apply to your approximate daily calorie intake, sex, and age.

TOTAL DAILY GOAL OR LIMIT			
Total energy	_____ calories	Cholesterol	__300__ mg
Protein	_____ grams	Sodium	__2300__ mg
Carbohydrate	_____ grams	Vitamin A	_____ RE
Dietary fibre	__23–38__ grams	Vitamin C	_____ mg
Total fat	_____ grams	Calcium	_____ mg
Saturated fat	_____ grams	Iron	_____ mg

This appendix contains information on the same nutrients found on most food labels, so you can make easy comparisons. On food labels, percent Daily Values without corresponding units are usually provided for vitamins and minerals. For reference, the Daily Values are as follows: 5000 IU of vitamin A, 60 mg of vitamin C, 1000 mg of calcium, and 18 mg of iron.

GRAIN PRODUCTS
Canada's Food Guide to Healthy Eating recommends 3–8 servings per day. One serving is equivalent to 1 slice of bread, about 1 cup of ready-to-eat cereal, or ½ cup of cooked cereal, rice, or pasta.

Name	Amount	Weight g	Energy calories	Protein g	Carb. g	Fibre g	Total fat g	Sat. fat g	Chol. mg	Sod. mg	Vit. A RE	Vit. C mg	Calc. mg	Iron mg
Bagel, plain	1 bagel, 10 cm dia.	89	245	9.3	47.5	2.0	1.4	0.2	0	475	0	0	66	3.2
Barley, pearled, cooked	½ cup	79	97	1.8	22.2	3.0	0.3	0.1	0	2	0	0	9	1.0
Bulgur, cooked	½ cup	91	76	2.8	16.9	4.1	0.2	0	0	5	0	0	9	0.8
Biscuit	1 biscuit, 6 cm dia.	35	127	2.2	17.0	0.5	5.8	0.9	0	368	0	0	17	1.2
Bread, corn	1 piece	60	188	4.3	28.9	1.4	6.0	1.6	37	467	26	0	44	1.1
Bread, French	1 slice	64	175	5.6	33.2	1.9	1.9	0.4	0	390	0	0	48	1.6
Bread, pita, white	1 pita, 16 cm dia.	60	165	5.5	33.4	1.3	0.7	0.1	0	322	0	0	52	1.6
Bread, pita, whole wheat	1 pita, 16 cm dia.	64	170	6.3	35.2	4.7	1.7	0.3	0	340	0	0	10	2.0
Bread, pumpernickel	1 slice	26	65	2.3	12.4	1.7	0.8	0.1	0	174	0	0	18	0.7
Bread, raisin	1 slice	32	88	2.5	16.7	1.4	1.4	0.3	0	125	0	0	21	0.9
Bread, rye	1 slice	32	83	2.7	15.5	1.9	1.1	0.2	0	211	0	0.1	23	0.9
Bread sticks	2 sticks	20	82	2.4	13.6	0.6	1.9	0.3	0	131	0	0	4	0.8
Bread stuffing	½ cup	100	178	3.2	21.7	2.9	8.6	1.7	0	543	118	0	32	1.1
Bread, white	1 slice	30	80	2.3	15.2	0.7	1.0	0.2	0	204	0	0	45	1.1

Name	Amount	Weight g	Energy calories	Protein g	Carb. g	Fibre g	Total fat g	Sat. fat g	Chol. mg	Sod. mg	Vit. A RE	Vit. C mg	Calc. mg	Iron mg
Bread, whole grain	1 slice	32	80	3.2	14.8	2.0	1.2	0.3	0	156	0	0.1	29	1.1
Bread, whole wheat	1 slice	28	69	2.7	12.9	1.9	1.2	0.3	0	148	0	0	20	0.9
Buckwheat groats, cooked	½ cup	84	77	2.8	16.8	2.3	0.5	0.1	0	3	0	0	6	0.7
Bun, hamburger/hot dog	1 roll	43	120	4.1	21.3	0.9	1.9	0.5	0	206	0	0	59	1.4
Cake, angelfood	1/12 of 25 cm cake	50	129	3.1	29.4	0.1	0.2	0	0	255	0	0	42	0.1
Cake, chocolate w/frosting	⅛ of 18 oz cake	64	235	2.6	34.9	1.8	10.5	3.1	27	214	16	0.1	28	1.4
Cake, yellow w/icing	⅛ of 18 oz cake	64	243	2.4	35.5	1.2	11.1	3.0	35	216	21	0	24	1.3
Cereal, All-Bran	⅓ cup	30	75	2.1	24.0	12.9	0.9	0.1	0	203	153	6.0	19	4.5
Cereal, Cheerios	1 cup	30	111	3.3	22.2	2.7	1.8	0.4	0	273	150	6.0	100	8.1
Cereal, Corn Flakes	1 cup	28	101	1.8	24.3	1.3	0.1	0	0	203	150	6.2	2	8.4
Cereal, Cream of Wheat	½ cup	126	63	1.9	13.8	0.5	0.3	0	0	168	0	0	56.5	4.8
Cereal, Frosted Flakes	¾ cup	31	114	1.0	28.0	1.0	0.2	0.1	0	148	160	6.2	2	4.5
Cereal, granola	½ cup	51	232	5.4	33.8	3.7	6.5	4.2	1	24	1	0.3	61	1.3
Cereal, Raisin Bran	1 cup	61	195	5.2	46.5	7.3	3.0	0.6	0	362	155	0.4	29	4.6
Cereal, Total	¾ cup	30	97	2.4	23.0	2.4	0.3	0.2	0	192	150	60.0	1000	18.0
Cereal, Wheat Chex	1 cup	30	104	3.0	24.3	3.3	0.6	0.1	0	267	90	3.6	60	8.7
Cereal, Wheaties	1 cup	30	106	3.0	24.3	3.0	0.3	0.2	0	218	150	6.0	0	8.1
Coffee cake w/topping	1 piece	63	263	4.3	29.4	1.3	14.7	3.7	20	221	21	0.2	34	1.2
Cookie, chocolate chip	1 medium cookie	16	78	0.9	9.3	0.4	4.5	1.3	5	58	26	0	6	0.4
Cookie, fig bar	1 cookie	16	56	0.6	11.3	0.7	1.2	0.2	0	56	1	0	10	0.5
Cookie, fortune	1 cookie	8	30	0.3	6.7	0.1	0.2	0.1	0	22	0	0	1	0.1
Cookie, oatmeal	1 large cookie	18	81	1.1	12.4	0.5	3.3	0.8	0	69	0	0.1	7	0.5
Cookie, sandwich	1 cookie	10	47	0.5	7.0	0.3	0.3	0.4	0	60	0	0	3	0.4
Corn meal, dry	¼ cup	35	126	2.9	26.8	2.6	0.6	0.1	0	1	14	0	2	1.4
Corn grits, cooked	½ cup	121	73	1.7	15.7	0.2	0.2	0	0	0	7	0	0	0.8
Couscous, cooked	½ cup	79	88	3.0	18.2	1.1	0.1	0	0	4	0	0	6	0.3
Cracker, crispbread, rye	3 crispbreads	30	110	2.4	24.7	5.0	0.4	0	0	79	0	0	9	0.7
Cracker, graham	3 squares	28	119	2.0	21.3	1.0	1.6	0.4	0	185	0	0	22	1.2
Cracker, matzo	1 matzo	28	111	2.8	23.4	0.8	0.4	0.1	0	1	0	0	4	0.9
Cracker, melba toast	6 pieces	30	117	3.6	23.0	1.9	1.0	0.1	0	249	0	0	28	1.1
Cracker, Ritz	5 crackers	16	79	1.2	10.3	0.3	3.7	0.6	0	124	0	0	24	0.6
Cracker, saltine	10 squares	30	130	2.8	21.5	0.9	3.5	0.9	0	390	0	0	36	1.6
Cracker, whole wheat	6 crackers	24	106	2.1	16.5	2.5	4.1	0.8	0	158	0	0	24	0.7
Croissant, butter	1 medium	57	231	4.7	26.1	1.5	12.0	6.6	38	424	106	0.1	21	1.2
Danish pastry, cheese	1 pastry	71	266	5.7	26.4	0.7	15.5	4.8	11	320	32	0	25	1.1
Doughnut, glazed	1 medium	45	192	2.3	22.9	0.7	10.3	2.7	14	181	1	0	27	0.5
English muffin, plain	½ muffin	29	67	2.2	13.1	0.8	0.5	0.1	0	132	0	0	50	0.7
French toast	1 slice	65	149	5.0	16.3	0	7.0	1.8	75	311	86	0.2	65	1.1
Macaroni, cooked	½ cup	70	99	3.3	19.8	0.9	0.5	0.1	0	1	0	0	5	1.0
Muffin, blueberry	5 cm by 7 cm	57	162	3.71	23.2	0	6.2	1.2	21	251	22	0.9	108	1.3
Muffin, oat bran	1 small	66	178	4.6	31.9	3.0	4.8	0.7	0	259	0	0	42	2.7
Noodles, chow mein	½ cup	23	119	1.9	12.9	0.9	6.9	1.0	0	99	2	0	5	1.1
Noodles, egg, cooked	½ cup	80	106	3.8	19.9	0.9	1.2	0.2	53	6	5	0	10	1.3
Noodles, Japanese soba	½ cup	57	56	2.9	12.2	0	0.1	0	0	34	0	0	2	0.3
Oat bran, raw	¼ cup	24	58	4.1	15.6	3.6	1.7	0.3	0	1	0	0	14	1.3
Oatmeal, instant	1 packet	28	103	4.3	17.9	3.1	1.7	0.3	0	80	300	0	100	8.1
Pancake	10 cm pancake	38	74	2.0	13.9	0.5	1.0	0.2	5	239	12	0.1	48	0.6
Pasta, cooked	2 oz.	57	75	2.9	14.2	0	0.6	0.1	19	3	3	0	3	0.7
Popcorn, air-popped	2 cups	16	61	1.9	12.5	2.4	0.7	0.1	0	1	3	0	2	0.4
Popcorn, oil-popped	2 cups	22	110	1.9	12.6	2.2	6.2	1.0	0	194	3	0	2	0.6
Pretzels	10 twists	60	229	5.5	47.5	1.9	2.1	0.5	0	1029	0	0	22	2.6
Quinoa, uncooked	¼ cup	43	159	5.6	29.3	2.5	2.5	0.3	0	9	0	0	26	3.9
Roll, dinner	1 roll, 5 cm square	28	84	2.3	14.1	0.8	2.0	0.5	0	146	0	0	33	0.8
Rice, brown, cooked	½ cup	98	108	2.5	22.4	1.8	0.9	0.2	0	5	0	0	10	0.4
Rice cake	1 cake	9	35	0.7	7.3	0.4	0.3	0	0	29	0	0	1	0.1
Rice, white, cooked	½ cup	79	103	2.1	22.3	0.3	0.2	0	0	1	0	0	8	0.9
Rice, wild, cooked	½ cup	82	83	3.3	17.5	1.5	0.3	0	0	3	0	0	2	0.5
Spaghetti, cooked	½ cup	70	99	3.3	19.8	1.2	0.5	0.1	0	70	0	0	5	1.0
Taco shell	1 medium	13	62	1.0	8.3	1.0	3.0	0.4	0	49	0	0	21	0.3
Tortilla chips	1 oz.	28	142	2.0	17.8	1.8	7.4	1.4	0	150	6	0	44	0.4

Name	Amount	Weight g	Energy calories	Protein g	Carb. g	Fibre g	Total fat g	Sat. fat g	Chol. mg	Sod. mg	Vit. A RE	Vit. C mg	Calc. mg	Iron mg
Tortilla, corn	1 medium	24	53	1.4	11.2	1.2	0.6	0.1	0	39	0	0	42	0.3
Tortilla, flour	20 cm tortilla	51	146	4.4	25.3	0	3.1	0.4	0	249	0	0	97	1.0
Wheat germ, toasted	¼ cup	28	108	8.3	14.1	3.7	3.0	0.5	0	1	0	1.7	13	2.6

FRUITS AND VEGETABLES

Canada's Food Guide to Healthy Eating recommends 4–10 servings per day. One serving is equivalent to 1 medium apple or banana; ½ cup chopped, cooked or canned fruit; ½ cup of fruit juice; 1 cup of raw leafy vegetables, ½ cup of other raw or cooked vegetables, or ¾ cup of vegetable juice.

Name	Amount	Weight g	Energy calories	Protein g	Carb. g	Fibre g	Total fat g	Sat. fat g	Chol. mg	Sod. mg	Vit. A RE	Vit. C mg	Calc. mg	Iron mg
Alfalfa sprouts	½ cup	17	5	0.7	0.6	0.4	0.1	0	0	1	1	1.4	5	0.2
Apple juice	¾ cup	179	284	0.3	20.7	0.2	0.2	0	0	13	0	44.8	11	0.5
Apple, raw, w/skin	1 medium	138	72	0.4	19.1	3.3	0.2	0	0	1	4	6.3	8	0.2
Apple sauce, unsweetened	½ cup	122	52	0.2	13.8	1.5	0.1	0	0	2	4	25.9	4	0.1
Apricots	2 medium	70	34	1.0	7.8	1.7	0.3	0	0	1	67	7.0	10	0.4
Apricots, dried	9 halves	32	75	1.2	19.7	2.3	0.1	0	0	3	228	0.8	14	1.5
Artichoke, cooked	1 medium	120	60	4.2	13.4	6.5	0.2	0	0	114	22	12.0	54	1.5
Arugula, raw	1 cup	20	5	0.5	0.7	0.3	0.1	0	0	3	24	3.0	16	0.1
Asparagus, cooked	6 spears	90	22	2.3	3.8	1.4	0.3	0	0	10	49	9.7	18	0.7
Avocado	1 medium	173	289	3.4	15.0	11.8	26.6	3.7	0	14	12	15.2	22	1.1
Bamboo shoots, canned	½ cup	66	13	1.1	2.1	0.9	0.3	0.1	0	5	1	0.7	5	0.2
Banana	1 medium	118	105	1.3	27.0	3.1	0.4	0.1	0	1	4	10.3	6	0.3
*Beans, baked (plain)	½ cup	127	118	6.1	26.0	6.4	0.6	0.1	0	504	22	3.9	64	0.4
*Beans, black, cooked	½ cup	86	114	7.6	20.4	7.5	0.5	0.1	0	1	1	0	23	1.8
*Beans, fava, raw	½ cup	63	55	4.9	11.1	0	0.5	0.1	0	16	11	2.3	23	0.9
Beans, green snap, cooked	½ cup	63	22	1.2	4.9	2.0	0.2	0	0	2	42	6.1	29	0.8
*Beans, kidney, cooked	½ cup	89	112	7.7	20.2	6.5	0.4	0.1	0	2	0	1.1	25	2.6
*Beans, lentils, cooked	½ cup	99	115	8.9	19.9	7.8	0.4	0.1	0	2	1	1.5	19	3.3
*Beans, lima, cooked	½ cup	94	108	7.3	19.6	6.6	0.4	0.1	0	2	0	0	16	2.2
*Beans, navy, cooked	½ cup	91	129	7.9	23.9	5.8	0.5	0.1	0	1	0	0.8	64	2.3
*Beans, pinto, cooked	½ cup	85.5	120	7.8	21.3	7.0	0.7	0.1	0	9	0	0.7	36	1.8
*Beans, refried	½ cup	126	118	6.9	19.6	6.7	1.6	0.6	10	377	0	7.6	44	2.1
Beans, yellow snap, cooked	½ cup	63	22	1.2	4.9	2.1	0.2	0	0	2	5	6.1	29	0.8
Beet greens, cooked	½ cup	72	19	1.9	3.4	2.1	0.1	0	0	174	276	17.9	82	1.4
Beets, cooked	½ cup	85	37	1.4	8.5	1.7	0.2	0	0	65	3	3.1	14	0.7
Blackberries, raw	½ cup	72	31	1.0	6.9	3.8	0.4	0	0	1	8	15.1	21	0.5
Blueberries	½ cup	73	41	0.5	10.2	2.0	0.3	0	0	1	2	7.0	4	0.2
Broccoli spears, cooked	2 spears	78	22	2.3	3.9	2.3	0.3	0	0	20	108	58.2	36	0.7
Brussels sprouts, cooked	4 sprouts	84	30	2.1	7.3	2.2	0.4	0.1	0	18	60	52.1	30	1.0
Cabbage, cooked	½ cup	75	17	0.8	3.3	1.7	0.3	0	0	6	10	15.1	23	0.1
Cabbage, raw	½ cup	45	11	0.6	2.4	1.0	0.1	0	0	8	6	14.3	21	0.3
Cantaloupe	¼ melon, 12 cm dia.	138	48	1.2	11.5	1.1	0.4	0.1	0	12	444	58.2	12	0.3
Carambola (starfruit)	1 small	70	23	0.4	5.5	1.9	0.2	0	0	1	34	14.8	3	0.2
Carrot, juice	¾ cup	177	71	1.7	16.4	1.4	0.3	0	0	51	1938	15.0	42	0.8
Carrots, cooked	½ cup	78	27	0.6	6.4	2.3	0.1	0	0	236	659	2.8	23	0.3
Carrots, raw	1 medium	61	21	0.6	5.8	1.8	0.2	0	0	42	367	3.6	20	0.2
Cauliflower, cooked	½ cup	62	14	1.1	2.5	1.7	0.3	0	0	9	1	27.4	10	0.2
Celery, raw	8 sticks	32	4	0.2	1.0	0.5	0	0	0	26	7	1.0	13	0.1
Chard, cooked	½ cup	88	18	1.6	3.6	1.8	0.1	0	0	156	275	15.8	51	2.0
Cherries, canned in syrup	½ cup	127	105	0.8	26.9	1.9	0.2	0	0	4	10	4.6	11	0.4
Cherries, sweet, raw	11 cherries	75	47	0.8	12.0	1.6	0.2	0	0	0	2	5.2	10	0.3
Coleslaw, homemade	½ cup	60	41	0.8	7.4	0.9	1.6	0.2	5	14	49	19.6	27	0.4
Collards, cooked	½ cup	95	25	2.0	4.7	2.7	0.3	0	0	9	297	17.3	113	0.4
Corn, yellow, cooked	½ cup	82	89	2.7	20.6	2.3	1.1	0.2	0	14	18	5.1	2	0.5
Cranberries, raw	½ cup	48	23	0.2	6.0	2.0	0.1	0	0	1	2	6.4	3	0.1
Cranberry juice cocktail	¾ cup	190	108	0	27.3	0.2	0.2	0	0	4	0	67.1	6	0.3
Cranberry sauce	½ cup	139	105	0.1	26.9	0.7	0.1	0	0	20	1	1.4	3	0.2
Cucumber, raw	½ cup	52	8	0.3	1.9	0.4	0.1	0	0	1	3	1.5	8	0.2
Currants, dried	¼ cup	36	102	1.5	26.7	2.4	0.1	0	0	3	3	1.7	31	1.2
Dates, dried	¼ cup	45	122	0.9	32.7	3.3	0.2	0.1	0	1	2	0	14	0.5

Name	Amount	Weight g	Energy calories	Protein g	Carb. g	Fibre g	Total fat g	Sat. fat g	Chol. mg	Sod. mg	Vit. A RE	Vit. C mg	Calc. mg	Iron mg
Eggplant, cooked	½ cup	50	17	0.4	4.3	1.2	0.1	0	0	0	1	0.6	3	0.1
Endive, raw	½ cup	25	4	0.3	0.8	0.8	0.1	0	0	6	51	1.6	13	0.2
Figs, raw	2 medium	100	74	0.8	19.2	2.9	0.3	0.1	0	1	7	2.0	35	0.4
Fruit cocktail, heavy syrup	½ cup	124	91	0.5	23.4	1.2	0.1	0	0	7	25	2.4	7	0.4
Fruit cocktail, juice	½ cup	119	55	0.5	14.1	1.2	0	0	0	5	18	3.2	9	0.3
Fruit cocktail, light syrup	½ cup	121	69	0.5	18.1	1.2	0.1	0	0	7	12	2.3	7	0.4
Grapefruit	½ medium	128	41	0.8	10.3	1.4	0.1	0	0	0	59	44.0	15	0.1
Grapes	12 grapes	60	41	0.4	10.9	0.6	0.1	0	0	1	2	6.5	6	0.2
Grapefruit juice	¾ cup	185	70	1.0	16.6	0.2	0.2	0	0	2	2	54.1	13	0.4
Guava	1 fruit	90	46	0.7	10.7	4.9	0.5	0.2	0	3	28	165.2	18	0.3
Hominy, canned	½ cup	83	59	1.2	11.8	2.1	0.7	0.1	0	173	0	0	8	0.5
Honeydew	⅛ melon, 13 cm dia.	125	44	0.6	11.5	1.0	0.1	0	0	13	5	22.5	8	0.2
Kale, cooked	½ cup	65	18	1.2	3.6	1.3	0.3	0	0	15	481	26.7	47	0.6
Kiwifruit	1 large	91	56	0.9	13.5	3.1	0.4	0	0	5	8	68.3	24	0.4
Kohlrabi, cooked	½ cup	83	24	1.5	5.5	0.9	0.1	0	0	17	2	44.5	21	0.3
Kumquats	5 fruits	95	67	1.8	15.1	6.2	0.8	0.1	0	10	14	41.7	59	0.8
Leeks, raw	½ cup	45	27	0.7	6.3	0.8	0.1	0	0	9	37	5.3	26	0.9
Lemon juice	2 tablespoons	31	8	0.1	2.6	0.1	0	0	0	6	0	14.0	2	0
Lemon, with peel	1 fruit	108	22	1.3	11.6	5.1	0.3	0	0	3	3	83.2	66	0.8
Lettuce, green leaf	1 cup	56	8	0.7	1.6	0.7	0.1	0	0	16	207	10.1	20	0.5
Lettuce, iceberg	1 cup	55	8	0.6	1.2	0.6	0.1	0	0	5	9	2.1	11	0.2
Lettuce, romaine	1 cup	56	10	0.7	1.8	1.2	0.2	0	0	4	162	13.4	18	0.5
Mango	½ medium	103	65	0.5	17.0	1.8	0.3	0.1	0	2	39	28.7	10	0.1
Mushrooms, cooked	½ cup	78	21	1.7	4.0	1.7	0.3	0	0	2	0	3.1	5	1.4
Mushrooms, raw	½ cup	35	8	1.1	1.1	0.4	0.1	0	0	1	0	0.8	1	0.2
Mustard greens, cooked	½ cup	70	10	1.6	1.5	1.4	0.2	0	0	11	212	17.7	52	0.5
Nectarine	1 fruit	136	60	1.4	14.4	2.3	0.4	0	0	0	23	7.3	8	0.4
Okra, cooked	½ cup	80	18	1.5	3.6	2.0	0.1	0	0	5	11	13.0	62	0.2
Olives, ripe	10 large	44	51	0.3	2.8	1.4	4.7	0.6	0	383	9	0.4	39	1.5
Onion, raw	½ cup	80	34	0.7	8.0	1.1	0.1	0	0	2	0	5.1	18	0.2
Orange juice	¾ cup	186	84	1.3	19.3	0.4	0.4	0	0	2	19	93	20	0.4
Orange	1 medium	131	62	1.2	15.4	3.1	0.2	0	0	0	14	69.7	52	0.1
Papaya	½ medium	152	59	0.9	14.9	2.7	0.2	0.1	0	5	84	93.9	36	0.2
Parsley, raw	2 tablespoons	8	3	0.2	0.5	0.3	0.1	0	0	4	32	10.1	10	0.5
Parsnip, raw	½ cup	67	50	0.8	12.0	3.2	0.2	0	0	7	0	11.3	24	0.4
Passion fruit	½ cup	118	114	2.6	27.6	12.3	0.8	0.1	0	33	76	35.4	14	1.9
Peach, canned in juice	½ cup	124	55	0.8	14.3	1.6	0	0	0	5	24	4.4	7	0.3
Peach, raw	1 medium	98	38	0.9	9.3	1.5	0.2	0	0	0	16	6.5	6	0.2
Pear, canned	½ cup	124	62	0.4	16.0	2.0	0.1	0	0	5	0	2.0	11	0.4
Pear, raw	1 medium	166	98	0.6	25.1	4.0	0.7	0	0	0	3	6.6	18	0.4
*Peas, blackeye, cooked	½ cup	86	100	6.6	17.9	5.6	0.5	0.1	0	3	1	0.3	21	2.2
*Peas, chickpeas (garbanzos)	½ cup	82	134	7.3	22.5	6.2	2.1	0.2	0	6	2	1.1	40	2.4
Peas, edible, podded	10 pea pods	34	14	1.0	2.6	0.9	0.1	0	0	1	5	20.4	15	0.7
Peas, green	½ cup	80	62	4.1	11.4	4.4	0.2	0	0	70	54	7.9	19	1.2
*Peas, split, cooked	½ cup	98	116	8.2	20.6	8.1	0.4	0.1	0	2	1	0.4	14	1.3
Pepper, green chili, canned	½ cup	70	15	0.5	3.2	1.2	0.2	0	0	276	9	23.8	25	0.9
Pepper, sweet green, raw	1 small	74	20	0.7	4.8	1.3	0.1	0	0	1	47	66.1	7	0.3
Pepper, sweet red, raw	1 small	74	20	0.7	4.8	1.5	0.1	0	0	1	422	140.6	7	0.3
Persimmon, raw	1 fruit	25	32	0.2	8.4	0	0.1	0	0	0	0	16.2	7	0.6
Pickle, dill	1 medium	65	12	0.4	2.7	0.8	0.1	0	0	21	833	1.2	6	0.3
Pineapple, canned in juice	½ cup	125	75	0.5	19.5	1.0	0.1	0	0	1	2	11.8	17	0.3
Pineapple, raw	1 slice	84	40	0.5	10.6	1.2	0.1	0	0	1	3	30.4	11	0.2
Plantain, raw	1 medium	179	218	2.3	57.1	4.1	0.6	0.3	0	7	100	32.9	5	1.1
Plums	1½ medium	99	46	0.7	11.3	1.4	0.3	0	0	0	17	9.4	6	0.2
Potato salad	½ cup	125	179	3.4	14.0	1.6	10.3	1.8	85	661	41	12.5	24	0.8
Potato, baked w/skin	1 medium	173	161	4.3	36.6	3.8	0.2	0.1	0	17	17	16.6	26	1.9
Potato, boiled	1 potato, 6 cm dia.	136	118	2.5	27.4	2.4	0.1	0	0	5	0	17.7	7	0.4
Potato, french fries	10 fries	50	100	1.6	15.6	1.6	3.8	0.6	0	15	0	5.0	4	0.6
Potato, mashed w/milk	½ cup	105	81	2.0	18.4	1.6	0.6	0.3	2	318	4	7.0	23	0.3
Prune juice	¾ cup	192	136	1.2	33.5	1.9	0.1	0	0	8	0	7.9	23	2.3

Name	Amount	Weight g	Energy calories	Protein g	Carb. g	Fibre g	Total fat g	Sat. fat g	Chol. mg	Sod. mg	Vit. A RE	Vit. C mg	Calc. mg	Iron mg
Prunes (dried plums)	5 prunes	42	101	0.9	26.8	3.0	1.2	0	0	1	16	0.3	18	0.4
Pumpkin, canned	½ cup	123	42	1.3	9.9	3.6	0.3	0.2	0	6	2702	5.1	32	1.7
Radish, raw	13 medium	56	9	0.4	2.1	0.9	0	0	0	23	0	8.7	15	0.2
Raisins	¼ cup	41	123	1.3	32.7	1.5	1.2	0	0	5	0	0.9	21	0.8
Raspberries	½ cup	62	32	0.7	7.3	4.0	0.4	0	0	1	1	16.1	15	0.4
Rhubarb, raw	1 stalk	51	11	0.5	2.3	0.9	0.1	0	0	2	3	4.1	44	0.1
Rutabaga, mashed	½ cup	120	47	1.5	10.5	2.2	0.3	0	0	24	67	22.6	58	0.6
Sauerkraut, drained	½ cup	121	13	0.6	3.0	1.8	0.1	0	0	469	1	10.5	21	1.0
Soybeans, green, boiled	½ cup	90	127	11.1	9.9	3.8	5.8	0.7	0	13	14	15.3	131	2.3
Spinach, cooked	½ cup	95	27	3.0	5.1	2.9	0.2	0	0	82	739	11.7	139	1.4
Spinach, raw	1 cup	30	7	0.9	1.1	0.8	0.1	0	0	24	202	8.4	30	0.8
Squash, summer, cooked	½ cup	90	18	0.8	3.9	1.3	0.3	0	0	1	26	5.0	24	0.3
Squash, summer, raw	½ small squash	59	12	0.7	2.6	1.1	0.1	0	0	1	12	8.7	12	0.3
Squash, winter	½ cup	100	39	0.9	8.8	2.8	0.6	0.1	0	1	356	9.6	14	0.3
Strawberries	5 large	90	27	0.6	6.3	2.1	0.3	0	0	1	1	51.0	13	0.3
Sweet potato, baked	½ cup	100	90	2.0	20.7	3.3	0.2	0	0	36	961	19.6	38	0.7
Sweet potato, canned w/syrup	½ cup	98	106	1.3	24.9	2.9	0.3	0.1	0	38	351	10.6	17	1.0
Tangerine	1 medium	84	37	0.5	9.4	1.9	0.2	0	0	1	29	25.9	12	0.1
Tomato juice	¾ cup	182	31	1.4	7.7	1.5	1.4	0	0	18	102	33.3	18	0.1
Tomato sauce	½ cup	123	39	1.6	9.0	1.8	0.3	0	0	642	21	8.6	16	1.3
Tomato, red, raw	1 medium	123	22	1.1	4.8	1.5	0.3	0.1	0	6	52	15.6	12	0.3
Turnip, cooked, mashed	½ cup	115	24	0.8	5.6	2.3	0.1	0	0	108	0	13.3	25	0.3
Vegetable juice	¾ cup	182	35	1.1	8.3	1.5	0.2	0	0	491	213	50.4	20	0.8
Vegetable soup	1 cup	241	72	2.1	12.0	0.5	1.9	0.3	0	822	301	1.4	22	1.1
Vegetables, mixed	½ cup	91	54	2.6	11.9	4.0	0.1	0	0	32	389	2.9	23	0.7
Water chestnuts	½ cup	70	35	0.6	8.7	1.8	0	0	0	6	0	0.9	3	0.6
Watermelon	1/16 melon	286	86	1.7	21.6	1.1	0.4	0	0	3	80	23.2	20	0.7

*Dry beans and peas (legumes) can be counted as servings of vegetables or as servings from the meat, poultry, fish, dry beans, eggs, and nuts group. They are listed here and marked with an asterisk.

MILK PRODUCTS

Canada's Food Guide to Healthy Eating recommends that Canadians consume from 2–4 servings of milk products per day. Requirements are based on both age and pregnancy status (women). One serving is equivalent to 1 cup milk or yogurt, 50 grams of natural cheese, or 65 grams of processed cheese.

Buttermilk, lowfat	1 cup	245	98	8.1	11.7	0	2.2	1.3	10	257	17	2.5	284	0.1
Cheese, American	65 g	57	188	11.1	4.7	0	13.9	8.8	36	548	90	0	282	0.5
Cheese, blue	50 g	43	150	9.1	1.0	0	12.2	7.9	32	593	84	0	225	0.1
Cheese, cheddar	50 g	43	171	10.6	0.5	0	14.1	9.0	45	264	113	0	307	0.3
Cheese, cottage, creamed	1 cup	210	216	26.2	5.6	0	9.5	6.0	32	850	92	0	126	0.3
Cheese, cottage, lowfat (1%)	1 cup	226	163	28.0	6.1	0	2.3	1.5	9	918	25	0	138	0.3
Cheese, cottage, non-fat	1 cup	145	123	25.0	2.7	0	0.6	0.4	10	19	13	0	46	0.3
Cheese, cream	65 g	57	198	4.3	1.5	0	19.8	12.5	62	168	208	0	45	0.7
Cheese, cream, fat free	65 g	57	55	8.2	3.3	0	0.8	0.5	5	311	159	0	105	0.1
Cheese, feta	50 g	43	112	6.0	1.7	0	9.0	6.4	38	475	54	0	210	0.3
Cheese, Mexican	50 g	43	151	9.6	1.2	0	12.0	7.6	45	279	23	0	281	0.2
Cheese, Monterey	50 g	43	159	10.4	0.3	0	12.9	8.1	38	228	84	0	317	0.3
Cheese, mozzarella (part skim)	50 g	43	108	10.3	1.2	0	6.8	4.3	27	263	54	0	333	0.1
Cheese, Parmesan, grated	2 tablespoons	10	43	3.9	0.4	0	2.9	1.7	9	153	12	0	111	0.1
Cheese, process spread	65 g	56	170	9.1	5.5	0	12.3	8.1	45	839	100	0.1	261	0.1
Cheese, provolone	50 g	43	149	10.9	0.9	0	11.3	7.3	29	373	100	0	321	0.2
Cheese, ricotta, part skim	½ cup	124	171	14.1	6.4	0	9.8	6.1	38	155	133	0	337	0.5
Cheese, Swiss	50 g	43	160	12.1	1.4	0	11.7	7.6	39	111	94	0	409	0.1
Ice cream, chocolate	1 cup	132	285	5.0	37.2	1.6	14.2	9.0	45	100	157	0.9	144	1.2
Ice cream, vanilla, rich	1 cup	214	533	7.5	47.7	0	34.7	22.1	197	131	389	0	250	0.7
Ice cream, vanilla, light	1 cup	146	241	7.8	39.0	0.4	5.8	3.8	36	108	201	0.3	169	0.1
Ice cream, vanilla, soft-serve	1 cup	172	382	7.0	1.2	1.2	22.4	12.9	157	105	279	1.4	225	0.4
Milk, chocolate	1 cup	250	208	7.9	25.9	2.0	8.5	5.3	30	150	65	2.3	280	0.6

Name	Amount	Weight g	Energy calories	Protein g	Carb. g	Fibre g	Total fat g	Sat. fat g	Chol. mg	Sod. mg	Vit. A RE	Vit. C mg	Calc. mg	Iron mg
Milk, fat free (skim)	1 cup	245	86	8.4	11.9	0	0.4	0.3	5	127	149	2.5	301	0.1
Milk, lowfat (1%)	1 cup	244	102	8.0	12.1	0	2.4	1.6	12	107	144	2.4	290	0.1
Milk, reduced fat (2%)	1 cup	244	122	8.1	11.7	0	4.7	2.9	20	122	139	2.4	298	0.1
Milk, whole	1 cup	244	146	7.9	11.0	0	7.9	4.6	24	98	68	0	276	0.1
Pudding, chocolate	½ cup	147	163	4.6	27.6	1.5	4.6	2.7	16	417	38	1.3	150	0.4
Yogurt, frozen, vanilla	1 cup	144	235	5.8	34.9	0	8.1	4.9	3	125	85	1.2	206	0.4
Yogurt, lowfat, plain	260 g container	227	143	11.9	16.0	0	3.5	2.3	14	159	32	1.8	415	0.2
Yogurt, lowfat, with fruit	260 g container	227	238	11.0	42.2	0	3.2	2.1	14	148	36	1.6	384	0.2
Yogurt, nonfat, plain	260 g container	227	127	13.0	17.4	0	0.4	0.3	5	175	5	2.0	452	0.2

MEAT AND ALTERNATIVES

Canada's Food Guide to Healthy Eating recommends 1–3 servings per day. One serving is equivalent to 75 grams of cooked lean meat, poultry, or fish. The following count as equivalents of 30 grams of meat: ½ cup of cooked dry beans or tofu, 80 grams of soyburger, 2 eggs, 2 tablespoons of peanut butter, ⅓ cup of nuts, or ¼ cup of seeds.

Name	Amount	Weight g	Energy calories	Protein g	Carb. g	Fibre g	Total fat g	Sat. fat g	Chol. mg	Sod. mg	Vit. A RE	Vit. C mg	Calc. mg	Iron mg
Bacon, back	2 slices	47	86	11.3	0.6	0	3.9	1.3	27	727	0	0	5	0.4
Beef, 1/20 fat	100 g	85	344	19.9	0	0	28.7	11.9	78	48	0	0	9	2.1
Beef, lean, fat trimmed	100 g	85	179	25.4	0	0	7.9	3.0	73	56	0	0	7	2.5
Beef, corned	100 g	85	213	23.0	0	0	12.7	5.3	73	856	0	0	10	1.8
Beef, ground, extra lean, broiled	100 g	85	218	21.6	0	0	13.9	5.5	71	60	0	0	6	2.0
Beef, ground, lean, broiled	100 g	85	231	21.0	0	0	15.7	6.2	74	65	0	0	9	1.8
Beef, ground, regular, broiled	100 g	85	246	20.5	0	0	17.6	6.9	77	71	0	0	9	2.1
Beef liver, braised	100 g	85	137	20.7	2.9	0	4.2	1.6	331	60	9011	19.6	6	5.8
Beef ribs, broiled	100 g	85	306	18.7	0	0	25.1	10.2	70	53	0	0	10	1.8
Chicken breast, w/skin, rst	½ breast	98	193	29.2	0	0	7.6	2.1	82	70	26	0	14	1.0
Chicken, dk mt, w/skin, rst	100 g	85	215	22.1	0	0	13.4	3.7	77	74	49	0	13	1.2
Chicken, dk mt, w/o skin, rst	100 g	85	168	22.2	0	0	7.9	2.2	76	76	18	0	12	1.1
Chicken, dk mt, w/skin, fried	100 g	85	253	18.6	8.0	0	15.8	4.2	76	251	26	0	18	1.2
Chicken, drumstick, w/skin, rst	1 drumstick	52	112	14.1	0	0	5.8	1.6	47	47	16	0	6	0.7
Chicken, lt mt, w/skin, rst	100 g	85	189	24.7	0	0	9.2	2.6	71	64	27	0	13	1.0
Chicken, lt mt, w/o skin, rst	100 g	85	147	26.3	0	0	3.8	1.1	72	65	8	0	13	0.9
Chicken, lt mt, w/skin, fried	100 g	85	235	20.0	8.1	0	13.1	3.5	71	243	20	0	17	1.1
Chicken, thigh, w/skin, rst	1 thigh	62	153	15.5	0	0	9.6	2.7	58	52	30	0	7	0.8
Chicken, wing, w/skin, rst	1 wing	34	99	9.1	0	0	6.6	1.9	29	28	16	0	5	0.4
Chicken liver, chopped	½ cup	70	110	17.1	0.8	0	3.8	1.3	442	36	3439	11.1	10	5.9
Egg white, large	1 egg white	33	17	3.5	0.3	0	0	0	0	55	0	0	2	0
Egg, whole, large	1 egg	50	75	6.2	0.6	0	5.1	1.6	213	63	97	0	25	0.7
Egg yolk, large	1 yolk	17	55	2.8	0.3	0	5.1	1.6	213	7	97	0	23	0.6
Fish, catfish, baked/broiled	100 g	85	129	15.9	0	0	6.8	1.5	54	68	13	0.7	8	0.7
Fish, cod, baked/broiled	100 g	85	89	19.5	0	0	0.7	0.1	47	66	9	2.6	7	0.3
Fish, halibut, baked/broiled	100 g	85	119	22.7	0	0	2.5	0.4	35	59	46	0	51	0.9
Fish, salmon, baked/broiled	100 g	85	175	18.8	0	0	10.5	2.1	54	52	13	3.1	13	0.3
Fish, salmon, canned	100 g	85	130	17.4	0	0	6.2	1.4	37	457	45	0	203	0.9
Fish, salmon, smoked	100 g	85	99	15.5	0	0	3.7	0.8	20	666	22	0	9	0.7
Fish, sardine, canned in oil	1 can (3.75 oz)	92	191	22.7	0	0	10.5	1.4	131	465	62	0	351	2.7
Fish, snapper, baked/broiled	100 g	85	109	22.3	0	0	1.5	0.3	40	48	30	1.4	34	0.2
Fish sticks	3 sticks	84	228	13.1	19.9	0	10.3	2.6	94	489	26	0	17	0.6
Fish, swordfish, baked/broiled	100 g	85	132	21.6	0	0	4.4	1.2	43	98	35	0.9	5	0.9
Fish, trout, baked/broiled	100 g	85	162	22.6	0	0	7.2	1.3	63	57	16	0.4	47	1.6
Fish, tuna, canned in oil	100 g	85	158	22.6	0	0	6.9	1.4	26	337	4	0	3	0.6
Fish, tuna, canned in water	100 g	85	109	20.1	0	0	2.5	0.7	36	320	5	0	12	0.8
Ham, extra lean	100 g	85	116	18.0	0.4	0	4.1	1.4	26	965	0	0	5	0.8
Ham, regular	100 g	85	192	17.5	0.4	0	12.9	4.3	53	800	0	11.9	7	1.2
Lamb, trimmed	100 g	85	218	20.8	0	0	14.3	6.7	74	65	0	0	14	1.6
Lunch meat, beef pastrami	100 g	85	297	14.7	2.6	0	24.8	8.9	79	1043	0	0	8	1.6
Lunch meat, beef, sliced	100 g	85	151	23.9	4.9	0	3.3	1.4	35	1224	0	0	9	2.3
Lunch meat, bologna (beef)	3 slices	85	265	10.4	0.7	0	24.2	10.3	49	834	0	0	10	1.4
Lunch meat, bologna (turkey)	3 slices	85	169	11.7	0.8	0	12.9	4.3	84	747	0	0	71	1.3

Name	Amount	Weight g	Energy calories	Protein g	Carb. g	Fibre g	Total fat g	Sat. fat g	Chol. mg	Sod. mg	Vit. A RE	Vit. C mg	Calc. mg	Iron mg
Lunch meat, chicken breast	100 g	85	108	14.3	1.9	0	4.7	1.2	50	1005	0	0	14	1.3
Lunch meat, franks (beef)	1 frank	57	180	6.8	1.0	0	16.2	6.9	35	585	0	0	11	0.8
Lunch meat, franks (chicken)	1 frank	45	116	5.8	3.1	0	8.8	2.5	45	617	17	0	43	0.9
Lunch meat, ham, lean, sliced	3 slices	85	111	16.5	0.8	0	4.2	1.4	40	1215	0	0	6	0.6
Lunch meat, liverwurst	100 g	85	277	12.0	1.9	0	24.2	9.0	134	731	7066	0	22	5.4
Lunch meat, salami, dry	8 slices	80	326	18.3	1.3	0	27.5	9.8	63	1808	0	0	10	1.2
Lunch meat, turkey, smoked	100 g	85	85	15.0	2.0	0	2.0	0.5	36	781	0	0	8	0.6
Meatloaf (80% lean meat)	100 g	85	216	21.5	0	0	13.7	5.2	76	57	0	0	20	2.2
Nuts, almonds	⅓ cup	47	274	10.1	9.3	5.6	24.0	1.8	0	0	0	0	117	2.0
Nuts, cashews, dry roasted	⅓ cup	46	262	7.0	14.9	1.4	21.2	4.2	0	7	0	0	21	2.7
Nuts, chestnuts, roasted	⅓ cup	48	117	1.5	25.2	2.4	1.0	0.2	0	1	1	12.4	14	0.4
Nuts, macadamia, dry roasted	⅓ cup	45	321	3.5	6.0	3.6	34.0	5.3	0	2	0	0.3	31	0.3
Nuts, pecans	⅓ cup	36	249	3.3	5.0	3.5	25.9	2.2	0	0	2	0.4	25	0.9
Nuts, pine	⅓ cup	45	300	6.1	5.8	1.6	30.5	2.2	0	1	0	0.4	7	2.5
Nuts, pistachios, dry roasted	⅓ cup	43	244	9.1	11.8	4.4	19.6	2.4	0	4	23	1.0	47	1.8
Nuts, walnuts	⅓ cup	41	255	9.9	4.1	2.8	24.3	1.4	0	1	1	0.7	25	1.3
Peanut butter, chunky	2 tablespoons	32	190	8.3	5.7	1.8	16.5	3.2	0	117	375	0	17	5.6
Peanut butter, smooth	2 tablespoons	32	190	8.1	6.2	1.9	16.3	3.3	0	149	0	0	12	0.6
Peanuts, dry roasted	⅓ cup	45	269	7.8	11.5	4.1	23.3	3.1	0	5	0	0.2	32	1.7
Pork chop, pan fried	100 g	85	190	23.5	0	0	10.0	3.7	60	44	2	0.3	4	0.7
Pork ribs, braised	100 g	85	252	20.3	0	0	18.3	6.8	74	50	2	0.6	25	1.0
Pork roast	100 g	85	214	22.9	0	0	12.9	4.5	69	41	3	0	5	0.8
Pumpkin seeds, roasted	¼ cup	57	296	18.7	7.6	2.2	23.9	4.5	0	10	22	1.0	24	8.5
Sausage, beef	1 sausage	43	134	6.1	1.0	0	11.6	4.9	29	486	0	0	3	0.8
Sausage, pork	1 link	68	265	15.1	1.4	0	21.6	7.7	46	1020	0	1.4	20	0.8
Sausage, smoked links	3 5 cm links	48	161	6.4	0.7	0	14.6	5.1	34	454	0	0	5	0.7
Shellfish, clams, canned	100 g	85	126	21.7	4.4	0	1.7	0.2	57	95	154	18.8	78	23.8
Shellfish, clams, steamed	10 clams	95	140	24.3	4.9	0	1.9	0.2	64	106	162	21.0	87	26.6
Shellfish, crab, steamed	100 g	85	82	16.4	0	0	1.3	0.1	45	911	8	6.5	50	0.6
Shellfish, oysters, fried	6 medium	88	173	7.7	10.2	0	11.1	2.8	71	367	79	3.3	55	6.1
Shellfish, shrimp, canned	100 g	85	102	19.6	0.9	0	1.7	0.3	147	144	15	2.0	50	2.3
Shellfish, shrimp, fried	4 large	30	73	6.4	3.4	0.1	3.7	0.6	53	103	17	0.5	20	0.4
Sunflower seeds, dry roasted	¼ cup	32	186	6.2	7.7	3.6	15.9	1.7	0	1	0	0.4	22	1.2
Tempeh	½ cup	83	160	15.4	7.8	0	9.0	1.8	0	7	0	0	92	2.2
Tofu, firm	½ cup	126	183	19.9	5.4	2.9	11.0	1.6	0	18	10	0.3	861	13.2
Turkey, dk mt, w/o skin, rst	100 g	85	138	24.5	0	0	3.7	1.2	95	67	0	0	22	2.0
Turkey, dk mt, w/skin, rst	100 g	85	155	23.5	0	0	6.0	1.8	99	65	0	0	23	2.0
Turkey, lt mt, w/o skin, rst	100 g	85	119	25.7	0	0	1.0	0.3	73	48	0	0	13	1.3
Turkey, lt mt, w/skin, rst	100 g	85	139	24.5	0	0	3.9	1.1	81	48	0	0	15	1.4
Veal, sirloin, roasted	100 g	85	172	21.4	0	0	8.9	3.8	87	71	0	0	11	0.8
Vegetarian bacon, cooked	30 g	16	50	1.7	1.0	0.4	4.7	0.7	0	234	1	0	4	0.4
Vegetarian franks	1 frank	51	118	12.1	1.5	1.5	7.1	0.8	0	224	0	0	10	1.0
Vegetarian patties	1 patty	67	119	11.2	10.2	4.0	3.8	0.5	0	382	76	0	48	1.2
Vegetarian sausage	1 patty	38	97	7.0	3.7	1.1	6.9	1.1	0	337	24	0	24	1.4

OTHER FOODS
Canada's Food Guide to Healthy Eating classifies foods that increase taste and enjoyment into Other Foods. Their higher fat and calorie contents require that Canadians be advised to consume these foods in moderation. The total amount of Other Foods you consume should be determined by your overall energy needs. Foods from this group should not replace foods from the other groups because they tend to provide calories but few nutrients.

Name	Amount	Weight g	Energy calories	Protein g	Carb. g	Fibre g	Total fat g	Sat. fat g	Chol. mg	Sod. mg	Vit. A RE	Vit. C mg	Calc. mg	Iron mg
Alcoholic beverage, beer	1 can or bottle	356	146	1.1	13.2	0.7	0	0	0	14	0	0	18	0.1
Alcoholic beverage, liquor	50 ml	42	97	0	0	0	0	0	0	0	0	0	0	0
Alcoholic beverage, wine	170 ml	148	106	0.3	2.5	0	0	0	0	7	0	0	12	0.6
Bacon	3 slices	24	126	9.1	0.4	0	9.6	3.2	27	575	3	0	3	0.3
Beverage, fruit punch	1 cup	247	114	0	28.9	0.2	0	0	0	10	2	108.4	10	0.2
Beverage, cola	1 can	370	155	0	39.7	0	0	0	0	15	0	0	11	0.1
Beverage, lemon-lime soda	1 can	368	147	0	38.3	0	0	0	0	40	0	0	7	0.3
Beverage, tea, bottled, sweetened	1 bottle	480	178	0	40.8	0	0	0	0	0	0	0	0	0

Name	Amount	Weight g	Energy calories	Protein g	Carb. g	Fibre g	Total fat g	Sat. fat g	Chol. mg	Sod. mg	Vit. A RE	Vit. C mg	Calc. mg	Iron mg
Butter	1 tablespoon	14	102	0.1	0	0	11.5	7.1	31	82	97	0	3	0
Candy, caramels	1 piece	10	39	0.5	7.8	0.1	0.8	0.7	1	25	1	0.1	14	0
Candy, fudge	1 piece	17	70	0.4	13	0.3	1.8	1.0	2	8	7	0	8	0.3
Candy, jelly beans	10 large	28	104	0	26.4	0	0.1	0	0	7	0	0	1	0.3
Candy, milk chocolate	1 bar	44	235	3.4	26.1	1.5	13.1	6.3	10	35	22	0	83	1.0
Chocolate syrup	2 tablespoons	39	109	0.8	25.4	1.0	0.4	0.2	0	28	0	0.1	5	0.8
Cream, half and half	2 tablespoons	30	39	0.9	1.3	0	3.5	2.2	11	12	29	0.3	32	0
Cream, heavy, whipped	½ cup	60	206	1.2	1.7	0	22.1	13.8	82	23	247	0.4	39	0
Cream, sour	1 tablespoon	12	26	0.4	0.5	0	2.5	1.6	5	6	21	0.1	14	0
Frosting, chocolate	2 tablespoons	41	163	0.5	25.9	0.4	7.2	2.3	0	75	0	0	3	0.6
Honey	1 tablespoon	21	64	0.1	17.3	0	0	0	0	1	0	0.1	1	0.1
Jam/preserves	1 tablespoon	20	56	0.1	13.8	0.2	0	0	0	6	0	1.8	4	0.1
Lard	1 tablespoon	13	115	0	0	0	12.8	5.0	12	0	0	0	0	0
Marmalade, orange	1 tablespoon	20	49	0.1	13.3	0	0	0	0	11	1	1.0	8	0
Margarine, regular stick	1 tablespoon	14	99	0	0.3	0	11.0	2.1	0	92	115	0	0	0
Margarine, liquid	1 tablespoon	14	102	0.3	0	0	11.4	1.9	0	111	113	0	9	0
Margarine, soft	1 tablespoon	14	101	0.1	0	0	11.3	2.0	0	152	113	0	4	0
Margarine-like spread	1 tablespoon	14	50	0.1	0.1	0	5.6	1.1	0	138	118	0	3	0
Mayonnaise, regular	1 tablespoon	15	57	0.1	3.5	0	4.9	0.7	4	105	12	0	2	0
Mayonnaise, fat free	1 tablespoon	16	11	0	2.0	0.3	0.4	6.1	2	120	1	0	1	0
Oil, canola	1 tablespoon	14	124	0	0	0	14.0	1.0	0	0	0	0	0	0
Oil, corn	1 tablespoon	14	120	0	0	0	13.6	1.7	0	0	0	0	0	0
Oil, olive	1 tablespoon	14	119	0	0	0	13.5	1.8	0	0	0	0	0	0.1
Popsicle	1 single stick	88	63	0	16.6	0	0	0	0	11	0	9.4	0	0
Salad dressing, blue cheese	2 tablespoons	31	154	1.5	2.3	0	16.0	3.0	5	335	20	0.6	25	0.1
Salad dressing, French	2 tablespoons	32	146	0.3	5.0	0	14.3	1.8	0	268	7	0	8	0.3
Salad dressing, Italian	2 tablespoons	29	86	0.1	3.1	0	8.3	1.3	0	486	1	0	2	0.2
Salad dressing, Italian, light	2 tablespoons	30	32	0	1.5	0	2.9	0.4	2	236	0	0	1	0.1
Sherbet	½ cup	74	107	0.8	22.5	0	1.5	0.9	0	34	7	2.3	40	0.1
Shortening, vegetable	1 tablespoon	13	115	0	0	0	12.8	5.2	0	0	0	0	0	0
Sugar, brown	1 tablespoon	14	52	0	13.4	0	0	0	0	5	0	0	12	0.3
Sugar, white	1 tablespoon	13	49	0	12.6	0	0	0	0	0	0	0	0	0
Syrup, corn	1 tablespoon	20	56	0	15.3	0	0	0	0	24	0	0	1	0
Syrup, maple	¼ cup	79	206	0	52.9	0	0.2	0	0	7	0	0	53	0.9

SOURCE: U.S. Department of Agriculture, Agricultural Research Service. 2004. *USDA Nutrient Database for Standard Reference, Release 16.1* (http://www.nal.usda.gov/fnic/foodcomp).

NUTRITIONAL CONTENT OF POPULAR ITEMS FROM FAST-FOOD RESTAURANTS

If you are developing a behaviour change plan to improve your diet, or if you simply want to choose healthier foods, you may want to know more about the nutritional content of common food items.

You can track your daily food intake and calculate your nutrient intake from foods with Health Canada's Canadian Nutrient File: www.hc-sc.gc.ca/fn-an/nutrition/fiche-nutri-data/index-eng.php. This database lists foods by both description and nutrient content to give you as precise as possible a calculation of the types and quantities of nutrients you are consuming.

Although most foods served at fast-food restaurants are high in calories, fat, saturated fat, cholesterol, sodium, and sugar, some items are healthier than others. If you eat at fast-food restaurants, knowing the nutritional content of various items can help you make better choices. Fast-food restaurants provide nutritional information both online and in print brochures available at most restaurant locations. To learn more about the items you order, visit the restaurants' websites. The following is a list of some common fast-food restaurants and URLs for accessing their nutrition guides:

- Arby's: www.arbys.ca/menu
- Burger King: www.burgerking.ca/en/View.aspx?uid=TopMenu_Nutrition
- Domino's Pizza: http://cache.dominos.com/ca021700/base/pdf/Canadian+Nutrition+Guide+Final+Secure.pdf
- KFC: www.kfc.ca/en/assets/pdf/KFC11834_NutritionalChart_Eng.pdf
- McDonald's: www.mcdonalds.ca/ca/en/food/nutrition_calculator.html
- Papa John's Pizza: www.papajohns.com/menu/nutritional_info.shtm
- Pizza Hut: www.pizzahut.ca/nutrition.aspx
- Subway: www.subway.com/Nutrition/Files/CanNutritionValues.pdf
- Taco Bell: www.tacobell.ca
- Tim Hortons: www.timhortons.com/ca/en/menu/menu-info.html
- Wendy's: www.wendys.ca/food/Nutrition.jsp?product_id=21&skip_update=true

MONITORING YOUR PROGRESS

C

NAME _____ SECTION _____ DATE _____

As you completed the 13 labs listed below, you entered the results in the Preprogram Assessment column of this lab. Now that you have been involved in a fitness and wellness program for some time, do the labs again and enter your new results in the Postprogram Assessment column. You will probably notice improvement in several areas. Congratulations! If you are not satisfied with your progress thus far, refer to the tips for successful behaviour change in Chapter 1 and throughout this book. Remember—fitness and wellness are forever. The time you invest now in developing a comprehensive, individualized program will pay off in a richer, more vital life in the years to come.

	Preprogram Assessment	Postprogram Assessment
LAB 2.2 Activity Profile	Sleep: _____ hours Light activity: _____ hours Moderate activity: _____ hours Vigorous activity: _____ hours Stairs climbed: _____ flights	Sleep: _____ hours Light activity: _____ hours Moderate activity: _____ hours Vigorous activity: _____ hours Stairs climbed: _____ flights
LAB 3.1 Cardiorespiratory Endurance 1.6-km walk test 3-minute step test 2.4-km run-walk test	$\dot{V}O_{2max}$: _____ Rating: _____ $\dot{V}O_{2max}$: _____ Rating: _____ $\dot{V}O_{2max}$: _____ Rating: _____	$\dot{V}O_{2max}$: _____ Rating: _____ $\dot{V}O_{2max}$: _____ Rating: _____ $\dot{V}O_{2max}$: _____ Rating: _____
LAB 4.1 Muscular Strength Maximum bench press test Maximum leg press test Hand grip strength test	Weight: _____ kg Rating: _____ Weight: _____ kg Rating: _____ Weight: _____ kg Rating: _____	Weight: _____ kg Rating: _____ Weight: _____ kg Rating: _____ Weight: _____ kg Rating: _____
LAB 4.2 Muscular Endurance Curl-up test Push-up test	Number: _____ Rating: _____ Number: _____ Rating: _____	Number: _____ Rating: _____ Number: _____ Rating: _____
LAB 5.1 Flexibility Sit-and-reach test	Score: _____ cm Rating: _____	Score: _____ cm Rating: _____

	Preprogram Assessment	Postprogram Assessment
LAB 5.3 Low-Back Muscular Endurance Side bridge endurance test Trunk flexors endurance test Back extensors endurance test	Right: _____ sec Rating: _____ Left: _____ sec Rating: _____ Trunk flexors: _____ sec Rating: _____ Back extensors: _____ sec Rating: _____	Right: _____ sec Rating: _____ Left: _____ sec Rating: _____ Trunk flexors: _____ sec Rating: _____ Back extensors: _____ sec Rating: _____
LAB 6.1 Body Composition Body mass index Skinfold measurements (or other method for determining percent body fat) Waist circumference Waist-to-hip-circumference ratio	BMI: _____ kg/m^2 Rating: _____ Sum of 3 skinfolds: _____ mm % body fat: _____ % Rating: _____ Circumf.: _____ Rating: _____ Ratio: _____ Rating: _____	BMI: _____ kg/m^2 Rating: _____ Sum of 3 skinfolds: _____ mm % body fat: _____ % Rating: _____ Circumf.: _____ Rating: _____ Ratio: _____ Rating: _____
LAB 7.1 Daily Diet Number of servings Number of servings Number of servings Number of servings	Milk products: _____ Meat and alternatives: _____ Fruits and vegetables: _____ Grain products: _____	Milk products: _____ Meat and alternatives: _____ Fruits and vegetables: _____ Grain products: _____
LAB 7.2 Dietary Analysis Percentage of calories Percentage of calories Percentage of calories Percentage of calories	From protein: _____% From fat: _____% From saturated fat: _____% From carbohydrate: _____%	From protein: _____% From fat: _____% From saturated fat: _____% From carbohydrate: _____%
LAB 8.1 Daily Energy Needs	Daily energy needs: _____ cal/day	Daily energy needs: _____ cal/day
LAB 10.1 Identifying Stressors	Average weekly stress score: _____	Average weekly stress score: _____
LAB 11.1 Cardiovascular Health CVD risk assessment Hostility assessment	Score: _____ Estimated risk: _____ Score: _____ Rating: _____	Score: _____ Estimated risk: _____ Score: _____ Rating: _____
LAB 12.1 Cancer Prevention Diet: Number of servings Skin cancer	Fruits/vegetables: _____ Score: _____ Risk: _____	Fruits/vegetables: _____ Score: _____ Risk: _____

BEHAVIOUR CHANGE WORKBOOK

This workbook is designed to take you step by step through the process of behaviour change. The first eight activities in the workbook will help you develop a successful plan—beginning with choosing a target behaviour and moving through the program planning steps described in Chapter 1, including the completion and signing of a behaviour change contract. The final seven activities will help you work through common obstacles to behaviour change and maximize your program's chances of success.

Part 1   Developing a Plan for Behaviour Change and Completing a Contract

1. Choosing a Target Behaviour
2. Gathering Information About Your Target Behaviour
3. Monitoring Your Current Patterns of Behaviour
4. Setting Goals
5. Examining Your Attitudes About Your Target Behaviour
6. Choosing Rewards
7. Breaking Behaviour Chains
8. Completing a Contract for Behaviour Change

Part 2   Overcoming Obstacles to Behaviour Change

9. Building Motivation and Commitment
10. Managing Your Time Successfully
11. Developing Realistic Self-Talk
12. Involving the People Around You
13. Dealing with Feelings
14. Overcoming Peer Pressure: Communicating Assertively
15. Maintaining Your Program over Time

ACTIVITY 1   CHOOSING A TARGET BEHAVIOUR

Use your knowledge of yourself and the results of Lab 1.2 (Lifestyle Evaluation) to identify five behaviours that you could change to improve your level of wellness. Examples of target behaviours include smoking cigarettes, not exercising regularly, eating candy bars every night, not getting enough sleep, getting drunk frequently on weekends, and not wearing a safety belt when driving or riding in a car. List your five behaviours below.

1. _____
2. _____
3. _____
4. _____
5. _____

For successful behaviour change, it's best to focus on one behaviour at a time. Review your list of behaviours and select one to start with. Choose a behaviour that is important to you and that you are strongly motivated to change. If this will be your first attempt at behaviour change, start with a simple change, such as wearing your bicycle helmet regularly, before tackling a more difficult change, such as quitting smoking. Circle the behaviour on your list that you've chosen to start with; this will be your target behaviour throughout this workbook.

ACTIVITY 2 GATHERING INFORMATION ABOUT YOUR TARGET BEHAVIOUR

Take a close look at what your target behaviour means to your health, now and in the future. How is it affecting your level of wellness? What diseases or conditions does this behaviour place you at risk for? What will changing this behaviour mean to you? To evaluate your behaviour, use information from this text, from the resources listed in the For Further Exploration section at the end of each chapter, and from other reliable sources.

Health behaviours have short-term and long-term benefits and costs associated with them. For example, in the short term, an inactive lifestyle allows for more time to watch TV and hang out with friends but leaves a person less able to participate in recreational activities. In the long term, it increases risk for cardiovascular disease, cancer, and premature death. Fill in the blanks below with the benefits and costs of continuing your current behaviour and of changing to a new, healthier behaviour. Pay close attention to the short-term benefits of the new behaviour—these are an important motivating force behind successful behaviour change programs.

Target (current) behaviour _____

Benefits   *Short-Term*   *Long-Term*

_____   _____

_____   _____

Costs   *Short-Term*   *Long-Term*

_____   _____

_____   _____

New behaviour _____

Benefits   *Short-Term*   *Long-Term*

_____   _____

_____   _____

Costs   *Short-Term*   *Long-Term*

_____   _____

_____   _____

ACTIVITY 3 MONITORING YOUR CURRENT PATTERNS OF BEHAVIOUR

To develop a successful behaviour change program, you need detailed information about your own behaviour patterns. You can obtain this information by developing a system of record keeping geared toward your target behaviour. Depending on your target behaviour, you may want to monitor a single behaviour, such as your diet, or you may want to keep daily activity records to determine how you could make time for exercise or another new behaviour. Consider tracking factors such as the following:

- What the behaviour was
- When and for how long it occurred
- Where it occurred
- What else you were doing at the time
- What other people you were with and how they influenced you
- What your thoughts and feelings were
- How strong your urge for the behaviour was (for example, how hungry you were or how much you wanted to watch TV)

Figure 1.6 shows a sample log for tracking daily diet. Below, create a format for a sample daily log for monitoring the behaviour patterns relating to your target behaviour. Then use this sample log to monitor your behaviour for a day.

Evaluate the log you've created as you use it. Ask yourself if you are tracking all the key factors that influence your behaviour; make any necessary adjustments to the format of your log. Once you've developed an appropriate format for your log, use a separate notebook (your health journal) to keep records of your behaviour for a week or two. These records will provide solid information about your behaviour that will help you develop a successful behaviour change program. Later activities in this workbook will ask you to analyze your records.

ACTIVITY 4   SETTING GOALS

For your behaviour change program to succeed, you must set meaningful, realistic goals. In addition to an ultimate goal, set some intermediate goals—milestones that you can strive for on the way to your final objective. For example, if your overall goal is to run a 5K road race, an intermediate goal might be to successfully complete 2 weeks of your fitness program. If you set a final goal of eating 7 servings of fruits and vegetables every day, an intermediate goal would be to increase your daily intake from 3 to 4 servings. List your intermediate and final goals below. Don't strive for immediate perfection. Allow an adequate amount of time to reach each of your goals.

Intermediate Goals   **Target Date**

_____   _____

_____   _____

_____   _____

_____   _____

Final Goal

_____   _____

ACTIVITY 5   EXAMINING YOUR ATTITUDES ABOUT YOUR TARGET BEHAVIOUR

Your attitudes toward your target behaviour can determine whether your behaviour change program will be successful. Consider your attitudes carefully by completing the following statements about how you think and feel about your current behaviour and your goal.

1. I like _____ because _____
           (current behaviour)
   _____

2. I don't like _____ because _____
                 (current behaviour)
   _____

3. I like _____ because _____
           (behaviour goal)
   _____

4. I don't like _____ because _____
                 (behaviour goal)
   _____

5. I don't _____ now because _____
            (behaviour goal)
   _____

6. I would be more likely to _____ if _____
                              (behaviour goal)
   _____

If your statements indicate that you have major reservations about changing your behaviour, work to build your motivation and commitment before you begin your program. Look carefully at your objections to changing your behaviour. How valid and important are they? What can you do to overcome them? Can you adopt any of the strategies you listed under statement 6? Review the facts about your current behaviour and your goals.

ACTIVITY 6   CHOOSING REWARDS

Make a list of objects, activities, and events you can use as rewards for achieving the goals of your behaviour change program. Rewards should be special, relatively inexpensive, and preferably unrelated to food or alcohol: for example, tickets to a hockey game, a CD, or a long-distance phone call to a family member or friend—whatever is meaningful for you. Write down a variety of rewards you can use when you reach milestones in your program and your final goal.

_____   _____

_____   _____

_____   _____

_____   _____

Many people also find it helpful to give themselves small rewards daily or weekly for sticking with their behaviour change program. These could be things like a study break, a movie, or a Saturday morning bike ride. Make a list of rewards for maintaining your program in the short term.

_____   _____

_____   _____

_____   _____

And don't forget to congratulate yourself regularly during your behaviour change program. Notice how much better you feel. Savour how far you've come and how you've gained control of your behaviour.

ACTIVITY 7   BREAKING BEHAVIOUR CHAINS

Use the records you collected about your target behaviour in Activity 3 and in your health journal to identify what leads up to your target behaviour and what follows it. By tracing these chains of events, you'll be able to identify points in the chain where you can make a change that will lead to your new behaviour. The following sample behaviour chain shows a sequence of events for a person who wants to add exercise to her daily routine—but who winds up snacking and watching TV instead. By examining the chain carefully, one can identify ways to break it at every step. After you review the sample, go through the same process for a typical chain of events involving your target behaviour. Use the blank behaviour chain , which follows the sample behaviour chain.

Some general strategies for breaking behaviour chains include the following:

- *Control or eliminate environmental cues that provoke the behaviour.* Stay out of the room where your television is located. Go out for an ice cream cone instead of keeping a half gallon of ice cream in your freezer.
- *Change behaviours or habits that are linked to your target behaviour.* If you always smoke in your car when you drive to school, try taking public transportation instead.
- *Add new cues to your environment to trigger your new behaviour.* Prepare easy-to-grab healthy snacks and carry them with you to class or work. Keep your exercise clothes and equipment in a visible location.

See also the suggestions in Chapter 1.

Chain of Events

Strategies for Breaking the Chain

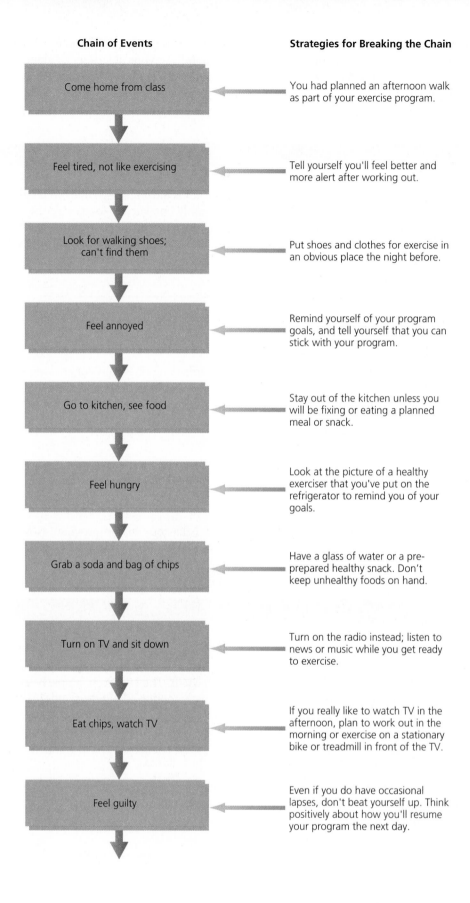

Chain of Events	Strategies for Breaking the Chain
Come home from class	You had planned an afternoon walk as part of your exercise program.
Feel tired, not like exercising	Tell yourself you'll feel better and more alert after working out.
Look for walking shoes; can't find them	Put shoes and clothes for exercise in an obvious place the night before.
Feel annoyed	Remind yourself of your program goals, and tell yourself that you can stick with your program.
Go to kitchen, see food	Stay out of the kitchen unless you will be fixing or eating a planned meal or snack.
Feel hungry	Look at the picture of a healthy exerciser that you've put on the refrigerator to remind you of your goals.
Grab a soda and bag of chips	Have a glass of water or a pre-prepared healthy snack. Don't keep unhealthy foods on hand.
Turn on TV and sit down	Turn on the radio instead; listen to news or music while you get ready to exercise.
Eat chips, watch TV	If you really like to watch TV in the afternoon, plan to work out in the morning or exercise on a stationary bike or treadmill in front of the TV.
Feel guilty	Even if you do have occasional lapses, don't beat yourself up. Think positively about how you'll resume your program the next day.

Chain of Events

Strategies for Breaking the Chain

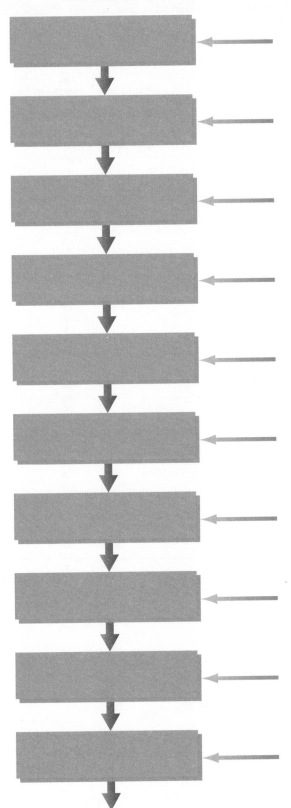

Your next step in creating a successful behaviour change program is to complete and sign a behaviour change contract. Your contract should include details of your program and indicate your commitment to changing your behaviour. Use the information from previous activities in this workbook to complete the following contract. (If your target behaviour relates to exercise, you may want to use the program plan and contract for a fitness program in Lab 9.1.)

1. I, _____ , agree to _____
   (name)   (specify behaviour you want to change)

   _____

2. I will begin on _____ and plan to reach my goal of _____
   (start date)   (specify final goal)

   _____ by _____

3. To reach my final goal, I have devised the following schedule of mini-goals. For each step in my program, I will give myself the reward listed.

   _____   _____   _____
   (mini-goal 1)   (target date)   (reward)

   _____   _____   _____
   (mini-goal 2)   (target date)   (reward)

   _____   _____   _____
   (mini-goal 3)   (target date)   (reward)

   _____   _____   _____
   (mini-goal 4)   (target date)   (reward)

   _____   _____   _____
   (mini-goal 5)   (target date)   (reward)

   My overall reward for reaching my final goal will be _____

4. I have gathered and analyzed data on my target behaviour and have identified the following strategies for changing

   my behaviour: _____

   _____

   _____

5. I will use the following tools to monitor my progress toward reaching my final goal:

   _____
                        (list any charts, graphs, or journals you plan to use)

   _____

   I sign this contract as an indication of my personal commitment to reach my goal.

   _____   _____
   (your signature)   (date)

   I have recruited a helper who will witness my contract and _____

   _____
                  (list any way in which your helper will participate in your program)

   _____   _____
   (helper's signature)   (date)

(See A Personal Fitness Program Plan and Contract in Chapter 9, Lab 9.1.)

Describe in detail any special strategies you will use to help change your behaviour (refer to Activity 7).

Create a plan below for any charts, graphs, or journals you will use to monitor your progress. The log format you developed in Activity 3 may be appropriate, or you may need to develop a more detailed or specific record-keeping system. Examples of journal formats are included in Labs 3.2, 4.3, 5.2, 9.1, and 10.1. You might also want to develop a graph to show your progress; posting such a graph in a prominent location can help keep your motivation strong and your program on track. Depending on your target behaviour, you could graph the number of push-ups you can do, the number of servings of vegetables you eat each day, or your average daily stress level.

Complete the following checklist to determine whether you are motivated and committed to changing your behaviour. Check the statements that are true for you.

_____ I feel responsible for my own behaviour and capable of managing it.

_____ I am not easily discouraged.

_____ I enjoy setting goals and then working to achieve them.

_____ I am good at keeping promises to myself.

_____ I like having a structure and schedule for my activities.

_____ I view my new behaviour as a necessity, not an optional activity.

_____ Compared with previous attempts to change my behaviour, I am more motivated now.

_____ My goals are realistic.

_____ I have a positive mental picture of the new behaviour.

_____ Considering the stresses in my life, I feel confident that I can stick to my program.

_____ I feel prepared for lapses and ups-and-downs in my behaviour change program.

_____ I feel that my plan for behaviour change is enjoyable.

_____ I feel comfortable telling other people about the change I am making in my behaviour.

Did you check most of these statements? If not, you need to boost your motivation and commitment. Consider these strategies:

- Review the potential benefits of changing your behaviour and the costs of not changing it (see Activity 2). Pay special attention to the short-term benefits of changing your behaviour, including feelings of accomplishment and self-confidence. Post a list of these benefits in a prominent location.
- Visualize yourself achieving your goal and enjoying its benefits. For example, if you want to manage time more effectively, picture yourself as a confident, organized person who systematically tackles important tasks and sets aside time each day for relaxation, exercise, and friends. Practise this type of visualization regularly.
- Put aside obstacles and objections to change. Counter thoughts such as "I'll never have time to exercise" with thoughts like "Lots of other people do it and so can I."
- Bombard yourself with propaganda. Take a class dealing with the change you want to make. Read books and watch television shows on the subject. Post motivational phrases or pictures on your refrigerator or over your desk. Talk to people who have already made the change.
- Build up your confidence. Remind yourself of other goals you've achieved. At the end of each day, mentally review your good decisions and actions. See yourself as a capable person, one who is in charge of her or his behaviour.

List two strategies for boosting your motivation and commitment; choose from the list above or develop your own. Try each strategy, and then describe how well it worked for you.

Strategy 1: _____

_____

How well it worked: _____

Strategy 2: _____

How well it worked: _____

_____

"Too little time" is a common excuse for not exercising or engaging in other healthy behaviours. Learning to manage your time successfully is crucial if you are to maintain a wellness lifestyle. The first step is to examine how you are currently spending your time; use the following grid broken into blocks to track your activities.

Time	Activity	Time	Activity
6:00 A.M.		6:00 P.M.	
6:30 A.M.		6:30 P.M.	
7:00 A.M.		7:00 P.M.	
8:00 A.M.		8:00 P.M.	
9:00 A.M.		9:00 P.M.	
10:00 A.M.		10:00 P.M.	
11:00 A.M.		11:00 P.M.	
12:00 P.M.		12:00 A.M.	
1:00 P.M.		1:00 A.M.	
2:00 P.M.		2:00 A.M.	
3:00 P.M.		3:00 A.M.	
4:00 P.M.		4:00 A.M.	
5:00 P.M.		5:00 A.M.	

Next, list each type of activity and the total time you engaged in it on a given day in the chart below (for example, sleeping, 7 hours; eating, 1.5 hours; studying, 3 hours; working, 3 hours; and so on). Take a close look at your list of activities. Successful time management is based on prioritization. Assign a priority to each of your activities according to how important it is to you: essential (A), somewhat important (B), or not important (C). Based on these priority rankings, make changes in your schedule by adding and subtracting hours from different categories of activities; enter a duration goal for each activity. Add your new activities to the list and assign a priority and duration goal to each.

Activity	Current Total Duration	Priority (A, B, or C)	Goal Total Duration

Prioritizing in this manner will involve tradeoffs. For example, you may choose to reduce the amount of time you spend watching television, listening to music, and chatting on the telephone while you increase the amount of time spent sleeping, studying, and exercising. Don't feel that you have to miss out on anything you enjoy. You can get more from less time by focusing on what you are doing. Strategies for managing time more productively and creatively are described in Chapter 10.

ACTIVITY 11   DEVELOPING REALISTIC SELF-TALK

Self-talk is the ongoing internal dialogue we have with ourselves throughout much of the day. Our thoughts can be accurate, positive, and supportive, or they can be exaggerated and negative. Self-talk is closely related to self-esteem and self-concept. Realistic self-talk can help maintain positive self-esteem, the belief that one is a good and competent person, worthy of friendship and love. A negative internal dialogue can reinforce negative self-esteem and can make behaviour change very difficult. Substituting realistic self-talk for negative self-talk can help you build and maintain self-esteem and cope better with the challenges in your life.

First, take a closer look at your current pattern of self-talk. Use your health journal to track self-talk, especially as it relates to your target behaviour. Does any of your self-talk fall into the common patterns of distorted negative self-talk shown in Chapter 10? If so, use the examples of realistic self-talk from Chapter 10 to develop more accurate and rational responses. Write your current negative thoughts in the left-hand column, and then record more realistic responses in the right-hand column.

Current Self-Talk About Target Behaviour

More Realistic Self-Talk

Your behaviour change program will be more successful if the people around you are supportive and involved—or at least are not sabotaging your efforts. Use your health journal to track how other people influence your target behaviour and your efforts to change it. For example, do you always skip exercising when you're with certain people? Do you always drink or eat too much when you socialize with certain friends? Are friends and family members offering you enthusiastic support for your efforts to change your behaviour, or do they make jokes about your program? Have they even noticed your efforts? Summarize the reactions of those around you in the chart below.

Target behaviour _____

Person	Typical Effect on Target Behaviour	Involvement in/Reaction to Program

It may be difficult to change the actions and reactions of the people who are close to you. For them to be involved in your program, you may need to develop new ways of interacting with them (for example, taking a walk rather than going out to dinner as a means of socializing). Most of your friends and family members will want to help you—if they know how. Ask for exactly the type of help or involvement you want. Do you want feedback, praise, or just cooperation? Would you like someone to witness your contract or to be involved more directly in your program? Do you want someone to stop sabotaging your efforts by inviting you to watch TV, eat rich desserts, and so on? Look for ways that the people who are close to you can share in your behaviour change program. They can help to motivate you and to maintain your commitment to your program. Develop a way that each individual you listed above can become involved in your program in a positive way.

Person	Target Involvement in Behaviour Change Program

Choose one person on your list to tackle first. Talk to that person about her or his current behaviour and how you would like her or him to be involved in your behaviour change program. Below, describe this person's reaction to your talk and her or his subsequent behaviour. Did this individual become a positive participant in your behaviour change program?

Longstanding habits are difficult to change in part because many represent ways people have developed to cope with certain feelings. For example, people may overeat when bored, skip their exercise sessions when frustrated, or drink alcoholic beverages when anxious. Developing new ways to deal with feelings can help improve the chance that a behaviour change program will succeed.

Review the records on your target behaviour that you kept in your health journal. Identify the feelings that are interfering with the success of your program and develop new strategies for coping with them. Some common problematic feelings are listed below, along with one possible coping strategy for each. Put a check mark next to those that are influencing your target behaviour and fill in additional strategies. Add the other feelings that are significant road-blocks in your program to the bottom of the chart, along with coping strategies for each.

✔	Feeling	Coping Strategies
	Stressed out	Go for a 10-minute walk.
	Anxious	Do one of the relaxation exercises described in Chapter 10.
	Bored	Call a friend for a chat.
	Tired	Take a 20-minute nap.
	Frustrated	Identify the source of the feeling and deal with it constructively.

Consider the following situations:

- Julia is trying to give up smoking; her friend Marie continues to offer her cigarettes whenever they are together.
- Emilio is planning to exercise in the morning; his roommates tell him he's being antisocial by not having brunch with them.
- Tracy's boyfriend told her that in high school he once experimented with drugs and shared needles; she wants him to have an HIV test, but he says he's sure the people he shared needles with were not infected.

Peer pressure is the common ingredient in these situations. To successfully maintain your behaviour change program, you must develop effective strategies for resisting peer pressure. Assertive communication is one such strategy. By communicating assertively—firmly, but not aggressively—you can stick with your program even in the face of pressure from others. Review your health journal to determine how other people affect your target behaviour. If you find that you often do give in to peer pressure, try the following strategies for communicating more assertively:

- Collect your thoughts, and plan in advance what you will say. You might try out your response on a friend to get some feedback.
- State your case—how you feel and what you want—as clearly as you can.
- Use "I" messages—statements about how you feel—rather than statements beginning with "You."
- Focus on the behaviour rather than the person. Suggest a solution, such as asking the other person to change his or her behaviour toward you. Avoid generalizations. Be specific about what you want.
- Make clear, constructive requests. Focus on your needs ("I would like . . .") rather than the mistakes of others ("You always . . .").
- Avoid blaming, accusing, and belittling. Treat others with the same respect you'd like to receive yourself.
- Ask for action ahead of time. Tell others what you would like to happen; don't wait for them to do the wrong thing and then get angry at them.
- Ask for a response to what you have proposed. Wait for an answer and listen carefully to it. Try to understand other people's points of view, just as you would hope that others would understand yours.

With these strategies in mind, review your health journal and identify three instances in which peer pressure interfered with your behaviour change program. For each of these instances, write out what you might have said to deal with the situation more assertively. (If you can't find three situations from your own experiences, choose one or more of the three scenarios described at the beginning of this activity.)

1. _____
   _____
   _____

2. _____
   _____
   _____

3. _____
   _____
   _____

Assertive communication can help you achieve your behaviour change goals in a direct way by helping you keep your program on track. It can also provide a boost for your self-image and increase your confidence in your ability to successfully manage your own behaviour.

If you maintain your new behaviour for at least 6 months, you've reached the maintenance stage and your chances of lifetime success are greatly increased. However, you may find yourself sliding back into old habits at some point. If this happens, there are some things you can do to help maintain your new behaviour.

• Remind yourself of the goals of your program (list them here).

_____

_____

_____

_____

• Pay attention to how your new pattern of behaviour has improved your wellness status. List the major benefits of changing your behaviour, both now and in the future.

_____

_____

_____

_____

• Consider the things you enjoy most about your new pattern of behaviour. List your favourite aspects.

_____

_____

_____

_____

• Think of yourself as a problem solver. If something begins to interfere with your program, devise strategies for dealing with it. Take time out now to list things that have the potential to derail your program and develop possible coping mechanisms.

Problem	Solution
_____	_____
_____	_____
_____	_____
_____	_____

• Remember the basics of behaviour change. If your program runs into trouble, go back to keeping records of your behaviour to pinpoint problem areas. Make adjustments in your program to deal with new disruptions. And don't feel defeated if you lapse. The best thing you can do is renew your commitment and continue with your program.

ENDNOTES

Chapter 1

1. Canadian Institite for Health Information. (2010, December). *Health Care in Canada*. Ottawa, CA: CIHI.
2. Heritage Canada (2004). Ministers Adopt New Canadian Policy on Doping in Sport. Proceedings of the Federal–Provincial–Territorial Conference of Ministers Responsible for Sport, Recreation and Fitness. Retrieved online at http://www.pch.gc.ca/newsroom/index_e.cfm?fuseaction=displayDocument&DocIDCd=4N0063.
3. Colley, R.C., Garriguet, D., Janssen, I., Craig, C.L., Clarke, J., & Tremblay, M.S. (2011). Physical activity levels of Canadian adults: Accelerometer results from the 2007 to 2009 Canadian Health Measures Survey. *Health Reports*, 22 (1).
4. Public Health Agency of Canada (2003). Healthy Living Unit. Physical Activity for Health–The Evidence (online). Retrieved online at http://www.phac-aspc.gc.ca/pau-uap/fitness/evidence.html#1.
5. Katzmaryzk, P.T., & Ardern, C.I. (2004). Overweight and obesity mortality trends in Canada, 1985–2000. *Canadian Journal of Public Health*, Jan/Feb, 2004.
6. Centers for Disease Control and Prevention (2004). NHANES Data on the Prevalence of Overweight and Obesity Among Adults: United States, 2003–2004. Retrieved online at www.cdc.gov/nccdphp/dnpa/obesity/trend/index.htm.
7. Canadian Centre on Substance Abuse. *The costs of substance abuse in Canada 2002: highlights*. Ottawa, Ontario: Canadian Centre on Substance Abuse, 2006.
8. Centers for Disease Control and Prevention. 2005. Annual smoking attributable mortality, years of potential life lost, and productivity losses—United States, 1997–2001. *Morbidity and Mortality Weekly Report* 54(5): 113–117.
9. Physicians for a smoke-free Canada (2002). Tobacco and the health of Canadians. Retrieved online at http://www.smoke-free.ca/Health/pscissues_health.htm.
10. Health Canada (2007). Reducing alcohol-related harm in Canada: Toward a culture of moderation. A report from the National Alcohol Strategy Working Group. Retrieved online at http://www.nationalframework-cadrenational.ca/uploads/files/FINAL_NAS_EN_April3_07.pdf.

Chapter 2

1. Canadian Fitness and Lifestyle Research Institute (2008). Bulletin 09: Attitudes towards physical activity. *Physical Activity Monitor*. Available online at: http://www.cflri.ca.
2. Lee, C.D., Blair, S.N., & Jackson, A.S. (1999). Cardiorespiratory fitness, body composition, and all-cause and cardiovascular disease mortality in men. *American Journal of Clinical Nutrition*, 69(3): 373–380.
3. Statistics Canada (2006). Prevalence of disability in Canada 2006. Available online at: http://www.statcan.gc.ca/pub/89-628-x/2007002/4125019-eng.htm.
4. Thomas, D.Q., Kotecki, J.E., & McCormack Brown, K. (2006). *Physical activity and health: An interactive approach* (2nd Ed), Toronto, CAN: Jones & Bartlett.
5. McArdle, W.D., Katch, F.I., & Katch, V.L. (2007). *Exercise physiology: Energy, nutrition, & human performance* (6th Ed), New York, USA:Lippincott Williams & Wilkins.

Chapter 3

1. Malina, R.M., Bouchard, C., & Bar-Or, O. (2004). *Growth, maturation, and physical activity*. Champaign, IL: Human Kinetics.
2. McTiernan, A., Yasui, Y., Sorensen, B., Irwin, M.L., Morgan, A., Rudolph, R.E., et al., (2006). Effect of a 12-month exercise intervention on patterns of cellular proliferation in colonic crypts: A randomized controlled trial. *Cancer Epidemiology Biomarkers and Prevention*, 15: 1588–1597.
3. Bernstein, L., Patel, A., Ursin, G., Sullivan-Halley, J., Press, M. F., Deapen, D., et al., (2005). Lifetime recreational exercise activity and breast cancer risk among black women and white women. *Journal of the National Cancer Institute*, 97(22): 1–9.
4. Shang, M., Lee, A.H., & Binns, C. W. (2003). Physical activity and epithelial ovarian cancer risk: A case-control study in China. *International Journal of Cancer*, 105(6): 838–843; Fang, C.Y., Miller, S.M., Bovjerg, D.H., Bergman, C., Edelson, M.I., & Rosenblum, N.G. (2008). Perceived stress is associated with impaired T-cell response to HPV16 in women with cervical dysplasia. *Annals of Behavioral Medicine*, 17(1): 87–96.
5. Canadian Diabetes Association (2007). Think diabetes can't affect you because you're young? Available online at: http://www.diabetes.ca/getserious/facts.htm.
6. Persinger, R., Foster, C., Gibson, M., Fater, D.C.W., & Porcari, J.P. (2004). Consistency of the Talk Test for exercise prescription. *Medicine and Science in Sport and Exercise* 36: 1632–1636.
7. Vetter, R.E. (2007). Effects of six warm-up protocols on sprint and jump performance. *Journal of Strength and Conditioning Research*, 21(3): 819– 823.

Chapter 4

1. Life in Canada a pain in the back: National survey (2003). *The Canadian Chiropractic Association*, June, 2003.
2. Lemmer, J.T., Martel, G.F., Hurlburt, D.E., Metter, J.E., Fozard, J.L., Fleg, J.L., & Hurley, B.F. (2001). Effects of strength training on resting metabolic rate and physical activity: Age and gender comparisons. *Medicine and Science of Sport and Exercise*, 33(4): 532–41.
3. Stump, T., Clark, D.O., Johnson, R.J., & Wolinsky, F.D. (1997). The structure of health status among Hispanic, African American, and White older adults. In W.W. Spirduso, K.L. Francis, & P.G. MacRae (Eds.), *Physical dimensions of aging* (pp. 109). Windsor, ON: Human Kinetics.
4. Osteoporosis Canada (2007). About osteoporosis. Available online at: http://www.osteoporosis.ca/english/About%20Osteoporosis/what-is/default.asp?s=1.
5. Heart and Stroke Foundation of Canada (n.d.). Types and amounts of physical activities. Available online at: http://www.heartandstroke.com/site/c.ikIQLcMWJtE/b.3484261/.

Chapter 5

1. Kiblmer, W.B., Chandler, T.J., Uhl, T., & Maddus, R.E. (1989). A musculoskeletal approach to the preparticipation physical examination. *American Journal of Sports Medicine*, 17: 525–531.
2. Shrier, I. (2004). Does stretching improve performance?: A systematic and critical review of the literature. *Clinical Journal of Sport Medicine*, 14(5): 267–273.
3. Gross, D.P., Ferrari, R., Russell, A.S., Battié, M.C., Schopflocher, D., Hu, R.W., et al. (2006). A population-based survey of back pain beliefs in Canada. *Spine*, 31(18): 2142–2145.
4. Shrier, I. (2004). Does stretching improve performance?: A systematic and critical review of the literature. *Clinical Journal of Sport Medicine*, 14(5): 267–273.

5. National Institute for Neurological Disorders and Stroke. Low back pain fact sheet. Available online at: http://www.ninds.nih.gov/disorders/backpain/detail_backpain.htm. Accessed December 2011.

6. Church, J., Schneider, M., Shipka, P., Triska, O., Smith, D., Slater, L., et al. (2004). *Review of current knowledge on the effectiveness and cost effectiveness of treatments for low back conditions*. Edmonton: Alberta Health Services Outcome Commission.

7. National Institute for Neurological Disorders and Stroke. Low back pain fact sheet. Available online at: http://www.ninds.nih.gov/disorders/backpain/detail_backpain.htm. Accessed December 2011.

Chapter 6

1. Statistics Canada. (2011). Overweight and obese adults (self-reported), 2010. *Health Facts Sheets* (Statistics Canada, Catalogue 82-625X). Available online at: http://www.statcan.gc.ca/pub/82-625-x/2011001/article/11464-eng.htm.

2. National Center for Health Statistics. 2006. 2003–2004 *National Health and Nutrition Examination Survey* (NHANES). Hyattsville, Md.: National Center for Health Statistics.

3. U.S. Department of Health and Human Services (2001). *The Surgeon General's call to action to prevent and decrease overweight and obesity*. Rockville, Maryland: U.S. Department of Health and Human Services, Public Health Service, Office of the Surgeon General.

4. Birmingham, C.L., Muller, J.L., Palepu, A., Spinelli, J.J., & Anis, A.H. (1999). The cost of obesity in Canada. *Canadian Medical Association Journal*, 160(4): 483–488.

5. Centers or Disease Control and Prevention. 2008. *Preventing Obesity and Chronic Diseases Through Good Nutrition and Physical Activity*. Available online at: http://www.cdc.gov/nccdphp/publications/factsheets/Prevention/obesity.htm.

6. Blackwell Publishing Ltd. (2007, March 12). Dialysis patients with metabolic syndrome show increased risk for heart disease. *ScienceDaily*. Available online at: http://www.sciencedaily.com-/releases/2007/03/070307152542.htm.

7. Pearl, B., & Moran, G.T. (2001). *Getting stronger: Weight training for men and women* [revised edition]. Bolinas, CA: Shelter Publications Inc.

Chapter 7

1. Garriguet, D. (2004). *Nutrition: Findings from the Canadian Community Health Survey*. Statistics Canada, Catalogue 82-620-MIE-No. 2.

2. Ibid.

3. Health Canada (2009). Food and nutrition: General questions and answers about trans fats. Available online at: http://www.hc-sc.gc.ca/fn-an/nutrition/gras-trans-fats/tfa-age_question-eng.php.

4. Ibid.

5. Ibid.

6. Ibid.

7. Messina, V., Melina, V., & Reed Mangels, A. (2003). A new food guide for North Americans. *Canadian Journal of Dietetic Practice and Research*, 64: 82-86.

Chapter 8

1. Canadian community health survey: Adult obesity in Canada: Measured height and weight (2008, November 18). Statistics Canada. Available online at: www.statcan.ca/english/research/82-620-MIE/2005001/articles/adults/aobesity.htm.

2. National Center for Health Statistics (2006). *Health, United States, with chartbook on trends in the health of Americans*. Hyattsville, Md: National Center for Health Statistics.

3. Roche Canada. (1997, December). Canadian national obesity survey. Toronto, ON: Pollara. Available online at: http://www.pollara.com/Library/News/news_1201.html.

4. King, S., & Hendricks, K. (2005, March). Addressing obesity and physical inactivity in Canadian children: National study shows it can be done. Available online at: http://www.activehealthykids.ca/Ophea/ActiveHealthyKids_v2/upload/Obesity-and-Physical-Inactivity.pdf.

5. Katzmarzyk, P.T., Gledhill, N, & Shephard, R.J. (2000) The economic burden of physical inactivity in Canada. *Canadian Medical Association Journal*, 163: 11, 1435–1440.

6. Agras, W.S., Hammer, L.D., McNicholas, F., & Kraemer, H.C. (2004). Risk factors for childhood overweight: A prospective study from birth to 9.5 years. *Journal of Pediatrics*, 145: 19–24.

7. Gray-Donald, K., Jacobs Starkey, L., & Johnson-Down, L. (2000). Food habits of Canadians: Reduction in fat intake over a generation. *Canadian Journal of Public Health*, 91(5): 381–385.

8. Canadian community health survey: Adult obesity in Canada: Measured height and weight (2008, November 18). Statistics Canada. Available online at: www.statcan.ca/english/research/82-620-MIE/2005001/articles/adults/aobesity.htm.

9. Ibid.

10. Schwartz, J., & Byrd-Bredbenner, C. (2006). Portion distortion: Typical sizes selected by young adults. *Journal of the American Dietetic Association*, 106(9): 1494–1495

11. Tjemkema, M. (2006). Adult obesity in Canada: Measured height and weight. Statistics Canada, Catalogue 82-620-MWE2005001.

12. Statistics Canada (2002). Mental health and well-being profile. (Table 105-1100).

13. Canadian Mental Health Association. About mental illness: Eating disorders. Available online at: http://www.cmha.ca/bins/content_page.asp?cid=3-98&lang=1.

14. Heweitt, P.L., Coren, S., & Steel, G.D. (2001). Death from anorexia nervosa: Age span and sex differences. *Aging and Mental Health*, 5(1): 41–46.

15. Canadian Mental Health Association. About mental illness: Eating disorders. Available online at: http://www.cmha.ca/bins/content_page.asp?cid=3-98&lang=1.

16. Hudson, J.I., Hiripi, E., Pope, H.G., Kessler, R.C. (2007). The prevalence and correlates of eating disorders in the National Comorbidity Survey replication. *Biological Psychiatry*, 61(3): 348–358.

17. Ross, R., Freeman, J. A., & Janssen, I. (2000). Exercise alone is an effective strategy for reducing obesity and related comorbidities. *Exercise and Sport Science Reviews*, 28(4): 165–170.

18. Curioni, C.C., & Lournco, P.M. (2005). Long-term weight loss after diet and exercise: A systematic review. *International Journal of Obesity*, 29: 1168–1174.

Chapter 9

1. Conference Board of Canada (2005). *Strengthening Canada: The Socio-economic Benefits of Sport Participation in Canada — Report August 2005*. Available at: http://www.conferenceboard.ca/documents.aspx?did=1340.

2. Active Healthy Kids Canada (2011). *Active Healthy Kids Report Card on Physical Activity for Children and Youth*. Available at: http://www.activehealthykids.ca/ReportCard/2011ReportCardOverview.aspx.

Chapter 10

1. Eliot, R.S. (1995). From stress to strength. *Stress Medicine*, 11(1): 139–140.

2. Landow, M.V. (ed). (2006). *Stress and mental health of college students*. Haupauge, NY: Nova Science Publishers.

3. Audet, C. (2009). *Executive summary: Student life survey (2002–2009)*. University of Alberta. Retrieved from http://www.uofaweb.ualberta.ca/counselling/execsummary.cfm on June 10, 2009.

4. Duxbury, L., Higgins, C., & Coghill, D. (2003). *Voices of Canadians: Seeking work-life balance* (Cat. No. RH54-12/2003). Hull, QU: Human Resources Development Canada.

5. Wallace, L.S., Buckworth, J., Kirby, T.E., & Sherman, W.M. (2000). Characteristics of exercise behaviour among college students: Application of social cognitive theory to predicting stage of change. *Preventative Medicine*, 31(5): 494–505.

6. Holt-Lunstad, J., Birmingham, W., & Jones, B.Q. (2008). Is there something unique about marriage? The relative impact of

marital status, relationship quality, and network social support on ambulatory blood pressure and mental health. *Annals of Behavioural Medicine*, 35(2): 239–44.

7. Crisis Intervention and Suicide Prevention Centre. Key suicide statistics. Available online at: http://www.crisiscentre.bc.ca/learn/stats.php.

Chapter 11

1. Heart and Stroke Foundation (2008). *Statistics*. Available online at: http://www.heartandstroke.com/site/c.ikIQLcMWJtE/b.3483991/k.34A8/Statistics.htm.

2. Linton, M. (2001). Healthy living a numbers game. Available online at: http://chealth.canoe.ca/columns.asp?columnistid=7&articleid=2387&relation_id=3224.

3. Canadian Stroke Network (2007). Reducing salt intake would eliminate hypertension in one million Canadians. Available online at: http://ww2.heartandstroke.ca/Page.asp?PageID=33&ArticleID=6207&Src=news&From=Category.

4. Health Canada (2007). Canadian Tobacco Use Monitoring Survey. Available online at: http://www.hc-sc.gc.ca/hl-vs/tobac-tabac/research-recherche/stat/ctums-esutc_2007-eng.php.

5. Statistics Canada. (2003). Community Health Survey (June 15, 2004). Available online at: http://www.statcan.ca/Daily/English/040615/d040615b.htm.

6. Physicians for a smoke-free Canada (nd). Tobacco and the health of Canadians. Available online at: http://www.smoke-free.ca/Health/pscissues_health.htm.

7. Qureshi, A.I., Suri, M.F., Kirmani, J.F., Divani, A.A., & Mohammad, Y. (2005). Is prehypertension a risk factor for cardiovascular diseases? *Stroke*, 36(9): 1859–63.

8. Grover, S.A., Coupal, L., Kaouache, M., & Lowensteyn, I. (2007). Preventing cardiovascular disease among Canadians: What are the potential benefits of treating hypertension or dyslipidemia? *The Canadian Journal of Cardiology*, 23(6): 467–473.

9. Public Health Agency of Canada (1997). Heart disease and stroke in Canada. Available online at: http://www.phac-aspc.gc.ca/publicat/hdsc97/s06_e.html.

10. Hu, G., Sarti, C., Jousilahti, J., Silventoinen, K., Barengo, N.C., & Tuomilehto, J. (2005). Leisure time, occupational, and commuting physical activity and the risk of stroke. *Stroke*, 36: 1994–1999.

11. Rosengren, A., Hawken, S., Ounpuu, S., Sliwa, K., Zubaid, M., Almahmeed, W.A., et.al. (2004). Association of psychosocial risk factors with risk of acute myocardial infarction in 11119 cases and 13648 controls from 52 countries (the INTERHEART study): Case-control study. *Lancet*, 364(9438): 953–62.

12. Stansfeld, S.A., Fuhrer, R., Shipley, M.J., & Marmot, M.G. (2002). Psychological distress as a risk factor for coronary heart disease in the Whitehall II Study. *International Journal of Epidemiology*, 31: 248–255.

13. Grover, S.A., Coupal, L., Kaouache, M., & Lowensteyn, I. (2007). Preventing cardiovascular disease among Canadians: What are the potential benefits of treating hypertension or dyslipidemia? *The Canadian Journal of Cardiology*, 23(6): 467–473.

14. Public Health Agency of Canada (1997). Heart disease and stroke in Canada. Available online at: http://www.phac-aspc.gc.ca/publicat/hdsc97/s06_e.html.

15. N.a. (2000). First Nations and Inuit regional health survey: National report 1999. St. Regis, QU: First Nations and Inuit Regional Health Survey Steering Committee.

16. Sheth, T., Nair, C., Nargundkar, M., Anand, S., & Yusul, S. (1999). Cardiovasular and cancer mortality among Canadians of European, south Asian, and Chinese origin from 1979 to 1993: An analysis of 1.2 million deaths. *Canadian Medical Association Journal*, 161(2): 132–8.

17. Heart and Stroke Foundation of Canada. (2003). *The growing burden of heart disease and stroke in Canada* 2003 (10896242-30-8). Ottawa, CAN: Author.

18. Anand S., Yi Q., Gerstein H., Loon E., Teo K., & Yusuf S., (2003). The study of health assessment and risk evaluation in Aboriginal people: Age-adjusted prevalence of metabolic syndrome in Canada. *Circulation*, 108: 420–425.

19. Heart and Stroke Foundation of Canada. (2003). *The growing burden of heart disease and stroke in Canada* 2003 (10896242-30-8). Ottawa, CAN: Author.

Chapter 12

1. Statistics Canada (2008), Health Statistics Division, Leading Causes of Death, by sex, 2008 (Table 102-0561).

2. Prostate Cancer Canada (2008). Statistics. Available online at: http://www.prostatecancer.ca/Prostate-Cancer/Prostate-Cancer/Statistics.aspx.

3. Prostate Cancer Canada (2008). Statistics. Available online at: http://www.prostatecancer.ca/Prostate-Cancer/Prostate-Cancer/Statistics.aspx.

4. Statistics Canada (2005). *Canadian Community Health Survey* (CCHS)–Cycle 3.1.

5. Ibid.

6. Canadian Cancer Society (2011). *Canadian Canadian Cancer Statistics 2011*. Available online at http://www.cancer.ca/Canada-wide/Publications/Alphabetical%20list%20of%20publications/Canadian%20Cancer%20Statistics.aspx?sc_lang=en.

7. Ibid.

8. Enger, S.M., Geif, J.M., Polokoff, J., & Press, M. (2004). Body weight correlates with mortality in early-stage breast cancer. *Archives of surgery*, 139(9): 954–960; Bianchini, F., Kaaks, R., & Vainio, H. (2002). Overweight, obesity, and cancer risk. *The Lancet Oncology*, 3(9): 565–574.

9. Bianchini, F., Kaaks, R., & Vainio, H. (2002). Overweight, obesity, and cancer risk. *The Lancet Oncology*, 3(9): 565–574.

Chapter 13

1. Broemeling, A-M., Weston, D.E., & Prebtani, F. (2008). Population patterns of chronic health conditions, comorbidity and healthcare use in Canada: Implications for policy and practice. *Healthcare Quarterly*, 11(3): 70–76.

2. Morrow-Howell, N., McCrary, S., Hong, S-I., & Blinne, W. (2008). *Experience Corps: Benefits of volunteering* (CSD Research Brief 08-23). St. Louis: Washington University, Center for Social Development.

SELECTED BIBLIOGRAPHY

Chapter 1

American Cancer Society. 2004. *Cancer Facts and Figures 2004*. Atlanta: American Cancer Society.

American Heart Association. 2004. *2004 Heart and Stroke Statistical Update*. Dallas, Tex.: American Heart Association.

Beers, M. H. 2004. *The Merck Manual of Med ical Information*. 2nd Home ed. New York: Pocket Books. Provides consumer-oriented advice for the prevention and treatment of common health concerns.

Calle, E. E., et al. 2003. Overweight, obesity, and mortality from cancer in a prospectively studied cohort of U.S. adults. *New England Journal of Medicine* 348(17): 1625–1638.

Canadian Fitness and Lifestyle Research Institute: 2008. Bulletin 02: Physical activity levels of Canadians. *Physical Activity Monitor* (http://www.cflri.ca; retrieved September 20, 2011).

Canadian Fitness and Lifestyle Research Institute: 2008. Bulletin 09: Attitudes towards physical activity. *Physical Activity Monitor* (http://www.cflri.ca; retrieved September 20, 2011).

Centers for Disease Control and Prevention. 2005. Racial/ethnic and socioeconomic disparities in multiple risk factors for heart disease and stroke, United States, 2003. *Morbidity and Mortality Weekly Report* 54(5): 113–117.

Centers for Disease Control and Prevention. 2005. Trends in leisure-time physical inactivity by age, sex, and race/ethnicity—United States, 1994–2004. *Morbidity and Mortality Weekly Report* 54(39): 991–994.

Centers for Disease Control and Prevention. 2006. Health behaviours of adults: United States, 2002–2004. *Vital and Health Statistics* 10(230).

Centers for Disease Control and Prevention. 2007. Prevalence of fruit and vegetable consumption and physical activity by race/ethnicity—United States, 2005. *Morbidity and Mortality Weekly Report* 56(13): 301–304.

Centers for Disease Control and Prevention. 2007. Prevalence of heart disease—United States, 2005. *Morbidity and Mortality Weekly Report* 56(6): 113–118.

Centers for Disease Control and Prevention. 2007. QuickStats: Prevalence of selected unhealthy behaviour characteristics among adults Aged ≥18 years, by race—National Health Interview Survey, United States, 2002–2004. *Morbidity and Mortality Weekly Report* 56(4): 79.

Centers for Disease Control and Prevention. 2008. Cigarette smoking among adults—United States, 2007. *Morbidity and Mortality Weekly Report* 57(45): 1221–1226.

Centers for Disease Control and Prevention. 2008. Smoking-attributable mortality, years of potential life lost, and productivity losses—United States, 2002–2004. *Morbidity and Mortality Weekly Report* 57(45): 1226–1228.

Chen, J., and W. Millar. 2001. Heart disease, family history and physical activity. *Health Report* 12(4): 23–32.

Department of Health and Human Services. 1996. *Physical Activity and Health: A Report of the Surgeon General*. Atlanta, Ga.: DHHS.

Ellison, L., H. Morrison, M. de Groh, and P. Villeneuve. (2000). Health consequences of smoking among Canadian smokers: An update. *Chronic Diseases in Canada* 20(3).

Finkelstein, E. A., et al. 2008. Do obese persons comprehend their personal health risks? *American Journal of Health Behaviour* 32(5): 508–516.

Gallagher, K. I., and J. M. Jakicic. 2002. Overcoming barriers to effective exercise programming. *ACSM's Health and Fitness Journal*, November/December.

Horneffer-Ginter, K. 2008. Stages of change and possible selves: Two tools for promoting college health. *Journal of American College Health* 56(4): 351–358.

Marcus, B. H., and L. H. Forsyth. 2003. *Motivating People to Be Physically Active*. Champaign, Ill.: Human Kinetics.

Martin, G., and J. Pear. 2007. *Behaviour Modification: What It Is and How to Do It*, 8th ed. Upper Saddle River, N.J.: Prentice-Hall.

Mokdad, A. H., et al. 2003. Prevalence of obesity, diabetes, and obesity-related health risk factors. *Journal of the American Medical Association* 289(1): 76–79.

Muller, A. 2002. Education, income inequality, and mortality: A multiple regression analysis. *British Medical Journal* 324(7328): 23–25.

National Center for Health Statistics. 2009. Deaths: Preliminary data for 2007. *National Vital Statistics Report* 58(1).

National Center for Health Statistics. 2009. *Health, United States, 2008*. Hyattsville, Md.: Public Health Service.

Ortlepp, J. R., et al. 2003. Relation of body mass index, physical fitness, and the cardiovascular risk profile in 3217 young normal weight men with an apparently optimal lifestyle. *International Journal of Obesity and Related Metabolic Disorders* 27(8): 979–982.

Prochaska, J. O., J. C. Norcross, and C. C. DiClemente. 1994. *Changing for Good: The Revolutionary Program That Explains the Six Stages of Change and Teaches You How to Free Yourself from Bad Habits*. New York: Morrow. Outlines the authors' model of behaviour change and offers suggestions and advice for each stage of change.

Ritchie, S. A., and J. M. Connell. 2007. The link between abdominal obesity, metabolic syndrome and cardiovascular disease. *Nutrition, Metabolism, and Cardiovascular Diseases* 17(4): 319–326.

Seals, J. G. 2007. Integrating the transtheoretical model into the management of overweight and obese adults. *Journal of the American Academy of Nurse Practitioners* 19(2): 63–71.

Sillence, E., et al. 2007. How do patients evaluate and make use of online health information? *Social Science & Medicine* 64(9): 1853–1862.

Smith, S. C. 2007. Multiple risk factors for cardiovascular disease and diabetes mellitus. *The American Journal of Medicine* 120(3 Suppl. 1): S3–S11.

Statistics Canada: Selected Leading Causes of Death by Sex (http://www40.statscan.ca/101/cst01/health36.htm; retrieved May 26, 2006).

Statistics Canada: Disability-free Life Expectancy, by Provinces and Territories (http://www40.statscan.ca/101/cst01/health38.htm; retrieved September 20, 2011).

Suminiski, R. R., and R. Petosa. 2002. Stages of change among ethnically diverse college students. *Journal of American College Health* 51(1): 26–31.

U.S. Department of Health and Human Services. 2000. *Healthy People 2010*, 2nd ed. Washington, D.C.: DHHS.

Chapter 2

American College of Sports Medicine. 2007. ACSM's Health/Fitness Facility Standards and Guidelines, 3rd ed. Champaign, Ill.: Human Kinetics.

American College of Sports Medicine. 2009. *ACSM's Guidelines for Exercise Testing and Prescription*, 8th ed. Philadelphia: Lippincott Williams and Wilkins.

American College of Sports Medicine. 2009. *ACSM's Resource Manual for Guidelines for Exercise Testing and Prescription*, 6th ed. Philadelphia: Lippincott Williams and Wilkins.

American College of Sports Medicine. 1998. The recommended quantity and quality of exercise for developing and maintaining cardiorespiratory and muscular fitness, and flexibility in healthy adults. ACSM position paper. *Medicine and Science in Sports and Exercise* 30(6): 975–991.

American College of Obstetrics and Gynecology Committee on Obstetric Practice. 2002. Exercise during pregnancy and the postpartum period. Committee Opinion No. 267. *International Journal of Gynaecology and Obstetrics* 77: 79–81.

American Diabetes Association. 2003. Physical activity/exercise and diabetes mellitus. *Diabetes Care* 26: S73–S77.

American Heart Association. 2003. Exercise and physical activity in the prevention and treatment of atherosclerotic cardiovascular disease. *Circulation* 107: 3109–3116.

Bouchard, C., et al. 2007. *Physical Activity and Health.* Champaign, Ill.: Human Kinetics.

Canadian Fitness and Lifestyle Research Institute. 2008 Physical Activity Monitor (http://www.cflri.ca/pub_page/98; retrieved September 20, 2011).

Canadian Society for Exercise Physiology 2003. *The Canadian Physical Activity, Fitness & Lifestyle Approach*, 3rd ed. Ontario, Canada: CSEP.

Centers for Disease Control and Prevention. 2007. Prevalence of regular physical activity among adults—United States, 2001 and 2005. *Morbidity and Mortality Weekly Report* 56(46): 1209–1212.

Centers for Disease Control and Prevention. 2008. Prevalence of self-reported physically active adults—United States, 2007. *Morbidity and Mortality Weekly Report* 57(48): 1297–1300.

Centers for Disease Control and Prevention. 2008. Self-reported pre-diabetes and risk-reduction activities—United States, 2006. *Morbidity and Mortality Weekly Report* 57(44): 1203–1205.

Ekelund, U., et al. 2007. Physical activity and metabolic risk in individuals with a family history of type 2 diabetes. *Diabetes Care* 30(2): 337–342.

Evans R. K., et al. 2002. Effects of warm-up before eccentric exercise on indirect markers of muscle damage. *Medicine and Science in Sports and Exercise* 34: 1892–1899.

Exercise for health: How much exercise is enough? ACSM works with others to avoid misunderstanding. 2003. *ACSM Fit Society Page*, Winter.

Garman, J. F., et al. 2004. Occurrence of exercise dependence in a college-aged population. *Journal of American College Health* 52(5): 221–228.

Go For Green: The Active Living and Environment Program Walking or biking for short trips saves our health and the environment (http://www.goforgreen.ca/at/eng/about/facts.aro; retrieved August 23, 2005).

Hu, F. B. 2003. Sedentary lifestyle and risk of obesity and type 2 diabetes. *Lipids* 38(2): 103–108.

Institutes of Medicine, National Academies. 2002. *Dietary, Reference Intakes for Energy, Carbohydrate, Fiber, Fat, Fatty Acids, Cholesterol, Protein, and Amino Acids.* Washington, D.C.: National Academy Press.

Is easy-does-it exercise enough? 2004. *Consumer Reports on Health*, February.

Katzmarzyk, P.T., Gledhill, N., & Shepard, R.J. (2000). The economic burden of physical inactivity in Canada, *Canadian Medical Association Journal*, 163 (11): 1435–1440.

Lee, I. 2003. Physical activity in women: How much is good enough? *Journal of the American Medical Association* 290(10): 1377–1379.

Le Masurier, G. C. 2004. Walk which way? *ACSM's Health and Fitness Journal*, January/February.

Lustyk, M. K., et al. 2004. Physical activity and quality of life: Assessing the influence of activity frequency, intensity, volume, and motives. *Behavioral Medicine* 30: 124–131.

Macfarlane, D. J., et al. 2006. Very short intermittent versus continuous bouts of activity in sedentary adults. *Preventive Medicine* 43(4): 332–336.

Malek, M. H., et al. 2002. Importance of health science education for personal fitness trainers. *Journal of Strength and Conditioning Research* 16: 19–24.

President's Council on Physical Fitness and Sports. 2000. Definitions: Health, fitness, and physical activity. *Research Digest* 3(9).

Public Health Agency of Canada. Physical Activity Guidlines (http://www.phac-aspc.gc.ca/hp-ps/hl-mvs/pa-ap/index-eng.php; retrieved September 10, 2011).

Saris, W.H.M., et al. 2003. How much physical activity is enough to prevent unhealthy weight gain? Outcome of the IASO 1st Stock Conference and consensus statement. *Obesity Reviews* 4: 101–114.

Shields M, Tremblay MS. Sedentary behaviour and obesity among Canadian adults. Health Reports (Statistics Canada, Catalogue 82-003) 2008; 19(2): 19-30.

Statistics Canada. Prevalence of disability in Canada, 2006 (http://www.statcan.gc.ca/pub/89-628-x/2007002/4125019-eng.htm;; retrieved September 10, 2011).

Statistics Canada. *Physical Activity During Leisure Time, 2009* (Catalogue 82-625) Ottawa: Statistics Canada, 2010. Available at: http://www.statcan.gc.ca/pub/82-625-x/2010002/article/11267-eng.htm, retrieved October 20, 1011.

Takahashi T., et al. 2002. Influence of cool-down exercise on autonomic control of heart rate during recovery from dynamic exercise. *Frontiers of Medical and Biological Engineering* 11: 249–259.

Wannamethee, S. G., et al. 2007. Decreased muscle mass and increased central adiposity are independently related to mortality in older men. *American Journal of Clinical Nutrition* 86(5): 1339–1346.

World Health Organization. 2008. *World Health Statistics 2008.* Geneva: World Health Organization.

Chapter 3

Achten, J., and A. E. Jeukendrup. 2003. Heart rate monitoring: Applications and limitations. *Sports Medicine* 33:517–538.

Adler, P. A., and B. L. Roberts. 2009. The use of Tai Chi to improve health in older adults. *Orthopedic Nursing* 25(2): 122–126

American Academy of Orthopaedic Surgeons. 2001. *Selecting Home Exercise Equipment* (http://orthoinfo.aaos.org/fact/thr_report.cfm; retrieved October 17, 2001).

American College of Sports Medicine. 2009. *ACSM's Guidelines for Exercise Testing and Prescription,* 8th ed. Philadelphia: Lippincott Williams and Wilkins.

American College of Sports Medicine. 2009. *ACSM's Resource Manual for Guidelines for Exercise Testing and Prescription,* 6th ed. Philadelphia: Lippincott Williams and Wilkins.

Brooks, G. A., et al. 2005. *Exercise Physiology: Human Bioenergetics and Its Applications,* 4th ed. New York: McGraw-Hill.

Canadian Society for Exercise Physiology. 2003. *The Canadian Physical Activity, Fitness & Lifestyle Approach (CPAFLA): CSEP-Health & Fitness Program's Health-Related Appraisal and Counselling Strategy,* 3rd ed.

Cheuvront, S. N., I. R. Carter, and M. N. Sawka. 2003. Fluid balance and endurance exercise performance. *Current Sports Medicine Reports* 2: 202–208.

Colcombe, S. J., et al. 2004. Cardiovascular fitness, cortical plasticity, and aging. *Proceedings of the National Academy of Sciences* 101(9): 3316–3321.

Courneya, K.S. 2009. Exercise for disease prevention and health promotion in cancer survivors. *European Journal of Cancer,* 7(2), 19, 65.

Friedenreich, C. M., et al. 2004. Case-control study of lifetime total physical activity and prostate cancer risk. *American Journal of Epidemiology* 159(8): 740–749.

Garcin, M., M. Wolff, and T. Bejma. 2003. Reliability of rating scales of perceived exertion and heart rate during progressive and maximal constant load exercises till exhaustion in physical education students. *International Journal of Sports Medicine* 24: 285–290.

Gleeson, M., D. C. Nieman, and B. K. Pedersen. 2004. Exercise, nutrition, and immune function. *Journal of Sports Science* 22(1): 115–125.

Goodwin, R. D. 2003. Association between physical activity and mental disorders among adults in the United States. *Preventive Medicine* 36(6): 698–703.

Humpel, N., N. Owen, and E. Leslie. 2002. Environmental factors associated with adults' participation in physical activity. A review. *American Journal of Preventive Medicine* 22(3): 188–199.

Karvonen, M.J., Kental, E., & Mustala, O. (1957). The effects of on heart rate: A longitudinal study. *Annales Medicinae Experimentalis et Biologiae Fenniae (Finnish Medical Society Duodecim)*,35(3): 307–15.

Ploughman, M. 2008. Exercise is brain food: The effects of physical activity on cognitive function. *Developmental Neurorehabilitation* 11(3): 236–240.

Reigle, B. S., and K. Wonders. 2009. Breast cancer and the role of exercise in women. *Methods in Molecular Biology* 472(1): 169–189.

Rixon K. P., et al. 2006. Analysis of the assessment of caloric expenditure in four modes of aerobic dance. *Journal of Strength and Conditioning Research* 20(3): 593–596.

Robinson, D. L. 2007. Bicycle helmet legislation: Can we reach a consensus? *Accident Analysis and Prevention* 39(1): 86–93.

Scott, S. 2005. Combating depression with exercise. *ACSM's Health & Fitness Journal* 9(4): 31.

Shaibi, G. Q., et al. 2006. Aerobic fitness among Caucasian, African–American, and Latino youth. *Ethnic Diseases* 16(1): 120–125.

Shaw, K., et al. 2006. Exercise for overweight or obesity. *Cochrane Database of Systematic Reviews Online* Oct. 18(4): CD003817.

Slentz, C. A., et al. 2005. Inactivity, exercise, and visceral fat. STRRIDE: A randomized, controlled study of exercise intensity and amount. *Journal of Applied Physiology* 99(4): 1613–1618.

Sui, X., et al. 2007. Cardiorespiratory fitness and adiposity as mortality predictors in older adults. *Journal of the American Medical Association* 298(21): 2507–2516.

Sui, X., et al. 2007. Cardiorespiratory fitness as a predictor of nonfatal cardiovascular events in asymptomatic women and men. *American Journal of Epidemiology* 165(12): 1413–1423.

Sui, X., et al. 2008. A prospective study of cardiorespiratory fitness and risk of type 2 diabetes in women. *Diabetes Care* 31(3): 550–555.

Suominen, H. 2006. Muscle training for bone strength. *Aging Clinical and Experimental Research* 18(2): 85–93.

Swain, D. P. 2005. Moderate or vigorous intensity exercise: Which is better for improving aerobic fitness? *Preventive Cardiology* 8: 55–58.

Tunceli, K., et al. 2006. Long-term effects of obesity on employment and work limitations among U.S. Adults, 1986 to 1999. *Obesity* 14(9): 1637–1646.

Winter, B., et al. 2007. High impact running improves learning. *Neurobiology of Learning and Memory* 87(4): 597–609.

Yung, L. M., et al. 2009. Exercise, vascular wall and cardiovascular diseases: An update (part 2). *Sports Medicine* 39(1): 45–63.

Chapter 4

American College of Sports Medicine. 2009. *ACSM's Resource Manual for Guidelines for Exercise Testing and Prescription*, 6th ed. Philadelphia: Lippincott Williams and Wilkins.

American College of Sports Medicine. 2009. American College of Sports Medicine position stand: Progression models in resistance training for healthy adults. *Medicine and Science in Sports and Exercise* 41(3): 687–708.

Bahrke, M., and C. Yesalis. 2002. *Performance-Enhancing Substances in Sport and Exercise*. Champaign, Ill.: Human Kinetics. Provides up-to-date coverage of the issues surrounding supplements as well as the current state of research on major types of supplements and their effects on athletic performance.

Burt, J., et al. 2007. A comparison of once versus twice per week training on leg press strength in women. *The Journal of Sports Medicine and Physical Fitness* 47(1): 13–17.

Canadian Society for Exercise Physiology. 2003. *The Canadian Physical Activity, Fitness & Lifestyle Approach (CPAFLA): CSEP-Health & Fitness Program's Health-Related Appraisal and Counselling Strategy*, 3rd ed.

Canadian Society for Exercise Physiology. 2008. Position Stand: Resistance training in children and adolescents. *Applied Physiology, Nutrition and Metabolism* 22: 547–561.

Caserotti, P., et al. 2008. Explosive heavy-resistance training in old and very old adults: Changes in rapid muscle force, strength and power. *Scandinavian Journal of Medicine and Science in Sports* 18(6): 773–782.

Cussler E. C., et al. 2003. Weight lifted in strength training predicts bone change in postmenopausal women. *Medicine and Science in Sports and Exercise* 35: 10–17.

Davis, W. J., et al. 2008. Concurrent training enhances athletes' strength, muscle endurance, and other measures. *Journal of Strength and Conditioning Research* 22(5): 1487–1502.

Delavier, F. 2010. *Strength Training Anatomy 3rd ed.*. Champaign, Ill.: Human Kinetics. Includes exercises for all major muscle groups as well as full anatomical pictures of the muscular system. A matching volume for women (Women's Strength Training Anatomy) was published in 2003.

Department of Justice Canada. 2003. *Natural Health Products Regulations* (http://http://gazette.gc.ca/archives/p2/2003/2003-06-18/html/sor-dors196-eng.html; retrieved November 27, 2011).

Durell, D. L., T. J. Pujol, and J. T. Barnes. 2003. A survey of the scientific data and training methods utilized by collegiate strength and conditioning coaches. *Journal of Strength and Conditioning Research* 17: 368–373.

Earle, R. W., and T. R. Baechle, eds. 2004. *NSCA's Essentials of Personal Training*. Champaign, Ill: Human Kinetics.

Fahey, T. D. 2010. *Basic Weight Training for Men and Women*, 7th ed. New York: McGraw-Hill. A comprehensive and practical guide to developing training programs, using free weights, tailored to individual needs.

Graham, M. R., et al. 2008. Anabolic steroid use: Patterns of use and detection of doping. *Sports Medicine* 38(6): 505–525.

Hoffman, J. R., et al. 2008. Nutritional supplementation and anabolic steroid use in adolescents. *Medicine and Science in Sports and Exercise* 40(1): 15–24.

Krentz, J.R., Quest, B., Farthing, J.P., Quest, D.W., & Chilibeck, P.D. (2008). The effects of Ibuprofen on muscle hypertrophy, strength and soreness during resistance training. *Applied, Physiology, Nutrition and Metabolism* 33: 470–475.

Nader, G. A. 2006. Concurrent strength and endurance training: From molecules to man. *Medicine and Science in Sports and Exercise* 38(11): 1965–1970.

Norrbrand, L., et al. 2008. Resistance training using eccentric overload induces early adaptations in skeletal muscle size. *European Journal of Applied Physiology* 102(3): 271–281.

Støren, O., et al. 2008. Maximal strength training improves running economy in distance runners. *Medicine and Science in Sports and Exercise* 40(6): 1087–1092.

Thiblin, I., and A. Petersson. 2005. Pharmacoepidemiology of anabolic androgenic steroids: A review. *Fundamental and Clinical Pharmacology* 19: 27–44.

Tsourlou, T., et al. 2006. The effects of a twenty-four-week aquatic training program on muscular strength performance in healthy elderly women. *Journal of Strength and Conditioning Research* 20(4): 811–818.

Wieser, M., and P. Haber. 2007. The effects of systematic resistance training in the elderly. *International Journal of Sports Medicine* 28(1): 59–65.

Willardson, J. M. 2006. A brief review: Factors affecting the length of the rest interval between resistance exercise sets. *Journal of Strength and Conditioning Research* 20(4): 978–984.

Willardson, J. M., and L. N. Burkett. 2005. A comparison of 3 different rest intervals on the exercise volume completed during a workout. *Journal of Strength and Conditioning Research* 19: 23–26.

Winchester, J. B., et al. 2008. Eight weeks of ballistic exercise improves power independently of changes in strength and muscle fiber type expression. *Journal of Strength and Conditioning Research* 22(6): 1728–1734.

Chapter 5

Alter, M. J. 2004. *Science of Flexibility*, 3d ed. Champaign, Ill.: Human Kinetics. An extremely well-researched book that discusses the scientific basis of stretching exercises and flexibility.

Amako, M., et al. 2003. Effect of static stretching on prevention of injuries for military recruits. *Military Medicine* 168: 442–446.

American College of Sports Medicine. 2009. *ACSM's Resource Manual for Guidelines for Exercise Testing and Prescription*, 6th ed. Philadelphia: Lippincott Williams and Wilkins.

Anderson, B., and J. Anderson. 2003. *Stretching*, 20th anniv. ed. Bolinas, Calif.: Shelter Publications. A best-selling exercise book, updated with more than 200 stretches for 60 sports and activities.

Armiger, P. and M. A. Martyn. 2010. *Stretching for Functional Flexibility*. Philadelphia: Lippincott, Williams & Wilkins. Presents stretching methods for fitness, athletics, and rehabilitation.

Barnett, A. 2006. Using recovery modalities between training sessions in elite athletes: Does it help? *Sports Medicine* 36(9): 781–796.

Barr, K. P., M. Griggs, and T. Cadby. 2005. Lumbar stabilization: Core concepts and current literature. Part 1. *American Journal of Physical Medicine and Rehabilitation* 84(6): 473–480.

Blahnik, J. 2004. *Full-Body Flexibility*. Champaign, Ill.: Human Kinetics. Presents a blend of stretching techniques derived from sports training, martial arts, yoga, and Pilates.

Buchbinder, R., and J. Hoving. 2002. Specific spinal exercise substantially reduces the risk of low back pain recurrence. *Australian Journal of Physiotherapy* 48: 55.

Canadian Society for Exercise Physiology 2003. *The Canadian Physical Activity, Fitness & Lifestyle Approach*, 3rd ed. Ontario, Canada: CSEP.

Costa, P. B., et al. 2009. The acute effects of different durations of static stretching on dynamic balance performance. *Journal of Strength and Conditioning Research* 23(1): 141–147.

Da Costa, B. R., and E. R. Vieira. 2008. Stretching to reduce work-related musculoskeletal disorders: A systematic review. *Journal of Rehabilitation Medicine* 40(5): 321–328.

Funk, D. C., et al. 2003. Impact of prior exercise on hamstring flexibility: A comparison of proprioceptive neuromuscular facilitation and static stretching. *Journal of Strength and Conditioning Research* 17: 489–492.

Grenier, S. G., C. Russell, and S. M. McGill. 2003. Relationships between lumbar flexibility, sit-and-reach test, and a previous history of low back discomfort in industrial workers. *Canadian Journal of Applied Physiology* 28:165–177.

Haldeman, S., Carroll, L.J., Cassidy, J.D., and the Scientific Secretariat. 2008. The bone and joint decade 2000-2010: Task force on neck pain and its associated disorders. Executive Summary. *The Spine Journal*, 33:(4S) Supplement to February 15, 2008.

Hart, L. 2005. Effect of stretching on sport injury risk: A review. *Clinical Journal of Sports Medicine* 15(2): 113.

Haskell, W. L., et al. 2007. Physical activity and public health: updated recommendation for adults from the American College of Sports Medicine and the American Heart Association. *Circulation* 116(9): 1081–1093.

Hayden, J. A., M. W. van Tulder, and G. Tomlinson. 2005. Systematic review: Strategies for using exercise therapy to improve outcomes in chronic low back pain. *Annals of Internal Medicine* 142(9): 776–785.

Hayes, P. R., and A. Walker. 2007. Pre-exercise stretching does not impact upon running economy. *Journal of Strength and Conditioning Research* 21(4): 1227–1232.

Henchoz, Y., and A. Kai-Lik So. 2008. Exercise and nonspecific low back pain: A literature review. *Joint Bone Spine* 75(5): 533–539.

Herbert, R. D., and M. de Noronha. 2007. Stretching to prevent or reduce muscle soreness after exercise. *Cochrane Database of Systematic Reviews* (4): CD004577.

Herman, S. L., and D. T. Smith. 2008. Four-week dynamic stretching warm-up intervention elicits longer-term performance benefits. *Journal of Strength and Conditioning Research* 22(4): 1286–1297.

Kovacs, F. M., et al. 2003. Effect of firmness of mattress on chronic non-specific low-back pain: Randomised, double-blind, controlled, multi-centre trial. *Lancet* 362(9396): 1594–1595.

McHugh, M. P., and M. Nesse. 2008. Effect of stretching on strength loss and pain after eccentric exercise. *Medicine and Science in Sports and Exercise* 40(3): 566–573.

Monteiro, W. D., et al. 2008. Influence of strength training on adult women's flexibility. *Journal of Strength and Conditioning Research* 22(3): 672–677.

Morse, C. I., et al. 2008. The acute effect of stretching on the passive stiffness of the human gastrocnemius muscle tendon unit. *Journal of Physiology* 586(1): 97–106.

Mortimer, M., et al. 2006. Low back pain in a general population. Natural course and influence of physical exercise—a 5-year follow-up of the Musculoskeletal Intervention Center–Norrtalje Study. *Spine* 31(26): 3045–3051.

Nieman, D. C. 2004. You asked for it: Low back pain. *ACSM's Health and Fitness Journal*, January/February.

Nieman, D. C. 2003. *Exercise Testing and Prescription: A Health-Related Approach*, 5th ed. New York: McGraw-Hill.

Palmer, K. T., et al. 2003. Smoking and musculoskeletal disorders: Findings from a British national survey. *Annals of Rheumatoid Diseases* 62:33–36.

Parks, K. A., et al. 2003. A comparison of lumbar range of motion and functional ability scores in patients with low back pain: Assessment for range of motion validity. *Spine* 28:380–384.

Rasmussen-Barr, E., et al. 2009. Graded exercise for recurrent low-back pain: A randomized, controlled trial with 6-, 12-, and 36-month follow-ups. *Spine* 34(3): 221–228.

Rassier, D. E. 2007. Stretching human muscles makes them stronger. *Journal of Applied Physiology* 102(1): 5–6.

Schur, P. E. 2001. Effectiveness of stretching to reduce injury. *British Journal of Sports Medicine* 35:138.

Tekur, P., et al. 2008. Effect of short-term intensive yoga program on pain, functional disability and spinal flexibility in chronic low back pain: A randomized control study. *Journal of Alternative and Complementary Medicine* 14(6): 637–644.

Ten nice-to-know facts about flexibility and stretching. 2003. *ACSM's Health & Fitness Journal*, July/August.

Thacker, S. B., et al. 2004. The impact of stretching on sports injury risk: A systematic review of the literature. *Medicine and Science in Sports and Exercise* 36(3): 371–378.

Weil, R. 2008. Exercising the aging body. Part 2: Flexibility, balance, and diabetes control. *Diabetes Self-Management* 25(1): 42–52.

Winchester, J. B., et al. 2008. Static stretching impairs sprint performance in collegiate track and field athletes. *Journal of Strength and Conditioning Research* 22(1): 13–19.

Witvrouw, E., et al. 2007. The role of stretching in tendon injuries. *British Journal of Sports Medicine* 41(4): 224–226.

Chapter 6

American College of Sports Medicine. 2009. *ACSM's Resource Manual for Guidelines for Exercise Testing and Prescription*, 6th ed. Philadelphia: Lippincott Williams and Wilkins.

Anderson, D. E. 2007. Reliability of air displacement plethysmography. *Journal of Strength and Conditioning Research* 21(1): 169–172.

Babcock, C. J., et al. 2006. A comparison of military circumference equations to skinfold-based equations to estimate body composition. *Military Medicine* 171(1): 60–63.

Blair, S. N. 2009. Physical inactivity: The biggest public health problem of the 21st century. *British Journal of Sports Medicine* 43(1): 1–2.

Dutton DJ, & McLaren L (2011). Explained and Unexplained Regional Variation in Canadian Obesity Prevalence. *Obesity (Silver Spring, Md.)* PMID: 21253004 Obesity advance online publication, January 20, 2011.

Ekelund, U., S. J. Griffin, and N. J. Wareham. 2007. Physical activity and metabolic risk in individuals with a family history of type 2 diabetes. *Diabetes Care* 30(2): 337–342.

Fang, J., et al. 2003. Exercise, body mass index, caloric intake, and cardiovascular mortality. *American Journal of Preventive Medicine* 25(4): 283–289.

Fenicchia, L. M., et al. 2004. Influence of resistance exercise training on glucose control in women with type 2 diabetes. *Metabolism* 53(3): 284–289.

Flegal, K. M., et al. 2007. Cause-specific excess deaths associated with underweight, overweight, and obesity. *Journal of the American Medical Association* 298 (17): 2028–2037.

Fontaine, K. R., et al. 2003. Years of life lost due to obesity. *Journal of the American Medical Association* 289(2): 187–193.

Frankenfield, D. C., et al. 2001. Limits of body mass index to detect obesity and predict body composition. *Nutrition* 17(1): 26–30.

Guida, B., et al. 2007. Bioelectrical impedance analysis and age-related differences of body composition in the elderly. *Nutrition, Metabolism, and Cardiovascular Disease* 17(3): 175–180.

Health Canada. 2003. Canadian guidelines for body weight classification in adults. (Catalogue no. H49-179/2003-1E).

Heyward, V. H., and D. R. Wagner. 2004. *Applied Body Composition Assessment*. 2nd ed. Champaign, Ill.: Human Kinetics. Describes different methods of measuring and assessing body composition.

Højgaard, B., et al. 2008. Waist circumference and body mass index as predictors of health care costs. *PLoS ONE* 3(7): e2619.

Jiang, R., et al. 2004. Body iron stores in relation to risk of type 2 diabetes in apparently healthy women. *Journal of the American Medical Association* 291(6): 711–717.

Liu, J., T. J. Wade, and H. Tan. 2007. Cardiovascular risk factors and anthropometric measurements of adolescent body composition: A cross-sectional analysis of the Third National Health and Nutrition Examination Survey. *International Journal of Obesity* 31(1): 59–64.

Malina, R. M. 2007. Body composition in athletes: Assessment and estimated fatness. *Clinics in Sports Medicine* 26(1): 37–68.

Mattsson, S., and B. J. Thomas. 2006. Development of methods for body composition studies. *Physics in Medicine and Biology* 51(13): R203–228.

Moon, J. R. 2008. Percent body fat estimations in college men using field and laboratory methods: A three-compartment model approach. *Dynamic Medicine* 7:7.

Murphy, M. H., et. al. 2009. Accumulated versus continuous exercise for health benefit: A review of empirical studies. *Sports Medicine* 39(1): 29–43.

Ode, J. J., et al. 2007. Body mass index as a predictor of percent fat in college athletes and nonathletes. *Medicine and Science in Sports and Exercise* 39(3): 403–409.

Plank, L. D. 2005. Dual-energy X-ray absorptiometry and body composition. *Current Opinion in Clinical Nutrition and Metabolic Care* 8: 305–309.

Romero-Corral, A., et al. 2008. Accuracy of body mass index in diagnosing obesity in the adult general population. *International Journal of Obesity* 32(6): 959–966.

Shields M. Overweight and obesity among children and youth. *Health Reports* (Statistics Canada, Catalogue 82-003) 2006; 17(3): 27–42.

Tjepkema M. Adult obesity. *Health Reports* (Statistics Canada, Catalogue 82-003) 2006; 17(3): 9–25.

Tjepkema, M. 2005. Measuring obesity. Adult obesity in Canada: Measured height and weight. (Catalogue no. 82-620-MWE).

Wang, X., et al. 2008. Weight regain is related to decreases in physical activity during weight loss. *Medicine and Science in Sports and Exercise* 40(10): 1781–1788.

Wong, S. L., et al. 2004. Cardiorespiratory fitness is associated with lower abdominal fat independent of body mass index. *Medicine and Science in Sports and Exercise* 36(2): 286–291.

Zanovec, M., et al. 2009. Self-reported physical activity improves prediction of body fatness in young adults. *Medicine and Science in Sports and Exercise* 41(2): 328–335.

Zhu, S., et al. 2005. Lifestyle behaviors associated with lower risk of having the metabolic syndrome. *Metabolism* 53(11): 1503–1511.

Chapter 7

Agriculture, Food and Rural Development. 2005. Canadian consumer trends in obesity and food consumption. (http://www1.agric.gov.ca/$department/deptdocs.nsf/all/sis8438; retrieved August 31, 2006).

American College of Sports Medicine. 2007. American College of Sports Medicine position stand: Exercise and fluid replacement. *Medicine and Science in Sports and Exercise* 39(2): 377–390.

American College of Sports Medicine and Dieticians of Canada 2009. American College of Sports Medicine Position Stand: Nutrition and Athletic Performance (http://www.acsm-msse.org/pt/pt-core/template-journal/msse/media/0309nutrition.pdf; retrieved December 10, 2011).

American Heart Association. 2008. Diet and Lifestyle Recommendations (http://www.americanheart.org/presenter.jhtml?identifier=851; retrieved December 10, 2011).

Bunyard, L. B., K. E. Dennis, and B. J. Nicklas. 2002. Dietary intake and changes in lipoprotein lipids in obese, postmenopausal women placed on an American Heart Association Step 1 diet. *Journal of the American Dietetic Association* 102(1): 52–57.

Centers for Disease Control and Prevention. 2009. Application of lower sodium intake recommendations to adults—United States, 1999–2006. *Morbidity and Mortality Weekly Report* 58(11): 281–283.

Centers for Disease Control and Prevention. 2009. Food Safety (http://www.cdc.gov/foodsafety/default.htm; retrieved April 30, 2009).

Duyff, R. L. 2002. *ADA Complete Food and Nutrition Guide,* 2d ed. Chicago, Ill.: Canadian Dietetic Association. An excellent review of current nutrition information.

Eat Well, Eat Safe. Foodborne illness (http://www.eatwelleatsafe.ca/illness/fdborne.htm; retrieved September 5, 2005).

Ervin, R. B., et al. 2004. Dietary intake of selected minerals for the United States Population: 1999–2000. *Advance Data from Vital and Health Statistics,* 341.

Food and Drug Administration. 2004. Fact Sheet: Carbohydrates (http://www.fda.gov/oc/initiatives/obesity/factsheet.html; retrieved April 28, 2004).

Food and Nutrition Board, Institute of Medicine. 2005. *Dietary Reference Intakes for Water, Potassium, Sodium, Chloride, and Sulfate.* Washington, D.C.: National Academies Press.

Food and Nutrition Board, Institute of Medicine. 2005. *Dietary Reference Intakes for Energy, Carbohydrate, Fiber, Fat, Fatty Acids, Cholesterol, Protein, and Amino Acids.* Washington, D.C.: National Academies Press.

Health Canada. 2001. New and improved nutrition labelling. (http://www.hc-sc.gc.ca/hppb/nutrition/labels/e_before.html; retrieved October 31, 2011).

Health Canada. 2004. Canada's food guide to healthy eating meets individual needs. (http://www.hc-sc.gc.ca/fn-an/food-guide-aliment/re/fg_background; retrieved Octobert 31, 2011).

Health Canada. 2005. Regulation of genetically modified foods. (http://www.hc-sc.gc.ca/sr-sr/pubs/biotech/reg_gen_mod-eng.php; retrieved December 10, 2011).

Health Canada. 2005. Canada's food guide to healthy eating rainbow. (http://www.hc-sc.gc.ca/fn-an/food-guide-aliment/fg-rainbow-arc_en_ciel_ga_e.html; retrieved October 31, 2011).

Health Canada. 2007. Trans Fats monitoring program. (http://www.hc-sc.gc.ca/fn-an/nutrition/gras-trans-fats/meth-eng.php; retrieved October 31, 2011).

Hites, R. A., et al. 2004. Global assessment of organic contaminants in farmed salmon. *Science* 303(5655): 226–229.

Insel, P., R. E. Turner, and D. Ross. 2004. *Nutrition,* 2d ed. Sudbury, Mass.: Jones and Bartlett. A comprehensive review of major concepts in nutrition.

Jacobs, D. R., H. E. Meyer, and K. Solvoll. 2001. Reduced mortality among whole grain bread eaters in men and women in the Norwegian Country Study. *European Journal of Clinical Nutrition* 55(20): 137–143.

Jacobson, M. F., and J. Hurley. 2002. *Restaurant Confidential.* New York: Workman Publishing. Provides information about restaurant foods, including tips for making healthier choices.

Joint WHO/FAO Expert Consultation. 2003. *Diet, Nutrition, and the Prevention of Chronic Diseases.* Geneva: World Health Organization.

Ludwig, D. S. 2002. The glycemic index: Physiological mechanisms relating to obesity, diabetes, and cardiovascular disease. *Journal of the American Medical Association* 287(18): 2414–2423.

Michaelsson, K., et al. 2003. Serum retinol levels and the risk of fracture. *New England Journal of Medicine* 348(4): 287–294.

Nanney, M. S., et al. 2004. Rationale for a consistent "powerhouse" approach to vegetable and fruit messages. *Journal of the American Dietetic Association* 104(3): 352–356.

National Center for Health Statistics. 2003. Dietary intake of ten key nutrients for public health, United States: 1999–2000. *Advance Data from Vital and Health Statistics* No. 334.

Of birds and bacteria. 2003. *Consumer Reports,* January.

Oomen, C. M., et al. 2001. Association between trans fatty acid intake and 10-year risk of coronary heart disease. *Lancet* 357(9258): 746–751.

Organic Trade Association. 2003. Update on Canada's coming organic regulation. (http://www.ota.com/standards/canadian/update.html; retrieved September 5, 2005).

Osteoporosis Society of Canada. 2005. About osteoporosis. (http://www.osteoporosis.ca/english.html; retrieved August 31, 2005).

Selkowitz, A. 2000. *The College Student's Guide to Eating Well on Campus.* Bethesda, Md.: Tulip Hill Press. Provides practical advice for students, including how to make healthy choices when eating in a dorm or restaurant and how to stock a first pantry.

Toborek, M., et al. 2002. Unsaturated fatty acids selectively induce an inflammatory environment in human endothelial cells. *American Journal of Clinical Nutrition* 75(1): 119–125.

U.S. Department of Health and Human Services and U.S. Department of Agriculture. 2005. Dietary Guidelines for Americans 2005 (http://www.health.gov/dietaryguidelines/dga2005/document/; retrieved April 30, 2009).

U.S. Department of Health and Human Services and U.S. Department of Agriculture. 2005. Finding your way to a healthier you: Based on the Dietary Guidelines for Americans. *Home and Garden Bulletin* No. 232-CP.

Vartanian, L. R., et al. 2007. Effects of soft drink consumption on nutrition and health: A systematic review and meta-analysis. *American Journal of Public Health* 97(4): 667–675.

Wardlaw, G. M. 2004. *Perspectives in Nutrition,* 6th ed. New York: McGraw-Hill. An easy-to-understand review of major concepts in nutrition.

Williams, M. H. 2005. *Nutrition for Health, Fitness, and Sport,* 7th ed. New York: McGraw-Hill. An overview of the role of nutrition in enhancing health, fitness, and sport performance.

Wong, S. H. S., and S. Chung. 2003. Glycemic index: An educational tool for health and fitness professionals? *ACSM's Health and Fitness Journal,* November/December.

Chapter 8

Adams, K. F., et al. 2006. Overweight, obesity, and mortality in a large prospective cohort of persons 50 to 71 years old. *New England Journal of Medicine* 355(8): 763–778.

Alinia, S., et al. 2009. The potential association between fruit intake and body weight—A review. *Obesity Reviews,* April (published online).

Baker, B. 2006. Weight loss and diet plans. *American Journal of Nursing* 106(6): 52–59.

Behn, A., and E. Ur. 2006. The obesity epidemic and its cardiovascular consequences. *Current Opinions in Cardiology* 21(4): 353–360.

Bowman, S. A, et al. 2004. Effects of fast-food consumption on energy intake and diet quality among children in a national household survey. *Pediatrics* 113(1 Pt. 1): 112–118.

Brownell, K. D. 2003. *Food Fight: The Inside Story of the Food Industry, America's Obesity Crisis, and What We Can Do About It.* New York: McGraw-Hill/Contemporary. An in-depth look at environmental factors supporting the North American lifestyle that contributes to obesity.

Bryan, S., et al. 2003. Women's health surveillance report—Physical activity and obesity (http://www.phac-aspc.gc.ca/publicat/whsr-rssf/chap_5_e.html; retrieved September 27, 2005).

Calle, E. E., et al. 2003. Overweight, obesity, and mortality from cancer in a prospectively studied cohort of U.S. adults. *New England Journal of Medicine* 348(17): 1625–1638.

Dahlman, I., and P. Arner. 2007. Obesity and polymorphisms in genes regulating human adipose tissue. *International Journal of Obesity* 31(11): 1629–1641.

Dhingra, R., et al. 2007. Soft drink consumption and risk of developing cardiometabolic risk factors and the metabolic syndrome in middle-aged adults in the community. *Circulation* 116(5): 480–488.

Dong, L., G. Block, and S. Mandel. 2004. Activities contributing to total energy expenditure in the United States: Results from the NHAPS Study. *International Journal of Behavioral Nutrition and Physical Activity* 1(4).

Donnelly, J. E., et al. 2009. American College of Sports Medicine Position Stand: Appropriate physical activity intervention strategies for weight loss and prevention of weight regain for adults. *Medicine and Science in Sports and Medicine* 41(2): 459–471.

Drewnowski, A., and F. Bellisle. 2007. Liquid calories, sugar and body weight. *American Journal of Clinical Nutrition* 85(3): 651–661.

Dong, L., G. Block, and S. Mandel. 2004. Activities contributing to total energy expenditure in the United States: Results from the NHAPS Study. *International Journal of Behavioral Nutrition and Physical Activity* 1(4).

Ephedra: Heart dangers in disguise. 2004. *Consumer Reports,* January.

Esposito, K., et al. 2003. Effect of weight loss and lifestyle changes on vascular inflammatory markers in obese women. *Journal of the American Medical Association* 289(14): 1799–1804.

Federal Trade Commission. 2002. *Weight Loss Advertising: An Analysis of Current Trends.* Washington, D.C.: Federal Trade Commission.

Ferguson, J. M., and C. Ferguson. 2003. *Habits Not Diets.* 4th ed. Boulder, Colo.: Bull Publishing. A behaviour-change approach to changing diet and activity habits that includes many practical tips, assessment worksheets, and tracking forms.

Finkelstein, E. A., I. C. Fiebelkorn, and G. Wang. 2004. State-level estimates of annual medical expenditures attributable to obesity. *Obesity Research* 12(1): 18–24.

Fontaine, K. R., et al. 2003. Years of life lost due to obesity. *Journal of the American Medical Association* 289(2): 187–193.

Food and Drug Administration. 2003. Questions and Answers about FDA's Actions on Ephedra Dietary Supplements (http://www.fda.gov/oc/initiatives/ephedra/december2003/qu.html; retrieved January 5, 2004).

Food and Nutrition Board, Institute of Medicine, National Academies. 2002. *Dietary Reference Intakes: Energy, Carbohydrate, Fiber, Fat, Fatty Acids, Cholesterol, Protein, and Amino Acids.* Washington, D.C.: National Academy Press.

Food for thought: Out-of-home dining. 2009. The Neilsen Company.

Graves, B. S., and R. L. Welsh. 2004. Recognizing the signs of body dysmorphic disorder and muscle dysmorphia. *ACSM's Health & Fitness Journal,* January/February.

Health Canada. 2010. Sugar substitutes (http://www.hc-sc.gc.ca/fn-an/securit/addit/sweeten-edulcor/index-eng.php; retrieved December 10, 2011).

Hutchinson, D. M., and R. M. Rapee. 2007. Do friends share similar body image and eating problems? The role of social networks and peer influences in early adolescence. *Behavior Research and Therapy* 45(7): 1557–1577.

Idelevich, E., et al. 2009. Current pharmacotherapeutic concepts for the treatment of obesity in adults. *Therapeutic Advances in Cardiovascular Disease* 3(1): 75–90.

Janiszewski, P. M., and R. Ross. 2007. Physical activity in the treatment of obesity: Beyond body weight reduction. *Applied Physiology, Nutrition and Metabolism* 32(3): 512–522.

Kirk, E. P., et al. 2009. Minimal resistance training improves daily energy expenditure and fat oxidation. *Medicine and Science in Sports and Exercise,* April (published online).

Katzmarzyk, P. 2002. The Canadian obesity epidemic, 1985–1998. *Canadian Medical Association Journal* 166(8): 1039–1040.

Kumanyika, S. K., et al. 2008. Population-based prevention of obesity: The need for comprehensive promotion of healthful eating, physical activity, and energy balance: A scientific statement from the American Heart Association Council on Epidemiology and Prevention, Interdisciplinary Committee for Prevention (formerly the Expert Panel on Population and Prevention Science). *Circulation* 118(4): 428–464.

Lake, H. (2005, March 08). What's eating us? A closer look at what we actually eat (http://www.lifewise.canoe.ca/FoodDrink/2005/03/08/pf-954229.html; retrieved December 10, 2011).

Leit, R. A., J. J. Gray, and H. G. Pope, Jr. 2002. The media's representation of the ideal male body: A cause for muscle dysmorphia? *International Journal of Eating Disorders* 31(3): 334–338.

Losing weight: More than counting calories. 2002. *FDA Consumer,* January/February.

Leone, J. E., and J. V. Fetro. 2007. Perceptions and attitudes toward androgenic-anabolic steroid use among two age categories: A qualitative inquiry. *Journal of Strength and Conditioning Research* 21(2): 532–537.

Ma, Y., et al. 2005. Association between dietary carbohydrates and body weight. *American Journal of Epidemiology* 161(4): 359–367.

Meunning, P., et al. 2006. Gender and the burden of disease attributable to obesity. *American Journal of Public Health* 96(9): 1662–1668.

Mitka, M. 2001. Magazine ideals wrong. *Journal of the American Medical Association* 286(4): 409.

Nash, J. D. 2003. *Maximize Your Body Potential: Lifetime Skills for Successful Weight Management.* Boulder, Colo.: Bull Publishing. A do-it-yourself guide that provides self-assessment tools and guidelines for setting realistic goals and creating a personal plan.

Nielsen, S. J., and B. M. Popkin. 2003. Patterns and trends in food portion sizes, 1977–1996. *Journal of the American Medical Association* 289(4): 450–453.

Nonas, C. 2002. *Outwit Your Weight.* Emmaus, Penn.: Rodale. Provides a behavioural-based program for weight management.

Pereira, M. A., et al. 2005. Fast-food habits, weight gain, and insulin resistance (the CARDIA study): 15-year prospective analysis. *Lancet* 365(9453): 36–42.

Ritchie, S. A., and J. M. Connell. 2007. The link between abdominal obesity, metabolic syndrome and cardiovascular disease. *Nutrition, Metabolism, and Cardiovascular Diseases* 17(4): 319–326.

Rubinstein, S., and B. Caballero. 2000. Is Miss America an undernourished role model? *Journal of the American Medical Association* 283(12): 1569.

Tate, D. F., R. R. Wing, and R. A. Winett. 2001. Using Internet technology to deliver a behavioral weight loss program. *Journal of the American Medical Association* 285(9): 1172–1777.

You underestimate calorie intake, but by how much? 2003. *Tufts University Health & Nutrition Letter,* November.

Weigle, D. S., et al. 2005. A high-protein diet induces sustained reductions in appetite, ad libitum caloric intake, and body weight despite compensatory changes in diurnal plasma leptin and ghrelin concentrations. *American Journal of Clinical Nutrition* 82(1): 42–48.

Whitlock, G. et al. 2009. Body-mass index and cause-specific mortality in 900,000 adults: Collaborative analysis of 57 prospective studies. *Lancet* 373(9669):1083–1096.

Chapter 9

Bernstein, M. S., M. C. Costanza, and A. Morabia. 2004. Association of physical activity intensity levels with overweight and obesity in a population-based sample of adults. *Preventive Medicine* 38(1): 94–104.

Canadian Fitness and Lifestyle Research Institute. 2010. Physical Activity Monitor. (http://72.10.49.94/pub_page/105; retrieved January 30, 2012).

Canadian Society for Exercise Physiology. 2003. *The Canadian Physical Activity and Lifestyle Approach Protocol* (CPAFLA), 3rd ed.

Colley, R.C., Garriguet, D., Janssen, I., Craig, C.L., Clarke, J. and Tremblay, M.S. 2011. Physical activity of Canadian children and youth: Accelerometer results from the 2007 to 2009 Canadian Health Measures Survey. *Health Reports*. Statistics Canada Catalogue no. 82-003-X. Available at http://www.statcan.gc.ca/access_acces/alternative_alternatif.action?l=eng&loc=11397-eng.pdf.

Finkelstein, E. A., et al. 2008. A randomized study of financial incentives to increase physical activity among sedentary older adults. *Preventive Medicine* 47(2): 182–187.

Hamer, M., and Y. Chida. 2008. Walking and primary prevention: A meta-analysis of prospective cohort studies. *British Journal of Sports Medicine* 42(4): 238–243.

Haskell, W. L., et al. 2007. Physical activity and public health: Updated recommendation for adults from the American College of Sports Medicine and the American Heart Association. *Circulation* 116(9): 1081–1093.

Hogan, M. 2005. Physical and cognitive activity and exercise for older adults: A review. *International Journal of Aging and Human Development* 60: 95–126.

Ingham, S. A., et al. 2008. Physiological and performance effects of low-versus mixed-intensity rowing training. *Medicine and Science in Sports and Exercise* 40(3): 579–584.

Kilpatrick, M. W., et al. 2009. Heart rate and metabolic responses to moderate-intensity aerobic exercise: A comparison of graded walking and ungraded jogging at a constant perceived exertion. *Journal of Sports Sciences* 27(5): 509–516.

Kokkinos, P. 2008. Physical activity and cardiovascular disease prevention: Current recommendations. *Angiology* 59(2 Supplement): 26S–29S.

Levine, J. A., et al. 2008. The role of free-living daily walking in human weight gain and obesity. *Diabetes* 57(3): 548–554.

Nichols, D. L., et al. 2007. Bone density and young athletic women. An update. *Sports Medicine* 37(11): 1001–1014.

Oken, E., et al. 2007. Television, walking, and diet: Associations with postpartum weight retention. *American Journal of Preventive Medicine* 32(4): 305–311.

Pascual, C., et al. 2009. Socioeconomic environment, availability of sports facilities, and jogging, swimming and gym use. *Health and Place* 15(2): 553–561.

Plisiene, J., et al. 2008. Moderate physical exercise: A simplified approach for ventricular rate control in older patients with atrial fibrillation. *Clinical Research in Cardiology* 97(11): 820–826.

Schneider, P. L., et al. 2006. Effects of a 10,000 steps per day goal in overweight adults. *American Journal of Health Promotion* 21(2): 85–89.

Suminski, R. R., et al. 2008. Observing physical activity in suburbs. *Health and Place* 14(4): 894–899.

Troped, P. J., et al. 2008. Prediction of activity mode with global positioning system and accelerometer data. *Medicine and Science in Sports and Exercise* 40(5): 972–978.

Walters, P. H. 2000. Sleep facts. *ACSM's Health and Fitness Journal* 4(6): 17–19, 28.

World Health Organization/FAO Expert Consultation. 2003. *Diet, Nutrition and the Prevention of Chronic Diseases*. WHO Technical Report Series 916. Geneva: World Health Organization.

Xu, D. Q., et al. 2008. Tai Chi exercise and muscle strength and endurance in older people. *Medicine and Sports Science* 52: 20–29.

Yabroff, K. R., et al. 2008. Walking the dog: Is pet ownership associated with physical activity in California? *Journal Physical Activity and Health* 5(2): 216–228.

Chapter 10

Abbott, R. B., et al. 2007. A randomized controlled trial of Tai Chi for tension headaches. *Evidence Based Complementary and Alternative Medicine* 4(1): 107–113.

Antoni, M. H. 2003. Stress management effects on psychological, endocrinological, and immune functioning in men with HIV infection: Empirical support for a psychoneuroimmunological model. *Stress* 6(3): 173–188.

Benson, H. 2000. *The Relaxation Response*. New York: Avon, Whole-care. An expanded and updated edition of the 1975 classic on relaxation techniques and their physical benefits.

Bovier, P. A., E. Chamot, and T. V. Perneger. 2004. Perceived stress, internal resources, and social support as determinants of mental health among young adults. *Quality of Life Research* 13(1): 161–170.

Carmody, J., et al. 2008. Mindfulness, spirituality, and health-related symptoms. *Journal of Psychosomatic Research* 64(4): 393–403.

Dingfelder, S. F. 2008. An insidious enemy: New research pinpoints the ways stress undermines our immune systems at the cellular level. *Monitor on Psychology* 39(9): 22.

Ditzen, B., et al. 2007. Effects of different kinds of couple interaction on cortisol and heart rate responses to stress in women. *Psychoneuroendocrinology* 32(5): 565–574.

Givens, J. L., et al. 2009. Personality traits of centenarians' offspring. *Journal of the American Geriatrics Society* 57(4): 683–685.

Greenberg, J. 2004. *Comprehensive Stress Management*. 8th ed. New York: McGraw-Hill. An easy-to-understand introduction to the physiology of stress and to many strategies for successful coping.

Health Canada. January 2008. Mental health: Coping with stress. *It's Your Health*. Retrieved from http://www.hc-sc.gc.ca/hl-vs/iyh-vsv/life-vie/stress-eng.php on June 10, 2009.

Kimata, H. 2001. Effect of humor on allergen-induced wheal reactions. *Journal of the American Medical Association* 285(6): 738.

Koenig, H. G., L. K. George, and P. Titus. 2004. Religion, spirituality, and health in medically ill hospitalized older patients. *Journal of the American Geriatrics Society* 52(4): 554–562.

Kivlighan, K. T., D. A. Granger, and A. Booth. 2005. Gender differences in testosterone and cortisol response to competition. *Psychoneuroendocrinology* 30(1): 58–71.

Lampert, R., et al. 2009. Anger-induced T-wave alternans predicts future ventricular arrhythmias in patients with implantable cardioverter-defibrillators. *Journal of the American College of Cardiology* 53(9): 774–778.

Lazarus, R. S., and S. Folkman. 1984. *Stress, Appraisal and Coping*. New York: Springer.

Lee, S. H., et al. 2007. Effectiveness of a meditation-based stress management program as an adjunct to Oman, D., et al. 2008. Meditation lowers stress and supports forgiveness among college students: A randomized controlled trial. *Journal of American College Health* 56(5): 569–578.

Redwood, S. K., and M. H. Pollak. 2007. Student-led stress management program for first-year medical students. *Teaching and Learning Medicine* 19(1): 42–46.

Schoonman, G. G., et al. 2007. Is stress a trigger factor for migraine? *Psychoneuroendocrinology* 32(5): 532–538.

Travis, F., et al. 2009. Effects of transcendental meditation practice on brain functioning and stress reactivity in college students. *International Journal of Psychophysiology* 71(2): 170–176

Wang, J., et al. 2009. Changes in perceived job strain and the risk of major depression: Results from a population-based longitudinal study. *American Journal of Epidemiology* 169(9): 1085–1091.

Warr, D. J., et al. 2007. Money, stress, jobs: Residents perceptions of health-impairing factors in poor neighborhoods. *Health & Place* 13(3): 743–756.

Chapter 11

Agency for Healthcare Research and Quality. 2002. *Task Force Issues Caution on Combined Hormone Therapy* (http://www.ahrq.gov/news/press/pr2002/hrtrecpr.htm; retrieved October 15, 2002).

American Heart Association. 2009. *Heart Disease and Stroke Statistics—2009 Update*. Dallas: American Heart Association.

Canadian Hypertension Education Program. 2006. *Canadian Recommendations for the Management of Hypertension*.

Canadian Hypertension Society. nd. *General information on hypertension* (http://www.hypertension.ca/factsOnHypertension_va.html; retrieved October 04, 2005).

Erkkila, A. T., et al. 2005. Cereal fiber and whole-grain intake are associated with reduced progression of coronary-artery atherosclerosis in post menopausal women with coronary artery disease. *American Heart Journal* 150(1): 94–101.

Gommans, J., et al. 2009. Preventing strokes: The assessment and management of people with transient ischemic attack. *New Zealand Medical Journal* 122 (1293): 50–60.

Greenland, P., et al. 2003. Major risk factors as antecedents of fatal and nonfatal coronary heart disease events. *Journal of the American Medical Association* 290(7): 891–897.

Gus, M., et al. 2004. Association between different measurements of obesity and the incidence of hypertension. *American Journal of Hypertension* 17(1): 50–53.

Hackam, D. G., and S. S. Anand. 2003. Emerging risk factors for atherosclerotic vascular disease. *Journal of the American Medical Association* 290(7): 932–940.

Hayden, M., et al. 2002. Aspirin for the primary prevention of cardiovascular events: A summary of the evidence for the U.S. Preventive Services Task Force. *Annals of Internal Medicine* 136(2): 161–172.

Heart and Stroke Foundation. 2008. *Stroke statistics* (http://www.heartandstroke.ca; retrieved January 30, 2012).

Kidambi, S., et al. 2009. Hypertension, insulin resistance, and aldosterone: Sex-specific relationships. *Journal of Clinical Hypertension* 11(3): 130–137.

Marshall, D. A., et al. 2009. Achievement of heart health characteristics through participation in an intensive lifestyle change program (Coronary Artery Disease Reversal Study). *Journal of Cardiopulmonary Rehabilitation and Prevention* 29(2): 84–94.

Matthews, C. E., et al. 2007. Influence of exercise, walking, cycling, and overall nonexercise physical activity on mortality in Chinese women. *American Journal of Epidemiology* 165(12): 1343–1350.

McSweeney, J. C., et al. 2003. Women's early warning symptoms of acute myocardial infarction. *Circulation* 108:2619–2623.

Moore, T., et al. 2003. *The DASH Diet for Hypertension*. New York: Pocket Books. Provides background information and guidelines for adopting the DASH diet; also includes recipes.

Müller, D., et al. 2006. How sudden is sudden cardiac death? *Circulation* 114(11): 1146–1150

National Center for Health Statistics. 2009. Deaths: Final Data for 2006. *National Vital Statistics Reports* 57(14): 1–80.

National Center for Health Statistics. 2009. *Health, United States, 2008*. Hyattsville, Md.: National Center for Health Statistics.

Nita, C., et al. 2008. Hypertensive waist: First step of the screening for metabolic syndrome. *Metabolic Syndrome and Related Disorders* 7(2): 105–110.

Physicians for a Smoke-Free Canada. 2005. *Tobacco and the health of Canadians* (http://www.smoke-free.ca/Health/pscissies_health.htm).

Reaven, G. M. 2001. *Syndrome X: Overcoming the Silent Killer That Can Give You a Heart Attack*. St. Louis, Mo.: Fireside. Provides information about syndrome X and insulin resistance, including lifestyle strategies for affected individuals.

Spencer, L. 2002. Results of a heart disease risk-factor screening among traditional college students. *Journal of American College Health* 50(6): 291–296.

Steffen, P. R., et al. 2003. Effects of perceived racism and anger inhibition on ambulatory blood pressure in African Americans. *Psychosomatic Medicine* 65(5): 746–750.

Sui, X., et al. 2007. Cardiorespiratory fitness and the risk of nonfatal cardiovascular disease in women and men with hypertension. *American Journal of Hypertension* 20(6): 608–615.

Wang, X., et al. 2007. Efficacy of folic acid supplementation in stroke prevention: A meta-analysis. *Lancet* 369(9576): 1876–1882.

Chapter 12

Agar, N. S., et al. 2004. The basal layer in human squamous tumors harbors more UVA than UVB fingerprint mutations: A role for UVA in human skin carcinogenesis. *Proceedings of the National Academy of Sciences* 101: 4954–4959.

American Cancer Society. 2009. *Cancer Facts and Figures, 2009*. Atlanta: American Cancer Society.

American Cancer Society. 2009. *Cancer Prevention and Early Detection Facts and Figures 2009*. Atlanta: American Cancer Society.

Betts, K. S. 2007. Secondhand suspicions: Breast cancer and passive smoking. *Environmental Health Perspectives* 115(3): A136–A143.

Brennan, P., et al. 2004. Secondhand smoke exposure in adulthood and risk of lung cancer among never smokers: A pooled analysis of two large studies. *International Journal of Cancer* 109(1): 125–131.

Canadian Cancer Society, et al. 2011. *Canadian cancer statistics 2011* (http://www.cancer.ca; retrieved January 30, 2012).

Chan, J. M., F. Wang, and E. A. Holly. 2005. Vegetable and fruit intake and pancreatic cancer in a population-based case-control study in the San Francisco Bay Area. *Cancer, Epidemiology, Biomarkers and Prevention* 14(9): 2093–2097.

Chao, A., et al. 2005. Meat consumption and risk of colorectal cancer. *Journal of the American Medical Association* 293(2): 172–182.

Cho, E., et al. 2004. Alcohol intake and colorectal cancer: A pooled analysis of 8 cohort studies. *Annals of Internal Medicine* 140(8): 606–613.

Dorn, J., et al. 2003. Lifetime physical activity and breast cancer risk in pre- and postmenopausal women. *Medicine and Science in Sports and Exercise* 35(2): 278–285.

Engeland, A., A. Tretli, and T. Bjorge. 2003. Height, body mass index, and ovarian cancer: A follow-up of 1.1 million Norwegian women. *Journal of the National Cancer Institute* 95(16): 1244–1248.

Flora, S. J. 2007. Role of free radicals and antioxidants in health and disease. *Cellular and Molecular Biology* 53(1): 1–2.

Fung, T., et al. 2003. Major dietary patterns and the risk of colorectal cancer in women. *Archives of Internal Medicine* 163(3): 309–314.

Gibbs, W. W. 2003. Untangling the roots of cancer. *Scientific American*, July.

Giovannucci, E., et al. 2002. A prospective study of tomato products, lycopene, and prostate cancer risk. *Journal of the National Cancer Institute* 94(5): 391–398.

Goldie, S. J., J. J. Kim, and T. C. Wright. 2004. Cost-effectiveness of human papillomavirus DNA testing for cervical cancer screening in women aged 30 years or more. *Obstetrics and Gynecology* 103(4): 619–631.

Goodwin, P. J., et al. 2002. The effect of group psychosocial support on survival in metastatic breast cancer. *New England Journal of Medicine* 345(24): 1719–1726.

International Agency for Research on Cancer. 2008. *World Cancer Report 2008*. Lyon, France: International Agency for Research on Cancer.

International Agency for Research on Cancer Working Group on Artificial Ultraviolet (UV) Light and Skin Cancer. 2007. The association of use of sunbeds with cutaneous malignant melanoma and other skin cancers: A systematic review. *International Journal of Cancer* 120(5): 1116–1122.

Lindberg, N. M., et al. 2009. A brief intervention designed to increase breast cancer self-screening. *American Journal of Health Promotion* 23(5): 320–323.

Martinez, M. E. 2005. Primary prevention of colorectal cancer: Lifestyle, nutrition, exercise. *Recent Results in Cancer Research* 166: 177–211.

McClay, E. F., and J. Smith. 2003. *101 Questions and Answers About Skin Cancer*. Sudbury, Mass.: Jones and Bartlett. Provides information about major types of skin cancer, including prevention and treatment.

Meadows, M. 2003. Don't be in the dark about tanning. *FDA Consumer*, November/December.

Michels, K. B., and A. Ekbom. 2004. Caloric restriction and incidence of breast cancer. *Journal of the American Medical Association* 291(10): 1226–1230.

Nelson, W. G., et al. 2003. Prostate cancer. *New England Journal of Medicine* 349(4): 366–381.

Paavonen, J., et al. 2003. Serum antibody response to the heat shock protein 60 of Chlamydia trachomatis in women with developing cervical cancer. *American Journal of Obstetrics and Gynecology* 189(5): 1287–1292.

Pelucchi, C., et al. 2004. Fibre intake and prostate cancer risk. *International Journal of Cancer* 109(2): 278–280.

Rose, S., and R. Hara. 2004. *101 Questions and Answers About Caring for Family or Friends with Cancer.* Sudbury, Mass.: Jones and Bartlett. Provides helpful practical advice about caring for patients and coping with emotional challenges.

Saraiya, M., et al. 2003. Preventing skin cancer: Findings of the Task Force on Community Preventive Services on reducing exposure to ultraviolet light. *MMWR Recommendations and Reports* 52(RR–15): 1–12.

Schatzkin, A., et al. 2007. Dietary fiber and whole-grain consumption in relation to colorectal cancer in the NIH-AARP Diet and Health Study. *American Journal of Clinical Nutrition* 85(5): 1353–1360.

Singletary, K. W., and S. M. Gapstur. 2001. Alcohol and breast cancer. Review of the epidemiologic and experimental evidence and potential mechanisms. *Journal of the American Medical Association* 286(17): 2143–2151.

Stein, C. J., and G. A. Colditz. 2004. Modifiable risk factors for cancer. *British Journal of Cancer* 90(2): 299–303.

Swaen, G. M., et al. 2007. Mortality study update of acrylamide workers. *Occupational and Environmental Medicine* 64(6): 396–401.

Troisi, R., et al. 2007. Cancer risk in women prenatally exposed to diethylstilbestrol. *International Journal of Cancer* 121(2): 356–360.

Valko, M., et al. 2007. Free radicals and antioxidants in normal physiological functions and human disease. *International Journal of Biochemistry and Cellular Biology* 39(1): 44–84.

Van Gils, C. H., et al. 2005. Consumption of vegetables and fruits and risk of breast cancer. *Journal of the American Medical Association* 293(3): 183–193.

Vineis, P., et al. 2004. Tobacco and cancer: recent epidemiological evidence. *Journal of the National Cancer Institute* 96(2): 99–106.

Widmark, A., et al. 2009. Endocrine treatment, with or without radiotherapy, in local advanced prostate cancer (SPCG-7/SFUO-3): An open randomized phase III trial. *Lancet* 373(9660): 301–308.

Chapter 13

Canadian HIV/AIDS Legal Network. 2006. *The use of complementary alternative health care* (http://www.aidslaw.ca/Maincontent/issues/cts/cam/useofcam.htm; retrieved June 28, 2006).

Cunningham, W. P., et al. 2004. *Environmental Science: A Global Concern.* 8th ed. New York: McGraw-Hill. A nontechnical survey of basic environmental science and key concerns.

DeGenova, M. K., and F. P. Rice. 2005. *Intimate Relationships, Marriages, and Families,* 6th ed. New York: McGraw-Hill.

Diener, E., and M. E. Seligman. 2002. Very happy people. *Psychological Science* 13(1): 81–84.

Eisenberg, D. M. 1997. Advising patients who seek alternative medical therapies. *Annals of Internal Medicine* 127: 61–69.

Goddard Institute for Space Studies. 2003. *Global Temperature Trends: 2002 Summation* (http://www.giss.nasa.gov/research/observe/surftemp; retrieved February 4, 2004).

Gottman, J. M. 2004. *The Seven Principles for Making Marriage Work.* New York: Three Rivers Press.

Heyn, P. C., et al. 2008. Endurance and strength training outcomes in cognitively impaired and cognitively intact older adults: A meta-analysis. *Journal of Nutrition, Health & Aging* 12(6): 401–409.

Houle, C., et al. 2007. What women want from their physicians: A qualitative analysis. *Journal of Women's Health* 16(4): 543–550.

Karasu, S. R. 2007. The institution of marriage: terminable or interminable? *American Journal of Psychotherapy* 61(1): 1–16.

Low, G., and A. E. Molzahn. 2007. Predictors of quality of life in old age: A cross-validation study. *Research in Nursing and Health* 30(2): 141–150.

Meadows, M. 2003. Strategies to reduce medication errors. *FDA Consumer,* May/June.

Olson, D., and J. DeFrain. 2006. *Marriages and Families: Intimacy, Diversity, and Strengths.* 5th ed. New York: McGraw-Hill.

Plante, T., and K. Sullivan. 2000. *Getting Together and Staying Together: The Stanford Course on Intimate Relationships.*

Singh-Manoux, A., M. Richards, and M. Marmot. 2003. Leisure activities and cognitive function in middle age: Evidence from the Whitehall II study. *Journal of Epidemiology and Community Health* 57(11): 907–913.

Slingerland, A. S., et al. 2007. Aging, retirement, and changes in physical activity: Prospective cohort findings from the GLOBE study. *American Journal of Epidemiology* 165(12): 1356–1363.

Tower, R. B., S. V. Kasl, and A. S. Darefsky. 2002. Types of marital closeness and mortality risk in older couples. *Psychosomatic Medicine* 64(4): 644–659.

United Nations Population Division. 2007. *World Population Prospects: The 2006 Revision.* New York: United Nations.

Worldwatch Institute. 2009. *Vital Signs 2009.* New York: Norton.

PHOTO CREDITS

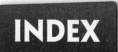

Boldface numbers indicate pages on which glossary definitions appear.